Explore

Self-Assessments!

In *MyHealthLab*, you have an opportunity to evaluate your behaviour and determine ways to improve your lifestyle—and ultimately your health.

Multidimer

Instructions:
Indicate your deg
the blank before it

Key	
1	strongly disag
2	disagree
3	neither agree r
4	agree
5	strongly agree

Subscale A: Internal

If I get sick, it is my own behavior that determines how soon I get well.	1○	2○	3○	4○	5○
I am in control of my health.	1○	2○	3○	4○	5○
When I get sick, I am to blame.	1○	2○	3○	4○	5○
The main thing that affects my health is what I myself do.	1○	2○	3○	4○	5○
If I take care of myself, I can avoid illness.	1○	2○	3○	4○	5○
If I take the right actions, I can stay healthy	1○	2○	3○	4○	5○

Self-Study Quiz: Case Studies in Health

To receive instant feedback for this self-study quiz, click the Check Answers button. Self-study quizzes are not recorded in your course gradebook, and you may take them as many times as you like. These questions are specific to your textbook and have been provided to reinforce chapter materials. Since this self-study quiz contains essay questions, please note:

- Feedback on essay questions may be limited to sample answers, as available.
- To save or share your essay, copy and paste the text into a Word document or an email.

This activity contains 1 question.

1.   Scenario

Kelly is spending the summer at home after finishing her first year of college. In returning home, she begins to notice that alcohol is a constant presence in her family. Kelly's father has used alcohol for as long as she can remember. He has never been arrested or been violent, but he spends almost every evening after supper down at the local bar with his friends. He drives to and from the bar and often gets home after everyone else has gone to bed. When Kelly came home this year during school vacations, she felt hurt that her father would choose to spend time at the bar rather than catch up with her, but she never said anything. Kelly's mother doesn't directly discuss his drinking, but she seems to give him the "cold shoulder" the day after a particularly long visit to the bar.

Addiction to a substance or behavior can be a powerful force. Psychological and physiological dependence to a substance can be a difficult pattern to break, and science suggests there is both a chemical process and a psychological dynamic that causes one to become addicted. When does a habit become an addiction? What symptoms are associated with an addiction?

Conclusions

Write an evaluation of the situation above. Is Kelly's father dependent on alcohol? How has his drinking affected Kelly? What communication patterns are present in the family that either help or hinder dealing with the issue? How might Kelly's family history affect her own decisions about alcohol?

To create paragraphs in your essay response, type <p> at the beginning of the paragraph, and </p> at the end.

Simulate

Case Studies!

Case Studies pursue and support topics introduced in the text.

Self-Study Quiz: Critical Thinking Activities

To receive instant feedback for this self-study quiz, click the Check Answers button. Self-study quizzes are not recorded in your course gradebook and you may take them as many times as you like. These questions are specific to your textbook and have been provided to reinforce chapter materials. Since this self-study quiz contains essay questions, please note:

- Feedback on essay questions may be limited to sample answers, as available.
- To save or share your essay, copy and paste the text into a Word document or an email.

This activity contains 12 questions.

1.   All of us go through difficult times. Refer to the basic elements of psychologically healthy people and identify which of those elements are most challenging for you. Think about a person or role model that you admire. Describe him/her and list the qualities that you admire in that person. Do you possess any of the same qualities? List similarities. List differences.

To create paragraphs in your essay response, type <p> at the beginning of the paragraph, and </p> at the end.

Practise

Critical Thinking!

Critical Thinking Exercises provide you with additional practice for topics introduced in the text.

From *MyHealthLab* you can link directly to *MySearchLab*, where you will have access to peer-reviewed articles on health and wellness, which will assist you in your research and broaden the scope of your knowledge.

Save Time. Improve Results.
www.pearsoned.ca/myhealthlab

Health the basics

FIFTH CANADIAN EDITION

Rebecca J. Donatelle
Oregon State University

Angela M. Thompson
St. Francis Xavier University

Pearson Canada
Toronto

Library and Archives Canada Cataloguing in Publication

Donatelle, Rebecca J., 1950–
    Health: the basics/Rebecca J. Donatelle, Angela M. Thompson.—5th Canadian ed.

Includes bibliographical references and index.
ISBN 978-0-321-60063-9

1. Health—Textbooks.   I. Thompson, Angela Maria, 1966–   II. Title.

RA776.H42 2011   613   C2009-904093-X

ISBN 978-0-321-60063-9

Vice-President, Editorial Director: Gary Bennett
Acquisitions Editor: Michelle Sartor
Sponsoring Editor: Carolin Sweig
Marketing Manager: Colleen Gauthier
Developmental Editor: Darryl Kamo
Production Editor: Andrea Falkenberg
Production Coordinator: Marisa D'Andrea
Copy Editor: Trish O'Reilly
Proofreader: Tara Tovell
Indexer: Jo-Anne Pelissier
Permissions and Photo Research: Sandy Cooke
Compositor: MPS Limited, A Macmillan Company
Art Director: Miguel Acevedo
Cover and Interior Designer: Opus House/Sonya Thursby
Cover Image: Corbis

1 2 3 4 5   14 13 12 11 10

Printed and bound in the United States of America.

To finding your perfect fit in all that you do.

Angie

BRIEF CONTENTS

CONTENTS

PREFACE

Today's university and college students know more than previous generations about their health, but understanding health issues also requires more critical analysis than ever before because of the constant flow of information issued from a growing variety of media sources. Students now make decisions about their health on a daily basis, and *Health: The Basics* is designed to help them use this information in the pursuit of positive health outcomes.

In setting out to revise the fifth Canadian edition, we listened to the comments and concerns of Canadian personal health educators and learned that we share the following goals for a personal health text:

- To prepare students to lead healthy lives, now and in the future by providing knowledge, tools, and strategies to make responsible health decisions, and to effect positive attitude and behaviour changes.

- To include "high-interest" topics not always included in health texts, such as multicultural and sex-specific perspectives on health.

- To include current Canadian research, material, and statistics.

- To recognize that students learn in many ways and require strong pedagogical elements to help them synthesize information and build healthy attitudes and behaviours.

- To include practical, real-life applications that encourage students to think critically and apply the material to their own lives.

New to the Fifth Canadian Edition

The new edition of *Health: The Basics* introduces MyHealthLab, Pearson Canada's online platform which connects students to self-assessments, critical thinking exercises, case studies, links to health on the net, and the Pearson eText.

MyHealthLab reaches beyond the covers of the text to provide additional material that will not only help students reach their goals for the course, but their goals for health and well-being as well.

The **self-assessments** on MyHealthLab provide students with opportunities to evaluate their behaviour and determine ways to improve their lifestyles and ultimately their health.

MyHealthLab contains **critical thinking exercises** that provide students with additional practice for topics introduced in the text.

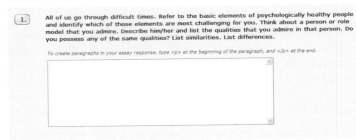

Self-Study Quiz: Critical Thinking Activities

Cases studies on MyHealthLab pursue and support topics introduced in the text.

Self-Study Quiz: Case Studies in Health

MySearchLab Exercises make use of peer-reviewed articles on health and wellness to provide students with an opportunity to broaden the scope of their knowledge of health issues directly affecting them.

Try It Now! sections encourage students to take action regarding specific health issues.

This new edition also includes the following:

- An overhaul of **physical fitness testing** in Chapter 4.
- The inclusion of **Canada's newest Food Guide** in Chapter 5, along with the rationale for changes made and recommendations given.
- The reorganization of Chapter 6 to present a lifelong approach to **managing weight**.
- The **Personal Fitness, Nutrition**, and **Managing Your Weight** chapters have been updated and reorganized to reflect the critical link among the three topics.
- Coverage of **diabetes** has been added to Chapter 11.
- The sequence of chapters has been changed to improve the organization of ideas and complement instructors' use.

As in previous editions, this fifth Canadian edition covers revisions made to update research and statistics, and to report on new developments in the field of health and wellness in Canada.

Inside the Book

- Beginning with the introduction of the **DECIDE model for decision making, Prochaska and DiClemente's Stages of Change model**, and **SuPeR SMART goal setting** in Chapter 1, decision making through critical thinking is a cornerstone of every chapter, including **Consider This . . .** scenarios and reflective questions, **What Do You Think?** boxed features throughout the chapter, and **Taking Charge** sections at the end of each chapter.
- The **Personal Fitness, Nutrition**, and **Managing Your Weight** chapters have been updated and reorganized to reflect the critical link among the three topics. Included in these chapters are the Canadian Society of Exercise Physiology– approved process for physical fitness testing, Canada's newest recommendations for healthy eating via "Eating Well with Canada's Food Guide," and a lifetime approach to maintaining a healthy body weight.
- Coverage of **heart disease, type 2 diabetes**, and **cancer** emphasizes prevention and treatment of the major killers in Canada. The section on type 2 diabetes is new to this edition.
- **Coverage of sex issues** in health is integrated throughout the text. Topics include sex bias in mental health treatment, women and heart disease, and how sex and gender roles may affect stress, stress management, and a person's ultimate health status.
- The book highlights **the role of the community** and how to improve a community's health. Community coverage appears throughout the text and in special community-focused "Checklists for Change" within the Taking Charge boxes.
- **Prevention** is emphasized in the context of making healthy lifestyle choices and changing not-so-good health attitudes and behaviours. For example, the text covers how early intervention allows more options, how prevention eases the burden on the health-care system, and how prevention can positively influence the quality and quantity of life.
- A **pedagogical framework** that stresses building health skills is integrated consistently throughout the text. Students will learn specific applications through the colourful Rate Yourself, Skills for Behaviour Change, Building Communication Skills, and Taking Charge boxes.

Healthy Decisions, Healthy Lives

Health: The Basics includes the following special feature boxes designed to help build health behaviour skills and to encourage students to think about and apply the concepts:

Rate Yourself (self-assessment) boxes give students the chance to evaluate their behaviours and determine ways to improve their lifestyle and ultimately their health.

Skills for Behaviour Change boxes suggest specific skills that students can develop and use in improving their lifestyle behaviours related to health and wellness.

Taking Charge sections encourage students to apply the chapter material to their own lives. This feature includes the following sections: "Making Decisions for You," which outlines steps and strategies for making and implementing health decisions; "Checklist for Change," which outlines specific actions to be taken to change unhealthy behaviours, on both a personal and a community level; and "Critical Thinking," which presents a hypothetical situation in which students must make a decision (we encourage the use of the DECIDE model to make this decision).

Spiritual and Emotional Health boxes introduce stories, practices, and techniques that will help students to understand, build, and strengthen their spiritual and emotional health.

Building Communication Skills boxes emphasize using communication as a tool to better health. These boxes provide practical suggestions for improving communication, interpersonal relationships, and social interactions—essential components of good health.

Focus on Canada boxes highlight health issues specifically related to Canadians.

Health in the Media boxes focus students' attention on issues of the day and raise their awareness of how these issues relate to each of them individually.

Additional Features

In addition to these boxes, *Health: The Basics* continues to improve upon the pedagogical features you've come to expect.

Learning Objectives: Each chapter begins with four or five learning objectives to emphasize important topics.

Consider This . . . Chapter-Opening Scenarios: These scenarios present practical, life-like scenarios that can be used to prompt stimulating discussions to introduce concepts presented in each chapter. End-of-chapter Application Exercises initiate further discussion of the topic after the information has been presented.

What Do You Think? Reflective Questions: These questions appear throughout each chapter to encourage students to think critically about the concepts presented and how they relate to them.

Try It Now! Feature (NEW): Specific suggestions made in each chapter encourage students to take action to improve their health and wellness.

MySearchLab Exercises (NEW): These exercises are linked to an online, peer-reviewed database. Students find an online resource and then respond to a series of questions or tasks based upon a specific article or topic.

Discussion Questions: These questions encourage critical thinking about important concepts presented from a variety of angles.

Application Exercises: These exercises are linked to the chapter-opening scenarios and expand discussion and critical reflection.

Running Glossary of Key Terms: Key terms are boldfaced in the text and defined in boxes on the page where they first appear.

MyHealthLab reaches beyond the covers of the text to provide additional material which will help students reach their goals for the course along with their goals for health and well-being. Some of the material includes self-assessments, chapter quizzes, videos, and animations, as well as links to health on the net and Pearson's eText.

✳ When you see this icon placed next to a heading, you'll know a related self-assessment can be found on MyHealthLab.

◉ This icon placed next to a heading indicates that a related case study exercise can be found on MyHealthLab.

✔ When you see this icon next to a heading, you'll know a related critical thinking exercise can be found on MyHealthLab.

myhealthlab This logo acts a reminder that the self-assessment can be completed on MyHealthLab, as well as any one of the many other self-assessments students will find there which are designed to help them assess their health.

MySearchLab provides students with peer-reviewed articles on health and wellness, broadening the scope of their knowledge of health issues which directly affect them.

Supplements

Available with *Health: The Basics*, Fifth Canadian Edition, is a comprehensive set of ancillary material designed to facilitate classroom preparation and enhance student learning.

Instructor Resource CD-ROM (ISBN 978-0-321-60982-3): The Instructor's Resource CD-ROM (IRCD) contains everything you need for efficient course preparation. All the supplements on the IRCD have been revised to reflect changes made to the Canadian edition. The Instructor's CD-ROM contains the following four supplements:

- **Instructor's Manual:** This comprehensive manual, filled with material to enhance the course, includes the following: what's new in this edition, chapter objectives, detailed chapter outlines, discussion questions, student activities including individual, community, and diverse population/non-traditional categories, solutions to the MySearchLab questions, additional references for further information, and a list of applicable media resources for classroom presentation.

- **Test Generator:** The Test Generator is composed of more than 1400 questions made up of multiple-choice, true/false, fill-in-the-blank, matching, and essay formats. Each question is rated for difficulty level and for skill type as factual, applied, or conceptual. Answers and page references to the text are also provided with each question as feedback. TestGen test-generating software allows instructors to custom design, save, and generate classroom tests. The test program permits instructors to edit, add, or delete questions from test banks; edit existing graphics and create new graphics; analyze test results; and organize a database of tests and student results. This new software allows for greater flexibility and ease of use.

- **PowerPoint Slides:** The PowerPoint Lecture Slides provide instructors with notes to supplement their in-class lectures. More than 400 PowerPoint presentation slides provide an indispensable teaching tool for instructors.

- **Image Library:** Almost all of the figures and tables from the text are available to instructors in the Image Library. Instructors can download these images to include in their own classroom presentations.

CBC Videos (DVD—ISBN 978-0-321-60981-6 and VHS 978-0-321-62154-2): Current information from such CBC series as *The National* and *Marketplace* complement the text and enhance learning by bringing to life practical applications and issues. With the latest news and information on health, these videos provide an excellent vehicle for launching lectures, showing additional examples, and sparking classroom discussion.

CourseSmart provides instant online access to the textbook and course material you need at a lower cost for students. And even as students save money, you can save time and hassle with a digital eText that allows you to search for the most relevant content at the very moment you need it. Whether it's evaluating textbooks or creating lecture notes to help students with difficult concepts, CourseSmart can make life a little easier. See how when you visit www.coursesmart.com/instructors.

Visit the Instructor Support page of the Pearson Education Canada website (http://vig.pearsoned.ca): The CBC videos are also available for viewing to both students and instructors on Pearson Education Canada's Video Central website.

Available to instructors only, the Instructor's Manual, PowerPoint Slides, and Test Generator are available for download from a password-protected site on the Pearson Education Online Catalogue. Follow the online instructions to create a password and download the available supplements.

MyHealthLab (www.pearsoned.ca/myhealthlab). This new online resource provides students with access to a wide range of resources that make studying convenient and fun. The addition of MyHealthLab includes "Getting Fit" self-assessments, an interactive eText, CBC videos, critical thinking questions, case studies, and chapter quizzes, as well as links to MySearchLab exercises.

Also Available—Student Supplements

CourseSmart goes beyond traditional expectations—providing instant online access to the textbook at an average savings of 50%. With instant access from any computer and the ability to search your text, you'll find the content you need quickly, no matter where you are. And with online tools like highlighting and note-taking, you can save time and study efficiently. See all the benefits at www.coursesmart.com/students.

Take Charge of Your Health! Worksheets: This pad of 50 self-assessment activities allows students to further explore their health behaviours and make steps towards positive change.

Behaviour Change Log Book and Wellness Journal: This assessment tool helps students track daily exercise and nutritional intake and create a long-term nutrition and fitness prescription plan. It also includes a Behaviour Change Contract and topics for journal-based activities.

Live Right! Beating Stress in College and Beyond: This book gives students useful tips for coping with stressful life challenges both during college and for the rest of their lives. Topics include sleep, managing finances, time management, coping with academic pressure, and relationships. This supplement also presents an objective overview of some of the health-oriented products on the market.

Eat Right! Healthy Eating in College and Beyond: This handy, full-colour 80-page booklet provides students with practical guidelines, tips, shopper's guides, and recipes that turn healthy eating principles into blueprints for action. Topics include healthy eating in the cafeteria, dorm room, and fast-food restaurants; planning meals on a budget; weight management; vegetarian alternatives; and effects of alcohol on health.

MyDietAnalysis: Powered by ESHA Research, Inc., MyDietAnalysis features a database of nearly 20 000 foods and multiple reports. This easy-to-use program allows students to track their diet and activity for up to three profiles and to generate and submit reports electronically.

Acknowledgments

We thank the following people at Pearson Canada for their part in the fifth Canadian edition of *Health: The Basics:* acquisitions editors Carolin Sweig and Michelle Sartor; developmental editors Darryl Kamo and Madhu Ranadive; production editor Andrea Falkenberg; production coordinator Marisa D'Andrea; copy editor Trish O'Reilly; proofreader Tara Tovell; and technical reviewer Anne MacLean.

We also thank the following reviewers:

Brenda Bruner, Queen's University

Penny Deck, Simon Fraser University

Joe Ellis, Sir Sanford Fleming College

Celine Homsy, John Abbott College

Gareth R. Jones, University of British Columbia–Okanagan

Jennifer Kuk, York University

Linda McDevitt, Algonquin College

Mary McKenna, University of New Brunswick

Chris Perkins, Lambton College

Deanna Schick, Trinity Western University

Tammy Whitaker-Campbell, Brock University

Sanni Yaya, University of Ottawa

CHAPTER 1

PROMOTING HEALTHY BEHAVIOUR CHANGE

◦ CONSIDER THIS . . .

Cameron is a 22-year-old fourth-year university student who engages in very little physical activity and is 35 kilograms overweight. A sensitive, caring young man, he has many close friends and volunteers at various agencies that help people in need. He enjoys nature and the inner peace he derives from sitting on the beach listening to the waves or a quiet night by a campfire in the wilderness. He is a strong advocate for human rights, animal rights, and the preservation of the environment.

Megumi is a 19-year-old first-year university student who lives off campus. She tries to eat well most of the time, thinks she is a few kilograms overweight, and walks two to four kilometres per day. She is shy and has not made many friends since coming to university. During a typical day, she goes to class, studies, watches TV or a movie, sends emails to her high-school friends and family, and spends time on the internet. She likes cycling and usually gets out for a short ride on the weekends.

Do you know people similar to either Cameron or Megumi? Who do you think is healthier? Why? What factors contribute to their current attitudes and behaviours? What actions could you take to help them achieve a more balanced "healthstyle"? Where could they go for help at your school? In your community?

CHAPTER OBJECTIVES

- Define health and wellness; identify and describe the seven dimensions of health.

- Describe the health status of Canadians and the factors that contribute to national health.

- Identify the leading causes of death and the lifestyle patterns associated with them.

- Describe the predisposing, enabling, and reinforcing factors that affect behaviour change.

- Compare and contrast behaviour-change techniques.

- Describe the role of decision making in making behaviour change.

If you and your close friends were to list the most important things in your lives, you might be surprised by the differences. Some would probably list family, love, financial security, significant others, and happiness. Others might list health. Raised on a steady stream of clichés and slogans—"If you have your health, you have everything," "Be all that you can be," "Use it or lose it," "Just do it!"—most of us readily acknowledge that good health is desirable. But what does it really mean to be healthy? How do you "get healthy"? How can you maintain and enhance the positive attitudes and behaviours you already have? How can you change your not-so-good, health-detracting attitudes and behaviours?

This text provides you with health information consistent with making positive lifestyle decisions that support who you are and what you want to be. Specifically, you can learn how to change attitudes and behaviours to significantly reduce your risk factors for a number of physical and mental health issues. For the risk factors beyond your control, you can learn to react, adapt, and make optimal use of the resources available to you to create the best situation for you. Further, by making informed, rational decisions, you will be able to improve the quality—and quantity—of your life.

WHAT IS HEALTH?

Although we use the term *health* widely, few people understand the broad scope of the word. For some, health simply means the antithesis of sickness or to be without disease. To others, it means being in good physical shape or having the ability to resist disease and illnesses. Still others include in the terms *wellness* or *well-being* a wide array of factors that lead to positive health status. Why all the definitions? Partly because of the different perceptions of an increasingly enlightened view of health that has evolved over time. As our understanding of illness has improved, so has our ability to understand the many nuances of health.

Health and Sickness: Defined by Extremes

Before the late 1800s, people viewed health simply as the absence of sickness. A person was healthy if he or she wasn't suffering from a life-threatening infectious disease. When deadly epidemics such as bubonic plague, pneumonic plague, influenza, tuberculosis, and cholera killed millions of people, survivors were considered healthy and congratulated themselves on their good fortune. In the late 1800s and early 1900s, researchers discovered that the victims of these epidemics were not simply unhealthy people but victims of microorganisms found in contaminated water, air, and human waste. Public health officials moved swiftly to sanitize the environment and, as a result, many people began to think of health as good hygiene. Practices such as sanitary disposal of wastes, hand washing, and other behaviours that promoted hygiene then became the harbingers of good health.

Health: More Than a Statistic

Once scientists learned about the microorganisms that caused infectious diseases, dramatic changes occurred in the sickness profile of the Canadian population. In the early 1900s, the leading causes of death were infectious diseases such as tuberculosis, pneumonia, and influenza, and the average life expectancy at birth was only 58.8 years for men and 60.6 years for women.[1] Improved sanitation brought about dramatic changes in life expectancy, and the development of vaccines and antibiotics added years to the average life span. According to **mortality** (death rate) statistics, people live longer now than at any other time in our history. Further, **morbidity** (illness) rates indicate that people are also sick less often from the common infectious diseases that devastated previous generations. Today, because most childhood diseases are curable and because multiple public health efforts are aimed at reducing the spread of infectious diseases, many people are living well into their 70s, 80s, and even 90s. The average Canadian child born in 2003 (the latest data

Responsiveness to the physical, social, mental, occupational, emotional, environmental, and spiritual dimensions of life—not merely the presence or absence of illness—determines health status.

available) has a life expectancy of 79.9 years—
77.4 years for boys and 82.4 years for girls.[2]

However, just because we are living longer and not getting sick as often does not necessarily mean we are healthier. If you and your classmates were asked "Are you healthy?" and "What do you base your response on?" your answers would vary according to your individual views of health.

In 1947, the World Health Organization (WHO), whose objective is "the attainment by all peoples of the highest possible level of health,"[3] defined **health** as " . . . complete physical, mental, and social well-being, not merely the absence of disease or infirmity."[4] For the first time, health was defined as more than the absence of disease or a vital statistic indicating low mortality or morbidity rates. But given the recognition of mental, occupational, environmental, and spiritual health contributions to quality and quantity of life, some critics argue that health includes even more than what is listed in the WHO's definition. Regardless of the number of components included, health can be limited by income, education, occupation, access to medical care, environmental pollution, age, and sex. In addition, since education is also a determinant of health, increasing your knowledge is one way to obtain an optimal level of health.

Health as Wellness: Putting Quality into Years

Biologist and philosopher Rene Dubos provides a multi-dimensional definition of health, noting that it "involves social, emotional, mental, spiritual, and biological fitness on the part of the individual, which results from adaptations to the environment."[5] The concept of adaptability or the ability to successfully cope with life's ups and downs is a key element of this definition. In recent decades, the term **wellness** has become popular. It includes the previously mentioned elements and implies as well that there are levels to obtain in each category: to achieve a high level of wellness, a person attempts to move progressively higher on a continuum of positive health indicators. Today, *health* and *wellness* are often used interchangeably to refer to the dynamic, ever-changing process of trying to achieve one's individual potential in each of the interrelated dimensions. These dimensions typically include those presented in Figure 1.1.

- **Physical health.** Includes physical characteristics such as body size and shape, sensory acuity, susceptibility to disease and disorders, body functioning, and recuperative ability. Newer definitions of

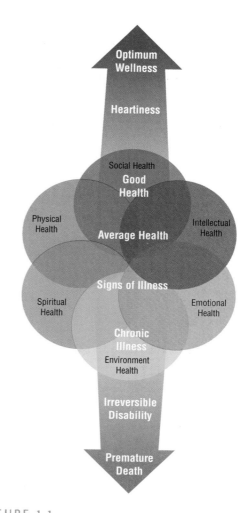

FIGURE 1.1

The Dimensions of Health and the Wellness Continuum

physical health include the ability to perform activities of daily living, such as getting out of bed in the morning, bending to tie up shoes, and shoulder checking while driving.

- **Social health.** Refers to the capacity for satisfying interpersonal relationships, interacting with others, and adapting to various social situations. It also includes communication skills and other daily activities.

Mortality: Death rate.

Morbidity: Illness rate.

Health: Dynamic, ever-changing process of trying to achieve individual potential in the physical, social, mental, occupational, emotional, environmental, and spiritual dimensions.

Wellness: Similar to health, a dynamic, ever-changing process in which a person attempts to reach his or her potential in each of health's components.

Having the motivation to improve the quality of life within the framework of your unique capabilities and limitations is crucial to achieving optimal health and wellness.

- **Mental health.** Refers to the ability to think clearly, reason objectively, analyze critically, and use brain power effectively to meet life's challenges. It includes learning from successes and failures and making responsible decisions.
- **Occupational health.** Refers to the satisfaction a person gets from his or her career or stage of career development. It also involves attaining and maintaining a satisfying balance between work and leisure.
- **Emotional health.** Refers to the "feeling" component of health and to the ability to effectively and appropriately express emotions. Feelings of self-esteem, self-confidence, self-efficacy, trust, love, and others are part of emotional health.
- **Environmental health.** Refers to an appreciation of the external environment and the role individuals play in preserving, protecting, and improving it. Biophilia specifically refers to the instinctive bond between people and their environment.[6] It also includes a student's personal studying environment—the desk, room, lighting, noise level, comfortable emotional atmosphere, and so on.

- **Spiritual health.** Your spirit refers to the deepest or innermost part of you, the part that helps you to understand the world and your role in it.[7] Spirituality is what we draw strength and hope from. It is through understanding our spiritual selves that we know who we are and what our specific purpose is. Spiritual health may involve a belief in a supreme being or a specified way of living prescribed by a particular religion or it may relate to personal relationships with others and/or being at peace with nature.

Whether the term used is *health* or *wellness*, the focus is on personal attempts to achieve optimal well-being within a realistic framework of individual potential. In Figure 1.1, a continuum from illness to optimal well-being describes health and wellness. Where you are on this continuum may vary from day to day, week to week, month to month, and year to year. That said, if you persist in your attempts to change attitudes and behaviours to reduce risk and/or improve health, your chances of remaining on the positive end of the continuum greatly improve. Each of us must try to achieve this optimal level of being in a sometimes hostile environment and come to terms with obstacles by focusing on our positive attributes whenever possible, changing what negative aspects we can, and learning to recognize and manage the aspects we can't change.

Individuals who are well take an honest look at their capabilities and limitations and make an effort to change what is within their control. They attempt to achieve balance in each health and wellness dimension while trying to achieve a positive position on the imaginary wellness continuum. Many people believe wellness can best be achieved by adopting a holistic approach in which emphasis is placed on integrating and balancing mind, body, and spirit. Persons on the illness and disability end of the continuum may have failed to achieve this integration and balance, and may be deficient in one or more of the wellness dimensions.

The disability component of the wellness continuum does not imply that a person with a physical and/or mental disability is not well or cannot achieve wellness. Such a person can be healthy in all aspects of wellness—within his or her potential, recognizing physical and/or mental limitations. In contrast, a person who spends hours in front of a mirror lifting weights to perfect the size and shape of each muscle may be less healthy in the other aspects of wellness—even though he or she is physically and mentally able. Appearance and physical performance are only two signs of a person's overall health and thus provide a limited indication of how well or healthy a person may be.

Breast Cancer Hope: Yukon River Quest

Many of us have heard of dragon boat races. More importantly, we are aware of the reasoning behind them. Participants of dragon boat races are most often survivors of breast cancer or individuals paddling in memory or support of a wife, mother, sister, daughter, aunt, grandmother, cousin, or friend who has had breast cancer. What do you do if you can't find a body of water that's available or suitable for a dragon boat race? What if you don't have a dragon boat? You adjust or adapt to your natural terrain and find a boat that works, just as the Yukon River Quest does for a number of breast cancer survivors in the Yukon.

Inaugurated in 1999 with kayaks and small canoes as the only participating vessels, the Yukon River Quest is the world's longest annual canoe and kayak race that begins in Whitehorse and ends approximately 740 kilometres later in Dawson City. Many of the 11 women who came together to compete in 2001 had never paddled before. They paddled in a Voyageur canoe under the team name Paddlers Abreast and finished their first race in just under 86 hours. In 2005, the team whittled their time down to 60 hours and 25 minutes, placing fourth behind the winning team that came in at just over 55 hours.

The teams that form the Yukon River Quest develop a camaraderie that goes beyond their similarities in experiences with breast cancer. This camaraderie reflects the hope these women have for their future—one without cancer. The women (and their friends) who choose to participate in the Yukon River Quest take part because of their need to share hope, to live beyond their experiences with breast cancer, and to grab hold of life again.

A Yukon filmmaker Werner Walcher created a documentary about the paddlers and their experiences. He tells the story of all breast cancer survivors who participated for five years in the Yukon River Quest. In this documentary, Walcher shows that women with breast cancer lead full and active lives. Further, he attempts to present the male partner's view because he feels that as a male, it is difficult to understand what a woman with breast cancer really goes through. Walcher's wife had a breast cancer scare, and experienced the procedures of being tested and waiting for results. It was this experience that fuelled his interest in a documentary on women's and their partners' experiences with breast cancer. He hopes that national interest will develop as a result of the film and that it will provide hope to those diagnosed with the disease in the future.

Source: Adapted from N. Reveler, "Paddlers Abreast–Yukon River Quest," *Network News: Essential News for Canadians Affected by Breast Cancer* 10 (Winter/Spring 2006). Retrieved on December 18, 2006, from www.cbcn.ca/en/ ?page=7181&section=4.

Typically, the closer you get to your potential in the seven wellness components, the healthier you are. Keep in mind that optimal health and wellness is not a static state that one achieves but rather an ongoing, active process that includes positive attitudes and behaviours in each dimension. Complete the appraisal in the Rate Yourself box, and get a better perspective on how you measure up in each of the wellness dimensions discussed in this section.

✓• Health Promotion: Helping You Stay Healthy

In discussions of health and wellness, the term **health promotion** is often used. Health promotion requires educational, organizational, environmental, and financial supports to help individuals and groups build positive health attitudes and behaviours and to change negative ones. In other words, health promotion does not just involve telling people to lose weight and to eat better. Efforts are also made to promote learning (*educational supports*), provide programs and services that encourage participation (*organizational supports*), establish rules governing attitudes and behaviours and supporting decisions to change (*environmental supports*), and provide monetary incentives to motivate them toward healthful decision making (*financial supports*). In short, health promotion enhances the likelihood that, once a person decides to change a behaviour, conditions are optimal for success. In health promotion, healthy people at risk for disease are identified and efforts made to motivate them to improve their health. Further, various health promotion efforts encourage those whose health and wellness are already sound to maintain and improve their relevant health-enhancing activities.

Health promotion: Combines educational, organizational, policy, financial, and environmental supports to enhance healthy lifestyle choices and to help people change negative health attitudes and behaviours.

How Healthy Are You?

Although many of us recognize the importance of healthy attitudes and behaviours, we often do not maintain a healthy regimen. Rate your health status in each of the following dimensions by circling the number of the response that best describes you.

	Very Unhealthy	Somewhat Unhealthy	Somewhat Healthy	Very Healthy
Physical Health	1	2	3	4
Social Health	1	2	3	4
Emotional Health	1	2	3	4
Environmental Health	1	2	3	4
Spiritual Health	1	2	3	4
Mental Health	1	2	3	4
Occupational Health	1	2	3	4

After completing the above section, how healthy do you think you are? Which area(s), if any, do you think you should work on improving? Respond to the following questions regarding each dimension of health by circling the number for the response that best describes you.

PHYSICAL HEALTH

	Rarely, If Ever	Sometimes	Most of the Time	Always
1. I maintain a desirable weight.	1	2	3	4
2. I engage in vigorous exercises such as brisk walking, jogging, swimming, or running for at least 30 minutes per day, 3–4 times per week.	1	2	3	4
3. I do exercises designed to strengthen my muscles and joints.	1	2	3	4
4. I warm up and cool down by stretching before and after vigorous exercise.	1	2	3	4
5. I feel good about the condition of my body.	1	2	3	4
6. I get 7–8 hours of sleep each night.	1	2	3	4
7. My immune system is strong and I am able to avoid most infectious diseases.	1	2	3	4
8. My body heals itself quickly when I get sick or injured.	1	2	3	4
9. I have lots of energy and can get through the day without being overly tired.	1	2	3	4
10. I listen to my body; when there is something wrong, I seek professional advice.	1	2	3	4

SOCIAL HEALTH

	Rarely, If Ever	Sometimes	Most of the Time	Always
1. When I meet people, I feel good about the impression I make on them.	1	2	3	4
2. I am open, honest, and get along well with other people.	1	2	3	4
3. I participate in a wide variety of social activities and enjoy being with people who are different from me.	1	2	3	4

	Rarely, If Ever	Sometimes	Most of the Time	Always
4. I try to be a "better person" and work on behaviours that have caused problems in my interactions with others.	1	2	3	4
5. I get along well with the members of my family.	1	2	3	4
6. I am a good listener.	1	2	3	4
7. I am open and accessible to a loving and responsible relationship.	1	2	3	4
8. I have someone I can talk to about my private feelings.	1	2	3	4
9. I consider the feelings of others and do not act in hurtful or selfish ways.	1	2	3	4
10. I consider how what I say might be perceived by others before I speak.	1	2	3	4

EMOTIONAL HEALTH

	Rarely, If Ever	Sometimes	Most of the Time	Always
1. I find it easy to laugh about things that happen in my life.	1	2	3	4
2. I avoid using alcohol as a means of helping me forget my problems.	1	2	3	4
3. I can express my feelings without feeling silly.	1	2	3	4
4. When I am angry, I try to let others know in non-confrontational and non-hurtful ways.	1	2	3	4
5. I am a chronic worrier and tend to be suspicious of others.	4	3	2	1
6. I recognize when I am stressed and take steps to relax through exercise, quiet time, or other activities.	1	2	3	4
7. I feel good about myself and believe others like me for who I am.	1	2	3	4
8. When I am upset, I talk to others and actively try to work through my problems.	1	2	3	4
9. I am flexible and adapt or adjust to change in a positive way.	1	2	3	4
10. My friends regard me as a stable, emotionally well-adjusted person.	1	2	3	4

ENVIRONMENTAL HEALTH

	Rarely, If Ever	Sometimes	Most of the Time	Always
1. I am concerned about environmental pollution and actively try to preserve and protect natural resources.	1	2	3	4
2. I report people who intentionally hurt the environment.	1	2	3	4
3. I recycle my garbage.	1	2	3	4
4. I reuse plastic and paper bags and tin foil.	1	2	3	4
5. I vote for pro-environmental candidates in elections.	1	2	3	4
6. I write my elected leaders about environmental concerns.	1	2	3	4
7. I consider the amount of packaging covering a product when I buy groceries.	1	2	3	4
8. I try to buy products that are recyclable.	1	2	3	4
9. I use both sides of the paper when taking class notes or doing assignments.	1	2	3	4
10. I try not to leave the tap running too long when I brush my teeth, shave, or bathe.	1	2	3	4

SPIRITUAL HEALTH

	Rarely, If Ever	Sometimes	Most of the Time	Always
1. I believe life is a precious gift that should be nurtured.	1	2	3	4
2. I take time to enjoy nature and the beauty around me.	1	2	3	4
3. I take time alone to think about what's important in life—who I am, what I value, where I fit in, and where I'm going.	1	2	3	4
4. I have faith in a greater power, be it a God-like force, nature, or the connectedness of all living things.	1	2	3	4
5. I engage in acts of caring and goodwill without expecting anything in return.	1	2	3	4
6. I feel sorrow for those who are suffering and try to help them through difficult times.	1	2	3	4
7. I feel confident that I have touched the lives of others in a positive way.	1	2	3	4
8. I work for peace in my interpersonal relationships, in my community, and in the world at large.	1	2	3	4
9. I am content with who I am.	1	2	3	4
10. I go for the gusto and experience life to the fullest.	1	2	3	4

MENTAL HEALTH

	Rarely, If Ever	Sometimes	Most of the Time	Always
1. I tend to let my emotions get the better of me and I act without thinking.	4	3	2	1
2. I learn from my mistakes and try to act differently the next time.	1	2	3	4
3. I follow directions or recommended guidelines and act in ways likely to keep myself and others safe.	1	2	3	4
4. I consider the alternatives before making decisions.	1	2	3	4
5. I am alert and ready to respond to life's challenges in ways that reflect thought and sound judgment.	1	2	3	4
6. I tend to act impulsively without thinking about the consequences.	4	3	2	1
7. I actively try to learn all I can about products and services before making decisions.	1	2	3	4
8. I manage my time well, rather than allowing time to manage me.	1	2	3	4
9. My friends and family trust my judgment.	1	2	3	4
10. I think about my self-talk (the things I tell myself) and then examine the real evidence for my perceptions and feelings.	1	2	3	4

OCCUPATIONAL HEALTH

	Rarely, If Ever	Sometimes	Most of the Time	Always
1. I am happy with my career choice.	1	2	3	4
2. I look forward to work.	1	2	3	4
3. My work responsibilities are consistent with my values.	1	2	3	4
4. The advantages in my career are consistent with my values.	1	2	3	4
5. I am happy with the balance between my work and leisure time.	1	2	3	4
6. I am happy with the amount of control I have in my work.	1	2	3	4
7. My work gives me personal satisfaction and stimulation.	1	2	3	4
8. I am happy with the professional and personal growth provided by my job.	1	2	3	4
9. I feel my work allows me to make a difference in the world.	1	2	3	4
10. My work contributes positively to my overall well-being.	1	2	3	4

PERSONAL CHECKLIST

Now, total your scores in each of the health dimensions and compare them to the ideal score. Which areas do you need to work on? How does your score compare with how you rated yourself in the first part of the questionnaire?

	Ideal Score	Your Score
Physical Health	40	_____
Social Health	40	_____
Emotional Health	40	_____
Environmental Health	40	_____
Spiritual Health	40	_____
Mental Health	40	_____
Occupational Health	40	_____

WHAT YOUR SCORES MEAN

Scores of 35–40: Outstanding! Your answers show you are aware of the importance of this component of your health. More important, you are putting your knowledge to work by practising good health habits. As long as you continue to do so, this component will not pose a serious health risk. It's likely that you are a role model for your family, friends, and classmates.

Scores of 30–35: Your health practices in this area are good, but there is room for improvement. Look again at the items where you scored one or two points. What changes could you make to improve your score? Even a small change in behaviour can help you achieve better health.

Scores of 20–30: Your health risks are showing! Do you need more information about the risks you are facing and

why it is important for you to change these behaviours? Perhaps you need help in deciding how to make the changes you desire. In either case, help is available from this book, from your professor, and from your student health services.

Scores below 20: You may be taking serious and unnecessary risks with your health. Perhaps you are not aware of the risks and what to do about them. Perhaps you are not sure what lifestyle attitudes and behaviours lead to good health and wellness. In this book, you will find the information you need to attain and maintain optimal health and wellness.

Source: Adapted from the U.S. Health and Human Services, "Health Style: A Self Test" (Washington, DC: Public Health Service, 1981).

In 2005, the Pan-Canadian Healthy Living Strategy was released (see the Focus on Canada box).[8] Actions proposed through this Strategy should improve the health status and health outcomes of the Canadian population.[9] Further, the proposed actions should reduce the current burden and contribute to the efficiency and sustainability of Canada's universal health-care delivery system. Rather than focusing on individual behaviour change, the Healthy Living Strategy takes a population health approach, recognizing that sustainable changes in individual behaviours are difficult to achieve without addressing living and working conditions. Thus, one of the key elements of the Strategy is to recognize and address linkages between lifestyle choices and the surrounding social, economic, and environmental influences.[10]

The Strategy primarily emphasizes healthy eating and physical activity, and their relationship to healthy weight. Other healthy living priorities will be addressed in upcoming initiatives. As mentioned, a population health approach guides the Healthy Living

Strategy. Using this approach, healthy living refers to the attitudes and behaviours that improve or maintain the health of the entire population and its subgroups.[11] When this approach is applied to individuals, healthy living refers to enhancing healthy behaviours, making healthy choices, and living in healthy ways. At all levels, the social, economic, political, cultural, and environmental conditions must be supportive of healthy living.

Whether we use the term *health* or *wellness*, we are talking about a person's overall responses to the challenges of living. Occasional dips into the ice cream bucket, a missed daily walk, an outburst of anger, or other deviations from optimal behaviours should not be viewed as major failures in attaining or maintaining your wellness. In fact, the ability to recognize that each of us is an imperfect being trying to adapt in an imperfect world signals individual well-being. Further, living life means that you savour some less healthy foods in smaller quantities, infrequently, and that there are times when your usual

The Integrated Pan-Canadian Healthy Living Strategy 2005

An extensive pan-Canadian consultation process resulted in the release of the *Integrated Pan-Canadian Healthy Living Strategy 2005*. The federal, provincial, and territorial Ministers of Health noted a need for a pan-Canadian healthy living approach in 2002. Various consultations followed across the country, and the Strategy is the culmination of these discussions. This first Strategy focused on healthy eating, physical activity, and their relationship to healthy weight; plans exist for future Strategies to cover topics such as mental health and injury prevention.

THE HEALTHY LIVING STRATEGY

The Healthy Living Strategy provides a conceptual framework for sustained action that focuses on improving the health of all Canadians as a group. With the population focus for the strategy, it is necessary to address the inequalities in health status among various groups. The Healthy Living Strategy visualizes Canada as a healthy nation, with conditions that support the attainment of optimal health and wellness for all. Thus, the goals of the Healthy Living Strategy are to improve overall health outcomes and to reduce health disparities.

HEALTHY LIVING TARGETS

Given the current overweight and obesity epidemic, along with Canadians' eating and physical activity habits, the proposed pan-Canadian Healthy Living targets "seek to obtain a 20 percent increase in the proportion of Canadians who are physically active, eat healthily, and are at healthy body weights." The year 2015 is considered the first marker for ongoing monitoring and evaluation to assess progress and allow for adjustments as appropriate. The specific targets of the Healthy Living Strategy are as follows:

Healthy Eating: By 2015, increase by 20 percent the proportion of Canadians who make healthy food choices according to the Canadian Community Health Survey (CCHS) and Statistics Canada (SC)/Canadian Institute for Health Information (CIHI) health indicators. This target would measure the food insecurity index and the consumption of vegetables and fruits, among other things.

Physical Activity: By 2015, increase by 20 percent the proportion of Canadians who participate in regular physical activity based on 30 minutes per day of moderate to vigorous activity as measured by the CCHS and the Physical Activity Benchmarks/Monitoring Program.

Healthy Weights: By 2015, increase by 20 percent the proportion of Canadians at a "normal" body weight based on a Body Mass Index (BMI) of 18.5 to 24.9, as measured by the National Population Health Survey (NPHS), CCHS, and SC/CIHI health indicators.

The *Integrated Pan-Canadian Healthy Living Strategy 2005* is available from www.phac-aspc.gc.ca/hl-vs-strat/pdf/hls_e.pdf.

Information about the *Canadian Community Health Survey* can be obtained from www.hc-sc.gc.ca/fn-an/surveill/nutrition/commun/index_e.html.

Information from Statistics Canada is available from www.statcan.gc.ca.

Information from the Canadian Institute for Health Information is available from www.cihi.ca.

Canadian Guidelines for Body Weight Classification in Adults, 2003 is available from www.hc-sc.gc.ca/fn-an/nutrition/weights-poids/guide-ld-adult/cg_quick_ref-ldc_rapide_ref_e.html.

QUESTIONS

1. Identify problems that affect the health of Canadians. How many of these problems are directly (or indirectly) a result of poor dietary practices, physical inactivity, or overweight?

2. Do you think the Healthy Living targets are reasonable? Why or why not? What targets would you choose? Why?

3. Why are integrated efforts among the various sectors a critical component in the pursuit of public health? What contributions to population health could these other sectors provide? How would these other sectors benefit from improvements in health and the conditions that influence health?

Source: Adapted from The Secretariat for the Intersectoral Healthy Living Network in partnership with the F/P/T Healthy Living Task Group and the F/P/T Advisory Committee on Population Health and Health Security (ACPHHS), "The Integrated Pan-Canadian Healthy Living Strategy 2005." Retrieved on May 31, 2006 from www.phac-aspc.gc.ca/hl-vs-strat/pdf/hls_e.pdf.

level of physical activity is not possible or you get a short night's sleep. This means that it is your *overall* approach to healthy eating, physical activity, and other lifestyle habits that is of greater importance than any one element in that approach, and this should be your focus in your efforts to attain and maintain optimal health and wellness.

We must also remember to be tolerant of others who are trying to improve their health. We need to be supportive, understanding, and nonjudgmental in our interactions with those attempting to make positive changes to their lifestyle. Further, health bashing—intolerance or negative feelings, words, or actions aimed at people who fail to meet our expectations of healthy attitudes and behaviours—indicates deficiencies in our psychological, social, or spiritual dimensions of health.

Prevention: The Key to Future Health

Prevention means taking action now to avoid becoming sick or less well later. Getting immunized against diseases such as polio, measles, mumps, and hepatitis, not smoking or chewing tobacco, practising safer sex, eating well, engaging in regular physical activity, and taking other preventive measures constitute **primary prevention**—actions designed to prevent health problems. **Secondary prevention** refers to the early recognition of a health problem and intervention to eliminate or reduce it before an even more serious illness develops. Attending health education seminars in order to stop smoking is an example of secondary prevention. Another example is modifying one's dietary intake and physical activity levels in response to a blood-cholesterol or blood-glucose test.

Two-thirds of deaths in Canada are a result of cardiovascular diseases, cancer, type 2 diabetes, and respiratory diseases.[12] These chronic diseases share common preventable risk factors: physical inactivity, poor dietary intake, and tobacco use. Further, these risk factors are influenced by income, employment, education, geographic isolation, and social exclusion. Common sense suggests that health promotion dollars should focus on the primary and secondary prevention of these and other lifestyle-related diseases. Instead, government money is primarily allocated for research and **tertiary prevention**—that is, treatment or rehabilitation efforts made after a person has become sick. (This is clearly a misnomer, since tertiary prevention is not really prevention but a response *after* illness has developed.) In addition, although the intent of tertiary prevention is to prevent the further development or progression of the disease (for example, chemotherapy and radiation therapy for individuals with cancer, or coronary bypass surgery for people with cardiovascular disease), it is more costly and less effective in promoting health than primary and secondary prevention.

thyroid disease, lupus, and Alzheimer's disease, for example—are far more common in women than in men. Further, diseases may manifest differently in women than in men—for example, symptoms of a heart attack in women are more vague than in men. Finally, although women live longer than men, they do not necessarily have a better quality of life.[13]

Sex bias has been identified as a serious weakness in medical research. In one study that reviewed medical journals in Canada and the United States, four factors reflecting bias were identified: androcentricity, overgeneralization, gender insensitivity, and double standards.[14] *Androcentricity* refers to viewing the world from a male perspective. *Overgeneralization* occurs when a study explores issues for one sex and generalizes the findings to both sexes. (The same thing can be said for age bias—that is, conducting research on 20-year-olds and applying the results to all adults.) In the past, studies that examined the precise effects of a drug or treatment did not include women because researchers did not want to deal with potential issues related to hormonal fluctuations. *Sex insensitivity* means overlooking sex as an important variable. An example of sex insensitivity is research on symptoms of heart disease in men and women where the data from both sexes is analyzed in combination, with disregard for potential similarities and differences. When differences do not exist between men and women, the data can be collapsed and analyzed together; otherwise, sex should be a controlled variable. The term *double standards* refers to the "evaluation, treatment or measurement of the identical behaviours, traits or situations by different means."[15] In 1996, a policy on clinical trials stated that if the product is likely to be used by women, then the testing must also be done on women. There has been increasing pressure placed on government to provide a more balanced approach to funding women's health programs. One example of increased activism is in the area of breast cancer. In Canada, one in nine women will be diagnosed with breast cancer,[16] yet it was not until the mid-1990s that much research was conducted on the causes, treatments, and social and psychological concerns of women diagnosed with it.

SEX DIFFERENCES

Although much of male and female anatomy is identical, it's clear that many major medical differences exist. Many diseases—osteoporosis, arthritis, headaches,

Primary prevention: Actions designed to stop problems before they start.

Secondary prevention: Intervention early in the development of a health problem to reduce symptoms or to halt its progression.

Tertiary prevention: Treatment or rehabilitation efforts aimed at limiting the effects of a disease.

IMPROVING YOUR HEALTH

Benefits of Achieving Optimal Health

Figure 1.2 provides an overview of the leading causes of death in Canada, and Figures 1.3 to 1.5 give estimated incidence and mortality rates for heart disease, stroke, and cancers in men and women. Heart disease and cancer continue to be the leading causes of death for both sexes.[17]

As Figure 1.3 shows, deaths from cardiovascular disease are declining among men and women. The Atlantic provinces have higher mortality rates than the western provinces, and these rates are consistent with the relative prevalence of smoking, high blood pressure, and obesity in these regions.

Figure 1.4 provides estimated new cases and deaths from cancer for men. (The Canadian Cancer Society updates its estimates each year; see www.cancer.ca.) Incidence rates have declined for most forms of cancer, but there have been sizeable increases in the detection of prostate cancer through PSA testing. New cases of lung cancer have been declining since the 1980s, likely because of the decrease in smoking.

Figure 1.5 shows estimated new cases and deaths from cancer for women. Similar to that for men, the incidence of new cancers in women has been relatively stable since the 1980s. Breast cancer is estimated to be the most common newly diagnosed cancer among women while the leading cause of cancer death is still expected to be lung cancer. The incidence of breast and lung cancer have been increasing among women since the 1970s. While prevention and control strategies are making an impact on death rates from breast cancer, the increasing number of women who smoke is related to the rates of lung cancer death.

While you cannot change your genetic history, and you may have little control over the medical services available in your area, you can influence your future health status by the attitudes and behaviours you choose today. Changing your lifestyle to improve your health status will reduce risk for cardiovascular disease, cancer, and other major diseases—as well as increasing your lifespan and improving your quality of life. Other equally important benefits include

- greater energy levels and increased capacity for and interest in having fun
- a stronger immune system, which enhances your ability to fight infections
- improved self-confidence, self-concept and self-esteem, and self-efficacy
- enhanced relationships with others due to better communication and "quality" time

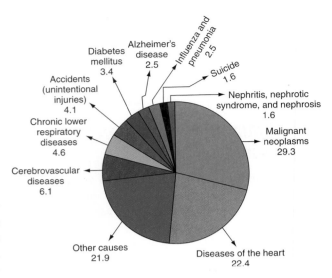

FIGURE 1.2

Leading Causes of Death in Canada, 2005

Source: Adapted from Table 102-0561 "Leading causes of death, total population, by age group and sex, Canada, annual," Statistics Canada. Retrieved on July 20, 2009 from http://cansim2.statcan.gc.ca/cgi-win/cnsmcgi.pgm.

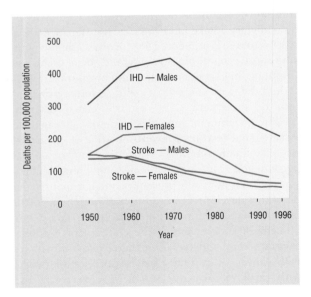

FIGURE 1.3

Death Rates Due to Ischemic Heart Disease and Stroke, Canada, 1950 to 1996*

* Age-standardized to the 1991 Canadian population.

Source: "Death Rates due to Ischemic Heart Disease and Stroke, Canada, 1950–1996," adapted from the Statistics Canada publication "Health Indicators," Catalogue No. 82-221, 1999.

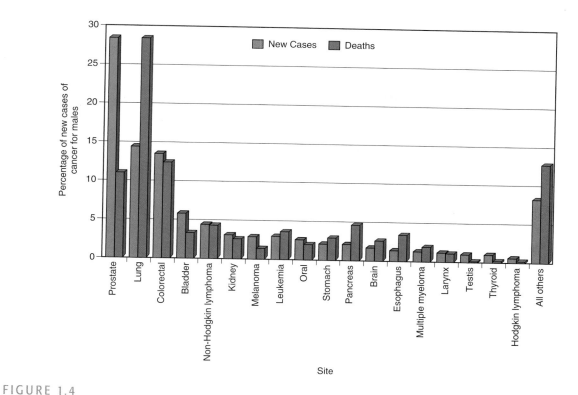

FIGURE 1.4

Percentage Distribution of Estimated New Cases and Deaths for Selected Cancer Sites, Males, 2008

Source: Canadian Cancer Society/National Cancer Institute of Canada, *Canadian Cancer Statistics 2008*, a report produced by Canadian Cancer Society; National Cancer Institute of Canada; Statistics Canada; Provincial/Territorial Cancer Registries; Public Health Agency of Canada. Toronto: CCS/NCIC, 2008.

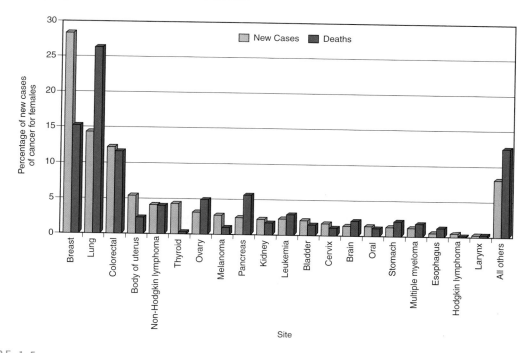

FIGURE 1.5

Percentage Distribution of Estimated New Cases and Deaths for Selected Cancer Sites, Females, 2008

Source: Canadian Cancer Society/National Cancer Institute of Canada, *Canadian Cancer Statistics 2008*, a report produced by Canadian Cancer Society; National Cancer Institute of Canada; Statistics Canada; Provincial/Territorial Cancer Registries; Public Health Agency of Canada. Toronto: CCS/NCIC, 2008.

- an improved ability to control and manage stress
- a reduced reliance on the health-care system
- improved cardiovascular functioning
- increased muscle tone, strength, flexibility, and endurance, which results in improved physical appearance, performance, and self-esteem
- a more positive outlook on life, fewer negative thoughts, and an ability to view life as challenging and to see negative events as an opportunity for growth
- improved environmental sensitivity, responsibility, and behaviours
- enhanced levels of spiritual health, awareness, and feelings of oneness with yourself, others, and the environment

✱ Making Health-Wise Choices

Although mounting evidence indicates significant benefits to being healthy, many people find it difficult to become and remain healthy. Most experts believe that several key behaviours will help people live longer, such as

- getting a good night's sleep (six to nine hours)
- maintaining healthy eating habits, which includes:
  - eating breakfast
  - spreading caloric intake throughout the day (at least 3–5 meals and snacks)
  - reducing intake of fat, salt, sugar, and processed foods; eating plenty of vegetables and fruit
- maintaining weight (within 2 to 5 kg of ideal)
- participating in regular physical activities (3–7 times per week)
- regular brushing and flossing of teeth
- practising safer sex
- avoiding tobacco products
- limiting intake of alcohol
- regular self-exams and medical checkups (including the dentist)
- wearing your seatbelt

Although health professionals can statistically assess the health benefits of the above behaviours, there are several other actions that, while perhaps not increasing quantifiable "years added to life," may significantly result in "life added to years." These include:

- controlling the real and imaginary stressors in life
- maintaining meaningful relationships
- making time for yourself and being as kind to yourself as you are to others

- participating in at least one fun activity each day
- respecting the environment and the people in it
- considering alternatives when making decisions and assessing how actions affect others
- valuing each day and making the best of each opportunity
- viewing mistakes as opportunities to learn and grow
- understanding the health-care system and using it wisely

While it's easy to list things that one *should* do and even things that one may really *want* to do, change is not easy. Still, all people, no matter where they are on the health and wellness continuum, have to start somewhere to improve their health. The key is to decide what needs to change, determine the actions necessary to make the change, set up a plan of action, put the plan into action, and then reinforce and maintain the plan. First, it is important to take a closer look at the factors that may contribute to current health attitudes and behaviours.

Preparing for Behaviour Change

In regard to behaviour change, Mark Twain said "habit is habit, and not to be flung out the window by anyone, but coaxed downstairs a step at a time." Changing negative attitudes and behaviours into healthy ones is a time-consuming and difficult process. The chances of successfully changing attitudes and behaviours improves when you make gradual changes that give you time to unlearn negative patterns and substitute positive ones. We have not yet developed a foolproof method for effectively changing attitudes and behaviours, and it may be, in fact, that different approaches work effectively for different individuals. To understand how the process of behaviour change works, we must first identify specific behaviour patterns and try to understand the reasons for them.

Factors Influencing Behaviour Change

Figure 1.6 identifies three categories of factors that influence attitudes, behaviours, and behaviour-change decisions.

---

what do you THINK?

Considering your lifestyle and the factors related to living a longer and better life, what attitudes and/or behaviours would you like to change?

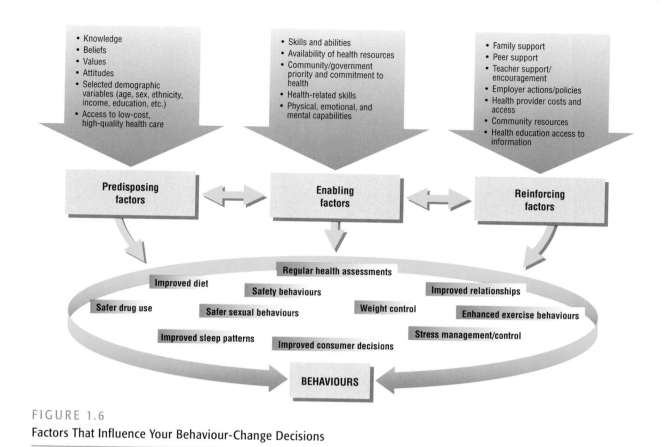

- Knowledge
- Beliefs
- Values
- Attitudes
- Selected demographic variables (age, sex, ethnicity, income, education, etc.)
- Access to low-cost, high-quality health care

- Skills and abilities
- Availability of health resources
- Community/government priority and commitment to health
- Health-related skills
- Physical, emotional, and mental capabilities

- Family support
- Peer support
- Teacher support/ encouragement
- Employer actions/policies
- Health provider costs and access
- Community resources
- Health education access to information

Predisposing factors ⟷ **Enabling factors** ⟷ **Reinforcing factors**

Regular health assessments

Improved diet

Safety behaviours

Improved relationships

Safer drug use

Safer sexual behaviours

Weight control

Enhanced exercise behaviours

Improved sleep patterns

Stress management/control

Improved consumer decisions

BEHAVIOURS

FIGURE 1.6

Factors That Influence Your Behaviour-Change Decisions

Predisposing Factors

Our life experiences, knowledge, cultural and ethnic inheritance, and current beliefs and values are *predisposing factors*. These are factors that are likely to lead to a particular behaviour. These factors that predispose us to certain conditions include our age, sex, ethnicity, income, family, education, environment, and access to health care. For example, if your parents smoked, you are 90 percent more likely to start smoking than someone whose parents did not. If your peers smoke, you are 80 percent more likely to smoke than someone whose friends do not.

Enabling Factors

Skills or abilities, physical, emotional, and mental capabilities, and resources and accessible facilities that make health decisions more convenient or difficult are *enabling factors*. Positive enablers encourage you to carry through on your intentions. Negative enablers work against your intentions to change. For example, if you would like to join a local fitness centre and discover that the closest one is 10 kilometres away and the membership fee is $1000, these factors may deter you from joining. On the other hand, if your school's fitness

centre is two blocks away, open until midnight, and has a reduced rate for students, these positive enablers might convince you to use it. Identifying the positive and negative enabling factors and devising alternative plans when the negative factors outweigh the positive ones is part of the necessary planning for behavioural change.

Reinforcing Factors

Reinforcing factors refer to the support and encouragement or discouragement that come from significant others or situations in your life that enable a particular behaviour. For example, if you decide to stop smoking and your family and friends smoke in your presence and ask if you would like a cigarette too, you may be tempted to start smoking again. In other words, your smoking behaviour is reinforced. If, however, you quit smoking and your family and friends tell you how great you are doing and attempt not to smoke in your presence, your positive behaviour change will be reinforced and you will be more likely to be successful. Reinforcing factors also include policies and services that make it easier for you to maintain a particular behaviour. Policies such as smoke-free public places and buildings reinforce the behaviour of individuals who stop smoking. Reinforcing factors that may influence

Are You "Staged" for Change?

Have you ever come up with a great New Year's (or Monday-morning) resolution about something you are going to "do differently" only to have your good intention forgotten or ignored a few days later? As most people discover, changing established behaviours is not an easy task. Much of what we do is influenced by a number of variables, including our history, reward systems, values, and culture. You have been doing the same sorts of things for years, and these behaviours become a part of who you are. Thus, changing that part of you will not be easy. Finding out where you are and how ready you are to change may help lead to success.

STAGES OF CHANGE, TRANSTHEORETICAL MODEL

A number of theories or models help explain the behaviour change process. One of these is the Stages of Change or Transtheoretical model created by James Prochaska and Carlo DiClemente in the early 1980s. Developed from research on smoking cessation and drug and alcohol addiction, the Stages of Change model has been applied to a wide range of health behaviours over the years, including HIV prevention. Essentially, the Stages of Change model asks

1. Are you ready for change? and

2. Where are you in terms of readiness to change?

This probably sounds a bit familiar to you; the Stages of Change model indicates that the readier you are to change and the greater your motivation to change, the more likely it is that you will succeed at change. From their research, Prochaska and DiClemente concluded that an individual proceeds through distinctive stages. These stages are

1. **Precontemplation.** People in the precontemplation stage have no intention at the moment of changing. They likely are not even aware of a need to change. They may also have tried to change a behaviour before and given up.

   Strategies for Change: Sometimes a few frank yet kind words may be enough to help people in this stage to take a closer look at themselves. Improving knowledge by recommending readings or making tactful suggestions may help people in the precontemplation stage consider a change.

   For Example: If increasing physical activity is the behaviour you want to change, you might learn more about the risks of inactivity and the benefits of regular physical activity. Consider the concerns you have—all of them. Your goal at this stage is simply to *think* about becoming more physically active.

2. **Contemplation.** In this phase, people recognize that they need to change and are thinking about doing it. Acknowledgment usually results from increased awareness, often due to feedback from family and friends or access to information or increased knowledge. People can languish in this stage for years, realizing that they have a problem but lacking the time, energy, or knowledge to make the change.

   Strategies for Change: Often, people in this stage need a little push to get them started. This may come in the form of helping set up a change plan (for example, an exercise routine), buying a helpful gift (such as a low-fat cook-

book), sharing articles about a particular problem, or inviting them to go with you to hear a speaker on a related topic. People often need time to think about a course of action or to build skill. Your assistance can help them move off the point of indecision.

   For example: At this stage you need to consider the obstacles or barriers to you becoming more physically active. You should also consider the benefits of an active lifestyle. You may even commit to *when* you will start to become more active and what steps you need to prepare.

3. **Preparation.** Most people at this point are close to taking action. They know they need to change, they have been thinking about it and are ready to come up with a plan. Rather than thinking about why they can't begin, they have started to focus on what they can do to move into the action phase.

   Strategies for Change: People in the preparation stage benefit from a few simple guidelines. Set realistic goals (large and small), take small steps toward change, change one thing at a time, and seek support from friends and family. Identify factors that enabled success or served as a barrier to success in the past, and modify them where possible.

   For example: Once again focus on the obstacles or barriers to you becoming more physically active. This time, think specifically about what has hindered you in the past. Set short and long term goals (for example, in the first week, I will walk twice to work; at the end of the year, I will run 5 kilometres). Focus on the positive, you can do it!

4. **Action.** In this stage, people actually make the change. Success comes to those prepared for change, specifically if you consider alternatives, engage social support, and make a realistic plan of action, you are more ready than those who give it little thought.

   Strategies for Change: Publicly stating the desire to change helps ensure success. Encourage friends making a change to share their plans with you. Offer to help, and try to remove potential obstacles from their intended action plan. Social support and the buddy system can provide a good source of motivation.

   For example: At this stage, you do the physical activity you planned. Be positive, stay focused, consider unexpected challenges and prepare for them.

5. **Maintenance.** Maintenance requires vigilance, attention to detail, and long-term commitment. Many people reach a goal, only to relax and slip back into the undesired behaviours. In this stage, it is important to be aware of

the potential for relapses and develop strategies for dealing with such challenges. Common causes of relapse include no longer planning for the change, overconfidence, daily temptations, stress or emotional distractions, and self-deprecation.

Strategies for Change: During maintenance, continue taking the same actions that led to success in the first place. Find fun and creative ways to maintain positive behaviours. This is where a willing and caring support group can be vital. Knowing where on campus to turn for help when you don't have a close support network is also helpful.

For example: Praise and reward yourself for your current success. Continue to plan for your physical activities. Focus on *how* you have achieved success. Again, consider unexpected challenges to your physical activity participation and prepare for them.

6. **Termination.** By this point, the behaviour is so ingrained that it is the "new" habit and the current level of vigilance may be unnecessary. The new behaviour has become an essential part of daily living.

For example: At this point, you simply are physically active each and every day; you look for ways to include physical activity in your daily life in addition to "working out."

HOW STAGED ARE YOU?

To understand the Stages of Change model, try the following exercise:

- Write down one health behaviour you would consider changing. Just the fact that you are aware of it puts you in the contemplative stage. Now take it a bit further.

- How serious are you about the change? What are the possible actions you could take to make it work? What are potential barriers that could interfere with success? What or who will motivate you?

- Have you identified ongoing reinforcements to help you follow the plan? List actions you will take on a daily basis. How will you reward yourself? What will you do if you slip and do not meet the goals for a particular day? What alternative actions can you take? What will you use as motivation to stay on target?

Source: J. O. Prochaska and C. C. DiClemente, "Stages and Processes of Self-Change of Smoking: Toward an Integrative Model of Change," *Journal of Consulting and Clinical Psychology* 51 (1983): 390–395.

you toward positive or negative behaviours include money, popularity, support and appreciation from friends, and family interest and enthusiasm for what you are doing.

The way you reward or punish yourself for your successes and failures may affect your chances of adopting healthy behaviours. Learning to accept small failures and to concentrate on your successes—regardless of how small they are—may foster further successes. Berating yourself because you ate ice cream, argued with a friend, or didn't jog may create an internal environment in which failure becomes inevitable. Telling yourself that you are worth the extra time and effort and giving yourself a pat on the back for small accomplishments is an often-overlooked factor in successfully changing your attitudes and behaviours.

It is not our intention to blame you if you are struggling with personal health behaviours or to suggest that all the variables that affect health are within your control. Our goal is to help you realize which factors are within your personal control and to help you to maximize your decision-making powers to take that control—to maintain or improve your current health or to prevent premature deterioration.

Major changes in health behaviours are not made by following easy, one-step recipes. Lasting behaviour changes that ultimately improve your overall health and well-being require careful thought, individual analysis, and considerable effort. Changing beliefs, attitudes, values, actions, and behaviours that have

been part of your life for a long time is difficult. Even the most strong-willed, disciplined people discover that willpower alone is not enough to get them through the many adjustments needed to make life-long behaviour changes.

Wanting to change is a prerequisite of the change process, but there is much more to the process than motivation. Motivation must be combined with common sense, commitment, and a realistic understanding of how best to move from point A to point B. *Readiness* is the state of being that precedes behaviour change. People who are ready to change possess the knowledge, attitudes, skills, and internal and external resources that make change a likely reality. For someone to be ready for change, certain basic steps and adjustments in thinking must occur. See also the Skills for Behaviour Change box.

Your Beliefs and Attitudes

Even if you know why you should make a specific behaviour change, your beliefs and attitudes about the value of your actions in making a difference (that is, whether or not making this change will have an impact) will significantly affect what you do. We assume that when rational people realize there is a risk in what they are doing, they will act to reduce that risk. But this is not necessarily true. Consider the number of physicians and other health professionals who continue to smoke, fail to manage their stress response, consume high-fat diets, are inactive, and act in other unhealthy ways. Surely they know better, but their "knowing" is disconnected from their "doing." In other words, knowledge does not equal behaviours. Why? Two strong influences on our actions are beliefs and attitudes.

what do you THINK?

What predisposing, enabling, and reinforcing factors will help you to change the attitudes and/or behaviours you most want to change? What predisposing, enabling, and reinforcing factors could make this change difficult? What can you do to avoid (or limit the effect of) these difficulties?

A **belief** is an appraisal of the relationship between some object, action, or idea (for example, smoking) and some attribute of that object, action, or idea (for example, smoking is expensive, dirty, and causes cancer—or, it is a sexy, cool, adult activity). Beliefs develop either from direct experience (for example, if you have trouble breathing after smoking for several years) or from secondhand experience or knowledge conveyed by other people (for example, if you see your grandfather, a pack-a-day smoker, die of lung cancer or emphysema).[18] Although most of us have a general idea of what constitutes a belief, we may be a bit uncertain about what constitutes an attitude. We often hear or make such comments as "He's got a rotten attitude" or "She needs an attitude adjustment," but may still be unable to define *attitude*. An **attitude** is a relatively stable set of beliefs, feelings, and behavioural tendencies in relation to something or someone.

Do Beliefs and Attitudes Influence Behaviours?

It seems logical to conclude that your beliefs will influence your behaviours. If you believe (make the appraisal) that taking drugs (an action) is harmful for you (an attribute of that action), you will choose not to use drugs. If you believe that drinking and driving are incompatible, you will choose not to drink and drive. Or will you? Psychologists studying the relationship between beliefs and health behaviours determined that although beliefs may subtly influence behaviours, they may not actually cause people to change them. The **health belief model (HBM)** explains how beliefs may or may not influence subsequent behaviours (see Figure 1.7).[19] According to this widely accepted model, several factors must support a belief in order for change to be likely:

- *Perceived seriousness of the health problem.* First, a person considers how severe the medical and social consequences would be if the health problem were to develop or be left untreated. The more serious a person believes the effects will be,

FIGURE 1.7
Health Belief Model

Source: Adapted by permission from Edward P. Sarafino, *Health Psychology: Biopsychosocial Interactions* (New York: John Wiley & Sons, 1990) 190. © 1990 by John Wiley & Sons.

the more likely he or she is to take action. For example, heart disease is the number-one killer of Canadians; therefore, a person is likely to perceive heart disease as a serious health problem.

- *Perceived susceptibility to the health problem.* Next, a person evaluates the likelihood of developing the health problem. Those who perceive themselves as more likely to develop the health problem are more likely to take preventive action. For example, if your mother and sister were recently diagnosed with breast cancer, you are likely to consider yourself highly susceptible.

- *Cues to action.* Those who are reminded or alerted about a potential health problem are more likely to take preventive action. For example, having your doctor tell you that your blood sugar levels are indicative of a prediabetic state may be the cue you need to get physically active and lose weight to prevent full-blown type 2 diabetes.

Three other factors are linked to perceived risk for health problems: *demographic variables,* including age, sex, ethnicity, and cultural background; *sociopsychological variables,* including personality traits, social class, and social pressure; and *structural variables,* including knowledge about or prior contact with the health problem.

The HBM is followed many times every day. Take smokers, for example. Older smokers are likely to know other smokers who developed serious heart or lung problems as a result of smoking. They are thus more likely to perceive a threat to their health connected with the behaviour of smoking than a young person who just started. The greater the perceived threat of health problems caused by smoking, the greater the chance a person will quit smoking. However, many chronic smokers know that they have serious health problems, yet they continue to smoke. Why do people fail to take actions to avoid further harm? Some people do not believe that they will be affected by a severe problem—they act as if they have some kind of immunity—and are unlikely to change their behaviours. In some cases, they think that, even if they get cancer or have a heart attack, the health-care system and improving technologies will be able to take care of them. For these individuals, a cue such as a friend or family member having a heart attack or being diagnosed with lung cancer may push them to realize their susceptibility to disease and move them into action.

Other factors from the HBM that affect the likelihood of behaviour change are assessments about whether the benefits outweigh the costs and whether proposed actions will actually make a difference (that is, reduce risk, improve health). If you are addicted to smoking, the thought of quitting may not be acceptable to you, and if you enjoy smoking too much, you will probably keep smoking—particularly if the consequences will not be felt for some time and the pleasure is instant. Similarly, you are not likely to make the effort to do something (for example, go for a jog) if you do not feel the health-related benefits right away.

---

what do you THINK?

Is there a health behaviour you should change? What could happen if you do not change this health behaviour (perceived seriousness)? How likely is the health problem to develop (perceived susceptibility)? What made you aware of this potential health problem (cues to action)? What steps will you take today to start the behaviour-change process?

Your Intentions to Change

Our attitudes tend to reflect our emotional responses and follow from our beliefs. According to the **theory of reasoned action**, our behaviours result from our intentions to perform actions. An intention is a result of our attitude toward an action and our beliefs about what others may want us to do.[20] A behavioural intention, then, is a written or stated commitment to perform an action.

If, for example, you are out of shape and your health is important to you, you may take steps to become more physically active. If your best friend also tells you that you really do need to get in shape and you value this person's opinion, your intention to become more physically active will become stronger. In brief, the more consistent and powerful your attitudes about an action and the more you are influenced by others to take that action, the greater will be your stated intention to do so—in this example, to get more physically active. Further, the more you verbalize your commitment to physical activity, the more likely it is that you will do it.

Significant Others as Change Agents

Many people are highly influenced by the approval or disapproval (real or imagined) of close friends and loved ones and of the social and cultural groups to

---

Belief: Appraisal of the relationship between some object, action, or idea and some attribute of that object, action, or idea.

Attitude: Relatively stable set of beliefs, feelings, and behavioural tendencies in relation to something or someone.

Health belief model (HBM): Model for explaining how beliefs may influence behaviours.

Theory of reasoned action: Model for explaining the importance of our intentions in regard to our behaviours.

which they belong. Such influences can offer support for health actions, making healthy behaviours more possible to attain; they can also affect behaviours negatively, interfering with even the best intentions of making a positive change.

Your Family

From the time of your birth, your parents have influenced your behaviours by giving you strong cues about which actions are socially acceptable and which are not. Brushing your teeth, bathing, wearing deodorant, and chewing food with your mouth closed are probably behaviours that your family instilled in you long ago. Your family culture influenced your food choices, your religious and political beliefs, and your other values and actions. If you deviated from your family's norms, a family member probably let you know fairly quickly. Good family units share unconditional love and trust, dedication to the healthy development of all family members, and a commitment to work out difficulties.

When a loving family unit does not exist, when it does not provide for basic human needs, or when dysfunctional, irresponsible individuals try to build a family under the influence of drugs or alcohol, it becomes difficult for a child to learn positive health behaviours. Healthy behaviours get their start in healthy homes; unhealthy homes breed unhealthy habits. Healthy families provide the foundation for a clear and necessary understanding of what is right and wrong, what is positive and negative. Without this fundamental grounding, many young people have difficulties.

The Influence of Others

Just as your family influences your actions during your childhood, your friends, your teachers/coaches, and significant others influence your behaviours as you grow older. Most of us desire to fit the "norm" and avoid hassles in our daily interactions with others. If you deviate from the actions expected in your hometown or among your friends, you may suffer ostracism, strange looks, and other negative social consequences. Understanding the subtle and not-so-subtle ways in which other people influence our actions is an important step in the process of changing our behaviours.

How others influence our behaviour choices is also explained in the *theory of planned behaviour*.[21] This theory outlines three reasons for how we choose to act:

- *Our attitudes toward the behaviour*—for example, what we think about the positive or negative effects of our actions and the importance of each.
- *Our level of perceived behavioural control,* or our beliefs about the constraints and opportunities we might have concerning the behaviour. More specifically, how much control we think we have over the particular behaviour we want to change.
- *Our subjective norms,* or whether or not we think our actions will be approved of by the people important to us.

For example, if you want to become more physically active to reduce your risk for type 2 diabetes, you will have strong intentions to a weight-loss program (*attitudes* toward the behaviour). Intentions are powerful indicators of successful behaviour change. If there is a convenient, affordable fitness centre near you, and if the schedule works for you, you will be more motivated and believe you can make the change (*control beliefs*). Finally, if friends offer encouragement (*subjective norms*), you are more likely to remain motivated to change your behaviours. On the other hand, if you perceive that your friends think you are a nerd for going to the gym, or if the gym is inconvenient (for instance, it is far away or has restricted hours of operation) or expensive, you may quickly lose your motivation. The opinions of key people play a powerful role in our motivation to change behaviours.

The influence of others can serve as a powerful social support for positive behaviour changes. Influential others can also play a role in our not-so-good health behaviours as we are influenced to drink too much, party too hard, eat too much, or engage in other negative actions because we don't want to be left out or because we fear criticism or being different. Learning to understand the subtle and not-so-subtle ways in which our families, friends, and others have influenced and continue to influence our behaviours is an important step toward making positive changes.

> ## try it NOW!
> Stay connected. A broad base of social support is an important part of ensuring overall health. Make an effort to strengthen social bonds. Call, email, or instant message a friend right now, and make a date for coffee, lunch, or "fun time" to catch up on each other's lives. Show you care.

If you are part of an abusive relationship, having friends you trust and can confide in can give you the strength to walk away—to change your behaviours. Someone who accepts you unconditionally and is there for you is a powerful asset to help deal with life's challenges. The more social support you have, and the closer the relationship or social bonds, the greater the chances that you will be able to deal with crises in healthy ways. If you expand your social support network to include counsellors, spiritual advisers, and others, you will further increase your likelihood of success. Whom would you call if you were stranded in the middle of a cold, snowy night on a remote road? Who would get out bed, without question, to come and get you? Surprisingly, many people have no one to call under any circumstances, let alone when they are in crisis. The importance of cultivating and maintaining close ties is an important part of overall health.

BEHAVIOUR CHANGE TECHNIQUES

Once you analyze the factors influencing your current behaviours, as well as the factors that may influence the direction and potential success of the behaviour change you are considering, you must decide which of several possible behaviour change techniques will work best for you.

Shaping: Developing New Behaviours in Small Steps

Regardless of how motivated and committed you are to change, some behaviours are almost impossible to change immediately because they require smaller steps/goals to reach the ultimate goal. Thus, to reach your goal, you may need to take a number of individual steps, each designed to change one small part of the overall behaviour. This process is known as **shaping.**

For example, suppose you have been physically inactive for a while. You decide that you want to become more physically active and physically fit. Your long-term goal is to be able to run 5 kilometres. You realize that it is not wise—and it will hurt—to simply start running, so you decide to build up your physical fitness gradually and have come up with a plan. During week one, you will walk for 20 minutes every other day at a moderate pace. During week two, you will walk four or five days. In week three, you will walk five days. Then in week four, you will increase the time to 25 minutes. Gradually, you will increase the time you walk, while maintaining a frequency of five days per week until you are ready to alternate five minutes of walking with five minutes of jogging. These gradual steps—and more like them—will help you to reach your goal.

Whatever the desired behaviour change, shaping involves:

- starting slowly to prevent or limit undue stress
- keeping the steps small and realistic/achievable
- being flexible/adaptable and ready to change if the original plan is not working

- refusing to skip steps or to move to the next step until the previous step has been mastered—or feels comfortable; your current lifestyle behaviours did not develop overnight, so they will not change overnight.
- rewarding yourself for meeting short- and long-term goals

Visualizing: The Imagined Rehearsal

Mental practice and rehearsal can help in the behaviour change process. Athletes and others often use a technique called **imagined rehearsal** to reach their goals. By visualizing their planned action ahead of time, they were better prepared—and able—when they actually engaged in the imagined behaviour. For example, suppose you want to ask a classmate out on a date. Imagine the setting (walking together to class). Then, in your mind and out loud, practise what you want to say ("There's a great concert this Sunday, and I was wondering if . . . "). Mentally anticipate different responses ("Oh, I'd love to, but . . . " or "That sounds like fun . . . ") and what you will say in response ("That's okay, maybe another time" or "How about I give you a call some time this week?"). Careful mental and verbal imagined rehearsal will greatly improve your likelihood of success.

Modelling

Modelling, or learning behaviours by carefully observing other people, is one of the most effective strategies for changing behaviours. If you carefully observe behaviours you admire, and isolate their components, you can model the steps of your behaviour-change strategy on a proven success. For example if you have trouble talking to people you don't know very well, one of the easiest ways for you to improve your communication skills is to observe someone whose skills you admire. Do they talk or listen more? How do they listen? How do people respond to them? What makes them good communicators? What is their body language like? Thus when you observe the behaviours you admire and isolate their components, you can model the steps in your behaviour change based on a proven success.

Shaping: Using a series of small steps to reach a particular goal gradually.

Imagined rehearsal: Practising a skill or behaviour through mental imagery.

Modelling: Learning specific behaviours by watching others perform them.

✿ Controlling the Situation

Sometimes, putting yourself in the right setting or with the right group of people will positively influence your behaviours directly or indirectly. Many situations and occasions trigger similar behaviours in different people. For example, in libraries, churches, and museums, most people talk softly. Few people laugh at funerals. The term **situational inducement** refers to an attempt to influence a behaviour by using situations and occasions structured to exert control over that behaviour. If you are trying to reduce the fat in your diet, an example could be choosing to eat at a vegetarian restaurant rather than a fast-food chain.

Reinforcement

A **positive reinforcement** seeks to increase the likelihood that a behaviour will occur by presenting something positive as a reward for that behaviour. Each of us is motivated by different reinforcers. While a special T-shirt may be a positive reinforcer for young adults entering a fun run, it may not be for someone who dislikes message-bearing T-shirts, or for someone with a drawer full of them. Most positive reinforcers can be classified under five headings:

- *Consumable reinforcers* are edibles such as candy, cookies, drinks, or gourmet meals.
- *Activity reinforcers* are opportunities to watch TV, go on a vacation, go swimming, or do something else enjoyable.
- *Manipulative reinforcers* are such incentives as lower rent in exchange for mowing the lawn or the promise of a better grade for doing an extra-credit project.
- *Possessional reinforcers* are tangible rewards such as a new TV or a sports car.
- *Social reinforcers* are such things as loving looks, affectionate hugs, and praise.

what do you THINK?

What types of consumable reinforcers (food or drink) would be healthy and appropriate rewards for your new behaviours? If you could choose one activity reinforcer to reward yourself for one day (or one week) of your new behaviours, what would it be? If you could obtain something for yourself (possessional reinforcer) after you reach your goal, what would it be? If you maintain your behaviours for one week, what type of social reinforcer would you like from your friends?

Changing Self-Talk

Self-talk, or the way you think and talk to yourself, also plays a role in your attempts at behaviour change. Rational-emotive therapy, Meichenbaum's self-instructional method, and blocking or thought stopping are examples.

Rational-Emotive Therapy

This form of cognitive therapy or self-directed behaviour change is based on the premise that a close connection exists between what people say to themselves and how they feel. Most everyday emotional problems and related behaviours stem from irrational statements that people make to themselves when events in their lives are different from what they expected or hoped for.[22]

Meichenbaum's Self-Instructional Methods

In Meichenbaum's behavioural therapies, clients are encouraged to give *self-instructions* ("Slow down, don't rush") and *positive affirmations* ("My speech is going fine—I'm almost done!") to themselves instead of thinking self-defeating thoughts ("I'm talking too fast—my speech is terrible") when a situation seems to be getting out of control. Meichenbaum is perhaps best known for a process known as *stress inoculation,* in which clients are subjected to extreme stressors in a laboratory environment. Before a stressful event (for example, going to the doctor), clients practise

The support and encouragement of friends with similar interests will strengthen your commitment to develop and maintain positive health behaviours.

Talking with friends or family can help you clarify your thinking about behaviours you want to change and provide ongoing support as you attempt to reach your goals.

individual coping skills (for example, deep breathing exercises) and self-instructions (for example, "I'll feel better once I know what's causing my pain"). Meichenbaum demonstrated that clients who practised coping techniques and self-instruction were less likely to resort to negative behaviours in stressful situations.

Blocking or Thought Stopping

By purposely blocking or stopping negative thoughts, a person can concentrate on taking positive steps toward necessary behaviour change. For example, suppose you are preoccupied with your ex-partner, who recently deserted you for someone else. In blocking or thought stopping, you consciously stop thinking about the situation and force yourself to think about something more pleasant (for example, dinner tomorrow with your best friend). By refusing to dwell on negative images and by forcing yourself to focus elsewhere, you can save wasted energy, time, and emotional resources and move on to positive change.

MAKING BEHAVIOUR CHANGE

Self-Assessment: Antecedents and Consequences

Behaviours, thoughts, and feelings always occur in a context—the situation. Situations can be divided into two components: the events that come before a behaviour and those that come after it. *Antecedents* are the setting events for a behaviour; they cue or

stimulate a person to act in certain ways. Antecedents can be physical events, thoughts, emotions, or the actions of other people. *Consequences*—the results of behaviours—affect whether a person will repeat a behaviour.[23] Consequences also include physical events, thoughts, emotions, or the actions of other people.

Learning to recognize the antecedents of your behaviours and acting to modify them is one method of changing them. A diary noting your undesirable behaviours and the settings in which they occur can be a useful tool. For example, if you are gaining weight, keep a diary of when, where, why, how, and with whom you eat. If you are eating potato chips while studying, you may need to study in the library, where food isn't allowed, or not have that kind of snack available in your house. If you eat more when you are angry, upset, depressed, or stressed, try to deal directly with your stressors or engage in an alternative activity, such as going for a walk or swim. The positive consequences of these changes will be that you will maintain your weight and feel better about yourself.

Analyzing the Behaviours You Want to Change

Successful behaviour change requires a careful assessment of exactly what it is that you want to change. All too often we berate ourselves by using

Situational inducement: Attempts to influence a behaviour by using situations and occasions structured to exert control over that behaviour.

Positive reinforcement: Presenting something positive following a behaviour being reinforced.

generalities: "I am not a good person; I'm lousy to my friend; I need to be a better person." Becoming a better person is a lofty goal, though difficult to define and measure. Before you can begin to change a negative behaviour, you must take a hard look at its specifics. Determining the specific behaviours you would like to change—as opposed to the general problem—will allow you to set clear goals for change. What are you doing that makes you a lousy friend? Are you gossiping about your friends? Are you lying to them? Have you been a "taker" rather than a "giver" in the friendship? Or are you really a good friend most of the time? What specifically do you do that makes you a not-so-good friend?

If the problem is gossiping, you can analyze your behaviour using the following:

- *Frequency.* How often do you gossip? In every conversation, once per day, less frequently?

- *Duration.* Have you been gossiping about your friend for a long period of time? A few weeks, a few months? Over the years?

- *Seriousness.* Is your gossiping idle chatter/sharing information, or are you really trying to injure the other person? What are the consequences for you? for your friend? for your friendship? for the person listening to you?

- *Basis for the problem behaviour.* Is your gossip based on facts, on your perceptions of facts, or on deliberate embellishments of facts? Are you trying to make yourself look or feel better? to discredit your friend?

- *Antecedents.* What kinds of situations trigger your gossiping? Do some settings or people bring out the gossip in you more than others? Why are you talking behind your friend's back?

✳ Decision Making: Choices for Change

So you've completed the background work and assessed the antecedents and consequences of the behaviour you want to change. Now comes the real crunch: deciding what to do when faced with choices that will assist or distract you from your intentions to change. Decision making is a skill you must consciously develop. Choosing among alternatives is difficult when you are consciously and unconsciously pressured by internal and external influences. For example, "just saying no" is, of course, one choice when you are handed a glass of beer or wine at a party. However, if you are trying desperately to fit in, if people with whom you identify all drink, or if you like the

taste of beer or wine, the decision becomes harder. By practising the following decision-making skills prior to having that drink put into your hands, you will increase your chances of making the choice you really want to make. This set of skills, referred to by the acronym DECIDE, can be applied to many decision-making situations.[24]

D *Decide in advance what the problem is.* By defining the problem in advance, you will have time to determine how important it is. If you decide that drinking is not for you, or that drinking in certain situations could put you at risk, you will have your basic criteria for acting in specific situations.

E *Explore the alternatives.* List the possible alternatives, ranging from not drinking to drinking heavily. If any of these alternatives is unacceptable to you, cross it off and work with those remaining.

C *Consider the consequences.* Think about each of the alternatives remaining. What are the possible positive and negative consequences of each? Think about what will probably happen, not just what may happen in the best and worst scenarios. How risky is each alternative? Are the consequences of losing the friendship of this particular group as serious as the risk of drinking heavily and getting into trouble sexually or drinking and driving? Is there another alternative that could reduce your risks?

I *Identify your values.* Your beliefs and feelings about certain behaviours represent your values, which then influence your behaviours. When choosing to drink or not to drink in a social setting, or when choosing how much to drink, you should base your choice on your values.

D *Decide and take action.* If you have seriously thought about the first four DECIDE components and determined that it's okay to have one or two drinks over the course of the evening and that is your absolute limit, this may be a reasonable decision for you. Then you must take action based upon this decision—you must actively take measures to ensure you stick to your limit.

E *Evaluate the consequences.* A key component of the decision-making process is a careful look backward at your decision, the decision making process followed, and your resulting behaviours, how you felt about them, and whether you want to do anything differently in the future. You may add alternatives at the second step, for instance. The secret to success is to think about the problem in advance, consider your values and desires, and anticipate the choices you will likely face.

Managing Your Behaviour: Change Strategies

From the information presented in this chapter, you should realize that health includes many dimensions and that changing negative health-related behaviours is a complicated, multifaceted process requiring commitment, personal insight, and knowledge. Few of us could ever "just do it" (at least not on the first try). As you continue to read this book, you will find that each chapter lists specific activities that enable you to choose to adopt or maintain healthy behaviours. The following activities and questions may help as you make decisions regarding your healthstyle.

MAKING DECISIONS FOR YOU

1. Identify a specific behaviour that you want to change. Although there may be many behaviours you would like to change, list only one to increase your chance of success.

2. Outline the steps you will take to achieve this change.

3. What reinforcers can you give yourself along the way? Whom could you call upon to help keep you motivated? Is that person willing to help?

4. What techniques do you think will be most useful (positive reinforcement, shaping, modelling, imagined rehearsal, situational inducement, changes in self-talk, others) in your preparations to change, when you make the change, and to maintain the change?

CHECKLIST FOR CHANGE: MAKING PERSONAL CHOICES

- Are you ready to make this change? Are you in a healthy emotional state? Is this change for you or to please someone else?

- Have you completed a personal health history to assess your risks?

- Have you developed an action plan with short- and long-term goals? Have you set priorities?

- Have you assessed your personal resources? Whom can you call on to help you? Where can you go for support and advice?

- Have you planned alternative actions in case you run into obstacles or begin to self-sabotage?

- Have you set up a list of reinforcers and supports that will keep you motivated along the way?

- Have you established a set of guidelines for success? Will you have small goals to achieve at selected intervals or will you consider yourself successful only if you have met your ultimate goal?

CHECKLIST FOR CHANGE: MAKING COMMUNITY CHOICES

- Have you taken time to become educated about issues or concerns affecting others in your community?

- Have you prioritized the actions that you can take to make a difference in changing community behaviours? Do you have a particular goal?

- Do you act responsibly to preserve the environment by consuming fewer resources? Using fewer packaged items? Do you reduce, reuse, and recycle whenever possible? Do you encourage others to?

- Do you analyze what is happening in your school, community, province, and nation by reading about issues, actively discussing problems and possible solutions, and developing personal opinions?

- Do you listen carefully to what your elected officials say and let them know in writing or by calling if you disagree with them?

- Do you volunteer your time to help less fortunate others at least once each term?

- Do you purchase products and services from companies that have proven records of protecting the environment, providing safe foods and products, and supporting the health and well-being of others through their organizational practices?

- Do you purchase Canadian-made products? Local-made products? Do you consider production/transportation costs of food before purchase?

CHECKLIST FOR CHANGE: MAKING CRITICAL THINKING CHOICES

Each chapter of this text will end with a decision-making situation. You may wish to use the DECIDE model introduced in this chapter to develop decision-making skills. For your first decision, we return to the situation described when we introduced the model: To drink or not to drink. Let's assume that you are attending a major party tonight where alcohol will be served—and you have a test tomorrow afternoon. Using the decision-making model, will you drink? If so, will you set a limit? How will you respond when pressured to drink more? Or pressured to stay later than you intended?

Goal Setting and Behaviour Change: SuPeR SMART

Goal setting is a critical part of the behaviour-change process. As noted previously, creating realistic short- and long-term goals provides a manageable target for your efforts. One practical method of goal setting is called SuPeR SMART.[25]

Self-controllable. The goals you set must be within your control, something that you can take action on. If eating more healthily is your goal, a more specific, appropriate goal within your control is to say you will consume at least four vegetables and three fruits each day. If becoming more physically active is something you would like to do, an example of a self-controllable goal is to plan for 15 minutes of walking each day after dinner.

Public. If you make your goal visible or known—for you and others to see—it will be a constant reminder of what you are trying to achieve. Using the examples above, put a calendar on the refrigerator or somewhere else in your kitchen where you can keep track of the number of vegetables and fruit you consume each day. Similarly, indicate on the calendar with a checkmark that you walked 15 minutes after dinner.

Rewards. Rewarding yourself for reaching your short- and long-term goals is important and motivates you to stay on track. The reward, however, should not contradict what you are trying to achieve (for example, treating yourself to a bag of chips when you are trying to eat more healthily). Instead, reward yourself with a new workout T-shirt or a new book. Rewards should occur frequently enough that they are attainable and provide the needed motivation.

Specific. Your goals should be clear and precise. "Eating more healthily" is not precise. Meeting the guidelines set out in Eating Well with Canada's Food Guide is more precise. You may even get more specific and say, I want to eat at least four vegetables and three fruits each day. "Getting more active" is also not very precise. Engaging in 30 minutes of physical activity every day is specific and measurable.

Measurable. Your goals should be measurable. Thus, a goal of meeting the guidelines set in the Food Guide (for a 19-year-old female consuming minimally, seven to eight servings from vegetables and fruits, six to seven servings from grain products two servings from milk and alternatives, and two servings from meat and alternatives) or of accumulating 30 minutes of physical activity every day, can be easily measured.

Adjustable. Your short- and long-term goals should be flexible. Life can be unpredictable, and if you start to fall behind because of one thing or another it is important to recognize that it's okay so long as you can get back on track as soon as possible. Using our examples, even though you did not meet all the Food Guide requirements over the holidays or engage in 30 minutes of physical activity every day, you can continue with your healthier eating or doing more physical activity starting today. You may also learn more about yourself and why it was that you were not able to stay on track so that you can adjust and manage the factors distracting you from your goals the next time.

Realistic. To successfully change your behaviours, your goals must be realistic. In determining the reality of your goals, evaluate your financial, environmental, physical, and emotional situations. A goal to climb Mount Everest although admirable, may not be realistic if you do not have the financial means to get there or networks to support your efforts. Similarly, a goal to lose 10 kg by the end of the month is not realistic either.

Time-based. Again, your goals should be quantifiable and include a specific date or timeline for achievement. Setting a realistic timeline requires accountability for your choices and actions. For example, in the first week of changing your behaviours you may add 10 minutes of physical activity each day. The next week you may increase the time to 15 minutes, and so forth until you reach your goal of 30 minutes each day. Be careful to set a realistic and achievable timeline to avoid failure and maintain motivation. Doing this realistically requires knowledge of not only the behaviour-change process, but also the behaviour you want to change. Overly ambitious, short timelines can lead to failure. But, on the other hand, if your timeline is too long, you may lose sight of your long-term goal.

Whether your chosen behaviour change is to become more socially active, eat more healthily, become more physically active, or enhance your spiritual health, your goal setting should be guided by the SuPeR SMART components and aimed at improving your overall well-being.

Go to MyHealthLab at **www.pearsoned.ca/myhealthlab**. Here you will find self-assessments, case studies, links to health on the net, and much more.

DISCUSSION QUESTIONS

1. Compare and contrast the terms *health* and *wellness*. What, components are included in the definitions of these terms?

2. In your opinion are Canadians healthy today? Why or why not?

3. How are men and women treated differently in the health-care system? Why do you think these differences exist? What can be done to change this?

4. What are the leading causes of death in Canada? How do the current efforts at health promotion address these leading causes of death at both an individual and population level? What lifestyle changes can you make to reduce your risk of these leading causes of death?

5. Briefly describe the health belief model, the theory of reasoned action, and the theory of planned behaviour. Which do you ascribe to the most? The least?

6. Explain the various factors (that is, predisposing, reinforcing, and enabling) that influence a young mother on social support to choose low-quality, high calorie foods (that is, potato chips and soda pop vs. fresh vegetables and milk) to feed herself and her children.

7. Describe what behaviour-change technique you would use to become physically active on a regular basis.

8. Why is it important that you are ready to change before attempting to start changing?

APPLICATION EXERCISE

Reread the Consider This. . . scenario at the beginning of the chapter and answer the following questions.

1. From what you learned in this chapter, what steps would Cameron and Megumi have to take to change their behaviours?

2. On your campus, where could students, like Cameron and Megumi go for help?

3. As a friend, what can you do to be more supportive of the health of someone you know who is trying to make a change?

MYSEARCHLAB EXERCISE

1. Log on to www.MySearchLab.com

2. Retrieve article AN 32549099 "E-mail at work: A cause for concern? The implications of the new communication technologies for health, wellbeing and productivity at work" by Howard Taylor, George Fieldman, and Yochanan Altman.

3. Read the article, then respond to the following questions:
   a. How has email helped/hindered communication in the work world?
   b. How has email helped/hindered personal communication?
   c. What is the influence of email on workplace stress?
   d. How do email, instant messaging, and other forms of rapid communication help/hinder students' academic development?
   e. What suggestions would you give your classmates to manage their email, instant messaging, and other forms of rapid communication?

CHAPTER 2

PSYCHOSOCIAL HEALTH

Achieving Mental, Emotional, Social, and Spiritual Wellness

CONSIDER THIS . . .

Marisol is a 19-year-old first-year student majoring in liberal arts. She has become increasingly bored with her classes, finds little excitement in her days, and doesn't have the energy or desire to go out with friends. One weekend, she stayed in bed for two days "resting," and when she got up on Monday, she was still so tired that she could barely stay awake in class. She has difficulty concentrating, finds herself lounging on the couch watching TV at every opportunity, and does not care whether her apartment is a mess. She has gone to the student health centre, and after several tests the doctor tells her that there is nothing physically wrong with her.

Have you ever felt like Marisol? What do you think is wrong with her? What do you think contributes to her condition? Do you have friends showing similar signs? Why might a typical student health professional miss such obvious symptoms? What do you think Marisol should do to help herself get better? As a friend, what could you do to help her? What services and programs are available on your campus and in your community to help her?

CHAPTER OBJECTIVES

- Define psychosocial health and its components mental, emotional, social, and spiritual health.

- Describe the external and internal factors influencing psychosocial health. Which of these factors can be changed?

- Identify common psychosocial problems, and explain their causes and available treatments.

- Describe the warning signs of suicide and the actions to take to help an individual contemplating suicide.

- Name the different types of mental health professionals and the most common types of therapy.

Most of us feel "down" occasionally; still, we get through the day in a reasonably productive, if not altogether exciting, way. We eventually sort through seemingly overwhelming problems, suppress our anxieties, and use our social support system (families, friends, and significant others) to help us through the low times. For some, though, these down times become persistent, nagging experiences that vary from small "downers" to "black holes" that are increasingly difficult to emerge from. Whether caused by temporary setbacks or major blows, these miserable moods sap our energy, reduce our physical reserves, waste our time, diminish our spirit, and take the joy out of our lives. They may even lead to a serious mental illness. Eventually, they may shorten our life span—reducing quantity as well as quality of life. How we feel and think about ourselves, those around us, and our circumstances can tell us a lot about our psychosocial health. Like our physical health, our psychosocial health can have a profound impact on the quality and quantity of our lives. We can enhance our psychosocial health just as we can our physical health, by becoming aware of relevant attitudes and behaviours and making changes where and when necessary.

DEFINING PSYCHOSOCIAL HEALTH

Psychosocial health encompasses the mental, emotional, social, and spiritual dimensions of health (see Figure 2.1). People who are psychosocially healthy develop these dimensions to optimal levels. They have an endless reserve for facing the normal ups and downs of life. They respond to challenges, disappointments, joys, frustrations, and pain by summoning up personal resources acquired through years of experience, and when a needed resource is not available, they find ways to develop it. Their resiliency is strong and they are actively involved in the process of living each day to the fullest.

Psychosocial health is the result of a complex interaction of a person's history and his or her conscious and unconscious thoughts about and interpretations of the past. Although definitions of psychosocial health vary, people who are psychosocially healthy share several basic characteristics:[1]

- *They feel good about themselves.* People who are psychosocially healthy are not overwhelmed by fear, love, anger, jealousy, guilt, or worry. They know who they are, have a realistic sense of their capabilities, and respect themselves even though they realize they are not perfect.
- *They feel comfortable with other people.* People who are psychosocially healthy have satisfying and

FIGURE 2.1

Psychosocial Health as a Complex Interaction of Mental, Emotional, Social, and Spiritual Health

lasting personal relationships and do not take advantage of others; nor do they allow others to take advantage of them. They give and receive love, consider others' interests, respect personal differences, and feel responsible for their fellow human beings.

- *They control tension and anxiety.* People who are psychosocially healthy recognize the underlying causes and symptoms of stress in their lives and consciously avoid illogical or irrational thoughts, unnecessary aggression, hostility, excessive excuse making, and blaming others for their problems. They use resources and learn skills to control reactions to stressful situations, including constructively expressing positive and negative feelings and learning to tolerate their frustrations.

- *They are able to meet the demands of life.* People who are psychosocially healthy try to solve problems as they arise, to accept responsibility for their thoughts and actions, and to plan ahead. They break down problems into manageable bits and work through them one piece or step at a time. They set realistic goals, think for themselves, and make independent decisions. Acknowledging that change is a normal part of life, they welcome new experiences.

- *They curb hate and guilt.* People who are psychosocially healthy acknowledge and combat their tendencies to respond with hate, anger, thoughtlessness, and selfishness. They do not take vengeance, nor do they allow feelings of inadequacy to build. They do not try to knock others aside to get ahead but rather reach out to help others—even those they may not be fond of.

Psychosocial health: The mental, emotional, social, and spiritual dimensions of health.

A joyful spirit and the resiliency to face life's ups and downs are measures of psychosocial health.

- *They choose a positive outlook.* People who are psychosocially healthy approach each day assuming it will go well. As Randy Pausch noted in *The Last Lecture* " . . . there's a decision we all have to make and it seems perfectly captured in the Winnie-the-Pooh characters created by A.A. Milne. Each of us must decide: Am I a fun-loving Tigger or am I a sad-sack Eeyore?"[2]

- *They enrich the lives of others.* People who are psychosocially healthy recognize that there are others whose needs may be greater than their own. They try to ease these people's burdens by doing simple things such as giving a ride to an elderly neighbour in need, bringing flowers to someone in pain, making dinner for someone who is grief-stricken, volunteering at a community agency, and making charitable donations. They generally trust others and themselves.

- *They cherish the things that make them smile.* People who are psychosocially healthy make a special place in their lives for memories of the past. Family pictures, high-school mementos, souvenirs of past vacations, and other reminders of good experiences brighten their day. Fun is an integral part of their lives. So is making time for themselves.

- *They value diversity.* People who are psychosocially healthy do not fear differences; they are not threatened by people of a different sex, religion, sexual orientation, ethnicity, or political party. They accept these differences. They are not judgmental and do not force their beliefs and values on others.

- *They appreciate and respect nature.* People who are psychosocially healthy enjoy and respect natural beauty and wonders. As mentioned in Chapter 1, the biophilia hypothesis refers to an instinctive bond between people and other living systems.[3] Psychosocially healthy people take the time to enjoy their surroundings—the environment and the living things within it—act responsibly, and are conscious of their place in the universe.

Of course, few of us ever achieve optimal levels in all these areas all the time. Attaining psychosocial health and wellness involves many complex processes and should be considered dynamic in nature, with ebbs and flows like the tide. This chapter will help you to understand not only what it means to be psychosocially healthy, but also the difficulties you may face in attaining and maintaining psychosocial health.

what do you THINK?

Which psychosocial qualities do you value most in your friends? Your family? Are these the same ones that you value most in yourself? Why or why not?

Mental Health: The Thinking You

The term **mental health** is used to describe the "thinking" or "rational" part of psychosocial health. It describes your ability to perceive things happening around you in realistic ways, to use reasoning in problem solving, to interpret what is happening, and to evaluate your situation effectively and react appropriately. In short, you are able to sort through the clutter of events, variety of messages (conflicting and corroborating), and uncertainties of a situation and attach meaning (either positive or negative) to it based upon your experiences, attitudes, behaviours, and the environmental cues. Your values, attitudes, and beliefs about your health, your relationships with your family and others, and your life in general are usually—at least in part—a reflection of your mental health.

A person who is mentally healthy enjoys life, the environment, and the people in it.[4] Such people tend to be creative, to learn, to try new things, and to take risks. They cope well in personal and professional situations of stress. They feel sad and angry when faced with the death of a loved one, a job loss or relationship problems, and other difficult events, but in time, with rational thinking and effective communication, are able to move forward and enjoy life again. They also take responsibility for their actions. For example, let's say that, knowing you have a major term paper and an exam when you return, you still decide to travel for spring break with friends. When you return and quickly throw together a paper and study hurriedly for your exam, there is no point in becoming distraught when you get a "D" for your efforts. Instead, the mentally healthy response would be to take responsibility for the choice made, learn from your mistake, and plan differently next time.

Similarly, people going through a difficult break-up often have difficulty picking themselves up and moving on in healthy ways. Learning to acknowledge that it is okay to feel sad, unhappy, disappointed, or frustrated and getting help through counselling or talking with trusted friends is part of a healthy process of adapting and coping. Unfortunately, too many of us get caught up in our emotional upheavals and are unable to pull ourselves out of the deep funk we find ourselves in. Further, many of us, particularly men, think it is a weakness to seek help—whether professional or just from our friends.[5]

When a person's mental health deteriorates, he or she may experience sharp declines in rational thinking and increasingly distorted perceptions. As a result, a person may become cynical and distrustful, experience volatile mood swings, or choose to be isolated from others. These negative reactions may threaten the quality and quantity of life of the person experiencing them, as well as the life and health of others. People showing such signs of extreme abnormal behaviours or mental disorders are classified as having mental illnesses, discussed later in this chapter.

❋ Emotional Health: The Feeling You

Emotional health is a term often used interchangeably with mental health. Although closely related, emotional health refers to the "feeling," or subjective, side of psychosocial health and includes our "feeling" reactions to life. **Emotions** are intensified feelings or complex patterns of feelings that we experience on a minute-by-minute, day-to-day basis. Love, hate, hurt, despair, release, joy, anxiety, fear, frustration, and anger are some of the many emotions we experience. Typically, emotions are described as the interplay of four components: *physiological arousal, feelings, cognitive (thinking) processes,* and *behavioural reactions.*

There are four basic types of emotions: (1) emotions resulting from harm, loss, or threats; (2) emotions resulting from benefits or rewards; (3) borderline emotions, such as hope and compassion; and (4) more complex emotions, such as grief, disappointment, bewilderment, and curiosity.[6] Each of us may experience these emotions in combination at any time. Each of us is also likely to experience a range in level of emotional responses from very intense to very little

reaction. Further, our emotional responses to various settings and situations will vary amongst and within individuals on a day-to-day basis. As rational beings, it is our responsibility to evaluate our emotional responses, the environment leading to these responses, and the appropriateness of our actions or reactions to these emotional responses.

People who are emotionally healthy are usually able to respond appropriately to upsetting or uplifting events. When threatened, they are not likely to react in an extreme fashion, behave inconsistently, or adopt an offensive attack. People who are emotionally healthy are less likely to let their feelings overpower them. How many times have you seen someone react with extreme anger by shouting, slamming a door, or punching a wall? Those are reaction of people who are emotionally unhealthy. These people may be highly volatile and prone to unpredictable emotional outbursts and to inappropriate, sometimes frightening, responses to events. An ex-boyfriend (or girlfriend) who becomes so angry that he or she hits and pushes you around or yells at you because he or she is jealous of you and/or your new relationship is demonstrating an unhealthy and dangerous emotional reaction.

try it NOW!

Seek change! Change is an inevitable part of life, and it can also be a challenge to your psychosocial health. Develop skills to cope with change by making change a regular part of your life. View changes as exciting chances for growth rather than negative events. Think of the positive things that change can create. Take a different route to class, study at the coffee shop instead of the library, or pick out the people you do not know in class as your project partners. Eat something different for dinner. Try a new physical activity. Do not get stuck in a "same old, same old" approach to life.

Poor emotional health often affects social health. Social isolation is one of the many potentially negative consequences of unstable emotional responses. People tend to avoid those who are feeling and/or acting hostile, withdrawn, moody, grumpy, nasty, or irritable, as well as those who are overly quiet, cry easily, or demonstrate other disturbing emotional responses. Since people in a poor emotional state are not much

Mental health: The "thinking" part of psychosocial health. Includes values, attitudes, and beliefs.

Emotional health: The "feeling" part of psychosocial health. Includes the "feeling" reactions to life.

Emotions: Intensified feelings or complex patterns of feelings we experience.

fun to be around, their friends, family, and colleagues tend to avoid them at the very time they most need support.

For students, a more immediate concern may be the impact of poor emotional health on academic performance. Imagine studying for an exam or trying to write a paper after a fight with a close friend, partner, or family member, or when someone close to you has recently died. Emotional turmoil seriously affects your ability to think clearly, reason, or act in a rational way. Many otherwise rational people do things they would not normally do when they are going through a major emotional upset. Mental functioning and emotional responses are intricately connected.

Social Health: Interactions with Others

Social health is the part of psychosocial health dealing with our interactions with others on an individual and group basis, our ability to use—and to provide—social resources and support in time of need, and our ability to adapt to a variety of social situations. People who are socially healthy have a wide range of social interactions with family, friends, and acquaintances, and are able to have healthy interactions with an intimate partner. They are able to listen, express themselves, form healthy relationships, act in socially acceptable and responsible ways, and find a best fit for themselves in society. Numerous studies document the importance of social health in promoting physical and mental health as well as enhanced longevity. Two factors, in particular, are important:[7]

- *Presence of strong social bonds.* **Social bonds**, or social linkages, reflect the general degree and nature of interpersonal contacts and interactions. Social bonds generally provide six major functions: (1) intimacy, (2) feelings of belonging to or integration with a group, (3) opportunities for giving or receiving nurturance, (4) reassurance of one's worth, (5) assistance and guidance, and (6) advice. In general, people more "connected" to others manage stress more effectively and are much more resilient when bombarded by life's crises.

- *Presence of key social supports.* **Social supports** refer to relationships that bring positive benefits to the individual. Social supports can be either expressive (emotional support, encouragement) or structural (housing, money). Social support can be provided informally by friends and family, or formally by professionals in various settings. People who are psychosocially healthy create a network of friends and family with whom they can give and receive informal support.

Social health also reflects the way we react to others around us. In its most extreme forms, a lack of social health is represented by acts of prejudice and bias toward other individuals or groups. **Prejudice** is a negative evaluation of an entire group of people typically based on unfavourable (and mistaken) ideas about the group.[8] In its most obvious manifestations, prejudice is reflected in acts of discrimination against others, in overt acts of hate and bias, and in purposeful intent to harm individuals or groups.

Spiritual Health: An Inner Quest for Well-Being

Although mental, emotional, and social health are key factors in overall psychosocial functioning, it is possible to be mentally, emotionally, and socially healthy and still not achieve optimal levels of psychosocial well-being. What is missing? For many people, that difficult-to-describe element that gives zest to life is the spiritual dimension. What does it mean to be spiritually healthy? As noted in Chapter 1, spiritual health reflects our values, beliefs, and perceptions of the world and all living things. Since spirituality is no longer believed to be rooted exclusively in religion, it is now more often defined as a search for meaning, connectedness, energy, and transcendence.[9] Spirituality refers to the deepest or innermost part of us, the part that helps us to make sense of the world and our part in it.[10] It is at the core of where we gather our strength and hope. It is that from which we determine who we are and what our purpose is. For some, spiritual health may involve a belief in a supreme being or a specified way of life as prescribed by a particular religion. For others, spiritual health may relate to personal relationships or being at peace with nature.

Many of us live on a rather superficial material plane throughout our formative years. We have basic human needs that must be satisfied according to a set hierarchical order. We tend to be rather egocentric, or self-oriented, during these formative years and to seek immediate material and emotional gratification while denying or ignoring the spiritual aspect of our lives. Worrying about the clothes you wear, the car you drive, the appearance of your apartment, and other material things are examples of this type of preoccupation. According to many psychologists and psychoanalysts, our materialistic Western civilization leads us to deny our spiritual needs. There comes a point, however, usually around midlife—or when a crisis occurs, such as a major illness or death of someone close to us—when we discover that the material world cannot bring a sense of happiness or self-worth.[11] We then recognize that material things like prestige, money, power, and fame count for little in the larger scheme of

FIGURE 2.2
Four Major Themes of Spirituality

life, and that if we were to die tomorrow these would not give meaning to our lives. Whatever the reason, the realization that there is more to life brings new opportunities for understanding ourselves and for spiritual growth. As we develop into people who are spiritually healthy, we come to recognize our uniqueness. We reach a better understanding of our strengths and weaknesses and our place in the universe. Many of us find that our families, the environment, animals, friends, strangers who are suffering, and religion assume greater significance in our lives. We become more willing to sacrifice for others or to improve the world around us. However, people do not have to wait until their middle years—or a crisis—to experience spiritual growth.

Attaining and maintaining spiritual health does take time and experience. The longer you live, the more you experience. The more you ponder the meaning of your experiences, the greater your chances of achieving spiritual health. In its purest sense, spirituality addresses four main themes: interconnectedness, mindfulness, spirituality as a part of everyday life, and living in harmony with the community (Figure 2.2).

- *Interconnectedness.* **Interconnectedness** refers to a sense of belonging and connecting with oneself, with others, and with a larger meaning or purpose of life. Connecting with oneself involves exploring feelings, assessing your reactions to people and experiences, and taking mental notes when things or people cause you to lose equilibrium. It also involves considering your values and achieving congruence between your goals and what you can do to achieve them without compromising your values.

- *Mindfulness.* **Mindfulness** refers to the ability to be fully present in the moment, to live in the now. It has been described as a way of nurturing greater awareness and clarity. It is a form of inner flow—a holistic sensation you feel when totally involved in the present.[12] You can achieve this inner flow

through an almost infinite range of opportunities for enjoyment and pleasure, either through the development and practice of physical and sensory skills in sport, music, dance, or yoga, or through the development of symbolic skills in areas such as poetry, philosophy, or mathematics.

- *Spirituality as a part of daily life.* Spirituality is embodied in the ability to discover and articulate our basic purpose in life; to learn how to experience love, joy, peace, and fulfillment; and to help ourselves and others achieve their full potential.[13] This ongoing process of growth fosters three convictions: faith, hope, and love. *Faith* is the belief that helps us realize our unique purpose in life; *hope* is the belief that allows us to look confidently and courageously to the future; and *love* involves accepting, affirming, and respecting oneself and others regardless of who they are.[14]

- *Living in harmony with our community.* Our values are an extension of our beliefs about the world and our attitude toward life. These values are formed over time from our experiences, and are reflected in our hopes, dreams, desires, goals, ambitions, and personal and community-oriented actions.[15] Although most people have some idea of what is important to them, many are largely unaware of how their values impact them or those around them until a crisis shakes up their perspective on life. Volunteering to help others, doing charitable work, and donating resources to help people in need are ways to "give back" to the community and the people who support you. These kinds of altruistic actions—that is, the giving of oneself out of genuine concern for others—also play a significant role in spiritual health.[16]

Spirituality: A Key to Better Health

Although the specific impact of spirituality on health remains elusive, many experts affirm the importance of this dimension in achieving health and wellness.

Social bonds: Degree and nature of interpersonal contacts.

Social supports: Structural and expressive aspects of social interactions.

Prejudice: A negative evaluation of an entire group of people typically based on unfavourable and often mistaken ideas about the group.

Interconnectedness: A web of connections, including our relationship to ourselves, to others, and to a larger meaning or purpose in life.

Mindfulness: Awareness and acceptance of the reality of the present moment.

A study of spirituality among post-secondary students from 46 diverse universities and colleges indicated that spirituality played a role in student health, grades, and other aspects of student life.[17] The researchers of this study found a correlation between spirituality and health achievement, with more spiritually oriented students having better health, higher grades, more involvement in charitable organizations or volunteerism, and more interest in helping others. Other studies also indicated a correlation between spirituality and positive health outcomes. For example, mindfulness therapies have been used effectively to treat depression, to reduce stress in outpatient therapy and in the nursing profession, with anxiety and heart disease treatments, and for other problems.[18]

A Spiritual Resurgence

An increase in spiritual awareness does not necessarily equate with an increase in beliefs in a god or supreme being of some kind. Some people find spiritual fulfillment in music, poetry, literature, art, nature, or intimate relationships.[19] For some, spirituality refers to a quest for self and selflessness—learning about oneself and learning how to willingly give of oneself to others. Understanding and appreciating oneself as a result of self-reflection can also help us to deepen or appreciate our life experiences more fully rather than just live through them. This topic has received much scholarly and popular attention. The fact that self-help books that focus on spirituality consistently top the bestseller lists demonstrates a renewed interest in spirituality within contemporary society.

✳ Putting Spirituality into Practice

How can you enhance the spiritual dimension of your psychosocial health? As noted, some people turn to a formal religion—for instance by attending religious services, engaging in prayer, or taking part in the organized study or discussion of religious texts (such as the Bible or the Koran). Others will find meaningful volunteer experiences or spend more time in personal reflection. Regardless of what you choose to do, keep in mind that enhancing your spiritual health is as time-consuming and requires as much effort as building your physical fitness or changing your dietary intake. The Skills for Behaviour Change textbox

---

SKILLS FOR BEHAVIOUR CHANGE

Strategies for Finding Your Spiritual Side

Spirituality involves connectedness to others and to the broader community, so it is important that we take time for meaningful interactions with our friends, family, and people within the community with whom we may not interact regularly. What types of actions foster connectedness?

VOLUNTEER

The ability to notice when others are in trouble, and reaching out to help them through volunteering, is an excellent way to feel connected with others and enhance your own health. In the aftermath of Hurricane Katrina, thousands of people volunteered their time, money, and effort to help an entire population that was suffering. Recognizing that we are all part of the greater system of humanity and that we have roles and responsibilities to help others in times of need is a key part of spirituality. Volunteering by helping your older neighbours clean their home, working at an animal shelter, or participating in a beach or highway cleanup is all a part of being responsible and finding a place to help in the greater scheme of things. Volunteering can be a huge boost for you when you are feeling down or wondering how you fit in.

TAKE TIME TO REFLECT

Connecting with your self is another method of finding your spiritual side. Make a ritual out of taking a few moments each day to think about who you are, what you value, why you feel good, or what things are troubling you. Setting aside this special time to reflect will become a sacred time meant just for you and can help you relieve tension, seek out answers to problems you are experiencing, or simply empty your mind and enjoy this time to yourself.

GET INVOLVED IN SERVICE LEARNING

Service learning involves making meaningful and productive relationships with the greater community. Community agencies and programs benefit from an enthusiastic, hardworking group of students. The students in turn have an opportunity to learn new skills and grow; they learn to look at the greater community and world around them, rather than remaining absorbed in college life and thoughts of papers due, the party on Friday night, and basketball practice.

features a few strategies you can implement to develop your spirituality.

❋ FACTORS INFLUENCING PSYCHOSOCIAL HEALTH

what do you THINK?

When you think of mental, emotional, social, and spiritual health, what do you think? What are your strengths and weaknesses in each? How can you enhance your strengths? How can you reduce the influence of your weaknesses?

Although it is relatively easy to define psychosocial health, it is much more difficult to explain why some people are psychosocially well almost all the time, others some of the time, and still others almost never. What factors influence your mental, emotional, social, and spiritual health? Are these factors changeable? What can you do to improve your psychosocial health? How can you enhance the positive qualities you already possess? See Table 2.1 for tips regarding mental fitness.

Most of our mental, emotional, social, and spiritual reactions to life are a direct outcome of our experiences, along with social and cultural expectations. Each of us is born with the innate capacity to experience emotions. Some of us apparently have a

TABLE 2.1
Mental Fitness Tips

- **Daydream** – Close your eyes and imagine yourself in a dream location. Breathe slowly and deeply. Whether it's a beach, a mountaintop, a hushed forest or a favourite room from your past, let the comforting environment wrap you in a sensation of peace and tranquility.

- **"Collect" positive emotional moments** – Make it a point to recall times when you have experienced pleasure, comfort, tenderness, confidence, or other positive emotions.

- **Learn ways to cope with negative thoughts** – Negative thoughts can be insistent and loud. Learn to interrupt them. Don't try to block them (that never works), and don't let them take over. Try distracting yourself or comforting yourself if you can't solve the problem right away.

- **Do one thing at a time** – For example, when you are out for a walk or spending time with friends, turn off your cellphone and stop making that mental "to do" list. Take in all the sights, sounds, and smells you encounter.

- **Exercise** – Regular physical activity improves psychological well-being and can reduce depression and anxiety. Joining an exercise group or a gym can also reduce loneliness, since it connects you with a new set of people sharing a common goal.

- **Enjoy hobbies** – Taking up a hobby brings balance to your life by allowing you to do something you enjoy because you want to do it, free of the pressure of everyday tasks. It also keeps your brain active.

- **Set personal goals** – Goals don't have to be ambitious. You might decide to finish that book you started three years ago; to take a walk around the block every day; to learn to knit or play bridge; to call your friends instead of waiting for the phone to ring. Whatever goal you set, reaching it will build confidence and a sense of satisfaction.

- **Keep a journal (or even talk to the wall!)** – Expressing yourself after a stressful day can help you gain perspective, release tension, and even boost your body's resistance to illness.

- **Share humour** – Life often gets too serious, so when you hear or see something that makes you smile or laugh, share it with someone you know. A little humour can go a long way to keeping us mentally fit!

- **Volunteer** – Volunteering is called the "win–win" activity because helping others makes us feel good about ourselves. At the same time, it widens our social network, provides us with new learning experiences and can bring balance to our lives.

- **Treat yourself well** – Cook yourself a good meal. Have a bubble bath. See a movie. Call a friend or relative you haven't talked to in ages. Sit on a park bench and breathe in the fragrance of flowers and grass. Whatever it is, do it just for you.

Source: Canada Mental Health Association.

predisposition toward more emotionality than others. How we express our emotions has a lot to do with our interpretations of what we experience. These interpretations are often learned reactions to environmental and social stimuli.

External Influences

Our psychosocial health is based on how we perceive our experiences. While some experiences are under our control, others are not. External influences refer to those factors that we do not control, such as who raised us and the physical environment in which we live.

Influences of the Family

Our families have a significant influence on our psychosocial development. Children raised in healthy, nurturing, happy families where they learn about being responsible and accountable are more likely to become well-adjusted, productive adults. Children raised in dysfunctional families in which violence, sexual, physical, or emotional abuse, negative behaviours, distrust, anger, dietary deprivation, drug abuse, parental discord, or other negative characteristics are present may have a harder time adapting to life. In dysfunctional families, security, unconditional love, and trust are lacking and the children are often confused and psychologically bruised. Yet not all people raised in dysfunctional families become psychosocially unhealthy. Conversely, not all people from healthy family environments are psychosocially healthy. Obviously more factors are involved in our "process of becoming" than just our family.

Influences of the Wider Environment

While isolated negative events may do little damage to psychosocial health, persistent stressors, uncertainties, and threats may cause significant problems. Children raised in environments where crime is rampant and daily safety is in question, for example, have an increased risk of psychosocial health issues among other things. Drugs, crime, violent acts, school failure, unemployment, and a host of other bad things can happen to good people. That said, it is believed that certain protective factors—such as having one or more positive role models in the midst of chaos, or a high level of self-esteem—may help children from even the worst environments be healthy and well adjusted.

Another important influence on psychosocial health is access to health services and programs designed to support the maintenance or enhancement of psychosocial health. Going to a support group or seeing a trained counsellor or therapist is often a crucial first step in prevention and intervention efforts. Unfortunately, individuals from a poor socioeconomic background (who often need the services most) may have more difficulty accessing such services.

Internal Influences

Although your life experiences influence you in fairly obvious ways, many internal factors also work subtly to shape who you are and who you become. Some of these factors include your traits, hormonal functioning, physical health status (including neurological or nervous system functioning), level of physical fitness, and selected elements of your mental and emotional health. If issues occur with any of these factors, overall psychosocial health can decline.

Self-Efficacy and Self-Esteem

During our formative years, our successes and failures in school, sports, friendships, intimate relationships, jobs, and in every other aspect of life subtly shape our perceptions and beliefs about our personal worth and ability to help ourselves. These perceptions and beliefs in turn become internal influences on our psychosocial health.

Self-efficacy describes our belief about whether or not we can successfully engage in and execute a specific behaviour. If we experience success in academics, sports, or popularity, we typically expect to be successful in these aspects in the future. If we fail an exam, were chosen last to be on a team, or have not been able to make friends easily, we may believe that failure is inevitable in this regard. In general, the more self-efficacious we are and the more our experiences have been positive, the more likely we are to keep trying to execute a specific behaviour successfully. People who have a high level of self-efficacy are also more likely to feel that they have **personal control** over situations or believe their internal resources allow them to control events. On the other hand, a person with low self-efficacy may give up easily or not even try to change his or her behaviours. Learning new skills and having successful experiences improves confidence and leads to the expectation of future success.

Self-esteem refers to our sense of self-respect or self-worth. It can be defined as an evaluation of ourselves and personal worth as individuals. People with high self-esteem tend to feel good about themselves and to express a positive outlook on life. People with low self-esteem tend to not be happy with themselves, to demean themselves, and to doubt their ability to succeed.

Past successes and happy experiences, often recalled through photos, mementos, and recollections, contribute to a person's psychosocial health.

Our self-esteem forms as a result of the relationships we have with our parents and family during our formative years, with our friends as we grow older, with our significant others as we form intimate relationships, and with our teachers, co-workers, and others important to us throughout our lives. If we feel loved and valued in each of these relationships, we believe that we are inherently loveable individuals and have a strong sense of self esteem.

Learned Helplessness versus Learned Optimism

People who continually experience failure may develop a pattern of responding known as **learned helplessness**, in which they give up and fail to take action to help themselves.[20] This attitude and resultant behaviours are due in part to society's tendency toward *victimology,* laying the blame for an individual's problems on other people and on the circumstances rather than placing responsibility on the individual. Although viewing ourselves as victims may help us to feel better temporarily, it does not address the underlying cause or causes of a problem. Ultimately, not taking responsibility for our actions erodes self-efficacy and fosters learned helplessness by developing an attitude that there is nothing we can do to improve the situation or the outcome, so we may as well give up.

Countering learned helplessness is the theory that we can also learn to be optimistic; this phenomenon is called, not surprisingly, **learned optimism**.[21] Scientists studying learned optimism have found that it is possible for an individual to make a conscious choice to take a more positive stance towards the world. By changing our self-talk, examining our reactions and the way we assess what happens to us in life, and blocking negative thoughts, replacing those thoughts with positive thoughts, we can actually "learn" how to be optimistic.

Personality

Our personality is the unique mix of characteristics that distinguishes us from others. Hereditary, environmental, cultural, and experiential factors influence how we develop our personality. For each of us, the amount of influence exerted by any of these factors differs. Our personality determines how we react to the challenges of life. It also determines how we interpret the feelings we experience and how we resolve the conflicts we feel about being denied the things we need or want.

It is believed that we have the power not only to understand our own behaviours but also to actively change them, and that we thus can shape our personalities. Although much has been written about the importance of a healthy personality, there is little consensus about what exactly it is. In general, however, people who possess the following traits appear to be psychologically healthy:[22]

- *Extroversion*: The ability to adapt to a social situation and demonstrate assertiveness as well as power or interpersonal involvement.

- *Agreeableness*: The ability to conform, be likeable, and demonstrate friendly compliance as well as love.

- *Openness to experience*: The willingness to demonstrate curiosity and independence (also referred to as *inquiring intellect*).

- *Emotional stability*: The ability to maintain control of feelings.

Self-efficacy: Belief in your ability to perform a task successfully.

Personal control: Belief that our efforts can and do influence situations and interactions with others.

Self-esteem: Sense of self-respect or self-worth.

Learned helplessness: An attitude of giving up and not trying because of past failures.

Learned optimism: Pattern of responding that focuses on the positive, because you choose to view each situation positively and with a sense of hope.

- *Conscientiousness*: The qualities of being dependable and demonstrating self-control, discipline, and a need to achieve.

what do you THINK?

Which factors of psychosocial health have the greatest positive impact on your life? What are the negative influences? Which are influencing your life most now? How resilient are you? How can you build resiliency?

Life Span and Maturity

Although the exact determinants of personality are impossible to define, we do know that our personalities are dynamic. Our temperament changes as we age, as illustrated by the extreme emotions experienced in adolescence as we search for our independence and experience an influx of hormones. Most of us learn to control our emotions as we advance toward adulthood.

The college or university years mark another critical transition period for young adults. This transition to independence is easier if students have successfully accomplished earlier developmental tasks such as learning how to solve problems, to make and evaluate decisions, to define and adhere to personal values, and to establish casual and intimate relationships. Management of personal finances, career management strategies, interpersonal communication skills, and parenting skills (for those who choose to become parents) are among the developmental tasks post-secondary students must accomplish. Older students often have to balance the responsibilities of family, career, and school.

If you have not fulfilled earlier tasks, you will continue to grow but may find your life interrupted by recurrent "crises" left over from earlier stages. For example, if you did not learn to trust others in childhood, you may have difficulty establishing intimate relationships in late adolescence or early adulthood.

Resiliency and Developmental Assets

It has become well established that some people are much better prepared to meet the challenges of life than others. The combination of certain personality traits coupled with a supportive environment can equip one to deal effectively with life's many challenges. Individuals with this set of traits and circumstances are able to cope and even thrive in times of great stress or pressure. **Resiliency**, or *protective factors*, is a term used to describe those traits or characteristics that protect an individual or community from threat or harm. In a sense, these traits may serve to inoculate one against potential ill health. People with assets, whether financial, emotional, spiritual, physical, mental, or social, and other positive forces in their lives are likely to be resilient and bounce back when facing life's challenges.

✓• ENHANCING PSYCHOSOCIAL HEALTH

You may believe that your psychosocial health is fairly well developed by the time you reach college or university. However, attaining self-fulfillment is a lifelong, conscious process that involves building self-efficacy and self-esteem, understanding and controlling emotions, maintaining support networks, and learning to solve problems and make decisions.

Developing and Maintaining Self-Esteem and Self-Efficacy

There are several ways to build self-esteem and self-efficacy. These include developing a support group, being a support for others, completing required tasks, forming realistic expectations, making and taking time for yourself, maintaining your physical health, and examining your problems and seeking help.

Developing a Support Group

One of the best ways to gain self-esteem and self-efficacy is through a support group—peers who share your values. A support group can make you feel good about yourself and help you to take an honest look at your actions and choices. Although you might seek support in a wholly new group, remember that old ties are often the strongest. Keeping in contact with old friends and family members can provide a foundation of unconditional love that will help you through the many life transitions ahead.

Being a Support for Others

Feel better about yourself by helping others to feel good about themselves. Write more "thank you" cards, postcards, and "thinking of you" notes. This will build your self-esteem and that of your friends. Become more interesting by being more interested (in people, current events, and so on). Send news clippings to friends. Join a discussion, political action, or recreational group.

Completing Required Tasks

Another way to boost your self-esteem or self-efficacy is to complete required tasks successfully and on time. You are not likely to succeed in your studies if you leave term papers until the last minute, fail to keep up with the reading for your courses, and do not ask for clarification of points confusing you. Some university and college campuses provide study groups for various content areas. Your school's student services department may offer tips for managing time, understanding assignments, dealing with professors, and preparing for test taking. Poor grades, or grades that do not meet a student's expectations, are major contributors to diminished self-esteem and to emotional distress among post-secondary students.

Forming Realistic Expectations

Having realistic expectations of yourself—and others—is another method of boosting self-esteem and self-efficacy. College or university is a time to explore your potential. If you expect perfect grades, a steady stream of Saturday-night dates and a Hollywood-type romantic involvement, a good job, and a beautiful home and car, you may be setting yourself up for failure. Assess your current resources and the direction in which you are heading. Set small, incremental goals that are possible for you to meet. Rather than suggesting, "I'm going to get better grades" without some realistic actions or achievable, definable goals to support your intentions, decide that tomorrow you will spend two hours studying or go to the library to do research on a paper, or decide to talk to your professor to see what he or she recommends to help you to better understand a particular topic.

Making and Taking Time for You

Taking time to enjoy yourself is another way to boost your psychosocial health. Making that time available is critical. For some people, participating in a sport improves self-esteem and self-efficacy via a sense of achievement and/or success. For others, meditating, doing volunteer work, getting a massage, or meeting a new challenge, such as successfully auditioning for a play, can enhance psychosocial health. Viewing each new activity as something to look forward to and an

opportunity to grow is an important part of keeping the excitement in your life.

Maintaining Physical Health

Maintaining physical health also contributes to self-esteem and to overall psychosocial health. Regular physical activity (see also Chapter 4) fosters a sense of well-being and improves mood.[23] Nourishing meals that provide variety, balance, and moderation (see also Chapter 5) help you to feel good about yourself. Combined, regular physical activity and healthy eating lead to weight maintenance (see also Chapter 6) rather than the usual weight gain, or "Frosh 15" (the 7 kilograms—or 15 pounds), experienced by many college or university students. Getting adequate sleep and managing your stress are two other behaviours critical to maintaining your physical and psychosocial health.

Examining Problems and Seeking Help

Examining your problems and seeking help when needed will also boost your self-esteem and self-efficacy. Facing and solving problems can be one of life's most satisfying experiences. You do not necessarily have to deal with your problems alone. Help can come in the form of a friend, a group, or a mental health professional.

✳ Getting Adequate Sleep

Getting adequate sleep is a key contributor to physical and psychosocial functioning. Many of us do not get enough sleep and some get too much sleep. Sleep serves at least two biological purposes: (1) conservation of energy, so that we are rested and ready to perform during high-performance daylight hours; and (2) restoration, so that neurotransmitters depleted during waking hours can be replenished. This process clears the brain of daily minutiae to prepare for a new day.

what do you THINK?

Considering the suggestions listed above and in Table 2.2, which are you actively engaged in to enhance your self-esteem and self-efficacy? How can you more actively work at enhancing your self-esteem and self-efficacy?

Resiliency: Those traits or characteristics that protect an individual or community from threat or harm.

TABLE 2.2

Tips for Building Self-Esteem

- **Pay attention to your own needs and wants.** Listen to what your body, your mind, and your heart are telling you.

- **Take good care of yourself.** Eat healthy foods, limit junk foods, exercise, and plan fun activities for yourself.

- **Take time to do things you enjoy.** Make a list of things you enjoy doing. Then do something from that list every day.

- **Do something that you have been putting off.** Cleaning out your closet, or paying a bill that you've been putting off will make you feel like you've accomplished something.

- **Give yourself rewards.** Acknowledge that you are a great person by rewarding yourself occasionally.

- **Wear clothes that make you feel good about yourself.** You don't have to spend a lot to find clothes that make you feel good. Check out local thrift stores and consignment shops for great bargains.

- **Spend time with people.** People who make you feel better about yourself are great self-esteem boosters. Avoid people who treat you badly or make you feel bad about yourself.

- **Display items that you like.** You may have items that remind you of your achievements, your friends, or special times. Keep those special items close by.

- **Make your meals a special time.** Get rid of distractions such as the television, and really concentrate on enjoying your meal, whether you are by yourself or with others.

- **Learn something new every day.** Take advantage of any opportunity to learn something new every day–you'll feel better about yourself and be more productive.

- **Do something nice for another person.** There is no greater way to feel better about yourself than to help someone in greater need. Check out local volunteer opportunities, or make a special effort to be nice to those around you, such as your parents or siblings.

Most of us can identify with that tired, listless feeling caused by sleep deprivation during periods of peak stress. Either we do not make enough time to sleep, we have difficulty falling asleep, or we do not stay asleep once we get there. Lack of sleep is especially common among post-secondary students given their relatively high workload and levels of anxiety and stress. Women, in particular, have problems with sleep.[24]

How much sleep do we need? That depends on a number of factors. There is a genetically based need for sleep and it differs for each person, though six to nine hours is generally recommended. Sleep duration is also controlled by *circadian rhythms*, which are linked to the hormone *melatonin*. People alter their sleep patterns by staying up late, drinking coffee, getting lots of exercise, eating a heavy meal, or using an alarm or other wake-up device. *Sleep inertia* is a term used to describe the cognitive impairment, disorientation, and grogginess we experience when we first get up in the morning. This sleep inertia may impair our ability to think clearly and function effectively in tasks that occur shortly after we wake up. To wake up effectively and well rested, you should go to bed and get up

regularly at the same time. Exercise and a healthy breakfast (that is, three of the four food groups, low in fat, high in fibre) also help us to feel awake. Further, a coffee or tea upon awakening may speed the wakefulness process and for some people who must wake up quickly and be alert—such as physicians, pilots, truck drivers, and students with an 8:00 a.m. exam—this "jump start" may be necessary in order to perform effectively.[25]

Most of us follow characteristic stages of sleep, ranging from wakefulness to drowsiness to light sleep, and then move to a deeper sleep. The most important period of sleep, a deeper sleep, is called "rapid eye movement" (REM) sleep and is essential to feeling rested and refreshed. In REM sleep, heart rate increases, respiration speeds up, and dreaming tends to occur. If we miss REM—which we do in an alcohol-induced sleep—we are left feeling groggy and sleep deprived.

Though many people turn to over-the-counter sleeping pills, barbiturates, or tranquillizers to get some sleep, the methods presented in Table 2.3 for conquering sleeplessness are less harmful.[26]

TABLE 2.3

Getting a Good Night's Sleep

- **Go to bed and rise on a regular schedule.** It is important to go to bed and get up at about the same time every day.

- **Ensure your sleep environment is conducive to sleep.** Remove excessive noises, darken the room, and ensure you have quality bed and bedding.

- **Limit caffeine and alcohol.** Caffeine can linger in your body for up to 12 hours and may relate to insomnia. Although alcohol may initially make you drowsy, it affects REM sleep and the sleep–wake cycle.

- **Avoid eating a heavy meal or drinking large amounts of liquids before bed.**

- **Engage in regular physical activity.** You sleep better when you have been physically active, particularly if the activity has been outdoors. Keep in mind, however, that it is best to not be physically active right before bed; physical activity acts as a stimulant, speeding the body's metabolism and making it harder to fall asleep immediately after.

- **Nap only in the afternoon.** This works in conjunction with your circadian rhythm, and if you do, make it a "cat-nap," no longer than 20 minutes so that you do not interfere with your night sleep.

- **Establish a relaxing nighttime ritual that puts you in the mood to sleep.** Take a warm shower, relax in a comfortable chair, read, listen to music, or do something else that is quiet. Doing this consistently will tell your mind and body it is time to wind down.

- **Do not bring work to bed.**

- **If you are unable to fall asleep after 30 minutes, get up and do something else.** If you wake up in the middle of the night and cannot return to sleep, get up and do something quiet to repeat your night time ritual. Do not make your sleeplessness a cause for additional worry. Insomnia is not a crime. Not everyone needs eight hours of sleep. You can feel well—and be quite healthy—on fewer.

Understanding the Mind–Body Connection

Can negative emotions and stress make us physically sick? Can positive emotions and happiness help us feel well? Do positive emotions boost the immune system? Although considerable research has attempted to answer these questions, much remains unknown. For decades, research focused primarily on negative emotions and disease; however, little is known about the role of positive emotions in preserving health and protecting against disease. Many believe that this end of the emotional continuum may hold the key to future advances in health, and that mind–body health science may expand into new areas and may be accorded a higher level of importance as a result. One emotion that appears to have particularly positive benefits is *happiness*.

✷ Happiness and Physical Health

Happiness refers to a number of positive states in which individuals actively embrace the world around them.[27] As researchers examined characteristics of happy people, they found that this emotion had a

profound impact on the body. Specifically, researchers found that happiness, or related mood states such as hopefulness, optimism, and contentment reduced the risk or limited the severity of cardiovascular disease, pulmonary disease, type 2 diabetes, hypertension, colds, and other infections. Laughter increases heart and respiration rates, and reduces stress hormones in the same way as physical activity. For this reason, it has been promoted as a possible risk reducer for those with hypertension and other forms of cardiovascular disease.[28]

If happiness is good for your health, how does one "get happy"? **Subjective well-being (SWB)** refers to that uplifting feeling of inner peace or overall "feel-good state," which includes happiness. SWB is defined by three central components:[29]

1. *Satisfaction with present life.* People high in SWB tend to like their work and are satisfied with their current personal relationships. They are sociable,

Happiness: Feeling of contentment created when expectations and physical, psychological, and spiritual needs are met and life is enjoyed.

Subjective well-being (SWB): An uplifting feeling of inner peace and/or an overall feel-good state.

outgoing, and willing to open up to others. They also like themselves and enjoy good health and self-esteem.

2. *Relative presence of positive emotions.* People with high SWB more frequently feel pleasant emotions, mainly because they perceive the world around them in a generally positive way. They have an optimistic outlook, and they expect success in what they undertake.

3. *Relative absence of negative emotions.* Individuals with a strong sense of SWB experience fewer and less severe episodes of negative emotions, such as anxiety, depression, and anger.

Researchers also suggest that people may be biologically predisposed to happiness. In fact, happiness may be related to actual differences in brain physiology: *neurotransmitters,* the chemicals that transfer messages between neurons, may function more efficiently in happy people.[30] Others suggest that we can develop happiness by practising positive psychological actions.[31]

You do not have to be happy all the time to achieve overall subjective well-being. It is normal or usual to experience disappointment, unhappiness, and times when life seems unfair. In these situations, people with SWB are typically resilient, able to look on the positive side, able to get themselves back on track fairly quickly, and less likely to fall into despair over setbacks. Happiness does not depend on age, sex, ethnicity, race, or socioeconomic status. Take the quiz on happiness and see how satisfied you are with life (Figure 2.3).

Humans are remarkably resourceful creatures. We respond to great loss, such as the death of a loved one or a traumatic event, with an initial period of grief, mourning, and sometimes anger. Yet, with time and the support of others, we move forward and find satisfaction and peace once again. Typically, we learn from suffering and emerge stronger and more capable of dealing with the next crisis. Most find some measure of happiness after the initial shock and pain of loss.

Does Laughter Enhance Psychosocial Health?

Remember the last time you laughed so hard that you cried or that your belly ached? Remember how relaxed you felt afterward? Researchers are beginning to understand the role and importance of humour in our lives and health, as noted in the following:

- Stressed people with a strong sense of humour become less depressed and anxious than those whose sense of humour is less well developed.

- Students who use humour as a coping mechanism report that it predisposes them to a positive mood.

- Telling a joke, particularly one that involves a shared experience, increases one's sense of belonging and social cohesion.

try it NOW!

Laugh for health! Laughing not only feels good, it also is good for you. Next time you are in a funk or feeling tired and out of sorts, seek out a laugh or two. Read a funny book, watch a favourite comedy, call a good friend, or play with a pet. You may be surprised how a few chuckles can make you feel better all over.

How happy are you?
Read the following statements, and then rate your level of agreement with each one using the 1–7 scale.

1	2	3	4	5	6	7
Strongly disagree	Disagree	Slightly disagree	Neither agree nor disagree	Slightly agree	Agree	Strongly agree

1. In most ways, my life is close to my ideal. _____
2. The conditions of my life are excellent. _____
3. I am satisfied with my life. _____
4. So far I have gotten the important things I want in life. _____
5. If I could live my life over, I would change almost nothing. _____

Total score: _____

Scoring:
31–35: You are very satisfied with your life 26–30: Satisfied 21–25: Slightly satisfied
20: You are neither satisfied nor dissatisfied 15–19: Slightly dissatisfied 10–14: Dissatisfied 5–9: Very dissatisfied

FIGURE 2.3

Satisfaction with Life Scale

Source: W. Pavot and E. Diener, "Review of the Satisfaction with Life Scale," *Psychological Assessment* 5 (1993): 164–172.

Clearly, laughter enhances mental and emotional health. It also promotes social health: people like to be around others who are fun and who laugh easily. Learning to laugh puts more joy into everyday experiences and increases the likelihood that people will keep company with us.

Positive emotions such as joy, interest, and contentment serve valuable life functions. Joy is associated with playfulness and creativity. Interest encourages us to explore our world, which enhances knowledge and cognitive ability. Contentment allows us to savour and integrate experiences, an important step in achieving mindfulness and insight. By building our physical, social, and mental resources, these positive feelings empower us to cope effectively with life's challenges. While the actual emotions may be transient, their effects can be permanent and provide lifelong enrichment.[32]

Psychosocial Health and Well-Being

In the 1970s and '80s, a number of widely publicized studies of the health of widowed and divorced people indicated higher rates of illness and death than those of married people. Moreover, tests revealed below-normal immune-system functioning with follow-up studies indicating unusually high rates of cancer among people who were depressed.[33] Are these studies conclusive evidence of the mind–body connection? Probably not, because they did not take into account other factors relevant to health and disease. For example, some researchers suggest that people who are divorced, widowed, or depressed are more likely to drink and smoke, use drugs, eat and sleep poorly, and fail to engage in regular physical activity—all of which negatively affect the immune system. Another possibly relevant factor is that such people may be less tolerant of illness and more likely to report their problems.[34]

Keep in mind that the immune system changes measured in various studies of the mind–body connection are relatively small. (They are nowhere near as large as what is found in people with AIDS, for example.) The health consequences of such minute changes are difficult to gauge because the body can tolerate a certain amount of reduced immune function without illness developing. The exact amount the body is able to tolerate and under what circumstances are still unresolved questions.[35] Thus, although there is a large body of evidence pointing to an association between emotions and physical health, there is still much to learn about this relationship. In the meantime, maintaining an optimistic mindset continues to be sound advice as it relates to improved quality of life, regardless of whether or not it also improves quantity of life.

A powerful strategy for maintaining psychosocial health is to make time for friends and activities you enjoy and that bring laughter into your life.

WHEN THINGS GO WRONG

In spite of our best efforts to remain psychosocially healthy, circumstances and events in our lives sometimes are more than we can handle. Abusive relationships, stress, anxiety, loneliness, financial upheavals, and other traumatic events can sap our spirits, causing us to turn inward or act in ways that are not healthy. Chemical imbalances, drug interactions, trauma, neurological disruptions, and other physical problems may also contribute to these not-so-healthy behaviours. **Mental illnesses** are disorders that disrupt thinking, feeling, moods, and behaviours, and cause a varying degree of impaired functioning in daily life.

Similar to a physical disease, mental illnesses can range from mild to severe and exact a heavy toll on the quality of life of the individual affected and those who come in contact with him or her. It is estimated that one in five Canadians will directly experience a mental illness at some point in his or her lifetime.[36]

Depression

Depression is the most common emotional disorder in Canada: 6 percent of Canadians aged 18 and over have experienced a major depressive episode. It was

Mental illnesses: Disorders that disrupt thinking, feeling, moods, and behaviours and cause a varying degree of impaired functioning in daily life.

estimated from the 2000/01 Canadian Community Health Survey that 9.9 percent of Canadians over the age of 12 had a possible or probable risk of depression.[37] Females have a greater risk of depression than males (12.3 versus 7.5 percent). Individuals between 20 and 24 years of age have the greatest possible and probable risk of depression (13.3 percent), while individuals over the age of 75 have the lowest risk (5.1 percent).

There are two acknowledged forms of depression: endogenous and exogenous depression. **Endogenous depression** is of biochemical origin. Neurotransmitters (chemicals that transmit nerve impulses across synapses) in the brain responsible for mood elevation become unbalanced for unknown reasons. A decrease in these neurotransmitters gives rise to outward expressions of depression. If not treated, endogenous depression may become chronic. **Exogenous depression**, on the other hand, is usually caused by an external event such as the loss of something or someone of great value. People who experience exogenous depression can slide into chronic depression if unable to work through the grieving process necessary for overcoming event-related depression.

Similar symptoms appear in the two types of depression: lingering sadness; inability to find joy in pleasure-giving activities; loss of interest in work and reduced concentration; diminished or increased appetite; unexplainable fatigue; sleep disorders, including insomnia or early-morning awakenings; loss of sex drive; withdrawal from friends and family; feelings of hopelessness and worthlessness; and a desire to die. A depressed person may be unable to get out of bed in the morning or may find it impossible to leave the house.

A depressed person usually suffers from low self-esteem. He or she may feel alone—separated from and unable to communicate with others. After a while, depression becomes a vicious circle. The person feels helpless and trapped, having no way out. He or she may feel that depression is a deserved punishment for real or imagined failings. Prolonged depression may cause a person to feel utterly worthless and to view suicide as the only way out.

Facts about Depression

Although depression appears to be one of the fastest-growing psychosocial health problems, the general public is uninformed and misinformed about many aspects of it. The following points may help you to understand it.[38]

- *Depression is not a natural reaction to crisis and loss.* Something has happened to the mood and thinking of people who are depressed such that they experience pervasive pessimism, helplessness, despair, and lethargy, sometimes coupled with

Without appropriate treatment, depression and anxiety can become overwhelming problems that affect psychosocial well-being and physical health.

agitation. Individuals who are depressed may have difficulty at work and they tend to have chronically negative interpersonal relationships. Symptoms may come and go, get worse, or stay stable; they do not get better without treatment. People who are depressed forget what it is like to feel normal.

- *People will not "snap out of" depression by using a little willpower.* Telling a depressed person to "snap out of it" is like telling a person with diabetes to produce more insulin. Medical intervention in the form of antidepressant drugs and therapy is often necessary. Depression also tends to recur—more than half of those afflicted once will experience a recurrence. Understanding the seriousness of the disease and supporting people in their attempts to recover is important.

- *Frequent crying is not a hallmark of depression.* Some depressed people do not cry at all. In fact, biochemists theorize that crying may actually ward off depression by releasing chemicals that the body produces as a positive response to distress.

- *Depression is not "all in the mind."* In fact, depressive illnesses originate with an inherited chemical imbalance in the brain. Depression-like symptoms can also be a side-effect of certain physiological conditions (or their treatment), such as thyroid disorders, Lyme disease, diabetes, multiple sclerosis, hepatitis, mononucleosis, rheumatoid arthritis, and pancreatic cancer.

- *No single psychotherapy method works for all cases of depression.* A variety of methods are available. What works best for each person is a treatment that is tailored to him or her and deals with his or her personal circumstances and experiences.

Treating Depression

Depression is one of the most treatable of mental health problems;[39] with various types of treatments available, including lifestyle modification (that is, engaging in regular moderate- to vigorous-intensity physical activity, eating well, managing stress, getting adequate sleep, developing a strong social support system, and so on); talking to a physician, counsellor, psychologist, or psychiatrist; attending a support group; or taking a medication. Selecting the best treatment for a specific person involves determining his or her type and degree of depression and its possible causes. Psychotherapeutic and pharmacologic modes of treatment are recommended for clinical (severe and prolonged) depression. Drugs often relieve the symptoms of depression, such as loss of sleep or appetite, while psychotherapy can improve the social and interpersonal functioning of a person who is depressed. Treatment may be weighted toward one or the other mode depending on the specific situation. In some cases, psychotherapy alone may be the most successful treatment. The two most common psychotherapeutic therapies for depression are cognitive and interpersonal therapy.

Cognitive therapy aims to help an individual look at life rationally and to correct habitually pessimistic thought patterns. It focuses on the here and now rather than analyzing the past. To pull a person out of depression, cognitive therapists usually need 6 to 18 months of weekly sessions comprising reasoning and behavioural exercises. *Interpersonal therapy* is sometimes combined with cognitive therapy. It also addresses the present but differs from cognitive therapy in that its primary goal is to manage chronic human relationship problems. Interpersonal therapists focus on individuals' relationships with their families and other people.

Antidepressant drugs relieve symptoms in nearly 80 percent of people with chronic depression. In recent years, drug therapies have become so common that it is not unusual to know someone taking them. Despite their commonness, caution is warranted regarding the use of antidepressants. Many emergency-room visits occur when people misuse their antidepressants, in particular when they try to quit "cold turkey" or when they have drug interactions. Clinics have been established in large metropolitan areas to offer group support for depressed people. Some clinics treat all types of depressed people; others restrict themselves to specific groups, such as widows, adolescents, or families and friends of people with depression.

Seasonal Affective Disorder

Seasonal affective disorder (SAD), a type of depression, affects approximately 2 to 3 percent of Canadians.[40] As much as 25 percent of the population in Canada experiences a milder form of the disorder known as the "winter blues." SAD strikes during the winter months and is associated with reduced exposure to sunlight. People with SAD suffer from irritability, apathy, carbohydrate craving and weight gain, increases in sleep time, and general sadness. Researchers believe that SAD is caused by a malfunction in the hypothalamus, the gland responsible for regulating responses to external stimuli. Stress may also play a role in SAD.

Certain factors seem to put people at risk for SAD. Women are four times more likely to suffer from SAD than men. Although SAD occurs in people of all ages, those between 20 and 40 years of age appear to be the most vulnerable. Certain families also appear to be at risk. People living in cities with cold, bright winters and with an active winter culture often have lower rates of SAD than expected. Vancouver has relatively high rates of SAD due to frequent overcast skies; Saskatchewan has lower rates due to the frequency of sunshine in the winter. Some people experience a reduction in symptoms if they move south.[41]

There are some simple but effective therapies for SAD. The most beneficial appears to be light therapy, in which an individual is exposed to lamps that mimic sunlight. In fact, following four days of daily light exposure, 80 percent of individuals experienced relief from their symptoms. Other forms of treatment include dietary modifications (eating more foods high in complex carbohydrates), increased physical activity, stress management, sleep restriction (limiting the number of hours slept in a 24-hour period), psychotherapy, and antidepressants.

✳ Anxiety Disorders

Anxiety disorders are the most common of mental health problems, occurring in about 1 in 10 people and more frequently in women than in men.[42] Anxiety disorders refer to a group of disorders that affect behaviour, thoughts, emotions, and physical health. These include obsessive-compulsive disorder, phobias, panic disorders, and post-traumatic stress disorder. People with anxiety disorders have intense, prolonged feelings of fright and distress for no apparent reason.

Endogenous depression: A type of depression with a biochemical basis.

Exogenous depression: A type of depression with an external cause, such as the death of a loved one or marital break up.

Seasonal affective disorder (SAD): A type of depression that occurs in the winter months, when sunlight levels are low.

Anxiety disorders: Disorders characterized by persistent feelings of threat and anxiety in coping with everyday problems.

It is believed that anxiety disorders are caused by a combination of genetics and personal circumstances. Anxiety disorders can be effectively treated with a combination of pharmaceutical intervention and cognitive-behavioural therapy.[43]

Obsessive-Compulsive Disorders

An **obsessive-compulsive disorder** (**OCD**) is an anxiety disorder that affects the thoughts, behaviours, emotions, and sensations of those who experience it.[44] Obsessions—intrusive and illogical—are persistent ideas, thoughts, impulses, or images. Common OCDs revolve around contamination (therefore the need to wash one's hands many times before eating), doubts (such as not being sure whether the lights were turned off), and disturbing sexual or religious thoughts. More harmful behaviours include pulling out one's hair, eyebrows, or eyelashes, and other forms of self-mutilation.

It is believed that OCDs have a neurological and genetic basis. They occur equally in men and women of all ages, though usually before 40 years of age, and most often begin during adolescence or early childhood.

Phobias

A **phobia** is an anxiety disorder that involves a deep and persistent fear of a specific object, activity, or social situation, and results in a compelling desire to avoid the source of fear.[45] Phobias are thought to be more prevalent in women than in men. Simple phobias, such as fear of spiders, flying, or heights, can be treated successfully with behavioural therapy. Social phobias (fears related to interaction with others), such as fear of public speaking, inadequate sexual performance, and eating in public places, require more extensive therapy.

Panic Disorders

Another type of anxiety disorder is panic disorders which are expressed via a **panic attack**, the sudden onset of disabling terror.[46] These attacks can happen at any time: while sleeping, sitting in traffic, or just before you deliver your class presentation. Suddenly and unexpectedly, your heart starts to race, your face turns red, you can't catch your breath, you feel nauseated, you start to perspire, and you may feel like you are going to pass out or are having a heart attack. Panic attacks may have no obvious link to environmental stimuli, or they may be learned responses to environmental stimuli. Researchers believe that panic attacks are caused by some physiological change or

Canadians are becoming more familiar with their psychosocial health, the risk factors for poor psychosocial health, and their treatment options, partly because of people like James Bartleman, who shared his story of depression at the National Canadian Mental Health Association Conference.

biochemical imbalance in the brain; they are still searching for the mechanisms that trigger such attacks.

Post-Traumatic Stress Disorder

Sometimes people experience something so unexpected and so shattering that is has a serious effect on them long after the danger has passed.[47] Examples of these experiences include traumas such as rape, abuse, assault, war, natural disasters (hurricanes, tornadoes, floods, forest fires), or airplane or car crashes. People who suffer serious after-effects of such experiences are afflicted by **post-traumatic stress disorder** (**PTSD**). Common symptoms include flashbacks in which the terrifying experience is relived, nightmares, depression, detachment, and feelings of anger and irritability.

Schizophrenia

Perhaps the most frightening of all mental disorders is **schizophrenia**, a disease that affects about 1 percent of the Canadian population. Schizophrenia is characterized by alterations of the senses (including auditory

CMHA Applauds Work of Senate Committee, Wants Recommendations to Move Forward

On May 9, 2006, the Canadian Mental Health Association (CMHA)* applauded the Senate Committee on Social Affairs, Science and Technology on the 118 recommendations it made in a report on mental health, mental illness, and addictions in Canada. This report (titled *Out of the Shadows at Last*) is the result of a three-year study of mental health and addiction. In the report, the Senate Committee recommends that a 5-percent tax be placed on alcoholic beverages to assist with the funding of the $5.4-billion plan to transform Canada's mental health system.

The CMHA looks forward to working with the government, its agencies, and other stakeholders across the country to make the recommendations a reality.

It should be noted that Canada is one of the only G-8 countries currently without a national strategy for mental health and mental illness. The CMHA actively supports the Senate Committee's recommendation for a call for a strategy on mental health and mental illness for the people of Canada. The organization recommends that the federal government work with the provincial and territorial governments and key stakeholders in the mental health community to develop and implement a national strategy

The CMHA also strongly supports the Senate Committee's recommendation for the establishment of a Mental Health Commission that will bring together key stakeholders to improve the quality of life of those affected directly and indirectly by

mental illness. Finally, the CMHA endorsed the Senate Committee's recommendation for the creation of a Mental Health Transition Fund, which would be used to assist individuals with mental illness in obtaining affordable housing.

The complete report can be downloaded from www.parl.gc.ca/ 39/1/parlbus/commbus/senate/com-e/soci-e/rep-e/ rep02may06-e.htm.

* The CMHA is a leading national, voluntary organization within the mental-health sector. For more than 90 years, it has existed to promote the mental health of Canadians and to serve mental-health consumers and their families and friends through education, public awareness, research, advocacy, and direct services.

Source: Adapted from Canadian Mental Health Association, "CMHA Applauds Work of Senate Committee, Wants Recommendations to Move Forward." Retrieved on May 26, 2006, from www.cmha.ca/bins/print_page.asp?cid=6-20-21-1229-1355&lang=1.

and visual hallucinations); the inability to sort out incoming stimuli and make appropriate responses; an altered sense of self; and radical changes in emotions, movements, and behaviours. Individuals with this disease often cannot function in society, unless treated pharmacologically.

Schizophrenia is now recognized as a biological brain disease. It has become evident that the brain damage involved occurs very early in life, possibly as early as in the second trimester of fetal development. However, the disease most commonly has its onset in late adolescence.

Schizophrenia is treatable but not curable. Treatments usually include some combination of hospitalization, medication, and supportive psychotherapy. Supportive psychotherapy, as opposed to psychoanalysis, is used to help the individual acquire skills for living in society.

Despite its genetic roots, a stigma remains attached to the disease. Families of individuals with schizophrenia often experience anger and guilt. They often need help in the form of information, family counselling, and advice on how to meet the needs for shelter, medical care, vocational training, and social interaction of the family member with schizophrenia.

SEX ISSUES IN PSYCHOSOCIAL HEALTH

Studies indicate that sex bias often gets in the way of correct diagnosis of psychosocial disorders. In one study, 175 mental health professionals of both sexes were asked to diagnose an individual on the basis of a summarized case history. Some were told that the individual was male, others female. The sex of the patient made a substantial difference in the diagnosis

Obsessive-compulsive disorder (OCD): A disorder characterized by obsessive thoughts or habitual behaviours.

Phobia: A deep and persistent fear of a specific object, activity, or situation that results in a compelling desire to avoid the source of the fear.

Panic attack: The sudden, rapid onset of disabling terror.

Post-traumatic stress disorder: A disorder characterized by terrifying flashbacks, detachment, and anxiety following a severe traumatic event.

Schizophrenia: A mental illness characterized by irrational behaviours, severe alterations of the senses (hallucinations), and, often, an inability to function in society.

(though the sex of the clinician did not). When clinicians thought the case history was from a female, they were more likely to diagnose hysterical personality, a "women's disorder." When they believed the case history was from a male, the more likely diagnosis was antisocial personality, a "male disorder."

Depression and Sex

For reasons not well understood, women are twice as likely to develop depression than men.[48] Researchers have proposed biological, psychological, and social explanations. The biological explanation relates to women's hormone level changes observed during the menstrual cycle, pregnancy, miscarriage, postpartum period, pre-menopause, and menopause. Women also face various stressors related to their multiple roles and responsibilities—work, child-rearing, household work, relationships, and caring for older parents—at rates much greater than men. Although men's hormone levels appear to remain relatively stable throughout life, they too experience depression. For men, depression is often masked by alcohol or drug use or by the socially acceptable habit of working excessively long hours. Typically, men who are depressed present as irritable, angry, and discouraged rather than hopeless and helpless.

Not only do researchers note different rates of depression in men and women, they also observe sex differences in coping strategies, or the response to certain events or stimuli, and thus propose that women's strategies put them at greater risk. Results indicate that men distract themselves from a depressed mood, whereas women tended to focus on it. If focusing on depressed feelings intensifies these feelings, women's response style then may make them more likely than men to become clinically depressed.

PMS: Physical or Mental Disorder?

A major controversy regarding sex bias is the inclusion of a diagnosis for premenstrual syndrome (PMS) and premenstrual dysphoric disorder (PMDD) in the American Psychiatric Association's *Diagnostic and Statistical Manual of Mental Disorders*, fourth edition (known as *DSM-IV*). PMS is characterized by depression, irritability, and other symptoms of increased stress typically occurring just prior to menstruation and lasting for a day or two. Whereas PMS is somewhat disruptive and uncomfortable, it does not interfere with daily function; PMDD does. To be diagnosed with PMDD, a woman must have at least five symptoms of PMS for a week to ten days, at least one of which is serious enough to interfere with her ability to function at work or at home. In these more severe cases, antidepressants may be prescribed.

SUICIDE: GIVING UP ON LIFE

Statistics Canada reported 3613 suicides in Canada for 2004 (2734 men and 879 women)—equivalent to a rate of 11.3 per 100 000 people,[49] lower than the worldwide rate of 14.5 per 100 000 people reported by the World Health Organization.[50] The pressures, joys, disappointments, challenges, and changes within the college or university environment are believed to be in part responsible for these rates. However, young adults who choose not to go to post-secondary school and who search for the directions to their career and relationship goals and other life aspirations are also at risk for suicide. Experts estimate that there may actually be more cases than are reported due to the difficulty in determining the causes of suspicious deaths. Suicide is often a consequence of poor coping skills, lack of social support, lack of self-esteem, and the inability to see one's way out of a bad or negative situation. Suicide can also be viewed as an extreme form of violence—anger, rage, and hopelessness turned inward rather than outward.

University or college students are more likely than the general population to attempt suicide; suicide is the second leading cause of death in people between the ages of 15 and 24. Although women attempt suicide at four times the rate of men, more than three times as many men as women actually succeed in ending their lives. Men may be more "successful" than women because they often choose more violent measures to kill themselves (that is, firearms versus an overdose of painkillers). The suicide rate among First Nations peoples is reported to be three to eight times that of non-Aboriginal Canadians.[51]

People likely to commit suicide include those who (1) are experiencing a serious physical or mental illness, (2) are abusing alcohol or drugs, (3) are experiencing a major loss—such as the death of a loved one, unemployment, or divorce, (4) are experiencing major changes in life—for example, teenagers and seniors, and (5) have made previous suicide attempts.[52]

Many of us will be touched by a suicide at some time. In most cases, the suicide does not occur unpredictably. In fact, it is estimated that 8 out of 10 people who attempt suicide or die by suicide hint or talk openly about it beforehand.[53] Further, suicide is considered a process, not an event, with most contemplating their fate over a relatively long period of time.

Warning Signals of Suicide

Common warning signals of suicide include[54]

- talk of suicide—for example, "no one cares if I live or die"

Prescribing Antidepressants for Depression in 2005: Recent Concerns and Recommendations

In 2005, a review was conducted after the safety of prescribed antidepressants (selective serotonin reuptake inhibitors [SSRIs], selective serotonin and noradrenalin reuptake inhibitors [SNRIs], and other novel antidepressants) was questioned as a first-line treatment for major depressive disorders (MDD) in adults and in children and adolescents because of the drugs' potential to cause or enhance aggression and suicide. Results from this review led to the following clinical recommendations for prescribing antidepressants:

- In adults, including the elderly, SSRIs, SNRIs, and other novel agents remain the best first-line treatments for MDD.
- In children and adolescents, only fluoxetine should be used as a first-line treatment for MDD.
- In children and adolescents, SSRIs other than fluoxetine can be used as a second-line treatment when depression is severe, chronic, and associated with other comorbid conditions or if psychosocial treatments have not worked. SNRIs

and other novel agents should be used only as a third-line treatment because of their greater risk of adverse events.

- It is essential to closely monitor patients for suicidality (emerging or worsening suicidal thoughts, behaviours, and attempts), particularly in the early phases of treatment—weekly contact in the first month of antidepressant treatment is recommended. It is also critical to inform the patients and families (when appropriate) of the potential side-effects that may increase suicidality (anxiety, agitation, hypomania, and activation syndrome).

Further research is recommended; specifically to determine risks and benefits to antidepressant use in children, adolescents, and the elderly.

Source: Adapted from R. W. Lam and S. H. Kennedy, "CPA Position Statement: Prescribing Antidepressants for Depression in 2005: Recent Concerns and Recommendations," *The Canadian Journal of Psychiatry*, 49.12, 1–6. Retrieved May 30, 2006 from www.canmat.org/suicidality_antidepressant/suicidality-antidepressant.html.

- making a plan or increased risk taking
- writing or drawing about suicide (in a diary, for example)
- a preoccupation with death; giving away valued possessions
- a withdrawal from friends and family and from activities once found pleasurable
- hero worship of people who have died by suicide
- increased use of alcohol or drugs
- recent loss of a friend, family member, or parent, especially if they died by suicide
- conflicting feelings or sense of shame about being gay or straight
- mood swings, emotional outbursts, high level of irritability or aggression
- feelings of hopelessness

Taking Action to Prevent Suicide

Suicide is often seen as the only way out of an intolerable situation. People who commit suicide are in such pain they cannot see any other way out. Crisis counsellors and help lines may help temporarily, but the only way to prevent suicide is to get rid of conditions, situations, and substances that may precipitate attempts, including alcohol, drugs, loneliness, isolation, and

access to guns. If someone you know threatens or displays warnings signs of suicide, take the following actions:[55]

- *Monitor the warning signals.* Ensure that there is someone around the person as much as possible.
- *Find a safe place to talk with the person.* Allow as much time as necessary. Talking about suicide can only decrease the likelihood that someone will act on suicidal feelings.
- *Take any threat seriously.* Don't brush them off.
- *Do not belittle the person's feelings or say that he or she doesn't really mean it or couldn't succeed at suicide.* To some people, these comments offer the challenge of proving you wrong.
- *Let the person know how much you care about him or her.* State that you are there if he or she needs help.
- *Listen.* Try not to discredit or be shocked by what the person says to you. Empathize, and keep the person talking. Talk about stressors and listen to responses.
- *Ask the person directly, "Are you thinking of hurting or killing yourself?"*
- *Help the person think about alternatives.* Go with the person for help.
- *Make a plan with the person for the next few hours or days.* Help this person make contact with an

appropriate health-care professional or make the contact yourself. Take this person to an appropriate health-care facility to meet with a counsellor.

- *If the person has a plan, remove any pills or guns; call 911 for help immediately.*
- *Tell your friend's spouse, partner, parents, brothers and sisters, or counsellor.* Do not keep your suspicions to yourself. Don't let a suicidal friend talk you into keeping your discussions confidential. Let your friend know you must share this information with a professional. If your friend is successful in a suicide attempt, you will have to live with the consequences of your inaction. Counselling services available on campus can help you talk with your friend and suggest options for you.

what do you **THINK?**

If your roommate showed warning signs of suicide, what would you do? Whom would you contact first? Where on campus might your friend get help? In your community?

SEEKING PROFESSIONAL HELP

Many Canadians feel that seeking professional help for psychosocial problems is an admission of personal failure. Typically, any physical health problem, such as an abscessed tooth or prolonged severe pain, sends us to the nearest dentist or physician. On the other hand, we tend to ignore psychosocial problems until they pose a serious threat to our well-being—and even then, we may refuse to ask for the help needed. Despite this custom, however, an increasing number of Canadians are turning to mental health professionals for help. Researchers believe that more people want help today because "normal" living has become more difficult. Breakdown in support systems, high expectations of the individual by society, and dysfunctional families are cited as the three major reasons more people ask for help.

You should consider seeking help under the following circumstances:

- you think you need help
- you experience wild mood swings
- a problem is interfering with your daily life
- your fears or feelings of guilt frequently distract you
- you begin to withdraw from others
- you have hallucinations
- you feel that life is not worth living
- you feel inadequate or worthless
- your emotional responses are inappropriate in various situations
- your daily life seems to be nothing but repeated crises
- you feel you can't "get your act together"
- you are considering suicide
- you turn to drugs or alcohol to escape your problems
- you feel out of control

Types of Mental Health Professionals

Several types of mental health professionals, or providers, are available to help you. The most important criterion when choosing a provider is whether you feel you can work well with that person, not how many degrees he or she has.

Psychiatrist

A **psychiatrist** is a medical doctor. After obtaining a medical degree, a psychiatrist spends up to 12 years studying psychosocial health and disease. As a licensed physician, a psychiatrist can prescribe medications for various mental or emotional problems and may have admitting privileges at local hospitals. Some psychiatrists are affiliated with hospitals, while others are in private practice. Psychiatric fees are normally covered by provincial or territorial health insurance.

Psychoanalyst

A **psychoanalyst** is a psychiatrist or a psychologist with special training in psychoanalysis. Psychoanalysis is a type of therapy in which a person is helped to remember early traumas that block personal growth. Facing these traumas helps the individual to resolve their conflicts and begin to lead a more productive life.

Psychologist

A **psychologist** usually has a PhD or doctorate in counselling or clinical psychology. In addition, all provinces require licensure. Psychologists are trained in various types of talk therapy. Most are trained to conduct individual and group counselling sessions. Psychologists may also be trained in certain specialties, such as family

Choosing a Therapist: Key Factors to Consider

When you are in emotional or psychological trouble, you are often in the most vulnerable of situations. The choices you make in times of desperation are often critical to your eventual health; yet, many people choose their therapists at random at their lowest emotional point. Like auto mechanics, physicians, and professors, all therapists are not created equal, nor are they equally skilled at what they do. A degree or credential does not ensure compatibility with you, or even general competence. Taking some time to check out the person you are going to see and evaluating that person during your first session are important first steps in taking care of yourself. While even the most thorough check does not guarantee satisfaction, assessing the following may help make your experience a positive and fulfilling one.

1. *Does the therapist have qualities you want in a close friend?* Early in your interaction with the therapist, you should find that the therapist is someone you like, admire, and respect—someone you relate to well and would be willing to trust with your most intimate thoughts. The therapist should convey a genuine interest in you and your problems, rather than watch the clock or check his or her book to schedule your next appointment. You should enjoy sitting in the room with this person and talking. In short, you need to "connect" with your therapist.

2. *Does the therapist act professionally?* Most therapists adhere to a very basic code of ethics. They set boundaries around their relationships with clients to ensure the clients' safety, to foster a feeling of trust, and to encourage confidence in their ability to help. There are exceptions, however. Signs of unprofessional behaviour include

   - suggestions of meetings or social interactions outside of your sessions, particularly if the therapist appears to be trying to be a personal friend or lover rather than maintaining a professional role
   - agreeing to counsel someone with whom there is a conflict of interest in the counselling situation. Former partners, business relationships, friends, and other clients should be off-limits
   - continually being late for sessions, seeming distracted in sessions, forgetting what you told them before and needing you to repeat things
   - spending too much time talking about him- or herself during the session rather than listening to you; identifying too much of what you are saying with him- or herself rather than your own situation
   - questionable billing practices, such as discrepancies in billing, billing errors to insurance companies, or seeming to

   want your business and the money rather than displaying a sincere desire to help
   - locking you into the therapist's own specialty; for example, a counsellor who specializes in alcoholism and adult children of alcoholics who continually tries to force you into the "adult child of alcoholic" box, even though this has little to do with your unique situation
   - continual interruptions of your session with phone calls, talking to the receptionist, or other diversions so that you do not get your full amount of time
   - never seeming to want to release you from therapy or encouraging an indefinite dependence on their help. Although the length of treatment varies with each client and his or her respective problems, one of the goals of therapy should be to get out of therapy

3. Does the therapist work with you to set your goals, thereby empowering you to get better at your pace? Good therapists will assess your general problem fairly early and set at least some provisional goals on which to work. These usually take the form of small steps that you can tackle each week between sessions, or things that you can do to help you think about your issues and problems. If therapy takes place only in the office, the therapist is not moving you toward recovery. A good therapist is not a detective there to solve your problem per se; his or her role is to provide insight into the things you are doing or to help you understand how your situation and personal actions contribute to your problem(s). A good therapist should serve as a catalyst for you to help yourself, rather than serving as your saviour. Good therapists help you find your answers and build on your strengths, rather than just focusing on getting rid of your weaknesses.

4. Is the therapist willing to let you conduct an interview before committing to his or her services? Good therapists will allow you at least one meeting (often at a minimal or reduced charge) to check out the aforementioned information and to find out about their credentials, their counselling style, their personality, and the general "fit."

Most therapy should result in at least minor improvements in six to eight weeks. If you find that you are getting nowhere, if you are repeating the same things over and over, or if you find problems with any of the above, do not be afraid to find another therapist.

Sources: "How to Choose a Therapist," *CBS This Morning*, July 24–26, 1996; David Meyers, *Psychology*, Chapter 16, "How to Choose a Therapist," Worth Publishing, 537–572; James W. Kalat, "Treatment of Psychologically Troubled People," in *Introduction to Psychology*, 4th ed., eds. Brooks/Cole (1996), 648–678.

counselling, sexual counselling, or counselling related to compulsive behaviours. Psychologists may work in private practice or in publicly funded organizations. Some employee assistance programs cover a certain number of psychologist visits annually, and the

Psychiatrist: A licensed physician who specializes in treating mental and emotional disorders.

Psychoanalyst: A psychiatrist or psychologist with special training in psychoanalysis.

Psychologist: A person with a PhD and training in psychology.

extended health plan through your university or college may have some coverage for these fees.

Clinical/Certified/Psychiatric Social Worker

A **social worker** has at least a master's degree in social work (MSW) and two years of experience in a clinical setting. Some provinces require an examination for accreditation in the College of Clinical Social Work. Some social workers work in clinical settings, whereas others have private practices. Certified clinical social workers (CSW) often work in private practices, and their clients are sometimes insured through employee assistance programs.

Counsellor

Persons having a variety of academic and experiential training call themselves counsellors. The **counsellor** often has a master's degree in counselling, psychology, educational psychology, or a related human service. Professional societies recommend at least two years of graduate coursework or supervised practice as a minimal requirement. Many counsellors are trained to do individual and group counselling. They often specialize in one type of counselling, such as family, marital, relationship, children, drug, divorce, behavioural, or personal counselling. Remember that in Canada anyone can use the title of therapist or counsellor. Before you begin treatment, you should consider the credentials of your counsellor, your desired outcomes, and both your and your counsellor's expectations.

Psychiatric Nurse Specialist

Although all registered nurses can work in psychiatric settings, some have chosen to continue their education and specialize in psychiatric practice. The psychiatric nurse specialist can be certified by the Registered Psychiatric Nursing Association in some provinces.

What to Expect When You Begin Therapy

The first trip to a therapist can be extremely difficult. Most of us have misconceptions about what therapy is and about what it can do. That first visit is a verbal and mental sizing up between you and the therapist. You may not accomplish much in that first hour. If you decide that the therapist is not for you, you will at least have learned how to present your problem and what qualities you need in a therapist. Some suggestions to get the most out of your visit:

1. Before meeting a therapist, briefly explain your needs to the therapist or to the individual whom you made the appointment with. Ask about the fee. Arrive on time. Wear comfortable clothing. Expect to spend about an hour with the therapist during your first visit.

2. The therapist may want to take down your history and details about the problems that brought you to therapy. Answer as honestly as possible. Many therapists will ask how you feel about aspects of your life. Do not be embarrassed to acknowledge your feelings.

3. Therapists are not mind readers. They cannot tell what you are thinking. It is therefore critical to the success of your treatment that you have enough trust in your therapist to be open and honest.

4. Do not expect the therapist to tell you what to do or how to behave. Very few hand out behavioural prescriptions.

5. Find out if the therapist will allow you to set your own therapeutic goals and timetables. Also, find out if, later in therapy, your therapist will allow you to determine what is and what is not helping you.

6. If, after your first visit (or even after several visits), you feel you cannot work with a therapist,

Managing Your Psychosocial Health

Psychosocial health is a complex concept. Finding the best way to help yourself achieve optimal psychosocial health requires careful introspection and planned action. Remembering the following points and acting upon them whenever possible may help you along the way.

MAKING DECISIONS FOR YOU

Psychosocial health is influenced by many factors.

- Why is being psychosocially healthy important to you? To the people close to you?
- What steps can you take to improve your mental health? What actions can you take today that will improve your emotional health? What steps can you take to improve your social health? What can you do to improve your spiritual health?
- If you thought you had a psychosocial problem, would you seek help? Why or why not? Who could you seek help from?

CHECKLIST FOR CHANGE

- Consider life an opportunity for discovery and learning.
- Accept yourself as the best that you are able to be right now.
- Remember that nobody is perfect.
- Remember that the most difficult times in life occur during transitions and can be opportunities for growth even though they may be painful.
- Remember that there are other perspectives than your own.
- Recognize the sources of your anxiety and act to reduce them.
- Ask for help when you need it; discuss your problems with others.

- Become sensitive to and aware of your body's physical and mental signals—take care of yourself.
- Find a meaning for your life and work toward achieving your goals.
- Develop strategies to get through problem situations.
- Remain open to emotional experiences—give yourself to today rather than waiting for tomorrow.
- Even when you fail, be proud of yourself for trying.
- Keep your sense of humour—learn to laugh at yourself.
- Never quit trying to grow, to experience, to love, and to live life to its fullest.

CRITICAL THINKING

Suppose that your roommate ended a long-term relationship last month. Ever since, your roommate no longer jogs every morning or attends religious services, and doesn't even want to attend school mixers to meet someone else. Worse yet, even minor mistakes lead your roommate to vicious self-berating.

You are concerned about your roommate's psychosocial health, but unsure of what to do. You know that your roommate has in the past said that anyone who needs therapy should be "locked up and the key thrown away." But your roommate's mood is beginning to affect you. Use the DECIDE model described in Chapter 1 to determine what you should do in this situation. Explain your decision. If the action you chose did not bring about the desired result, what would you do next? Then list some ways you can show support for a friend who shows signs of psychosocial illness.

you must summon up the courage to say so. Do not worry about hurting the therapist's feelings. If there is a personality conflict or if you do not feel comfortable, the therapy will not be effective.

Social worker: A person with a master's degree and clinical training.

Counsellor: A person with a variety of academic and experiential training who deals with the treatment of emotional problems.

PEARSON
myhealthlab

Go to MyHealthLab at **www.pearsoned.ca/myhealthlab.** Here you will find self-assessments, case studies, links to health on the net, and much more.

DISCUSSION QUESTIONS

1. What is psychosocial health? What are the indicators of psychosocial health?

2. Discuss the factors that influence your overall level of psychosocial health. Why do you think the university or college environment may provide a challenge to your psychosocial health? What factors can you change? Which ones may be more difficult to change? How do you cope with factors you cannot change?

3. What steps could you take today to improve your psychosocial health? Which steps require long-term effort?

4. What factors contribute to psychosocial difficulties and illnesses? Which of the more common psychosocial illnesses are likely to affect people in your age group?

5. What are the warning signs of suicide? What would you do if you heard a stranger in the cafeteria say to no one in particular that he was going to "do the world a favour and end it all"? What if this person was a friend; how would you react then?

6. Describe the different types of health professionals and therapies. What services are provided by your student health centre? Which service/professional would you recommend for which service?

APPLICATION EXERCISE

Reread the "Consider This..." scenario at the beginning of the chapter and answer the following questions.

1. How psychosocially healthy is Marisol?

2. What factors contribute to Marisol's current health status?

3. What services on your campus would be available to help Marisol improve her psychosocial health?

4. As a friend, what could you do to help Marisol?

MYSEARCHLAB EXERCISE

1. Log on to www.MySearchLab.com.

2. Retrieve article AN 22533583, "Gender Differences In Spiritual Well-Being: Are Females More Spiritually Well Than Males?" by Jon Hammermeister, Matt Flint, Amani El-Alayli, Heather Ridnour, and Margaret Peterson.

3. Read the article, then provide responses to the following:
   a. What sex differences exist in regard to spiritual well-being?
   b. What sex differences exist in regard to religiosity?
   c. Briefly describe the study conducted by Hammermeister et al.
   d. What were the main findings?
   e. What other sex differences do you think exist for psychosocial health?

CHAPTER 3

MANAGING STRESS

Toward Prevention and Control

CONSIDER THIS . . .

Rhett is taking a full load of classes in his first year of post-secondary studies. He is living with his best friend from high school in a residence on campus and goes home one weekend each month. He is involved in several student organizations and plays intramural sports. He is doing well in his science courses, but struggling in his arts courses. Although he tries to study in his room, he finds residence life too distracting and as a result has been forced to find somewhere else to study. The library is often overcrowded and he has difficulty finding a spot. He tries to get to bed by midnight; however, the noise level in residence often keeps him awake until 1 or 2 a.m. Since being on campus, he's eaten fewer fruits and vegetables and more pasta, pizza, burgers, and fries. Unlike many of his friends who say they know what they are planning to do when they graduate, Rhett is still searching for his career path.

Are Rhett's experiences common for first-year university or college students? What components of first-year post-secondary studies may cause him to feel stressed? What advice would you give to him as a first-year student?

CHAPTER OBJECTIVES

- Define stress, stressors, and stress reaction.

- Explain the three phases of the general adaptation syndrome and describe what happens physiologically and psychologically when you perceive a threat. How and when is your immune system affected?

- Discuss psychosocial, environmental, and self-imposed sources of stress. Describe the stressors particularly relevant to university and college students.

- Identify stress management techniques.

Stress: it's hard to live with and it's almost impossible to live without. We are bombarded by a host of subtle and not-so-subtle internal and external factors that may lead us to feel stressed from the moment we wake until we finally fall asleep. Even during our sleep, noise, temperature changes, and other activities can lead to a stress response. Rarely does a day go by without someone you know talking about being under stress—from homework, part-time or full-time job responsibilities, financial pressures, relationship demands, volunteer-related responsibilities, technology, or other problems. Despite our best efforts to ignore it, stress-inducing factors cannot be run from, hidden from, or wished away. For some people, these factors provide the stimulus for growth and higher levels of achievement. Yet for others, they increase the likelihood of dysfunctional or abnormal behaviours or illness.

Stress in itself is neither positive nor negative. Rather, it is our reactions to it that can be described as positive or negative. Whether we are aware of it or not, our reactions to stress can become the habits that lead us either to health-enhancing personal growth or to debilitation in the form of migraines, substance misuse and abuse, circulatory disorders, asthma, gastrointestinal problems, and hypertension (high blood pressure). In addition, our responses to stress can lead to psychological and social problems, including dysfunctional relationships. In this chapter, we explore why and how these reactions take place and how we may be able to control them and channel our efforts more effectively such that our health and wellness is not compromised.

WHAT IS STRESS?

Many things that have contributed to making you who you are also influence how you respond to potentially stress-inducing events in your life. Stress responses—such as breaking out in a cold sweat before asking someone to go out on a date, becoming anxious or irritated around people who speak too slowly or drive too cautiously, feeling nervous when meeting new people, a racing heart rate when you are called upon to make a response in class, feeling edgy or pumped when it is time to play a game—are all unique by-products of past experiences. Your family, friends, environmental conditions, general health status, drug use, personality, and support systems influence how you respond to a given event.

Stress means different things to different people. Often, we think of **stress** as an externally imposed factor that threatens or makes a demand on our minds and bodies.[1] If your hard-nosed instructor tells you that you have to do a 10-page paper in the next week,

that's an external stressor. However, most stress is actually self-imposed and is usually the result of an internal state of emotional tension that occurs in response to the various demands of living. Stress may manifest itself in physiological and psychological responses to the demands placed upon us, and many researchers define stress as these responses.[2] Most current definitions state that stress is the mental and physical response of our bodies to the various demands or expectations in our lives. It is our thoughts about the situation we are in that are the critical factor; if we decide the demands of the situation outweigh the skills we have, then we are likely to judge he situation as stressful and react with a stress response.[3]

A **stressor** is any physical, social, or mental event or condition that forces our minds and bodies to react or adjust. Stressors may be tangible, such as an angry parent or a disgruntled roommate, or intangible, such as the mixed emotions associated with meeting your significant other's parents for the first time. Adjustment is our attempt to cope with a given situation.[4] As we try to adjust to the various stressors in our lives, strain may develop. Strain is the wear and tear our bodies and minds sustain during the process of adjusting to or resisting a stressor.

Most of our daily activities involve situations or events that may elicit a stress response. Positive stress, or stress that results from generally positive situations, is called **eustress**. Getting married, starting school, beginning a career, developing new friendships, and learning a new physical skill can lead to eustress. **Distress**, or negative stress, is caused by things such as financial problems, injury or illness, the death of a loved one, trouble at work, academic difficulties, the unexpected ending of a relationship, and not being sure of your purpose in life. Both types of stress provide an opportunity for personal growth and can lead to personal satisfaction.

Although the mind and body each react to eustress and distress, most of us only worry about our reactions to distress. We cannot prevent distress; like eustress, it is simply a part of life. However, we can learn to recognize the events likely to cause stress and to anticipate our reactions to them by learning to practise prestress coping skills and develop post-stress management techniques. Developing these skills depends on our understanding of the major components of stress.

The Mind–Body Connection: Physical Responses

Although much has been written about the negative effects of stress, researchers have only recently begun to untangle the complex web of physical and emotional interactions that actually cause the body to wear down over time. As a result, stress is often described generically as a "disease of prolonged arousal" that often leads to other negative health effects. Nearly all systems of the body become potential targets for this onslaught, and the long-term effects may be devastating.

Much of the initial impetus for studying the health effects of stress came from prospective observations. Specifically, researchers in the Framingham Study noted that highly stressed individuals were significantly more likely to experience cardiovascular diseases.[5] Monkeys exposed to high levels of unpredictable stressors in studies also showed significantly increased levels of disease and mortality.[6] In a study of susceptibility to cold viruses, subjects who reported recent high levels of stressors were much more likely to catch a cold after inhaling large doses of a cold virus through their nose than their counterparts who reported fewer stressors.[7] While the battle over the legitimacy of these observations continues to be waged in research labs, the correlation of too much stress over long periods of time to selected ailments has gained credibility. What do repeated experiences of the stress response actually do to the body? Why are health and wellness experts concerned about repeated responses or reactions to stress? What are the short- and long-term health implications of the stress response?

Stress and Impaired Immunity

Although the health effects of prolonged stress responses provide dramatic evidence of the direct and indirect impact of stress on body organs, researchers continue to seek more definitive answers about the exact physiological and psychological mechanisms that lead to specific diseases. The science of **psychoneuroimmunology (PNI)** analyzes the relationship between the mind's response to stress and the functioning of the immune system.

Much of the preliminary PNI data on stress and immune functioning focused on the hypothesis that during periods of prolonged stress elevated levels of adrenal hormones, including cortisol, destroy or reduce the ability of the white blood cells known as "natural killer T cells." Killer T cells aid in the immune response, and when they are suppressed the body is less effective at combatting illnesses. In addition to killer T suppression, many other body processes are disrupted and overall disease-fighting capacity is reduced. Although several studies have supported the hypothesis of a relationship between increased stress levels and greater risk of disease in times of grief, social disruption, poor mood, and so

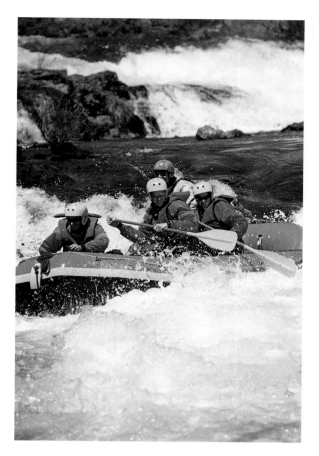

Stress is a positive factor in life when it creates opportunities for personal growth and satisfaction rather than psychological or physiological wear and tear.

forth, there is still much to be learned about possible mediating factors.[8] Other studies have shown no increased risk for disease among people suffering from prolonged arousal by stressors.[9] These conflicting findings also emphasize the need to further examine the relationships of physical and mental health and wellness to stressors, stress responses, and coping mechanisms.

Stress: Our mental and physical responses to the demands placed upon us.

Stressor: A physical, social, or mental event or condition that forces us to adjust to it.

Eustress: Stress perceived as "good" because it results in positive change.

Distress: Stress perceived as "bad" because it potentially results in negative change.

Psychoneuroimmunology (PNI): Science that focuses on the relationship between the mind's response to stress and the functioning of the immune system.

✳ THE GENERAL ADAPTATION SYNDROME

Every living organism attempts to achieve a state of balance known as **homeostasis**. In homeostasis, all physiological and psychological systems function smoothly, and equilibrium is maintained. When a stress is perceived, the mind and body adjust with an **adaptive response**, or an attempt to restore homeostasis. This adaptive response varies in intensity and physical manifestation from person to person and from stressor to stressor. Further, this response can vary within an individual from time to time, even in reaction to the same stressor.

The physiological and psychological responses to stress follow a pattern first recognized in 1936 by Hans Selye.[10] The three-stage response to stress is called the **general adaptation syndrome (GAS)**. The phases of the GAS are alarm, resistance, and exhaustion (see Figure 3.1).

Alarm Phase

During the alarm phase, a stressor disturbs homeostasis. The brain subconsciously perceives the stressor and prepares the body either to fight or to run away, a response sometimes called the "fight or flight response." The subconscious perceptions and appraisal of the stressor stimulate the areas in the brain responsible for emotions. Emotional stimulation, in turn, starts the physical reactions that we associate with stress

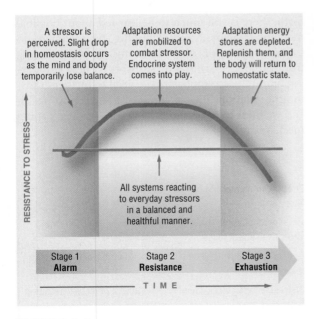

FIGURE 3.1

The General Adaptation Syndrome

FIGURE 3.2

The General Adaptation Syndrome: Alarm Phase

(see Figure 3.2). This entire process usually takes only a few seconds.

When the mind perceives a stressor (either real or imaginary), such as a potential attacker, the cerebral cortex, the region of the brain that interprets the nature of an event, is called to attention. If the cerebral cortex consciously or unconsciously perceives a threat, it triggers an instantaneous **autonomic nervous system (ANS)** response that prepares the body for action (that is, fight or flight). The ANS is the portion of the central nervous system that regulates bodily functions that we do not normally consciously control, such as heart rate, breathing, and glandular function. When we are stressed, the rate of these bodily functions increases dramatically to give us the physical strength to protect ourselves against an attack, or to mobilize internal forces. The ANS has two branches. One branch, the **sympathetic nervous system (SNS)**, energizes the body for either fight or flight by signalling the release of several stress hormones that increase heart and breathing rates, as well as many other responses. The other branch, the **parasympathetic nervous system (PNS)**, slows all the systems stimulated by the stress response. In other words, the PNS works in opposition to the SNS and attempts to restore homeostasis. In a healthy person, these two systems work together to maintain balance or homeostasis. Long-term stress can cause this balance to become strained, resulting in chronic physical and mental problems.

The response of the SNS to various stressors involves a complex series of biochemical exchanges between different parts of the body. The **hypothalamus**, a section of the brain, functions as the control centre and determines the overall reaction to stressors. When the hypothalamus perceives that extra energy is needed to fight or flee a stressor, it stimulates the adrenal glands, located near the top of the kidneys, to release the hormone **epinephrine**, also called adrenaline.

Epinephrine causes more blood to be pumped with each beat of the heart, dilates the alveoli (air sacs in the lungs) to increase oxygen intake, increases the rate of breathing, stimulates the liver to release more glucose (which fuels muscular contractions), and dilates the pupils to improve visual sensitivity. The body is then poised to act immediately. As epinephrine secretion increases, blood is diverted away from the digestive system, which can cause nausea and cramping if it occurs shortly after eating. Further, epinephrine dries nasal and salivary tissues, resulting in a dry mouth.

The stress response of the alarm phase also leads to longer-term reactions to stress. The hypothalamus triggers the pituitary gland, which in turn releases another powerful hormone, **adrenocorticotrophic hormone (ACTH)**. ACTH signals the adrenal glands to release **cortisol**, a hormone that facilitates the release of stored nutrients to meet energy demands. Finally, other parts of the brain and body release endorphins, the body's naturally occurring opiates, which relieve pain that may be caused by a stressor or the body's response to the stressor.

Resistance Phase

The resistance phase of the GAS begins almost immediately after the alarm phase kicks in. In this phase, the body has reacted to the stressor and adjusted in a way that begins to allow the system to return to homeostasis. As the sympathetic nervous system is working to energize the body via the hormonal action of epinephrine, norepinephrine, cortisol, and other hormones, the parasympathetic nervous system is working to keep these energy levels under control and attempting to return the body to a normal level of functioning.

Exhaustion Phase

In the exhaustion phase of the GAS, the physiological and psychological energy used to respond to a stressor (that is, the fight or flight impulse) has been depleted. Short-term response to stress would probably not deplete all a person's energy reserves, but chronic stressors may create continuous states of alarm and resistance. When a person no longer has the adaptation energy stores for responding to a distressor, burnout and serious illness may result.

what do you **THINK?**

How do you typically react to stressors? What happens to your body? To your mind? Do your responses cause you discomfort? Can you control your responses?

◄● SOURCES OF STRESS

Eustress and distress have many sources, including psychosocial factors, such as change, pressure, inconsistent goals and behaviours, conflict, overload, and

Homeostasis: A balanced physical and mental state in which all the body's systems function smoothly.

Adaptive response: Form of adjustment in which the mind and body attempt to restore homeostasis.

General adaptation syndrome (GAS): The pattern followed by our physiological and psychological responses to stress, consisting of the alarm, resistance, and exhaustion phases.

Autonomic nervous system (ANS): The portion of the central nervous system that regulates bodily functions and is not normally consciously controlled.

Sympathetic nervous system (SNS): Branch of the ANS responsible for stimulating the stress response.

Parasympathetic nervous system (PNS): Part of the ANS responsible for slowing systems stimulated by the SNS.

Hypothalamus: A section of the brain that controls the SNS and directs the stress response.

Epinephrine: Also called adrenaline, a hormone that stimulates body systems.

Adrenocorticotrophic hormone (ACTH): A pituitary hormone that stimulates the adrenal glands to secrete cortisol.

Cortisol: Hormone released by the adrenal glands that facilitates the release of stored nutrients to meet energy demands.

burnout; environmental stressors, such as natural and human-made disasters; and self-imposed stressors including factors related to self-concept.

Psychosocial Sources of Stress

As you learned in the previous chapter, psychosocial health refers to the social, mental, emotional, and spiritual dimensions of health. These components combined define how we perceive our lives, relate to one another, and react to stress. Many psychosocial factors in our daily lives cause us to feel stressed. Our interactions with others, the subtle and not-so-subtle expectations we have for ourselves and others, the expectations others have for us, and the social conditions we work, play, and live in force us to adjust and readjust continually. Some of these stressors present real threats to our mental or physical well-being; others cause us to worry about things that may never happen. Still other stressors result from otherwise good psychosocial events—being around someone you are attracted to, meeting new friends, moving to a new and better apartment, celebrating a win or successful paper or exam.

Change

There is the potential to experience stress any time there is change, whether good or bad, in your normal daily routine. The more changes you experience and the more adjustments you must make as a result, the greater the stress response may be. In 1967, Holmes and Rahe analyzed the social readjustments experienced by more than 5000 patients, noting which events seemed to occur just before the onset of disease.[11] They determined that certain events (positive and negative) were predictive of increased risk for illness. They called their scale for predicting stress overload and the likelihood of illness the Social Readjustment Rating Scale (SRRS).[12] The SRRS has since been modified for certain groups, including university or college-aged students. Although many other factors must be considered, it is generally believed that the more stressors you have, the more likely you are to experience negative effects on your health and wellness and the more important it is to address your behaviours or situations before health problems occur. (See the Rate Yourself box.)

While Holmes and Rahe focused on such major sources of stress as a death in the family, psychologists such as Richard Lazarus focused on petty annoyances, irritations, and frustrations—collectively referred to as hassles—as sources of stress.[13] Minor hassles—losing your keys, having the grocery bag rip on the way to the door, slipping and falling in front of everyone as you walk to your seat in class, finding that you went through a whole afternoon with a big chunk of spinach stuck in your front teeth—may seem unimportant, but Lazarus's research found that the cumulative effects of these minor hassles may be harmful in the long run.

Pressure

Pressure occurs when we feel forced to speed up, slow down, intensify, or shift the direction of our behaviours to meet a higher standard of performance.[14] Pressures can be based on our personal goals and expectations or on a concern about what others may think of us. Pressure can also come from outside influences. Among the most significant and consistent of these are seemingly relentless demands from society that we look a certain way, compete in all that we do, and be all that we can be. The forces that push us to attempt to shape our bodies into an image that may not even be physiologically realistic for us or to compete for the best grades, the nicest cars, the most attractive partners, and the highest paying jobs create a lot of pressure to be the personification of success.[15] Being pressured into doing something we do not want to do (for example, being pressured to go to a movie or party because everyone else is going, when you really need and want to be studying) can also be a source of frustration.

Inconsistent Goals and Behaviours

For many of us, negative stress effects are magnified when there is a conflict between our goals (what we value or hope to obtain in life) and our behaviours. For instance, you want good grades and your family expects them, yet you party and procrastinate throughout the term, spending very little time studying. Thus, your behaviours are inconsistent with your goals. On the other hand, if you choose to use your time well, study hard, and are committed to your school work, your goals and behaviours are congruent and you will not experience this kind of negative stress. Thwarted goals may lead to frustration, and frustration has been shown to be a significant disrupter of homeostasis (see Figure 3.3).

Determining whether our behaviours are consistent with the goals we want to reach is an essential component of our efforts to maintain a balance in our lives. If we consciously strive to attain our goals in a very direct manner, our chances of success are greatly improved. If we deviate from the plan, or if we act in a manner that is inconsistent with our goals, significant stress may result that makes achieving our goals impossible, and they may then become negative sources of stress.

BEHAVIOURS   GOALS

Work ethic
Priorities
Perseverance
Commitment
Dedication
Consistency
Interpersonal interactions

Health
Grades
Love
Career success
Financial gain
Expectations/ desires
Achievement levels
Values/beliefs
Relationship satisfaction

HOMEOSTASIS

FIGURE 3.3

Homeostatic Balance Requires Actions Related to Goals and Values

try it NOW!
Write it down! Journal writing is a great way to cleanse the mind, release emotions, and draft strategies for resolution. The next time an event or situation activates your stress response, identify the emotions that accompany it and then list several options to bring closure to the event. You might also consider journaling a little every day—write about the good things that happened as well as the challenges and your feelings associated with each.

Conflict

Of all life's difficulties, **conflict** is probably the most common. Conflict occurs when we are forced to make challenging decisions concerning two or more competing motives, behaviours, or impulses, or when we are forced to face two incompatible demands, opportunities, needs, or goals.[16] What if your best friends choose to smoke marijuana and you don't want to, yet you fear rejection? Such conflicts occur every day for most of us. Worrying about the alternatives, fretting, stewing, and becoming overly anxious are common responses when conflict occurs.

Overload

Overload occurs when we experience excessive time pressure, excessive responsibility, lack of support, or excessive expectations of ourselves and those around us. Have you ever felt that you had so many responsibilities that you could not possibly begin to fulfill them all? Have you longed for a weekend when you could just curl up and read a good book or take time out with friends and not feel guilty? These feelings typically occur when a person has been under continuous pressure for some time and as a result experiences overload. Students who are overloaded may experience anxiety about tests and assignments, poor self-concept, thoughts about dropping classes or dropping out of school, and other problems. In severe cases, in which they are unable to see any solutions to their problems, students may suffer from depression or resort to overeating or consuming alcohol or drugs.

Burnout

People who regularly feel overload, frustration, and disappointment may eventually experience **burnout,** a state of physical and mental exhaustion caused by an excessive and continuous response to stress. People involved in the helping professions, such as teaching, social work, drug counselling, nursing, and psychology, appear to experience high levels of burnout, as do police officers, firefighters, and air-traffic controllers, who work in high-pressure, dangerous jobs.

Other Forms of Psychosocial Stress

Other forms of psychosocial stress include problems with adaptation (difficulty in adapting to life's changes), frustration (the thwarting or inhibiting of natural or desired behaviours or goals), overcrowding (the presence of too many people in one's space), discrimination (the unfavourable actions taken against people based on prejudices concerning race, ethnicity, religion, social status, gender, sex, sexual orientation, lifestyle, national origin, or physical characteristics), and socioeconomic events (inflation, unemployment, or poverty). People of different ethnic backgrounds and individuals who are homosexual may face disproportionately heavy impacts from these sources of stress.

Conflict: Simultaneous existence of incompatible demands, opportunities, needs, or goals.

Overload: A condition in which we feel pressured by constant and overwhelming demands made upon us.

Burnout: Physical and mental exhaustion as a result of the continuous experience of overload.

How Stressed Are You?

Each of us reacts differently to life's little challenges. Faced with a long line at the bank, most of us will get heated up for a few seconds before we shrug and move on. But for others—the one in five of us whom researchers call *hot reactors*—such incidents are an assault on good health. That's why rating your stress requires you to tally your life's stressors (Part One) and to figure out whether you are particularly susceptible to stress (Part Two). (As university or college students, you should consider your job as being a student.) You can then read the interpretation and make efforts to manage your stress response more effectively in the future.

PART ONE

The Stress in Your Life

How often are the following potentially stressful situations a part of your daily life?

1. Never
2. Rarely
3. Sometimes
4. Often
5. All the time

I work long hours.	1 2 3 4 5
There are signs my job is not secure.	1 2 3 4 5
Doing a good job goes unnoticed.	1 2 3 4 5
It takes all my energy just to make it through the day.	1 2 3 4 5
There are severe arguments at home.	1 2 3 4 5
A family member is seriously ill.	1 2 3 4 5
I am having problems with child care.	1 2 3 4 5
I do not have enough time for fun.	1 2 3 4 5
I am on a diet.	1 2 3 4 5
My family and friends count on me to solve their problems.	1 2 3 4 5
I'm expected to keep up a certain standard of living.	1 2 3 5 5
My neighbourhood is crowded or dangerous.	1 2 3 4 5
My home is a mess.	1 2 3 4 5
I cannot pay my bills on time.	1 2 3 4 5
I cannot save money.	1 2 3 4 5

Your Total Score

Below 38: You have a lower-stress life.

38 and above: You have a high-stress life.

PART TWO

Your Stress Susceptibility

Try to imagine how you would react in these situations:

1. You have been waiting 20 minutes for a table in a crowded restaurant, and the host seats a party that arrived after you. You feel your anger rise as your face gets hot and your heart beats faster.

   True or False

2. Your sister calls you out of the blue and starts to tell you how much you mean to her. Uncomfortable, you change the subject without expressing what you feel.

   True or False

3. You come home to find the kitchen looking like a disaster area and your partner (or roommate) lounging in front of the TV. You tense up and can not seem to shake your anger.

   True or False

4. Faced with a public-speaking event (such as a class presentation), you get keyed up and lose sleep for a day or more, worrying about how you will do.

   True or False

5. On Thursday, your repair shop promises to fix your car in time for a weekend trip. As the hours go by, you become increasingly worried that something will go wrong and your trip will have to be cancelled.

   True or False

Two or Fewer True: You are a Cool Reactor, someone who tends to roll with the punches when a situation is out of your control.

Three or More True: You are a Hot Reactor, someone who responds to mildly stressful situations with a "fight-or-flight" adrenaline rush that drives up blood pressure and can lead to heart rhythm disturbances, accelerated clotting, and damaged blood vessel linings. Some hot reactors can seem cool as a cucumber on the outside, but inside their bodies are silently killing them.

WHAT YOUR SCORES MEAN

Combine the results from Parts One and Two to get your total stress rating.

Lower-Stress Life/Cool Reactor

Whatever your problems, stress is not one of them. Even when stressful events do occur—and they will—your health is not likely to suffer.

Lower-Stress Life/Hot Reactor

You are not under stress—at least for now. Though you tend to overreact to problems, you have wisely managed your life to avoid the big stressors. Before you honk at the guy who cuts you off in rush-hour traffic, remember that getting angry can destroy thousands of heart muscle cells within minutes. Robert S. Eliot, author of *From Stress to Strength,* says hot reactors have no choice but to calm themselves down with rational thought. Ponder the fact that the only thing you will hasten by reacting is a decline in health. "You have to stop trying to change the world," Eliot advises, "and learn to change your response to it."

High-Stress Life/Cool Reactor

You are under stress, but only you know if it is hurting. Even if you normally thrive with a full plate of challenges, now you might be biting off more than you can chew. Note any increase in headaches, backaches, or insomnia; that is your body telling you to lighten your load. If your job is the main source of stress, think about reducing your hours. If that is not possible, find a way to make your job more enjoyable, and stress will become manageable.

High-Stress Life/Hot Reactor

You are in the danger zone. Make an extra effort to engage in physical activity, get enough sleep, and keep your family and friends close. Unfortunately, even being physically active and physically fit does little to protect you if your body is in perpetual stress mode. To survive, you may need to make major changes—walking away from a life-destroying job or relationship, perhaps—as well as to develop a whole new approach to life's hourly obstacles. Such effort will be rewarded, too. In one experiment, 77 percent of hot reactors were able to cool down—lower their blood pressure and cholesterol levels—by training themselves to stay calm.

Source: Reprinted by permission of the Health Publishing Group, a division of Time Publishing Ventures, Inc., from "How Stressed Are You?" *Health* (October 1994): 47. Researched by Lora Elise Ma. © 1994.

Environmental Stress

Environmental stress results from events occurring in our physical environment. Environmental stressors include natural disasters, such as floods, earthquakes, hurricanes, tornadoes, hail storms, blizzards, ice storms, and forest fires, and industrial disasters, such as chemical spills, accidents at nuclear power plants, and explosions. Often as damaging as one-time disasters are **background distressors**, such as noise, air, and water pollution or heat, humidity, cold, and wind-chills—although we may be unaware of them, and their effects may not become apparent for decades. As with other distressors, our bodies respond to environmental distressors with the GAS. People who cannot escape background distressors may exist in a constant resistance phase, which may also contribute to the development of stress-related disorders.

Self-Imposed Stress

Self-Concept and Stress

How we feel about ourselves, our attitudes toward others, and our perceptions and interpretations of the stressors in our lives are part of the psychological component of stress. Also included are the defence or coping mechanisms we have learned to use in various situations in response to stress.

The psychological system that governs our stress responses is called the **cognitive stress system**.[17] It recognizes stressors; evaluates them on the basis of self-concept, past experiences, and emotions; and makes decisions about how to best cope with them. Our sensory organs serve as input channels for information reaching the brain. From that point on, attention to the problem, memory, reasoning, and problem solving

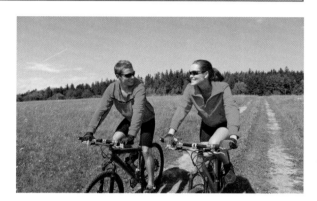

Moderate and vigorous intensity aerobic exercise is an effective stress management tool.

processes are organized in various parts of the brain before we respond to the stressor. Because learning and memory involve the changing of various proteins in brain neurons, the emotions we experience during the stress response also "tickle" the memory-storage neurons and contribute to our responses. Behaviourally, we respond to the stressor in ways consistent with our memories of similar situations.

Self-esteem is closely related to the emotions engendered by past experiences. People with low self-esteem are more likely to feel helpless anger, an emotion experienced by people who have not learned to express anger in appropriate ways. People with helpless anger have usually learned that they are wrong to feel angry; therefore, instead of expressing their anger in healthy

Background distressors: Environmental stressors, such as heat, humidity, noise, etc. that result in the GAS even though we may be unaware of them.

Cognitive stress system: The psychological system that governs our emotional responses to stress.

Expressing Anger Effectively

Expressing anger constructively is an important skill involved in learning to cope with intimate relationships, family interactions, and other stressful situations. Suggestions for constructively expressing anger are included in this textbox.

1. *Determine the reason behind your anger.* Is it due to a real event (for example, someone you trusted is spreading malicious gossip) or to a perception you have about a situation (friends are avoiding you, so you think someone may be gossiping)?

2. *Do not let your anger build.* When you become angry, take control, and decide what actions you need to take. Try not to act rashly, and do not stew for too long. Employ the 24–48 hour rule. Allow 24 hours to pass; if you are still angry, take action to manage the situation. If more than 48 hours pass and you do not do anything, let it go; it was not that important to you.

3. *If you decide to confront a person, select an appropriate time and place for the meeting.* Do not attack your target unexpectedly or in the presence of others: the person may become defensive. Give the person a general idea of what you want to discuss ahead of time and choose the appropriate time and location together.

4. *Stick to the main reason for your anger.* Bringing up a whole list of things that have made you angry over the last year will complicate the issue and make the other person want to create his or her own list of wrongs that you have committed. Plan in advance which issue you want to discuss. Be careful of using all inclusive statements such as "You always . . . " or "You never . . . ."

5. *Attack the problem rather than the person.* ("It made me angry that we had to leave early" instead of "You made me angry because you made us leave early.") Do not get into a battle over personal characteristics. Use "I" statements to communicate resentment or disappointment ("I feel angry that we had to leave the party so early"). "You" statements often put people on the defensive.

6. *Listen carefully to what the other person has to say.* Do not interrupt; give the other person a chance to speak. Listen rather than planning what you are going to say next. If the other person starts wandering from the issue, gently bring him or her back to the point. If the other person attacks you personally, stay in control and do not allow yourself to fight back.

7. *Treat the other person with respect.* Even though you may say the right things, your gestures and body language can reveal that you do not value what the other person has to say, that you are hostile, or that you are losing patience. Drumming your fingers, sighing, or rolling your eyes while the other person is talking often increases friction. Remember, communication is 90 percent non-verbal.

8. *Recognize when to quit.* Sometimes even the best-laid plans go awry. No matter what you do, the problem may appear impossible to resolve. In such situations, knowing when to quit, either temporarily or permanently, is a key factor in controlling anger and the stress that results from it. Agree to disagree. Nobody has to "win" the argument.

9. *When it is over, let it be over.* After you have done all that you can do, let go of your anger. Do not dwell in the past. Acknowledge your right to be angry, recognize it for what it was, and move on.

ways, they turn it inward. They "swallow" their anger in food, alcohol, or other drugs, or act in other self-destructive ways. See the Building Communication Skills box for a series of questions concerning expressing your anger effectively.

Self-esteem significantly affects various disease processes. People with low self-esteem create a self-imposed distressor that can impair the immune system's ability to combat disease. Some researchers believe that chronic distress can depress the immune system and thus increase the symptoms of such diseases as acquired immune deficiency syndrome (AIDS), herpes, multiple sclerosis, and Epstein-Barr syndrome.

Personality Types and Hardiness

A person's personality may contribute to the kind and degree of self-imposed stress he or she experiences.

The coronary-disease-prone personality was first described by physicians Friedman and Rosenman in their book *Type A Behavior and Your Heart.*[18] Although their work is now considered controversial, it is the basis for much current research.

Friedman and Rosenman identified two stress-related personality types: Type A and Type B. Type A personalities are hard-driving, competitive, anxious, time-driven, impatient, angry, and perfectionistic. Type B personalities are relaxed and non-competitive. According to Rosenman and Friedman, people with Type A characteristics are more prone to heart attacks than their Type B counterparts.

Researchers today believe that more needs to be discovered about Type A and Type B personalities before we can say that all people with a Type A personality will have greater risks for heart disease than those with a predominantly Type B personality. First

Taming Technostress

Cellphones that ring or vibrate constantly with incoming calls or text messages; email lists that grow on your computer desktop like an out-of-control fungus; laptop computers that somehow end up in your luggage when you go on vacation; voice message systems that do not allow you to talk to a live person; and slow, slow, slow downloading of information. Can you feel your heart rate speeding up just thinking about these situations? On campuses across the country, students, faculty, and administrators are using electronic organizers, the internet, and other forms of technology. Email, the World Wide Web, and personal digital assistants (PDAs) are no longer flashy new tools but are now as commonplace as the backpack. Unfortunately, many people feel frustrated and distressed in their struggle to adapt to increasingly complex technology. As many as 85 percent of us have at least some level of discomfort around technology. If you are like millions of people today, you find that technology is often a daily terrorizer that raises your blood pressure, frustrates you, and prevents you from ever really getting away from it all. In short, you may be a victim of stressors that previous generations only dreamed (or had nightmares) about. Known as "technostress," this problem is defined as "personal stress generated by reliance on technological devices . . . a panicky feeling when they fail, and a state of near-constant stimulation, or being perpetually 'plugged in.'" When technostress grabs you, it may interact with other forms of stress to create a synergistic, never-ending form of stimulation that keeps your stress response reverberating all day.

Part of the problem, ironically, is that technology enables us to be productive. Because it encourages polyphasic activity, or "multitasking," people are forced to juggle multiple thoughts and actions at the same time, such as driving and talking on cellphones or checking handheld devices for appointments. People who multitask, however, are actually less efficient than those who focus on one project at a time. Moreover, there is clear evidence that multitasking contributes to auto accidents and other harmful consequences, including short-term memory loss. What is less clear is what happens to someone who is always plugged in. What are the symptoms of technology overload? It evokes typical stress responses by increasing heart rate and blood pressure and causing irritability and memory disturbances. Over time, many stressed-out people lose the ability to relax and find that they feel nervous and anxious when they are supposed to be having fun. Headaches, stomach and digestive problems, skin irritations, frequent colds, difficulty in wound healing, lack of sleep, ulcers, and other problems may result. Other red flags include gaps in your attentiveness and changes in your ability to concentrate. One study indicates that chronic stress may even thicken the waistline. Authors Michelle Weil and Larry Rosen describe *technosis*, a syndrome in which people get so immersed in technology that they risk losing their own identity. If you answer yes to questions such as, "Do you rely on preprogrammed systems to contact others?", "Do you feel stressed if you haven't checked your email within the last couple of hours?", or "Are you lost without your cellphone or PDA?" you may be too dependent on technology.

TIPS FOR FIGHTING TECHNOSTRESS

- *Enjoy the natural environment.* Take some time away from all forms of technology. Try to find a place that has few people and little noise—that usually means outdoors.
- *Become aware of what you are doing.* Log the time you spend on email, voice mail, etc. Set up a schedule to limit your use of technology. For example, spend no more than an hour per day answering emails or interacting on Facebook or MSN.
- *Give yourself more time for everything you do.* If you are surfing the web for resources for a term paper, start early rather than the night before the paper is due.
- *Manage the telephone—do not let it manage you.* Rather than interrupting what you are doing to answer, screen calls with an answering machine or caller ID. Get rid of call waiting, which forces you to juggle multiple calls, and subscribe to a voice mail service that takes messages when you are on the phone.
- *Set "time out" periods when you do not answer the phone, listen to the stereo, use the computer, or watch TV.* Switch off email notification systems so you are not notified of an incoming message during these periods.
- *Take regular breaks.* Even when working, take a short break every hour; get up, walk around, stretch, do deep breathing, get a glass of water, use the washroom, etc.
- *If you are working on the computer, look away from the screen and focus on something far away every 30 minutes.* Stretch your shoulders and neck hourly as you work. Play soft background music to help you relax.
- *When working on the computer, focus on one task at a time.* If you are working on a paper, close your email and instant messaging so that you can focus on your paper and not feel pressured to respond because "you've got mail" or someone has logged on to instant messaging.
- *Resist the urge to buy the newest and fastest technology.* Such purchases not only cause financial stress but also add to stress levels with the typical glitches that occur when installing and adjusting to new technology.
- *Do not take laptops, hand-held devices, or other technological gadgets on vacation.* If you must, take a cellphone for emergencies, turn it and your voice messaging system off, and use the phone only in true emergencies.
- *Back up materials on your computer at regular intervals.* Writing a term paper only to lose it during a power outage will send you into hyperstress very quickly.

of all, most people are not one personality type or the other all the time. Second, there are many other unexplained variables that must be explored, such as why some Type A personalities seem to thrive in stress-filled environments. Now labelled Type C personalities, these individuals appear to succeed more often than Type B personalities and have good health even while displaying Type A patterns of behaviour.

Critics of the supposed links between these personality types and risk of disease argue that attempts to explain ill health by means of personal behavioural patterns have so far been crude. For example, Ragland and Brand contend that the Type A personality may be more complex than previously described.[19] These researchers identified a "toxic core" in some Type A personalities. People with this toxic core are angry, distrustful of others, and have above-average levels of cynicism. Generally, people who are angry and hostile also have below-average levels of social support and other increased risks for ill health. It may be this toxic core rather than the hard-driving nature of the Type A personality that makes people more prone to self-imposed stress and its consequences.

Psychological hardiness has been identified as a characteristic that helps some people cope with the self-imposed stress associated with Type A behaviours.[20] Psychologically hardy people are characterized by control, commitment, challenge, choices, and connectedness (sometimes called the "Type C personality"). People with a sense of control take control of their actions and are able to accept responsibility for their behaviours. People with a sense of commitment have good self-esteem and understand their purpose in life. These individuals choose to commit themselves to the things that matter to them and say no when the situation is not of personal importance. People with a sense of challenge see changes or struggles in life as stimulating opportunities for personal growth. Psychologically hardy people also make lifestyle choices that enhance their health, such as eating well, being physically active regularly, getting adequate sleep, developing meaningful relationships, making time for

themselves, and so on. Finally, these individuals are connected to others in meaningful ways. This connectedness provides a level of social support that is health enhancing.

Modification of the Type A personality is possible when particular "learned" behaviours are modified. For example, some people with a Type A personality are able to reduce their hurried behaviours and become more tolerant, more patient, and better-humoured. Unfortunately, many people do not decide to modify their Type A habits until after they have become ill or suffered a heart attack or other circulatory system distress. Prevention of heart and circulatory disorders resulting from stress entails recognizing and changing dangerous behaviours before damage is done.

Self-Efficacy and Control

Whether people are able to cope successfully with stressful situations often depends on their level of self-efficacy, or belief in their skills and performance abilities.[21] If people have been successful in mastering similar problems in the past, they are more likely to believe in their own effectiveness in future situations. Similarly, people who have repeatedly tried and failed may lack confidence in their abilities to deal with life's problems. In some cases, this insecurity may prevent them from even trying to cope; this is the sense of learned helplessness that was discussed in Chapter 2.

In addition, people who believe they lack control in a situation may become easily frustrated and give up quickly. Those who feel they have little to no personal control over their life and what happens to them tend to have an external locus of control (that is a belief that an outside power—fate or destiny—controls one's life) and a low level of self-efficacy. People who are confident that their behaviours will influence the ultimate outcome of life's events tend to have an internal locus of control (that is, the belief that one is in control of one's own life). People who feel that they have limited control over their lives tend to have higher levels of stress.

what do you THINK?

What type of personality do you think you have? Do you think it is possible to change your personality type? Why or why not? Which of the Type C personality traits do you already possess? Which ones do you lack? What are you willing to do to become more like a Type C personality? Why?

✳ STRESS AND THE POST-SECONDARY STUDENT

Stress related to university or college life is more far-reaching than simply the pressure to excel academically. Post-secondary students experience numerous distressors, including changes related to being away from home for the first time, climatic differences between home and school, pressure to make friends in a new and sometimes intimidating setting, the feeling of anonymity imposed by larger classes, test-taking anxiety, and pressures related to time management. Some students are stressed by athletic team requirements, on-campus food selection, roommates' habits, peers' expectations, new questions about personal values and beliefs, relationship problems, fraternity or sorority demands, financial worries, changed sleeping habits (including reduced sleep), and the need to be technologically savvy. For older students, worries about competing with 18-year-olds may also be distressful, in addition to the pressure of determining their future career path and managing responsibilities regarding their family and home. Technological advances have created new pressures for students to be engaged in computer and computer-related tasks for longer time periods, which may cause mental as well as physical duress (that is, anxiety about not finding required information, sifting through the abundance of materials discovered to find credible information, and repetitive strain injuries related to overuse and poor body mechanics). Most colleges and universities offer stress management workshops through their health centres or student counselling departments.

You should not ignore the following symptoms of stress overload. If you experience one or more of these symptoms, act promptly to reduce their impact:

- difficulty keeping up with classes or difficulty concentrating on and finishing tasks
- frequent clashes with close friends, family, or intimate partners about trivial issues such as housekeeping
- frequent mood changes or overreaction to minor problems

- lethargy caused by lack of sleep or excessive frustration
- lack of interest in social activities or tendency to avoid others
- avoidance of stressors through use of drugs or alcohol or through other extreme behaviours
- sleep disturbances, TV or computer/technology-related addiction, free-floating anxiety, or an exaggerated sense of self
- difficulty in maintaining an intimate relationship
- lack of interest in sexual relationships or inability to participate in satisfactory sexual relationships
- tendency to be intolerant of minor differences of opinion
- hunger and cravings or tendency to overeat or to eat while thinking of other things
- lack of awareness of sensory cues
- inability to listen or tendency to jump from subject to subject in conversation
- stuttering or other speech difficulties
- accident-proneness
- difficulty finding the right words to say or misspeaking quite frequently

what do you THINK?

What are your signs and symptoms of stress? What about your university or college life causes you to react with a stress response? What can you do about these factors?

✔ STRESS MANAGEMENT

Stress can be challenging or defeating depending upon how we learn to view it. The most effective way to avoid defeat is to develop a number of skills known collectively as stress management. Stress management consists primarily of finding balance in our lives. We balance rest, relaxation, physical activity, dietary intake, work, school, family, community responsibilities, finances, and social activities. As we balance our lives, we make the choice to react constructively to our stressors. Robert Eliot, a cardiologist and stress researcher, offers two rules for people trying to cope

Psychological hardiness: A personality characteristic characterized by control, commitment, challenge, choices, and connectedness.

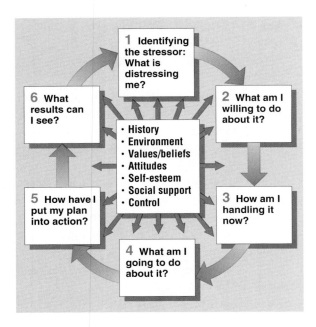

FIGURE 3.4

A Decision-Making Model for Stress Management

Source: Adapted from Lester A. Lefton, *Psychology,* 5th ed., 485 (Figure 13.5). © 1994 by Allyn & Bacon. Reprinted by permission.

with life's challenges: "Don't sweat the small stuff," and remember that "it's all small stuff."[22]

Dealing with Stress

The first step of stress management is to examine thoroughly any problem involving stress. Figure 3.4 shows a decision-making model for managing your response to stress. As the model shows, dealing with stress involves assessing all aspects of a stressor, examining how you currently respond to it and how you may be able to change your response, and evaluating various methods of coping with stress. Some stressors we cannot change, such as professors' assignments or unexpected distressors like car accidents or storm damage. Inevitably, we will take classes that bore us and for which we find no application to real life. And, of course, we feel powerless when a loved one has died. These facts themselves cannot be changed; only our reactions or responses to these situations can be altered.

Assessing Your Stressors

After recognizing a stressor, you need to assess it. Can you alter the circumstances in any way to reduce the amount of distress you are experiencing, or must you change your behaviours and reactions? For example, if five term papers for five different courses are due during the semester, you will probably quickly assess that you cannot alter the circumstances: your professors are unlikely to change their requirements. You can, however, alter your behaviours by working on one or two of the papers well before the due dates and spacing the others over time to avoid last-minute stress from trying to write them all in the week before they are due. Another example is your boss being vague about directions for assignments. You cannot change the boss; you can, however, ask the boss to clarify what is expected of you—in writing, if an oral response is insufficient.

Recognizing and Changing Your Responses

Recognizing and changing your responses to stressors requires self-reflection, practice, and emotional control. It is important to recognize your typical physical and mental responses to stress so that you can manage these responses more effectively in future situations. If your roommate is habitually messy and this causes you stress, you can choose from several responses. For example, you can express your anger by yelling, you can pick up the mess and leave a nasty note, or you can defuse the situation with humour. The first response that comes to mind is not always the best response. Stop before you react, to gain the time you need to find an appropriate response. Ask yourself, "What is to be gained from my response?" or "How will my response mediate this type of behaviour in the future?" Many people change their responses to potentially stressful events through cognitive coping strategies. These strategies help them prepare for stressors through gradual exposure to increasingly higher stress levels.

Learning to Cope

Everyone copes with stress and their stress responses in different ways.[23] For some people, drinking and taking drugs helps them to cope. Others choose to get help from counsellors. Still others try to get their minds off stress by engaging in physical activity or relaxation techniques. *Stress inoculation,* a newer technique, helps people prepare for stressful events ahead of time. For example, if you are petrified about speaking in front of your class, practising in front of a friend or a mirror may inoculate you and prevent you from freezing up on the day of your presentation. Some health experts compare stress inoculation to a vaccine. Stress inoculation

- increases the predictability of stressful events
- fosters coping skills
- generates self-talking

- encourages confidence about successful outcomes
- builds a commitment to personal action and responsibility for an adaptive course of action

Regardless of how you cope with a given situation, your conscious effort to deal with it is an important step in stress management.

Downshifting

Today's lifestyles are hectic and pressure-packed, with self-imposed stress often a result of trying to keep up. Many people are wondering if "having it all" is worth it, and as a result are taking a step back and simplifying their lives. This simplification is known as "downshifting." Moving from a big city to a small town or moving from a big house to a smaller home and a host of other changes typify downshifting. Some dedicated downshifters have given up television, phones, and even computers.

Downshifting involves a fundamental alteration in values and honest introspection about what is important in life. When you consider any form of downshift or perhaps even start your career this way, it's important to move slowly and consider the following:

- *Determine your ultimate goal.* What is most important to you, and what will you need to reach that goal? What can you do without? Where do you want to live? Where do you want to work?
- *Make a short- and long-term plan for simplifying your life.* Set up your plan in doable steps, and work slowly toward each step. Determine those people and organizations to whom it is important to give your time and say no to those requests from people and organizations that do not share your same values.
- *Complete a financial inventory.* How much money will you need to do the things you want to do? Will

you live alone or share costs with roommates? Do you need a car, or can you rely on active transportation, such as walking or cycling, or public transportation? Pay off credit cards and eliminate existing debt, or consider debt consolidation. Get used to paying with cash. If you don't have the cash, don't buy. Remember, your lifestyle may be different as a student compared to when you were working or living at home.

- *Select the right career.* Look for work that you enjoy; salary should not be the deciding factor. Can you be happy in a lower-paying job that is less stressful and provides you with sufficient challenge and the opportunities for the personal and professional growth that you consider important?
- *Consider options for saving money.* Downshifting doesn't mean you renounce money; it means you choose not to let money dictate your life. It's still important to save. If you are just getting started, you need to prepare for emergencies and future plans.
- *Clear out/clean out.* A cluttered life can be distressing. Take an inventory of material items, and get rid of things you haven't worn or used the last year or so. Donate these items to appropriate charities.

Managing Emotional Responses

Have you ever gotten all worked up about something you thought was happening only to find that your perceptions were totally wrong or that a communication problem resulted in a misinterpretation of events? This happens to most of us. We often get upset by our faulty perceptions rather than reality. For example, imagine you find out that your friends were invited to a party but you were not. You are likely to become angry as well as disappointed. Self-doubt will likely follow, and you will wonder if anybody likes you. Yet the reality may be that you were invited, but your invitation got lost or misplaced.

Stress management requires that you examine your emotional responses, including your self talk and explanatory style. With any emotional response to a distressor, you are responsible for your emotions and resulting behaviours. Learning to tell the difference between normal emotions and those based on irrational beliefs can help you to express them in a healthy and more appropriate way. Admitting your feelings and allowing them to be expressed either through communication or action is a stress management technique that can help you get through many difficult situations. Talking yourself through the situation—in a positive way—and explaining yourself to others, accepting

try it NOW!

A penny for your thoughts! Negative self-talk can contribute to feelings of stress. Try this idea to see how often you have negative emotional responses. Place a handful of pennies in your right-hand pocket, and each time you catch yourself having a negative thought about yourself, remove a penny from your right pocket and place it in your left pocket. Once you have an idea of how extensive your negative self-talk is, you can take steps to replace negative thoughts with positive ones.

responsibility when appropriate, and avoiding blaming others for your mistakes or setbacks are also part of managing your emotional responses and behaviours. It is also important in this regard to develop appropriate expectations for yourself and others.

Learning to Laugh and Cry

For some people, learning to express emotions freely is a difficult task. However, it is a task worth learning. Have you ever noticed that you feel better after a good laugh or cry? It was not your imagination. Laughter and crying stimulate the heart and temporarily invigorate many body systems. Heart rate and blood pressure then decrease significantly, allowing the body to relax.

Managing Social Interactions

The importance of social interaction should not be underestimated in your stress management plans. Consider the nature and extent of your friendships. Do you have a friend or several friends with whom you can share intimate thoughts and feelings? Is there someone you can call for help or in the case of an emergency? Do you trust your friends to be supportive? Do you think your friends will be honest and tell you if you are doing something risky or inappropriate? Having someone to listen to you when needed and to give helpful advice is an invaluable stress management tool. It is less important to have a wide circle of acquaintances than it is to have a few really good friends. Different friends often serve different needs, so having more than one friend is beneficial. In university and college, friends often fulfill roles that family members held in the past. As you continue to develop and cultivate friendships, look for individuals who:

- have values similar to your own
- have similar interests that you can enjoy together
- have different interests that force you to grow and explore new ideas
- are good listeners, give and share freely, are tolerant, and do not rush to judgment
- are trustworthy
- consider your needs in addition to theirs
- are not unusually critical, negative, selfish, or pessimistic.
- are responsible and value doing well in school
- know when and how to have fun
- are willing to be physical activity buddies or study partners with a mutual interest in a healthy lifestyle
- know how to laugh, cry, engage in meaningful conversation, and feel comfortable with silence

Just as it is important to find these characteristics in your friends, it is also important for you to bring these qualities to your friendships. Sometimes, focusing on others can help you get your problems into perspective and control.

Making the Most of Support Groups

Support groups can also be an important part of stress management. Friends, family members, and co-workers can provide us with emotional and physical support. Although the ideal support group differs for each of us, you should have one or two close friends in whom you are able to confide and neighbours with whom you can trade favours. You should participate in community activities at least once a week. Part of your support group may also involve a significant other; a healthy, committed relationship can provide vital support.

If you do not have a close support group, you should know where to turn when the pressures of life seem overwhelming. Family members are often a steady base of support on which you can rely. Most colleges and universities have counselling services available at no cost for short-term crises. Members of the clergy, instructors, and residence supervisors may also be supportive resources. You should also be able to find counselling services in the local community. All services are confidential.

Taking Mental Action

Stress management calls for mental action in two areas. First, positive self-esteem, which can help you cope with stressful situations, comes from learned habits. If you have the mental habit of assuming you can handle the challenges that come your way, you will be less likely to feel overwhelmed. Successful stress management involves mentally developing and practising self-esteem skills. For example, when things seem overwhelming, remind yourself of situations you have handled well in the past and challenges you have already overcome; do not assume the situation is beyond your control. Second, because you can not always anticipate what the next distressor will be, you need to develop the mental skills necessary to manage your reaction to stresses when they happen. The ability to think about and react quickly to stress comes with time, practice, experience with a variety of stressful situations and coping methods, and patience. Most of all, you must strive to become more aware of situations that potentially induce stress and act quickly to deal with them. Rather than seeing stressors as adversaries, learn to view them as exercises in life, challenges to be overcome, or obstacles to be cleared.

❋ Changing the Way You Think

Once you realize that some of your thoughts or self-talk may be negative, irrational, or overreactive, making a conscious effort to reframe or change the way you've been thinking and focusing on more positive ways of thinking is a key element of stress management. Here are some specific actions you can take to develop these mental skills.

- *Worry constructively.* Do not waste time and energy worrying about things you can not change or things that may never happen. For example, do not fret over the weather forecast even if rain or a storm is predicted for when you want to travel for the week end. Wait until the week end comes to adjust your plans accordingly.

- *Look at life as being fluid.* Accept change as a natural part of living and growing rather than resisting it. For example, if your roommate decides to move out, see that as an opportunity to live with someone different, to experience a new friendship.

- *Consider alternatives.* Remember that there is seldom only one appropriate action. Anticipating options will help you plan for change and adjust more rapidly. For example, when faced with several assignments or mid-term exams scheduled for the same day, there are a variety of approaches you can take. You might speak to each professor and outline your situation hoping for some rescheduling, or you may simply start each assignment right away and plan your time accordingly.

- *Have moderate expectations.* Aim high, but be realistic about your circumstances and capabilities. Be realistic about your grades—90s are rare in college and university! Aiming to maintain honours status may be more appropriate for you.

- *Weed out trivia.* Do not sweat the small stuff, and remember that most of it is small stuff. So, if someone took the last piece of pizza ahead of you in the food line, do not sweat about it; move on to your next option or wait until more pizza is brought out.

- *Do not rush into action.* Think before you act. You can use the 24–48 hour rule. If something happens that angers or disappoints you; leave it for 24 hours. If you are still disturbed, address the situation. If you leave it for 48 hours, it must not be important enough for you to follow up.

- *Keep things in perspective.* Try not to exaggerate the importance of what has happened. Yes, failing an exam or a paper is not a good thing. Still, consider how much it is actually worth—and in the whole scheme of things, how significant is it?

- *Focus on the positive.* Become selectively aware of the positive aspect of negative or unplanned situations.

For example, if you get caught up in traffic, plan your day ahead. Or if your partner ends your relationship, think about the extra time you will have to yourself or for your friends and family.

- *See stumbling blocks as challenges rather than barriers.* Expect challenges and difficulties rather than resisting them. So, when your schedule becomes full with many papers to write, exams to prepare for, and classes to attend, see that as the opportunity to learn how to organize your time well and to follow a planned agenda versus just seeing it as "stressful."

- *When you think "I can't do it," break the task into smaller pieces and work on one small part at a time.* For example, if you have a paper and a laboratory report due on the same day, break each down into logical pieces and work on one piece at a time.

- *Reframe.* Rather than seeing the situation as a stumbling block, see it as a challenge and an opportunity. For example, if your date is no longer available to go out, see the unexpected evening alone as an opportunity to unwind and indulge in a bath rather than getting angry or frustrated.

Taking Physical Action

Learning to use physical activity to prevent, alleviate, and manage stress will complement the emotional strategies you employ in stress management.

Physical Activity

Moderate and vigorous intensity physical activities play a critical role in stress management. When engaged in moderate or vigorous intensity physical activity, the body releases endorphins (mood-enhancing, pain-killing hormones) in the bloodstream. Being physically active also increases energy, reduces hostility, and improves mental alertness. Vigorous physical activity is particularly effective as an immediate response to stress because it can immediately alleviate or reduce the stress symptoms/response. Engaging in physical activity on a regular basis yields even more substantial benefits. Try to get at least 20 to 30 minutes of aerobic exercise 3 or 4 times a week for the added benefits to the hormonal regulation of stress. A quiet walk can also refresh your mind, calm your stress response, and replenish your adaptation energy stores. Plan walking breaks alone or with friends. In fact, walking and talking is often an effective way to manage stress—physically and emotionally. Stretch after prolonged periods of study at your desk. A short period of physical activity may provide the break you really need. For more information about physical activity, see Chapter 4.

Relaxation Techniques for Stress Management

You probably experience stressful situations every day—at school, at work, at home, even at play. Stress results from a combination of many factors often beyond our control. While stress cannot be eliminated completely, you can learn how to manage your responses in a positive way. Take steps to manage your response to stressful situations by using the following simple techniques:

1. **Diaphragmatic or deep breathing:** Typically, we breathe only using the upper chest and thoracic region rather than involving the abdominal region. Diaphragmatic breathing refers to deep breathing that maximally expands the chest by including the lower abdomen. This technique is commonly used in yoga exercises. Diaphragmatic breathing process occurs in three stages:

   • *Stage 1:* Assume a comfortable position. Whether sitting or lying down on your back, find the most natural position to be in. Close your eyes, unbutton your shirt or binding clothes, remove your belt, or unbutton your pants. Often it works best to hold your hands over your abdomen and get used to feeling the rise and fall of your stomach.

   • *Stage 2:* Concentrate on the act of breathing. Shut out external noise. Focus on inhaling, exhaling, and the route the air is following. Try saying to yourself, "Feel the warm air coming into your nose, warming your windpipe, and flowing into your lungs, expanding first your chest and then your belly."

   • *Stage 3:* Visualize. The above stages seem to work best when combined with visualization. A common example is to visualize clean, fresh, invigorating air slowly entering the nose and then being exhaled as grey, stale air. Such processes, particularly when they involve the whole body, seem to help individuals become refreshed from their experience.

2. **Progressive muscle relaxation:** Progressive muscle relaxation involves systematically contracting and relaxing each of several muscle groups; breathing deeply and concentrating on the muscles being contracted and relaxed are part of this process. Again, find a comfortable position and begin a deep-breathing cycle. The difference from diaphragmatic breathing is that, as you concentrate on inhaling, you will also contract a particular muscle group (for example, the hand and fingers). Hold that position for a short period and then, as you exhale, slowly release the muscles that you have been contracting. Repeat and add more muscle groups. You might start with the hands, then move to the forearms, the entire arms, the neck, then move to the shoulders, back, buttocks, thighs, lower legs, and finish with the feet. You can add components of other relaxation techniques to this experience by saying, "My hands are getting warmer, my arm is getting warmer," and so on as you work to gain maximum control of blood flow and muscle tension in a region.

Source: Paragraph on qigong from C. Dold, "The New Yoga," *Health* (May 2004): 73–77.

Relaxation

Like physical activity, relaxation can help you to cope with stressful feelings, preserve adaptation energy stores, and dissipate the excess hormones associated with the GAS. Relaxation may involve a warm bath, or some time sitting quietly and listening to music, or it may involve sitting comfortably repeating a mantra (a word to help you relax). There are various forms of relaxation that can be undertaken. Generally, relaxation helps you to refocus your energies and should be practised daily. When you begin to feel your body respond to stress—eustress or distress—make time to relax to give yourself added strength and to alleviate the negative physical effects of the GAS. As your body relaxes, your heart rate lowers, your blood pressure and metabolic rate decrease, and many other body-calming effects occur, allowing you to channel energy more effectively. See also the Your Spiritual and Emotional Health box.

Eating Well

Is food a destressor? Do Mom's chocolate chip cookies or Grandma's apple pie really make you feel better? Whether foods can calm us and nourish our psyches is a controversial question. Much of what has been published about hyperactivity and its relation to the consumption of sweets has been shown to be scientifically invalid. And high-potency stress-tabs that are supposed to provide you with resistance against stress-related ailments are nothing more than gimmicks. However, what is clear is that having a balanced, healthy dietary intake will provide you with the stamina needed to get through problems and may stress-proof you in ways not fully understood. It is also known that undereating, overeating, emotional eating, and a dietary intake that is insufficient in variety, balance, and moderation can create distress in the body. For more information about the benefits of healthy eating for overall health and wellness, see Chapter 5.

Learning Time Management

Time—everybody needs more of it, especially students trying to balance the demands of classes, social life, part-time jobs, family obligations, and time needed for relaxation and physical activity. The following tips regarding time management should become a part of your stress management program:

- *Clean off your desk.* According to Jeffrey Mayer, author of *Winning the Fight between You and Your Desk,* most of us lose time looking for things that are lost on our desks or in our homes. Go through the things on your desk, recycle the unnecessary papers, and organize the remaining papers in "to do" piles.

- *Never handle papers more than once.* When bills and other papers come in, take care of them immediately. Write out a cheque and hold it for mailing. Get rid of the envelopes. Read your mail and file it or toss it. If you haven't looked at something in over a year, recycle it. The same can be said for your email. Read it, handle it, and then delete it. Do not open and read your email unless you are ready to manage each message.

- *Prioritize your tasks.* Make a daily "to do" list and stick to it. Categorize the things you must do today, the things that you have to do but not immediately, and the things that it would be nice to do. Prioritize the Must Do Now and Have to Do Later items and put deadlines next to each. Only consider the Nice to Do items if you finish the others or if the Nice to Do list includes something fun for you.

- *Avoid interruptions.* When you've got a project that requires your total concentration, schedule uninterrupted time. Unplug the phone or let your voice mail get it. Turn off the instant messaging and email software on your computer. Close your door and post a Do Not Disturb sign. Go to a quiet room in the library or student union where no one will find you. Protect your time so you can use it well.

- *Do not be afraid to say no.* Too often, we overcommit ourselves. It is okay to say "No, I am too busy," "No, I am not really interested," or "I would like to help out; however, I am already committed to too many projects at this time."

- *Reward yourself for being efficient.* If you planned to take a certain amount of time to finish a task and you finish early, take some time for yourself. Have a cup of coffee or hot chocolate. Go for a walk. Read for pleasure. Differentiate between rest breaks and work breaks. Work breaks simply mean

Being able to talk comfortably to someone close to you is part of stress management.

that you switch tasks for a while. Rest breaks get you away from work and let you spend time for yourself.

- *Use time to your advantage.* If you are a morning person, plan your work to take advantage of that time. If you know that by Friday afternoon you will be tired and worn out, plan to work on tasks that require minimal concentration. Take breaks when needed. Use physical activity as an energizer.

- *Become aware of your own time patterns.* For many of us, minutes and hours drift by without us even noticing them. Chart your daily schedule, hour by hour, for one week. Note the time that was wasted, when it was wasted, and think of the reasons that may have led to that. Note also the time spent in productive work or restorative pleasure. Determine how you could be more productive and make more time for yourself.

- *Remember that time is precious.* Many people learn to value their time only when they face a terminal illness. Value each day. Time spent not enjoying life is a tremendous waste of potential.

Using Alternative Stress Management Techniques

The popularity of stress management has increased the amount of advertising for various "stress fighters" such as hypnosis, massage therapies, and meditation. Some universities and colleges may provide these services through extended health coverage. Most should also be available in your local community.

Managing Stress Behaviours

Stress is not something that you can run from or wish into non-existence. To control stress, you must meet it head-on and use the resources needed to ensure that your coping skills are fine-tuned and capable of helping you. In planning your personal strategies for coping with stress, consider the following:

MAKING DECISIONS FOR YOU

Following a few simple guidelines may help you not only to enjoy more guilt-free time but also to become more productive during work hours.

- *Plan life, not time.* Determining what you want from life rather than what you can get done may help change the way you use time. Evaluate all your activities, even the most trivial, to determine whether they add to your life. If they don't, get rid of them.

- *Decelerate.* Rushing is part of the Canadian work ethic and mindset that says "Busy is better." It can be addictive. When rushed, ask yourself if you really need to be. What is the worst that could happen if you slow down? Tell yourself at least once a day that failure seldom results from doing a job slowly or too well. Failures happen when rushing causes a lack of attention to detail.

- *Learn to delegate and share.* The need to feel in control is powerful. If you are unusually busy, leave details to someone else. Do not be afraid to ask others to help or to share the workload and responsibilities.

- *Learn to say no.* Give priority to what is most critical to your life, your job, or your current situation. Decide what things you can do, what things you must do, and what things you want to do, and delegate the rest to someone else either permanently or until you complete some of your priority tasks. Before you take on a new responsibility, finish or drop an old one.

- *Schedule time alone.* Find time each day for quiet thinking, reading, physical activity, or other enjoyable activities.

CHECKLIST FOR CHANGE: ASSESSING YOUR LIFE STRESSORS

- Have you assessed the major stressors in your life? Are they people, events, or specific activities?

- Have you thought about what you may be doing to elevate your stress levels? Do you often worry about things that never happen?

- Have you thought about what you could change to reduce your stress response?

- Do you have a network of friends and family members who can help you reduce your stress levels? Do you know how and where to access professional advice if needed?

- Have you thought about what changes you would like to work on first? Have you developed a plan of action? When do you plan to start?

CHECKLIST FOR CHANGE: ASSESSING COMMUNITY STRESSORS

- Have you considered what in your environment may be perceived as stressful for you and those around you?

- Do you have control over these stressors? How could they be changed? How would changing them make a difference?

- What on your campus or in your living situation is perceived as stressful for you or your friends? What could you do to manage these stressors?

- What advice might you give to your school administrators to help them reduce unnecessary stress among students?

CRITICAL THINKING

You just scraped by to pay your tuition bill in January, and then your university announced a large tuition hike for next year. You already work a part-time job, and seem to spend all your "free time" studying. The stress you have now is beginning to get to you, and you realize that you will have to work another 5 to 10 hours per week just to pay your bills next year. And tuition is likely to go up in your final year as well. How can you manage your time and finances so you can complete your degree?

Use the DECIDE model described in Chapter 1 to decide what you should do. Begin with your current situation: How can you make better use of your time? Could you prioritize your week in such a way that you could find the extra time to work? Finally, even if you make enough money, you need to deal with the increased stress. What will you do to keep the stress under control?

Massage Therapy

If you have ever had someone massage your stiff neck or aching feet, you know that massage is an excellent means of relaxation and thus a potential form of stress management. Massage therapists use techniques that vary from the aggressive methods typical of Swedish massage to more gentle methods such as acupressure and Esalen massage. Before selecting a massage therapist, check his or her credentials carefully. He or she should have training from a reputable program that teaches scientific principles for anatomical manipulation. Each province and territory has different requirements to become a registered massage therapist—check out the Canadian Massage Therapy Alliance website at www.cmta.ca for specific information.

Meditation

Another way to relax and to manage stress is through meditation. **Meditation** generally focuses on visualization and deep breathing, allowing tension to leave the body with each exhalation. There is no "right" way to meditate. Although there are several common forms of meditation, most involve sitting quietly and comfortably for 15 to 20 minutes, focusing on a particular word or symbol, controlling breathing, and getting in touch with your inner self. The deep breathing typically used is described in the Your Spiritual and Emotional Health textbox. Visualization can be added to this deep breathing. Visualization, or the creation of mental scenes, works by engaging your imagination of the physical senses of sight, sound, smell, taste, and feel to replace stressful stimuli with peaceful or pleasurable thoughts. Your choice of mental images is unlimited and should reflect a scene that brings you peace; this might be a beach or mountain lake, a mountain range, or a field of flax or grain blowing in the wind.

Meditation: A relaxation technique that involves deep breathing and potentially visualization.

Go to MyHealthLab at **www.pearsoned.ca/myhealthlab.** Here you will find self-assessments, case studies, links to health on the net, and much more.

DISCUSSION QUESTIONS

1. Compare and contrast distress and eustress. In what way are both types of stress harmful?
2. Describe the alarm, resistance, and exhaustion phases of the general adaptation syndrome. Discuss the physiological and psychological responses that take place during your stress response. At what point could you intervene with some form of stress management?
3. What are the major factors that seem to influence the nature and extent of a person's stress susceptibility? Explain how social support, self-esteem, and personality type may make you more or less susceptible to stress.
4. Why are university and college students often susceptible to overload and burnout? What services are available on your campus and in your community to help you deal with excessive stress?
5. What can university and college students do to build resilience against negative stress effects? What actions can you take to manage your stressors? How can you help others to manage their stressors more effectively?

APPLICATION EXERCISE

Reread the "Consider This . . ." scenario at the beginning of the chapter and answer the following questions.

1. How common is it for first-year students like Rhett to experience stress? Why?
2. If you were Rhett, what would you do to manage your arts courses? What kind of help is available on your campus if you had a similar problem? How do you access these services?
3. Are Rhett's experiences with residence life similar to what you might experience on your campus? What suggestions could you make to him so that he enjoys this part of campus life and still does well academically?
4. Is it important for Rhett to know precisely what career he is headed for? Why or why not?

MYSEARCHLAB EXERCISE

1. Log on to www.MySearchLab.com
2. Use the keywords "stress" and "stress management" to perform a search in the Education, Psychology, or Sociology data bases.
   a. How many articles did you find?
   b. Scan the titles; what themes emerge?
3. Choose one article. Create a one-page summary that you can share with your classmates.

CHAPTER 4

PERSONAL FITNESS

*Improving Your Health
through Physical Activity*

CONSIDER THIS . . .

While in high school, Magda participated in many school sports and physical activities, including dance, basketball, soccer, and track. Among the many lifestyle changes she encountered during her first year of post-secondary studies was the need to spend time alone in sedentary activities such as reading and writing. Magda had seen some of her older friends struggle to include any physical activity or exercise in their student lives. Despite the academic demands of her first semester at school, Magda was determined to make time for exercise and worked out daily, alternating cardiorespiratory endurance and muscular strength training each day. She studied for long solitary hours and got good grades, though she averaged less than six hours of sleep a night. By the end of each week, Magda usually felt lonely and tired and was not sure she could continue.

Was Magda overdoing it? What potential problems can you foresee if she continues her first-semester schedule? What changes should Magda make in her lifestyle to feel less lonely and tired?

CHAPTER OBJECTIVES

- Compare and contrast physical activity for health, physical fitness, and performance.

- Describe the components of a health-related physical fitness program and the exercise frequency, intensity, time, and type to build and/or maintain fitness in each component.

- Identify the recommendations for physical activity promoted in Canada's Physical Activity Guide for Healthy Active Living.

- Describe common physical fitness–related injuries as well as methods to reduce your risk of these injuries.

Regular physical activity results in a wide range of physical, social, and mental health benefits.[1] These health benefits are a result of an increased energy expenditure that relates to an overall improvement in the quality and quantity of life.[2] Regular physical activity reduces the likelihood of coronary artery disease, high blood pressure, type 2 diabetes, obesity, and other chronic diseases.[3] Further, regular physical activity helps to control stress, increases self-esteem, and contributes to that "feel-good" feeling. Thus, it is no wonder that physical activity is often viewed as the key to health and considered a tool for disease prevention.[4]

Most Canadians are aware of the health benefits of physical activity and that they should be more physically active, yet almost half the population is considered physically inactive—that is, expends less than 3 kcal/kg/day in physical activity.[5] Even more disturbing is that only 21 percent of Canadian teenagers are sufficiently physically active to meet the international physical activity recommendations for optimal growth and development, with boys twice as likely to obtain the recommendations as girls (27 versus 14 percent).[6] At all ages, men are more active than women. Further, children are more active than adolescents,[7] and adolescents are more active than adults. Research also indicates that your physical activity level as a child and adolescent influences your attitudes and behaviours toward your physical activity as an adult.[8] If your physical activity experiences as a child or adolescent were negative, don't despair! Your years at university or college provide an excellent opportunity to make a break with the past and develop positive physical activity attitudes and behaviours that can increase the quality and quantity of your life. Keep in mind that changes in physical activity level are not uncommon, with most people regularly cycling through more and less physically active times. For example over a 10-year span, 26.8 percent of Canadians over the age of 12 became more physically active while 21.5 percent became less active.[9]

what do you THINK?

Why do the physical activity levels of Canadians, on average, change from year to year or decade to decade? Check out the facts online at the Canadian Fitness and Lifestyle Research Institute (www.cflri.ca) and Statistics Canada (www.statcan.ca).

PHYSICAL ACTIVITY FOR HEALTH, FITNESS, AND PERFORMANCE

Physical activity refers to all body movements produced by skeletal muscles resulting in energy expenditure.[10] Walking, swimming, gardening, and housework are examples of physical activity. Physical activities can vary by intensity. For example, walking to class typically requires little effort, while walking up hill is more intense. There are three general categories of physical activity defined by the purpose for which they are done: physical activity for health, physical activity for fitness, and physical activity for performance.

what do you THINK?

Have you had your physical fitness assessed recently? Which components of your physical fitness would you like to improve? What exercises will you do to improve this component of your physical fitness?

Physical Activity for Health

Canadian researchers Warburton, Nicol, and Bredin[11] concluded from their review of the research on physical activity and health that "there is irrefutable evidence of the effectiveness of regular physical activity in the primary and secondary prevention of several chronic diseases (e.g., cardiovascular disease, diabetes, cancer, hypertension, obesity, depression and osteoporosis and premature death)" (801). Furthermore, the risk of breast cancer in women 40 years of age and younger is significantly reduced when they participated in regular physical activity (four or more hours accumulated over a week) beginning in adolescence and continuing into adulthood.[12]

Just adding more physical activity to your day can benefit your health. In fact, if *all* Canadians followed the physical activity recommendations in Canada's Physical Activity Guide for Healthy Living (CPAG), about one-third of deaths related to coronary heart disease, one-quarter of deaths related to stroke and osteoporosis, one-fifth of deaths related to colon cancer, high blood pressure, and type 2 diabetes, and one-seventh of deaths related to breast cancer could be prevented.[13] Unfortunately, few

Physical activity: Body movements produced by skeletal muscles resulting in energy expenditure.

Reduced risk of chronic disease and improved quality of life are among the many benefits of regular physical activity for people of all ages and capabilities.

Canadians are aware of CPAG (that is, 20.7 percent) and even fewer (that is, 5.5 percent) actually follow the recommendations.[14]

A physically active lifestyle might include choices such as walking or cycling to school, parking further away from your destination, taking movement breaks while studying, or taking the stairs instead of the elevator. You can also choose to be more physically active in your leisure or "down" time by dancing, playing Frisbee, or walking your dog. Every little bit helps, so get out of your seat and move more, more often. For additional information on putting together a physical activity program, download or view CPAG at www. phac-aspc.gc.ca/pau-uap/paguide/index.html.

Physical Activity for Fitness

Exercise refers to a particular kind of physical activity. Although all exercise is physical activity, not all physical activity would be considered exercise. For example, walking from your car to class is physical activity, whereas going for a brisk 30-minute walk is exercise. **Exercise** is defined as planned, structured, and repetitive bodily movements done to improve or maintain one or more components of physical fitness, such as cardiorespiratory endurance, muscular strength and endurance, or flexibility.[15] **Physical fitness** refers to a set of attributes that are either health- or performance-related. The health-related attributes—cardiorespiratory endurance, muscular

strength and endurance, and flexibility—allow you to perform moderate- to vigorous-intensity physical activity on a regular basis without undue fatigue and with energy left over to handle physical or mental emergencies.[16]

To become physically fit, you will need to do more than simply make physically active lifestyle choices. You will need to do particular exercises for a particular length of time, at a specific intensity, and for a certain number of times each week. Specific to cardiorespiratory endurance exercises, the Public Health Agency of Canada, along with the Canadian Society for Exercise Physiology, recommends 60 minutes of light-effort physical activity or exercise every day to maintain or improve your health.[17] Physical activities of a light effort—for example, light walking, easy gardening—result in the body feeling warm and a slight increase in breathing rate. As the intensity of your physical activity increases to a moderate level—where you are feeling warmer and have a noticeable increase in breathing rate—you can exercise for 30 minutes, four days a week. Examples of moderate-intensity physical activities include brisk walking, cycling, dancing, etc. Further, if the intensity of your exercise increases to a vigorous effort, you can exercise for 20 to 30 minutes, three days per week. Vigorous-intensity physical activities make you quite warm and breathing quite quickly, as you would while jogging, or playing basketball. In other words, the intensity of your exercise dictates the length and frequency of your exercise sessions. Further, your exercise can be accumulated in 10-minute time periods.

Some people have physical limitations that might be viewed as preventing them from being able to get the exercise recommended for them to achieve and/or maintain physical fitness. In fact, these individuals can and should be physically active and, in particular, should exercise to obtain the health-related benefits. For example, a woman with arthritis in her knee and hip joints might not be able to play soccer, but she can participate in water exercises, since the water may help relieve the stress on her joints. Similarly, a man who uses a wheelchair may not be able to jog, but he can meet the exercise recommendations by playing wheelchair basketball or rugby.

what do you THINK?

What type of physical fitness training do you think Canadian triathlete Simon Whitfield completes? How would his training and approach to exercise compare to yours? Which of the key aspects of physical fitness would you like to improve or develop? What types of physical activities (exercises) could you do to improve these key aspects?

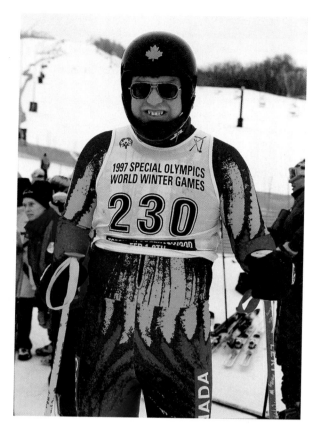

It is important for all people, including those with disabilities, to develop optimal levels of physical fitness to participate in physical activities they enjoy—including competitive sports.

Physical Activity for Performance

People who participate in athletics use physical activity to improve their performance. As such, specific exercises are undertaken to increase power, agility, speed, coordination, and the other performance-related attributes of physical fitness. Plyometrics are often used in training to improve performance. Plyometrics are exercises that contract muscles in a certain order to increase power. An example is doing push-ups with a hand-clap between each one. In addition to developing power, plyometrics help to improve body control and the speed at which you change directions.

Although many recreational exercisers use interval training to improve their speed as well as their cardiorespiratory fitness, performance training is safest for individuals who already have a high level of physical fitness. Generally, those who engage in performance training will achieve a higher level of physical fitness, but careful monitoring of one's training plan is essential, since there is an increased risk of injury and overtraining.

✳ BENEFITS OF REGULAR
✓ PHYSICAL ACTIVITY

Improved Cardiorespiratory Endurance

A regular program of moderately intense aerobic physical activity improves the efficiency of your cardiovascular and respiratory systems: it enables the heart to pump more blood with each stroke, thus lowering resting heart rate; it improves the body's capacity to take in and distribute oxygen to working muscles; and it strengthens the muscles responsible for respiration. See also Chapter 11 for more details.

Reduced Risk of Heart Disease

Your heart is a muscle made up of highly specialized tissue. Because muscles become stronger and more efficient with use, regular physical activity of sufficient intensity strengthens the heart, enabling it to pump more blood with each beat. This increased efficiency means that your heart requires fewer beats per minute to circulate blood throughout your body to maintain function. In this way, a stronger, more efficient heart is better able to meet the demands of life.

Prevention of Hypertension

Hypertension is the medical term for chronic high blood pressure. It is a cardiovascular disease itself and, in addition, increases the risk of coronary heart disease and stroke. Hypertension causes the heart to work harder with each beat because of increased resistance due to less pliable arterial walls.

Regular moderate-intensity physical activity lowers systolic and diastolic blood pressure by about 10 mmHg in people with mild to moderate hypertension.[18] Regular physical activity can also reduce systolic and diastolic blood pressure in people with normal blood pressure.[19]

Improved Blood Lipid and Lipoprotein Profile

Lipids are fats that circulate in the bloodstream and are stored in various places in your body. A high level of blood lipids (cholesterol and triglycerides) increases risk of coronary heart disease.[20] Risk increases for heart

Exercise: Planned, structured, and repetitive bodily movements done to improve or maintain one or more components of physical fitness.

Physical fitness: A set of attributes that are either health- or performance-related.

How Physically Fit Are You?

EVALUATING YOUR AEROBIC FITNESS: THE MODIFIED CANADIAN AEROBIC FITNESS TEST (MCAFT)

In this test endorsed by the Canadian Society for Exercise Physiology (CSEP), you complete one or more 3-minute sessions of stepping on double 20.3 cm steps at a predetermined pace based on your age and sex. Heart rate is measured 5 to 10 seconds after each 3 minutes of stepping. Depending upon your heart rate, you will proceed to the next step or terminate the test. Your final exercising heart rate, along with your age and sex, are used to determine your aerobic fitness score, which is then compared to the established health benefit zone. For complete details, refer to MyHealthLab.

EVALUATING YOUR MUSCULAR STRENGTH AND ENDURANCE

A number of tests are proposed by the CSEP for determining these parameters of physical fitness. The most commonly used tests are partial curl-ups and push-ups. Other tests include grip strength and vertical jump.

An alternative to the two-step approach in the mCAFT, is using a single step; participants step up onto a 40.6-cm (18") box or step completely with one foot (a), then the other (b), and then step down with one foot (c) and then other (d) to measure their cardiorespiratory endurance.

Female push-up.

Male push-up.

Partial curl-up.

Trunk flexibility is usually evaluated using the sit and reach test.

The partial curl-up measures the muscular endurance of the abdominal musculature. In the partial curl-up, the trunk is raised no more than 30 to 40 degrees above the mat so that the shoulders are raised about 15 to 25 cm. A full sit-up is not used because of the stress placed on the lower back when performed and because they also require hip flexor action when performed. Curl-ups are timed and performed at a slow and controlled cadence of 25 curl-ups per minute to a maximum of 25.

Push-ups provide a measure of the muscular endurance of the upper body, including the shoulders, arms, and chest. There is no time or ceiling limit for the measurement of push-ups.

Complete instructions for these two tests, as well as the tests for grip strength and vertical jump and the applicable health benefit zones, are included in MyHealthLab.

EVALUATING YOUR FLEXIBILITY

The most commonly used test to measure flexibility is the sit and reach test or trunk forward flexion. Another test endorsed by CSEP is back extension. The sit and reach test measures the ability of the back to flex, which involves the muscles of the lower back and of the back of the legs (that is, hamstrings).

Complete details on how to perform this test as well as the back extension test, along with the normative tables, are presented in MyHealthLab.

EVALUATING YOUR BODY COMPOSITION

Your body composition can be measured in a number of ways. One method involves determining your Body Mass Index (BMI) from your height and weight. Although widely used in population studies as an indicator of overweight and obesity, BMI does not actually provide a measure of fatness. Waist circumference is a simple measure that provides a relatively valid measure of abdominal fatness. Sum of five skinfolds is the final measurement of body composition advocated by the CSEP. Skinfold measurements provide an indication of subcutaneous fat (that is, fat that lies directly below the skin). Five measurements (triceps, biceps, subscapular, iliac crest, and medial calf) are taken, totalled, and compared to the health benefit zones. Complete details on these methods of body composition assessment, as well as the health benefits zones, are included in MyHealthLab.

Source: Adapted from: The Canadian Physical Activity, Fitness, and Lifestyle Approach Protocol (CPAFLA). Retrieved on August 28, 2008 from www.csep.ca.

disease because the heart has to work harder with each beat as a result of the reduced blood flow caused by the narrowing of the arteries that occurs with high blood fats as they "build up" on the artery walls. Regular aerobic exercise reduces low-density lipoproteins (LDLs— "bad cholesterol"), total cholesterol, and triglycerides (a blood fat), thus reducing plaque build-up in the arteries while increasing high-density lipoproteins (HDLs— "good cholesterol").[21] Higher HDL levels are associated with lower risk for coronary artery disease because they remove some of the "bad cholesterol," thus reducing fatty plaque accumulation from coronary artery walls and easing the work effort of the heart.

Improved Bone Health

Osteoarthritis is a nonfatal but incurable disease characterized by degeneration of joint cartilage and irritation of surrounding bone and soft tissues. Affecting 1 in 10 Canadians, osteoarthritis is the most prevalent chronic joint condition in Canada. Women are afflicted more frequently than men.[22] Supervised walking and weight-loss programs can improve physical capacity while reducing knee-joint osteoarthritis symptoms.[23]

A common affliction for the older population is osteoporosis, a disease characterized by low bone mass and deterioration of bone tissue, which increases fracture risk. Although men and women are both negatively affected by osteoporosis, the prevalence is greater in women. Weight-bearing and strength-building physical activities are recommended to maintain bone health and to prevent osteoporotic fractures. Bone, like other human tissues, responds to the demands placed upon it (the overload principle), and unless the mechanical stresses placed on bone by a particular physical activity exceed the level of stress the bone has adapted to, bone mass and structure will not adapt.[24] Women (and men) have much to gain by remaining physically active as they age—bone mass levels have been found to be significantly higher among physically active women than among those who are sedentary.[25] However, it appears that the full bone-related benefits of physical activity can be achieved only with sufficient hormone levels (estrogen in women, testosterone in men) and adequate calcium, vitamin D, and total calorie intakes.

Improved Weight Management

For many people, the desire to lose weight is the main reason for their physical activity. Physical activity has a direct positive effect on metabolic rate and keeps it elevated for a few hours following vigorous physical activities. As previously noted, research suggests that 60 minutes of moderate intensity physical activity each day should help in maintaining body weight. An effective method for losing weight should combine regular endurance-type physical activities with a moderate decrease (about 500 calories per day) in dietary intake. Decreasing daily caloric intake beyond this may decrease metabolic rate by as much as 20 percent, making short- and long-term weight loss more difficult.

Improved Health and Life Span

Prevention of Type 2 Diabetes

Diabetes is a complex metabolic disorder that affects many Canadians. It is believed that a healthy dietary intake combined with sufficient physical activity could prevent many of the current cases of type 2 diabetes.[26] A recent large epidemiological study found that for every 2000 calories of energy expended during leisure-time physical activities, the incidence of diabetes was reduced by 24 percent. Perhaps the most encouraging finding was that the protective effect of physical activity was greatest among individuals at the highest risk.[27]

Increased Longevity

Experts have long debated the relationship between physical activity and longevity. For decades, most research failed to show an increase in life expectancy through physical activity alone. Then, a classic prospective study of the Harvard alumni of more than 30 years reported that inactive men were at a greater risk of premature death from all causes than men who engaged in regular physical activity.[28] How much physical activity was required to produce this effect? Inactive men who included a brisk 30- to 60-minute walk each day experienced the most significant increases in their life expectancies.[29]

Improved Immunity to Disease

Will regular physical activity improve your immunity? Research suggests that regular moderate-intensity physical activity makes people less susceptible to disease, but that this potential benefit depends upon whether the physical activity was perceived as pleasurable or stressful.[30] Often the relationship of physical activity to immunity, or more specifically to disease susceptibility, is described as a J-shaped curve. In other words, susceptibility to disease decreases as you move from sedentary to moderately active, then increases again as you move to more extreme levels of physical activity or exercise. Athletes engaging in marathon-type events or very intense physical training programs have been shown to be at a greater risk for upper respiratory tract infections (colds and flu).[31] In a study of 2300 marathon runners, those who ran more than 100 kilometres per week suffered twice as many upper respiratory tract infections as those who ran fewer than 35 kilometres per week.[32]

Just how physical activity alters immunity is not well understood. We do know that moderate-intensity physical activity temporarily increases our white blood cells (WBCs), the blood cells responsible for fighting infection. How long does one have increased immunity? It is suggested that after 30 minutes or more of physical activity, WBCs may be elevated for 24 hours or more before returning to normal levels.[33]

Improved Mental Health and Stress Management

Although most people who engage in regular physical activity are not aware of the beneficial physiological changes of their activity apart from those that are most noticeable, such as weight loss or weight maintenance, most do notice the psychological benefits. While these psychological benefits are difficult to quantify, they are frequently mentioned as reasons for continuing to be physically active.

Regular vigorous physical activity has been shown to "burn off" the chemical byproducts released by our nervous system during its normal response to stress. Elimination of these biochemicals reduces our stress response by accelerating the neurological system's return to a balanced state. For this reason, regular physical activity of moderate to vigorous intensity should be an integral component of your stress management plan.

Regular physical activity can improve physical appearance by toning and developing muscles and, combined with a healthy dietary intake, reducing (or maintaining) body fat. Feeling good about personal appearance is an integral component of self-esteem. Other improvements to physical self-esteem result from learning new skills, developing increased ability and capacity in recreational activities, and "sticking with" a physical activity plan.

what do you THINK?
What makes you feel good about being physically active? How does it make you feel, physically and mentally, during and after the activity?

IMPROVING CARDIORESPIRATORY ENDURANCE

Cardiorespiratory endurance, or cardiovascular fitness, refers to the ability of the heart, lungs, and blood vessels to function efficiently. Our lives depend on our cardiorespiratory system's ability to deliver oxygenated blood and nutrients to our body tissues and to remove carbon dioxide and other metabolic waste products. The primary category of physical activity known to improve cardiorespiratory fitness is aerobic exercise. The term *aerobic* means "with oxygen" and describes any type of exercise, typically performed at moderate to vigorous intensity for extended periods of time. Aerobic activities such as brisk walking, jogging, bicycling, skating, and swimming are among the best exercises for improving or maintaining cardiorespiratory fitness.

Aerobic power is the term used to describe the current functional status of the cardiovascular system (that is, the heart, lungs, blood vessels) and refers specifically to the volume of oxygen consumed by the muscles during exercise, maximal aerobic power (often referred to as VO_2max). Maximal aerobic power refers to the maxi-

mal capacity of the cardiorespiratory system. The most common measure of maximal aerobic capacity is determined from a walk or run on a treadmill. In this test, you will walk or run at an easy pace, and then, at set time intervals gradually increase the workload (that is, a **graded exercise test** in which a combination of running speed and the angle of incline is used) to arrive at your point of maximal exertion. The higher your cardiorespiratory endurance, the more oxygen you can transport to exercising muscles and the longer you can maintain a high intensity of exercise before exhaustion. Other less valid, but reliable and safer, methods of measuring aerobic capacity are frequently employed and then used to estimate VO_2max. These submaximal tests may use stationary bicycles, walk/run tests, shuttle runs, or walk tests to quantify the aerobic fitness levels in people of all ages and of all abilities. You may have performed one of these aerobic capacity tests in a physical education class.

It is important for you to complete the Physical Activity Readiness Questionnaire (PAR-Q; available at www.csep.ca) prior to engaging in physical activity or any tests to measure your physical fitness.[34] If you answer yes to any of the questions on the PAR-Q or if you have certain medical conditions, such as asthma, diabetes, heart disease, or obesity, you should consult a physician to ensure that physical activity is safe for you. Further, you should engage in a walking/jogging program at low intensity before you attempt to measure your maximal aerobic capacity.

CARDIORESPIRATORY FITNESS PROGRAMS

When creating a cardiorespiratory fitness program, there are many variables to consider. Generally, what is needed is an aerobic physical activity you enjoy that works your heart at a moderate intensity (approximately 70 to 90 percent of your maximum heart rate, which corresponds to a workload of between 55 and 85 percent of your VO_2max[35]) for a continuous length of time (20 to 30 minutes) at least three days per week.

The most effective aerobic exercises for building cardiorespiratory endurance are total body activities involving large muscle groups of your body. If you have

Cardiorespiratory endurance: The ability of the heart, lungs, and blood vessels to function efficiently.

Aerobic power: The current functional status of a person's cardiorespiratory system; measured as VO_2max and referring specifically to the volume of oxygen consumed by the muscles during exercise.

Graded exercise test: A test of aerobic capacity administered by a physician, exercise physiologist, or other trained person.

Palpation of the radial (wrist) or carotid (neck) artery is a simple means of determining heart rate.

been sedentary for quite a while, initiating a physical activity program may be a challenge. The key is to begin slowly at a low intensity in a physical activity that you like and is easily accessible for you to do. To start slowly, for example, if jogging is the physical activity you choose, you should alternate jogging and walking (1 minute of jogging, 1 minute of walking; progress to 2 minutes of jogging, 1 minute of walking, and so on) until you develop a cardiorespiratory fitness level that enables you to jog continuously for 20 to 30 minutes.

Determining Exercise Frequency

If you have been physically inactive for the past few months or longer, the frequency of your aerobic exercise should begin at 3 times per week. If you exercise less frequently (that is, once or twice per week), you will achieve fewer health benefits. Exercising 3 to 5 times per week is the general recommendation for improving cardiorespiratory endurance. Your ultimate goal should be to exercise 5 times a week. To avoid overuse injuries and monotony, vary your physical activities and take a day off when needed.

Determining Exercise Intensity

An aerobic exercise program must employ sustained, moderate- to vigorous-intensity physical activity to improve cardiorespiratory endurance. A common measure of exercise intensity is your heart rate. The exercise intensity required to improve cardiorespiratory endurance is a heart rate between 70 and 90 percent of your maximum heart rate. To calculate your **target heart rate**, subtract your age from 220 (for males) or 226 (for females). The result is your maxi-

mum heart rate (HRmax). You then determine your target heart rate by calculating the desired percentage of maximum heart rate—that is, 70 to 90 percent. If you are a 20-year-old male, your estimated maximum heart rate is 200 ($220 - 20 = 200$). Your target heart rate would be somewhere between 140 ($200 \times 0.70 = 140$) and 180 ($200 \times 0.90 = 180$) beats per minute. Those who have been sedentary for a long time should set a lower target heart rate, somewhere between 50 and 60 percent of their maximum. As their cardiorespiratory fitness improves, these previously sedentary individuals can gradually increase their target heart rate using small increments—for example, from 50 to 55 percent, then from 55 to 60 percent. It is not recommended for people engaging in aerobic exercise for health benefits to exceed 90 percent of maximum heart rate.

Once you know your target heart rate, you can determine how close you are to this value during your workout. You'll need to stop exercising briefly to measure your heart rate. To take your pulse, lightly place your index and middle fingers (not your thumb) over one of the major (carotid) arteries in your neck, along either side of your Adam's apple, or on the artery on the inside of your wrist. Be sure to start counting your pulse immediately—the first count is "0"—after you stop exercising, as your heart rate decreases quickly. Using a watch or clock, take your pulse for 6 seconds and multiply this number by 10 (just add a zero to your count) to get the number of beats per minute. If necessary, increase or decrease the pace or intensity of your workout to achieve your target heart rate.

A target heart rate of 70 percent of maximum is sometimes called the "conversational level of exercise" because you are able to talk with a partner while exercising.[36] If you are breathing so hard that talking is

TABLE 4.1

Health- and Performance-Related Components of Physical Fitness

Health	
Cardiorespiratory endurance	Ability to sustain moderate-intensity whole-body activity for extended time periods
Muscular strength	Ability to apply maximum force with a single muscle contraction
Muscular endurance	Ability to perform muscle contractions repeatedly
Flexibility	Range of motion in a joint or series of joints
Body composition	Ratio of fat to total body weight
Performance	
Agility	Speed in changing direction or in changing body positions
Power	Combination of strength and speed
Balance	Maintenance of a stable body position
Coordination	Ability to have things work together
Reaction time	Ability to adjust or "react" to stimuli
Speed	Ability to move quickly

Source: Adapted from T. Baranowski, et al., "Assessment, Prevalence, and Cardiovascular Benefits of Physical Activity and Fitness in Youth," *Medicine and Science in Sports and Exercise* 24 (June 1992): supplement, S238.

difficult, the intensity of your exercise is too high. Conversely, if you are able to sing or laugh heartily while exercising, the intensity of your exercise is insufficient for improving or maintaining cardiorespiratory endurance.

Determining Exercise Time

Time refers to the number of minutes of exercise performed at the specified intensity during any one session. As previously mentioned, the length of your exercise session depends on the intensity. If the intensity is 70 to 90 percent HRmax, then only 20 to 30 minutes are needed. Although many individuals engage in exercise sessions lasting longer than 30 minutes, greater improvements to cardiorespiratory fitness are not realized.

Frequency, Intensity, or Time?

You will need to adjust the frequency, intensity, and time of your aerobic exercise program to accommo-

date your improving cardiorespiratory endurance. As you progress and are able to exercise for 20 minutes at 70 percent of your HRmax for three days per week, increase the frequency, time, or intensity of your exercise—but not all three at the same time. Generally, it is recommended to first increase the frequency of your workouts from 3 to 4 days per week, then from 4 to 5 days per week. Once you have adjusted to that change, it is recommended to increase the length of your exercise period in gradual amounts (usually a 10 percent increase in the volume or total amount of exercise). Once you have adjusted to those changes, it is recommended to increase the intensity of your workout gradually from 70 to 90 percent of HRmax.

> ## what do you THINK?
> Consider a type (or several types) of physical activity that you like doing and create a workout plan for a month, to improve your cardiorespiratory fitness using the principles discussed in this chapter. What will it take to get you to follow this plan? What will make it challenging? Easier?

Your goal should be to expend 300 to 500 calories per day through leisure-time physical activity, with an eventual weekly goal of 1500 to 2100 calories. The lower the intensity of the activity, the longer the time you will need to obtain the same caloric expenditure. If your preference is for lower-intensity physical activity, the recommendation changes to 60 minutes every day of the week.[37] It should be pointed out that whether the recommendation is for 30 minutes of moderate-intensity physical activity most days of the week or 60 minutes of light-intensity physical activity every day of the week, it is possible to accumulate these activities in 10-minute spurts. See the Focus on Canada box.

A physical activity program over several months or years—exercise training—improves the way your cardiorespiratory system meets your body's oxygen requirements at rest and during exercise and helps you to feel good about yourself. Keep in mind that the physiological health benefits associated with cardiorespiratory endurance activities (reduced blood pressure, decreased resting heart rate, improved blood flow, etc.) take about one year of regular exercise to achieve.[38] However, any physical activity, even if it does not meet all the exercise characteristics mentioned in this chapter, will benefit your overall health and help you to feel better about yourself almost immediately.

Target heart rate: The desired intensity of aerobic exercise for improving or maintaining cardiorespiratory fitness; calculated as a percentage of maximum heart rate (220 [for males] 226 [for females] minus age).

Physical Activity for Healthy Living: How Much Is Enough?

Similar to Eating Well with Canada's Food Guide (see Chapter 5), Canada's Physical Activity Guide to Healthy Active Living uses a rainbow approach to describe the amount and type of physical activities Canadians need for optimal health benefits (see Figure 4.1).

The outside of the rainbow includes physical activities we need the most of—endurance activities. These activities should be engaged in 4 to 7 days per week, depending upon the intensity of the activity, and are continuous in nature, thus providing benefits to the heart, lungs, and circulatory system. Examples include cross-country skiing, taking the stairs instead of the elevator, cycling, walking, and mowing the lawn.

The intensity of the physical activities engaged in for cardiorespiratory endurance significantly influences the frequency and time needed for health benefits. If your preferred physical activities involve light effort such as slow-paced walking, stretching, or easy gardening, you need 60 minutes 7 days a week. If the physical activities you engage in are of a moderate effort, such as brisk walking, biking, raking leaves, swimming, or dancing, you need 30 to 60 minutes at least 4 days per week. If your preference is for "workout" kinds of physical activities, then you need 20 to 30 minutes 3 days per week. Examples of workout activities include fitness classes, jogging, fast swimming, or fast dancing. Combinations of physical activities of various intensities can also lead to optimal health benefits.

The next arc of the rainbow describes the type of physical activity that we need the next most of—flexibility activities. It is also recommended that we obtain these types of activities 4 to 7 times per week. These types of physical activities are described as "gentle reaching, bending, and stretching activities to keep your muscles relaxed and joints mobile." Examples include various stretches that are often done after other types of physical activities.

The third arc of the rainbow is for strength activities, which should be done 2 to 4 days per week. These activities will strengthen muscles and bones as well as improve posture. Examples include weight training with hand-held weights, body-weight resistance exercise (curl-ups and push-ups), as well as walking with backpacks.

The last arc of the rainbow describes activities we should try to reduce. Examples included in this arc of the rainbow are sedentary activities such as watching television or movies, and working or playing on a computer.

STUDY QUESTIONS

1. Identify the practical, economic, and environmental roadblocks that make it difficult to attain and maintain a physically active lifestyle in Canada. Suggest potential solutions.

2. Describe ways that Canadians of all ages—children, adolescents, adults, and older adults—could begin to incorporate more physical activity into their lives. When answering this question, consider each demographic group in a rural, urban, and suburban environment.

3. What could the various levels of government (federal, provincial/territorial, municipal) do to enhance the physical activity level of Canadians? Should the private sector also get involved? How?

4. What is the role of education in promoting physical activity? How can this role be better played?

FIGURE 4.1

Canada's Physical Activity Guide to Healthy Active Living

Source: Canada's Physical Activity Guide to Healthy Active Living, Cat. No. H39-429/1998-1E ISBN 0-662-86627-7, Health Canada, 2003; available online at: www.phac-aspc.gc.ca/pau-uap/fitness/pdf/guideEng.pdf.

Source: Adapted from Public Health Agency of Canada, Canada's Physical Activity Guide to Healthy Living, Cat. No. H39-429/1998-2E. Canada's Physical Activity Guide to Healthy Living can be downloaded from www.phac-aspc.gc.ca/pau-uap/paguide/index.html.

IMPROVING MUSCULAR STRENGTH AND ENDURANCE

Musculoskeletal health (that is, strength, endurance, and flexibility) also significantly impacts health and overall wellness. Specifically, musculoskeletal health is associated with a reduced risk for coronary heart disease and osteoporosis as well as improved glucose tolerance and ease of completing tasks of daily living.[39] **Muscular strength** refers to the maximal amount of force a muscle or group of muscles is capable of exerting in one contraction. The most common way to measure strength is to determine the maximum amount of weight you can lift once. This value is called **one repetition maximum (1RM)**. Your 1RM can also be predicted from a 10RM test.[40] **Muscular endurance** is defined as a muscle's or group of muscles' ability to exert force repeatedly without fatiguing or the ability to sustain a muscular contraction. The more repetitions you can perform successfully (for example, push-ups) or the longer you can hold a certain position (for example, flexed arm hang), the greater your muscular endurance. Muscular endurance is often measured from the number of curl-ups or push-ups an individual can do.

Principles of Strength Development

There are three key principles—tension, overload, and specificity—to follow to increase your muscular strength and endurance.[41]

The Tension Principle

The key to developing strength is to create sufficient tension within a muscle. The most common way to create tension in a muscle is the use of external resistance such as that found in weight lifting. While weight lifting is one method of producing tension in a muscle, many other types of physical activity have the same effect—for example, lifting your own body weight (push-ups or pull-ups) or riding a bicycle up a steep hill. It really does not matter what type of resistance you choose to develop tension in your muscles; what matters is that you use sufficient resistance to improve muscular strength and/or endurance.

The Overload Principle

The overload principle is the most important of the three key principles for improving muscular strength.

FIGURE 4.2

The overload principle must be followed to increase strength or endurance. Notice that once the muscle has adapted to the original overload, a new overload must be placed on the muscle for subsequent gains in strength or endurance to occur.

Source: From Philip A. Sienna, *One Rep Max: A Guide to Beginning Weight Training,* Fig. 2.1, 8. © 1989. Wm. C. Brown Communications, Inc., Dubuque, Iowa. Reprinted by permission of Times Mirror Higher Education Group, Inc., Dubuque, Iowa. All rights reserved.

Everyone begins a resistance training program with an initial level of strength. To increase strength, you must then regularly create tension in your muscles greater than what you are accustomed to. This overload forces your muscles to adapt by getting larger (**hypertrophy**), stronger, and thus capable of generating more tension. Figure 4.2 illustrates a continual process of overload and adaptation resulting in improved strength. If you do not create an overload—if you "underload" your muscles—you will not increase strength. Conversely, if you create too great an overload, you may experience muscle injury, muscle fatigue, and even a loss of strength. Once you reach your strength goal, no further overloading is necessary. Your next challenge is to maintain that level of strength by continuing to engage in a regular (once or twice per week) total-body resistance exercise program.

Musculoskeletal health: The combination of strength, endurance, and flexibility and their influence on various components of health.

Muscular strength: The maximal amount of force that a muscle or groups of muscles is capable of exerting.

One repetition maximum (1RM): The maximum amount of weight/resistance that can be lifted/moved only once.

Muscular endurance: A muscle's or group of muscles' ability to exert force repeatedly or to sustain a contraction without fatiguing.

Hypertrophy: Increased size (girth) of a muscle.

These photographs illustrate concentric and eccentric muscle actions. In A, the abdominal muscles shorten, a concentric muscle action, while producing tension in the lifting phase of a curl-up. In B, the abdominal muscles lengthen, an eccentric muscle action, while producing tension as the body returns to its starting position.

The Specificity of Training Principle

This principle refers to the manner in which a specific body system responds to the physiological demands placed upon it. According to the specificity principle, you get a very specific response to the exercises you do. If the specific overload you impose is designed to improve strength in the muscles of your chest and back, the response to that demand (overload) will be improved strength in the chest and back, not in the overall body. Therefore, to improve overall or total body strength, you must include exercises for all the major muscle groups. You must also ensure that your overload is sufficient to increase strength and not only endurance.

The Recovery Principle

Allow 48 hours for the body to "recover" from and adapt to the resistance training undertaken (that is, to become stronger). This does not mean that you cannot resistance train daily, but rather that you need to design your work out so that you alternate which muscles you concentrate on when resistance training. Keep in mind that your core body is always involved in your training and you may need to take a day off to ensure that it too has sufficient time to heal and adapt to the overloads undertaken.

Types of Muscle Contractions

When your skeletal muscles receive a stimulus from your nervous system to contract, they respond by developing tension and producing a measurable force. Your skeletal muscles contract in three different modes—isometric, concentric, and eccentric—to produce this force.[42] In an **isometric muscle contraction**, force is produced by the muscle without movement. Isometric muscle actions do not create joint motion. Muscles act isometrically to stabilize a particular body

part while another body part is moving, or when a maximal resistance is met and the force produced cannot overcome the resistance. One example is the unsuccessful attempt to push a car out of a snow bank. Although you push with all your might, the car does not move (and neither do your joints). The muscles involved are producing force in an isometric way. Another example related to resistance training is trying to lift a barbell that is too heavy for you. The more you try, the more tired your muscles become, but the barbell never leaves the floor. Isometric muscle contractions are important because they are involved in maintaining body stability. Maintaining your balance and body alignment while holding a push-up is another example of isometric muscle contractions.

A **concentric muscle contraction** is one in which force is produced while the muscle shortens. Joint movement is always produced during concentric muscle actions. Raising the body in a curl-up is an example of a concentric action of the abdominal muscles. Usually, but not always, concentric muscle contractions produce movement in a direction opposite to the downward pull of gravity.

Eccentric muscle contraction describes a muscle's ability to produce force while lengthening. Typically, eccentric muscle actions occur when movement is in the same direction as the pull of gravity. If you want to be sure that a given resistance exercise has an eccentric phase, you must use the type of resistance that requires you to achieve the starting position before your next repetition. For example, in a curl-up, you lower your upper body slowly to the starting point of the exercise in an eccentric contraction of the abdominal muscles.

All factors being equal, the greatest amount of force is produced during eccentric muscle contractions, followed by isometric and then concentric muscle contractions. Changes in muscle size and strength are affected by the type of resistance exercise and by the type of muscle contraction(s) you use during your workout. When using free weights (barbells, dumbbells), the typical sequential pattern of concentric–eccentric muscle contractions during resistance training contributes to improved muscle strength and muscle fibre size. If your resistance exercise program uses only concentric muscle actions, you'll need to perform at least twice as many repetitions to achieve the same results as you would attain by using concentric–eccentric combinations.[43]

Methods of Providing Resistance

There are four commonly used methods of applying resistance for muscular strength and endurance training: body weight resistance, and fixed, variable, and accommodating resistance devices.

Body Weight Resistance

Muscular strength and endurance can be improved without exercise equipment, using your body weight as the resistance. For many individuals, using their body weight as resistance in a variety of exercises can be as effective as external resistance in developing and maintaining muscular strength and endurance. Exercises such as curl-ups, push-ups, and pull-ups require your muscles to lift and return your body weight off the floor, involving concentric and eccentric muscle contractions.

Fixed Resistance

Fixed resistance exercises provide a constant resistance throughout a full range of movement. Barbells and dumbbells provide fixed resistance because their weight or the amount of resistance applied does not change as you exercise. However, due to the biomechanics of human motion, the muscle forces that must be exerted to move the weight are lower at some joint angles and higher at others. Any given muscle generates the least amount of force at the beginning and ending positions of a resistance exercise, and the most force when the joint involved in the exercise approximates a right angle (90 degrees). As a result, the disadvantage of fixed resistance exercises is that the extent to which a muscle is overloaded varies throughout the exercise, and the exercise may not fully develop the muscle.

Variable Resistance

Whether found at a health club or in your home workout area, variable resistance equipment alters the resistance encountered by a muscle at all joint angles so that the effort by the muscle is consistent throughout the full range of motion. Variable resistance machines are typically single-station devices (for example, Nautilus), but some have multiple stations at which

muscles of the upper and lower extremities can be exercised (for example, Soloflex).

Accommodating Resistance

Accommodating resistance devices (isokinetic machines), maintain a constant speed through the range of motion. The exerciser performs at a maximal level of effort, while the exercise machine controls the speed of the exercise and does not allow any faster motion. The body segment being exercised must move at a rate faster than or equal to the set speed to encounter resistance.

Getting Started

You will find some general principles useful whatever your strength training goals. If sufficient tension is generated within a muscle, it will respond by becoming stronger regardless of the type of muscle action or resistance used. To design your program, first determine your 1RM for each muscle or muscle group you plan to exercise. Then, develop specific training goals as well as the strategies to achieve those goals.

Strength Training

There are almost as many ways to develop muscular strength as there are participants in strength training programs. Given the specificity principle, it is important to select at least one resistance exercise for each major muscle group in the body to develop total body strength. Generally, strength training exercises are done in a set, or series, of multiple repetitions using the same resistance. For increases in muscular strength, the amount of resistance should be at least 60 percent or greater of your 1RM for a given exercise, with 8 to 12 repetitions of the exercise performed per set.[44] Generally, a resistance that you can move or lift only 8 to 10 times is a good place to start. It is further recommended that 1 to 3 sets be performed.

Since resistance training exercises cause microscopic damage (tears) to muscle fibres and the rebuilding process takes about 24 to 48 hours, resistance training programs should incorporate at least one day of rest (and recovery) between workouts to allow the muscle or muscle groups to adapt. Thus, the recommended frequency of programs to build muscular strength is 2 to 4 days per week.[45]

Isometric muscle contraction: Force produced without muscle movement.

Concentric muscle contraction: Force produced while shortening the muscle.

Eccentric muscle contraction: Force produced while lengthening the muscle.

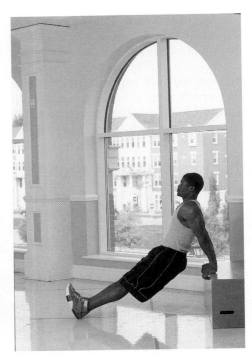

Using your body weight can be an effective way to build or maintain muscular strength and endurance.

To summarize, you should perform each strength building exercise at an intensity greater than 60 percent of your 1RM for 1 to 3 sets of 2 to 6 repetitions, 2 to 4 days per week. See also Table 4.2.

Muscular Endurance Training

In contrast to improvements in strength, increases in muscular endurance are achieved by performing a relatively high number of repetitions with a relatively low resistance. For endurance, instead of traditional resistance exercise equipment, consider adding variety to your training program with devices equipped with an ergometer, such as a stationary bicycle, rowing machine, or stair-climbing machine. With these and other devices, you can control the cadence of the activity and/or adjust the amount of resistance you encounter. Performing thousands of repetitions during a 20-minute (or longer) workout using a relatively low resistance will quickly develop muscular endurance in the muscles exercised. Other activities that build muscular endurance include hiking, wall climbing, jogging, and cycling. These latter types of exercises also provide cardiorespiratory benefits if you select an intensity that allows you to reach your target heart rate.

TABLE 4.2

Guide to Manipulating Training Variables to Achieve Different Strength Training Goals

	Endurance	Strength
Sets	2–6	1–3
Repetitions	10–15	2–6
Resistance (% of maximum)	< 60	> 60
Rest between sets (seconds)	30–60	120
Frequency per week (days)	2–4	2–4
Rest between workouts (days)	1–2	1–2

what do you THINK?

In regard to daily living, why is it important to develop your muscular strength and endurance? What type of resistance training program would work best for you? Do you require access to equipment and facilities to engage in this type of program? If so, do you know where to go and how to use this equipment?

You can also build muscular endurance through resistance training by performing 2 to 6 sets of 10 to 15 repetitions of a resistance less than 60 percent of your 1RM 2 to 4 days per week.[46] See also Table 4.2.

Lifting free weights to build muscular strength and endurance has many advantages.

IMPROVING YOUR FLEXIBILITY

Flexibility refers to the range of motion, or the amount of movement possible, at a particular joint or series of joints. Although this component of physical fitness is often overshadowed by muscular strength and cardiorespiratory endurance, it should not be overlooked because inflexible muscles are susceptible to injury. Improving your range of motion through stretching exercises will enhance the efficiency of your movements as well as your posture. A regular stretching program may also enhance psychological well-being.

Types of Stretching Exercises

Flexibility is most often enhanced by controlled stretching of muscles. The primary strategy is to

try it NOW!

Give yourself a break and stretch! Stretching and improved flexibility are just as important in the classroom and library as they are in the gym. Sitting hunched over a pile of books or leaning in toward your computer for extended periods of time can be a pain in the neck and/or back! When studying, be sure to stretch every 20 minutes or so by doing shoulder rolls, shrugs, and neck stretches (tilt ear to shoulder on both sides, chin to chest) to help work out the kinks. It is also a good idea to stand up and move the whole body a little. These mini-stretch breaks will ease your muscles and your mind.

decrease the resistance to stretch (tension) within a tight muscle targeted for increased range of motion.[47] To do this, you repeatedly stretch the muscle and its two tendons of attachment to elongate them.

The safest exercises for improving flexibility involve **static stretching**. Static stretching techniques slowly and gradually lengthen a muscle or group of muscles. In this regard, various positions and postures are used with the "stretch" held to a point where tension (mild discomfort) is felt within the muscle. This end position is then held for 10 to 30 seconds, and is repeated 2 or 3 times in close succession. With each repetition of a static stretch, your range of motion improves temporarily and when done regularly, range of motion increases for longer periods of time. Stretching regularly (at least four, and preferably seven, days a week) will effectively result in a more permanent elongation of the targeted muscle or muscle group and thus permit a greater range of motion at a given joint.

In regard to athletic performance, static stretching immediately prior to performance reduces the athlete's efforts.[48] Thus it is recommended that if static stretching is part of the warm-up, that it be followed immediately by more dynamic movements.

YOGA, TAI CHI, AND PILATES

Three popular styles of exercise that include stretching are yoga, tai chi, and Pilates. In addition to improving flexibility, these types of exercise may increase muscular strength and endurance as well as focus on the mind body connection through concentration on breathing and body position. Some people see these three activities strongly connected to the development of their spiritual health, particularly when time is spent relaxing, breathing deeply, and trying to clear the mind.

Yoga

Although yoga originated in India about 5000 years ago, it is currently one of the most popular physical activities that involves static stretching. Yoga blends the mental and physical aspects of exercise, a union of mind and body that provides a relaxing and satisfying experience that many find enhances their spiritual

Flexibility: The range of motion, or the amount of movement possible, at a particular joint or series of joints.

Static stretching: Assuming a "stretching" position—at the point of tension—for 10 to 30 seconds in which there is a gradual lengthening of a muscle.

health. If done regularly, the combination of mental focus and physical effort improves flexibility, vitality, posture, agility, and coordination.

The practice of yoga focuses attention on controlled breathing as well as purely physical exercise. In addition to its mental dimensions, yoga incorporates a complex array of static stretching exercises expressed as postures—or asanas. Over 200 postures/asanas exist with about 50 most commonly practiced. During a session, participants move to different asanas and hold them for 30 seconds or more. Asanas, singly or in combination, can be changed and adapted for young and old or to accommodate physical limitations or disabilities. Asanas can also be combined to provide well-conditioned athletes with a challenging workout!

A typical yoga session will move the spine and joints through their full range of motion. Yoga postures lengthen, strengthen, and balance musculature, leading to increased flexibility, stamina, and strength—and many people report a psychological sense of general well-being too. Table 4.3 details three popular types of yoga.

Tai Chi

Tai chi is an ancient form of exercise that combines stretching, balance, coordination, and meditation. It is designed to increase range of motion and flexibility while reducing muscular tension. Based on Chi Kung, a Taoist philosophy dedicated to spiritual growth and good health, tai chi was developed about 1000 CE by monks to defend themselves against bandits and warlords. It involves a series of positions called "forms," based on Chinese martial arts, performed continuously. Further, tai chi is often described as "meditation in motion" because it promotes serenity through gentle movements—connecting the mind and body.

TABLE 4.3

Popular Yoga Styles

- **Iyengar yoga** focuses on precision and alignment in the poses. Standing poses are basic to this style and are often held longer than in other styles.

- **Ashtanga yoga** in its pure form is based on a specific flow of poses with an emphasis on strength and agility that creates internal heat. *Power yoga,* a style growing in popularity, is a derivative of ashtanga yoga.

- **Bikram yoga**, or hot yoga, is similar to power yoga but does not incorporate a specific flow of poses. Literally the hottest yoga going, it is performed in temperatures of 38°C, or even a bit higher. Proponents say that the heat increases the body's ability to move and stretch without injury.

Pilates

Pilates was developed by Joseph Pilates in 1926. It teaches body awareness, good posture, and easy, graceful body movements. Further, Pilates improves flexibility, agility, coordination, strength, tone, and economy of motion. It may even alleviate back pain. Pilates combines stretching with movement against resistance aided by devices such as tension springs or heavy rubber bands. Pilates differs from yoga and tai chi in that it includes a component specifically designed to increase strength. The method consists of a sequence of carefully performed movements. Some are carried out on specially designed equipment, while others are performed on mats. Each exercise strengthens the muscles involved and has a specific breathing pattern associated with it.

BODY COMPOSITION

Body composition is the final component of a comprehensive health-related physical fitness program. As noted in Chapter 6, body composition describes the relative portions of fat and lean tissues in the body. Body composition parameters are influenced by regular physical activity and exercise in terms of total body mass, fat mass, fat-free mass, and regional fat distribution. Generally, aerobic physical activities improve body composition because they expend calories and contribute to weight maintenance and/or loss. For more details on body composition, including its measurement, refer to Chapter 6.

* PLANNING YOUR PHYSICAL FITNESS TRAINING PROGRAM

Identifying Your Physical Fitness Goals

Before you start a physical fitness training program, determine your personal health and physical fitness needs, limitations, exercise likes and dislikes, daily schedule, and goals. Whatever your primary reason for starting a training program, your most important goal should be to commit to regular physical activity, exercise, and physical fitness.

Once committed, you must decide what program is best suited to your needs. The amounts and types of exercises required to yield beneficial results vary with the age and physical condition of the exerciser. Regardless of age, first complete the Physical Activity Readiness Questionnaire (available at www.csep.ca) and consult your physician if you respond yes to any of the questions.

It is useful to map your journey by identifying your current physical fitness level and your end goal. Your program should reflect your initial positioning while addressing your individual strengths and weaknesses so that you can move along the chart stage by stage as you pursue your short- and long-term goals.

Designing Your Physical Fitness Program

To optimize your physical fitness training, develop a workout schedule that is both challenging and realistic. An important step in adopting a new behaviour is developing a new routine. Care must be taken to ensure that you do not set yourself up for failure before you begin by choosing an overly ambitious schedule. If you decide to walk 6 times per week, but are able to complete only four sessions, you might feel you failed to achieve your goal. It is very important to set yourself up for success by making your goals realistic and achievable—success in meeting and exceeding your short-term goals will give you the positive energy and confidence to move forward with your program and reach your long-term goals.

For many people, it is also important to keep a record of their workouts. Something as simple as checkmarks on the calendar for the days you exercised may help to keep you motivated from the visual signs of success. More detailed records provide positive feedback and motivation by allowing you to look back to see where you started and how much you have progressed over time. It is also important to regularly evaluate your progress—about every six to eight weeks—and adjust your program accordingly. As previously mentioned, the body adapts quickly to an overload and unless you keep overloading your body your progress will quickly plateau. You must consciously increase the intensity, volume (quantity), or frequency of your workouts over time to continue to make gains.

Your training program can be as simple as outlining which days you will exercise each week, and for how long—leaving the decision as to what type of activity you will do, or where, for that day. Alternately, you can develop a long-term program where each set of variables is carefully calculated and managed. Whatever your approach, all good fitness programs should address the major components of physical fitness—cardiorespiratory endurance, muscular strength and endurance, and flexibility.

Warm-up and Cool-Down

Every exercise session should begin with a warm-up and finish with a cool-down. Your warm-up should include 5 to 15 minutes of large body movements that increase your body temperature, followed by light stretching for the muscle groups you are about to use. The length of your warm-up is dependent upon how psychologically prepared you are to move; if you are geared up and ready to go, the warm-up may not take as long (approximately 5 minutes), whereas if you are not quite in the mood to exercise the warm-up may take longer (approximately 15 minutes). A warm-up should gradually increase heart rate and core body temperature, improve joint lubrication, increase muscles' and tendons' elasticity and flexibility, and enhance your performance during the workout that follows.

The cool-down should be similar to the warm-up, with 5 to 10 minutes of moderate- to low-intensity cardiorespiratory activity, followed by 5 to 10 minutes of stretching exercises. The purpose of the cool-down is to gradually reduce your heart rate, blood pressure, and body temperature to pre-exercising levels. In addition, a cool-down reduces the risk of blood pooling in the extremities, and facilitates quicker recovery between exercise sessions. Because of the body's increased temperature, the cool-down is an excellent time to stretch and increase flexibility.

Cardiorespiratory Endurance

It is important to spend a good portion of your exercise time developing your aerobic fitness. Choose physical activities that you like. Many people find cross training—alternating participation in two or more activities (such as jogging and swimming)—more enjoyable than long-term participation in only one activity. Cross training is also beneficial in that it strengthens a variety of muscles and reduces your risk of overuse injuries. Jogging, brisk walking, swimming, cycling, rowing, step aerobics, and cross country skiing are excellent activities for developing cardiovascular fitness.

Resistance Training

It is important to include strengthening exercises in your training plans as well. Although regular aerobic exercise will contribute to building and maintaining muscular endurance, it will not build or maintain muscular strength. Different exercises using free weights, your own body weight, or machines can be combined in many ways to create an effective resistance-training workout. As previously mentioned, physical activities such as yoga, tai chi, and Pilates are also effective at building strength.

Flexibility

For optimal flexibility, static stretching exercises should be performed every day following a general warm-up to raise the core body temperature and increase the elasticity of muscles and tendons. Many people find that stretching between sets during their resistance training sessions is quite effective. The target muscles are already warm, and since the stretches are performed during the rest time between sets, no additional time for stretching is required at the beginning or end of the workout.

FITNESS-RELATED INJURIES

There are two basic types of injuries stemming from participation in fitness training–related activities: overuse and traumatic.

Causes of Fitness-Related Injuries

Overtraining is the most frequent cause of injuries associated with physical fitness training. **Overuse injuries** occur because of cumulative, day-after-day stresses placed on body parts (tendons, bones, and ligaments). The forces that occur normally during physical activity are not enough to result in an injury, but when applied on a daily basis for weeks or months, they can result in an injury. That is why people who sustain this type of injury typically cannot pinpoint a particular time or day when they were injured. Common sites of overuse injuries are the leg, knee, shoulder, and elbow joints. While participating in your personal fitness program, listen to your body's warning signs. Muscle stiffness and soreness, bone and joint pains, and whole-body fatigue are common warning signs of an overuse injury. To minimize your risk of an overuse injury, vary your physical activities throughout the week. Further, set appropriate and realistic short- and long-term training goals.

Traumatic injuries, which occur suddenly and violently, typically by accident, are the second major type of fitness training–related injuries. Typical traumatic injuries are broken bones, torn ligaments and muscles, contusions, and lacerations. Most traumatic injuries are unavoidable—for example, spraining your ankle by landing on another person's foot after jumping up for a rebound in basketball. If your traumatic injury causes a noticeable loss of function and immediate pain or pain that does not go away after 30 minutes, you should have a physician examine it.

Prevention

To minimize your risk of injuries, it is important to examine the equipment you use—the actual exercise equipment you use and the shoes you wear.

Appropriate Footwear

When you purchase running shoes or sneakers, look for several key components. Proper footwear can decrease the likelihood of foot, knee, or back injuries. Biomechanics research suggests that running is a "collision" sport—that is, the runner's foot collides with the ground with a force three to five times the runner's body weight with each stride.[49] The force not absorbed by the running shoe is transmitted upward into the foot, leg, thigh, and back. Our bodies are able to absorb forces such as these, but may be injured by the cumulative effects of repetitive impacts (for example, running 65 kilometres per week). Therefore, the ability of running shoes to absorb shock is a critical factor to consider when you purchase footwear for your physical activities. Proper fit is also important. In addition, it is crucial to replace footwear regularly (after running approximately 1000 kilometres) to ensure that the shock absorbency is still effective. Other physical activities or sports (basketball, soccer, cycling, mountain climbing) require different footwear performance, and the requirements of the physical activity or sport should be considered when you prepare yourself to engage in those activities or sports.

Appropriate Protective Equipment

It is essential to use well-fitted, appropriate equipment for your physical activities. For some activities, there is specialized protective equipment to reduce your chances of injury. In tennis, for example, the use of the "right" racquet with the "right" tension helps prevent the general inflammatory condition known as "tennis elbow."

Eye injuries can occur in virtually all physical activities, though the risk of injury is much greater in some activities than others. As many as 90 percent of eye injuries resulting from racquetball and squash are preventable with appropriate eye protection—for example, goggles with polycarbonate lenses.[50]

While appropriate clothing and equipment help prevent injuries in any physical activity, a workout partner is also an important safeguard.

According to the Canadian Cycling Association, cycling is one of the most popular recreational activities in Canada and continues to grow every year. The selection of the right-sized bicycle frame and correct seat height, coupled with the use of a bicycle helmet, padded grips/handlebars, and padded cycling gloves, can significantly reduce injuries. In the past, head injuries accounted for 85 percent of all deaths attributable to bicycle accidents; however, the wearing of bicycle helmets has significantly reduced the number of skull fractures and facial injuries among recreational cyclists.[51] Cyclists should wear bicycle helmets that meet the criteria established by the Canadian Standards Association.

what do you THINK?

In what way do your physical activities put you at risk of injury? What changes can you make in terms of your training program, equipment, or footwear to reduce these risks?

Common Overuse Injuries

The three most common overuse injuries are plantar fasciitis, "shin splints," and "runner's knee."

Plantar Fasciitis

Plantar fasciitis is an inflammation of the plantar fascia, a broad band of dense, inelastic tissue (fascia) that runs from the heel to the toe on the bottom of your foot. The main function of the plantar fascia is to protect the nerves, blood vessels, and muscles of the foot from injury. In repetitive, weight-bearing activities such as walking and running, the plantar fascia may become inflamed. Common symptoms include pain and tenderness under the ball of the foot, at the heel, or at both locations. The pain of plantar fasciitis is particularly noticeable during your first steps out of bed in the morning. If not treated properly, this injury may progress in severity to the point that weight-bearing exercise is too painful to endure. Uphill running is not advised since each uphill stride severely stretches (and thus irritates) the already inflamed plantar fascia. Plantar fasciitis can be prevented by regular stretching of the plantar fascia prior to exercise and by wearing footwear with good arch support and shock absorbency. Stretching the plantar fascia involves slowly pulling all five toes upward toward your head, holding for 10 to 15 seconds, and repeating this 3 to 5 times on each foot before exercising.

Shin Splints

Shin splints is a general term for any pain that occurs on the front part of the lower legs. More than 20 different medical conditions have been identified within the broad description of shin splints. Problems range from stress fractures of the tibia (shinbone) to severe inflammation in the muscular compartments of the lower leg, which can interrupt the flow of blood and nerve conduction to the foot. The most common type of shin splints occurs along the inner side of the tibia and is usually a combination of muscle irritation and irritation of the tissues that attach the muscles to the bone. Typically, there is pain and swelling along the middle one-third of the postero-medial tibia in the soft tissues.

Sedentary people who start a new weight-bearing physical activity program are at the greatest risk for shin splints, though well-conditioned aerobic exercisers who rapidly increase their distance or pace may also be at risk.[52] Running and exercise classes are the most frequent cause of shin splints, but those who do a great deal of walking (for example, postal carriers or restaurant staff) may also develop shin splints.

To minimize your risk, wear shoes with good arch support and shock absorbency. If the severity of your shin splints increases to the point that you cannot comfortably complete your desired physical activity,

Overuse injuries: Injuries that result from the cumulative effects of day-after-day stresses placed on tendons, muscles, and joints.

Traumatic injuries: Injuries that are usually accidental in nature and occur suddenly and violently (for example, fractured bones, ruptured tendons, and sprained ligaments).

Evaluating Sources of Health Information

A quick glance at national newspaper headlines, magazine cover stories, nightly television news programs, and the internet shows how popular it has become to engage in exercise not only to improve health but also to shape one's body. Led by the desire of our aging population to remain physically fit and healthy, there is seemingly no end to the information available. However, the quality of information runs the gamut from physical activity trends, exercise fads, and weight-loss gadgets to scientifically sound research regarding the triangular relationship among physical activity, physical fitness, and health. Take time to carefully consider the original source of the information and the context in which it is presented.

Popular health and fitness magazines can be good sources of information about exercise techniques, program design variables, and training regimens for individuals at all skill levels. However, you must closely examine a magazine's masthead to identify whether or not the editors, staff, and writers have relevant qualifications. A high-quality, reputable health and fitness magazine will complement its staff of professional journalists with a variety of experts in the field—exercise editors, science editors, medical editors, and/or health editors—who hold advanced degrees in their fields and maintain their credentials through membership in respected professional associations. The same goes for television, newspapers, and the internet. The quality of the experts associated with each story or media outlet will be a fairly accurate indicator of the quality of the information. Are the "experts" celebrities and/or consumers who have experienced tremendous results from a particular product? Or are they researchers and scientists with recognized credentials from universities, colleges, and professional associations?

Look for these credentials when assessing the expertise of a source on physical activity and exercise:

BSc or BA—Bachelor of Science or Bachelor of Arts degree in human kinetics, kinesiology, human movement, or related exercise science fields

MSc (MS if US source)—Master of Science in an exercise science–related field

PhD—Doctor of Philosophy in an exercise science–related field

MD—Medical doctor

CSCS—Certified Strength and Conditioning Specialist (National Strength and Conditioning Association www.nsca-cc.org)

ACSM (American College of Sports Medicine)—Exercise Specialist (www.acsm.org)

CSEP (Canadian Society of Exercise Physiology)—Exercise Specialist (www.csep.ca)

---

see your physician. Specific pain on the tibia or on the fibula (the adjacent, smaller bone) should be examined for possible stress fracture. Reducing the frequency, intensity, and time of weight-bearing exercises may be required. You may also be advised to substitute a non–weight bearing exercise such as swimming, cycling, or rowing during your recovery period.

Runner's Knee

Runner's knee describes a series of problems involving the muscles, tendons, and ligaments of the knee. The most common problem is abnormal movement of the patella or kneecap.[53] Women are more commonly affected than men because of their anatomical structure. Specifically, their wider pelvis results in a lateral pull on the patella by the muscles that act on the knee. In women (and some men), this causes irritation to the cartilage on the back of the patella as well as to the nearby tendons and ligaments. The main symptom is the pain experienced when downward pressure is applied to the patella after the knee is straightened fully. Additional symptoms include swelling, redness, and tenderness around the patella, and a dull, aching pain in the centre of the knee.[54] With these symptoms,

your physician will probably recommend that you stop running for a few weeks and reduce daily physical activities that put compressive forces on the patella (for example, exercise on a stair-climbing machine or doing squats with heavy resistance) until you no longer feel any pain around your kneecap.

Treatment

Treatment for virtually all fitness training-related injuries involves **RICE:** rest, ice, compression, and elevation. Rest is required to eliminate the risk of further irritating the injured body part. Ice is applied to relieve pain and to constrict the blood vessels to reduce internal or external bleeding associated with the injury. To prevent frostbite or other irritation to the skin, do not apply directly to your skin; instead, place a layer of wet towelling between the ice and your skin. Ice should be applied to a new injury for approximately 20 minutes every hour for the first 24 to 72 hours. Compression of the injured body part can be accomplished with a 10- or 15-centimetre-wide elastic bandage; this applies indirect pressure to damaged blood vessels to help stop bleeding. Be careful that the compression wrap is not on so tight that it interferes with normal blood flow. A throbbing hand or foot indicates that the compression wrap was applied too tightly and should be loosened. Elevation of the injured extremity above the level of the heart also helps to control internal or external bleeding by making the blood flow uphill to reach the injured area.

Exercising in the Heat

For physical activities outside, the function of your exercise clothing is far more important than how you look in them. For some physical activities, you will need clothing that allows maximal body heat dissipation—for example, light-coloured nylon shorts and a mesh tank top while running in hot weather. For other physical activities, you will need clothing that permits significant heat retention without allowing you to become sweat-soaked—for example, layers of polypropylene and/or wool clothing while cross-country skiing.

---

what do you THINK?

Given what you've read about the symptoms of common fitness training–related injuries, are you currently at risk for overuse injuries? If so, what specific actions can you take to prevent these problems from getting more serious? If not, how can you minimize your risk of developing them?

Exercising in hot or humid temperatures increases your risk of a heat-related injury. However, if you are in good physical condition, wear appropriate clothing, and drink plenty of fluids, you can safely withstand a wide range of temperatures and humidity when engaged in physical activity. Heat stress, which includes several potentially fatal illnesses resulting from an elevated core body temperature, should be a concern when exercising in warm, humid weather. In these conditions, your body's rate of heat production often exceeds its ability to cool. You can prevent heat stress by following certain precautions. First, acclimatize yourself properly to hot and/or humid climates. The process of heat acclimatization, which increases your body's cooling efficiency, requires about 10 to 14 days of gradually increased exercise in a hot environment. Second, reduce your risk of dehydration by replacing fluids before, during, and after exercise. Third, wear clothing appropriate for the activity and the environment. Finally, use common sense—for example, when the temperature is 30°C and the humidity 90 percent, postpone your usual lunchtime run until the evening or reschedule for the early morning.

The three different heat stress illnesses, progressive in their level of severity, are heat cramps, heat exhaustion, and heat stroke. The least serious problem, **heat cramps**, is easily prevented by adequate fluid replacement and a dietary intake that includes the electrolytes lost during sweating (sodium and potassium). **Heat exhaustion** is most often caused by excessive water loss because of intense or prolonged exercise or physical work in a hot and/or humid environment. Symptoms of heat exhaustion include nausea, headache, fatigue, dizziness and faintness, and, paradoxically, "goosebumps" and chills. When suffering from heat exhaustion, your skin will be cool and moist. Heat exhaustion is actually a mild form of shock, in which the blood pools in the arms and legs away from the brain and major organs of the body. **Heat stroke**, often called sunstroke, is a life-threatening emergency condition with a 20- to 70-percent death rate.[55] Heat stroke occurs during vigorous exercise when the body's heat production significantly exceeds its cooling capacity. Core body temperature can rise from normal (37°C) to 40.5°C to 43°C within minutes after the body's cooling mechanism shuts down. A rapid increase in core body temperature can cause brain damage, permanent disability, and death. Common signs of heat stroke are dry, hot, and usually red skin, very high body temperature, and a very rapid heart rate.

Heat stress illnesses may occur in situations in which the danger is not obvious. Serious or fatal heat stroke may result from prolonged sauna or steam baths, prolonged total immersion in a hot tub or spa, or by exercising in a plastic or rubber head-to-toe "sauna suit." If you experience any of the symptoms mentioned here while exercising, stop immediately, move to the shade or a cool spot to rest, and drink plenty of cool fluids.

Exercising in the Cold

When you are physically active in cool or cold weather, especially in windy conditions, your body's heat loss is frequently greater than its heat production. Under these conditions, **hypothermia**—a potentially fatal

---

RICE: Acronym for the standard first-aid treatment for injuries: rest, ice, compression, and elevation.

Heat cramps: Muscle cramps that occur during or following exercise in warm/hot conditions.

Heat exhaustion: A heat stress illness caused by significant dehydration resulting from exercise in hot and/or humid conditions; frequent precursor to heat stroke.

Heat stroke: A deadly heat stress illness resulting from dehydration and overexertion in hot conditions; can cause body core temperature to rise rapidly from normal to 43°C in just a few minutes.

Hypothermia: A potentially fatal condition resulting from abnormally low body core temperature.

Managing Your Physical Activity Behaviours

The decision to become physically active is easy to make but not always easy to put into action. Physical activity should be enjoyable, so in addition to considering the health benefits you should choose activities that you like.

MAKING DECISIONS FOR YOU

Begin by making a list of your favourite physical activities. Which of these increases cardiorespiratory efficiency, strength, endurance, and flexibility? Your list may include walking, gardening, or mowing the lawn, as well as exercises such as weight lifting, cycling, and swimming. Which would you like to make part of your program? Next, you need to find time to exercise and be physically active. Do you have extra time you could set aside? If not, how could physical activity become part of your daily activities? Could you, for example, leave for class a few minutes earlier and walk a few blocks instead of taking the bus all the way; or rather than watch TV or have a coffee for a study break, do some stretching activities? Could your social time include physical activities?

CHECKLIST FOR CHANGE: MAKING PERSONAL CHOICES

- *Start slowly.* For the sedentary, first-time exerciser, any type and amount of physical activity is a step in the right direction. If you have been inactive for a long time or are extremely overweight, 5 minutes of walking may be all that you can do. Don't be discouraged: start there and progress as your fitness improves.

- *Make only one lifestyle change at a time.* Attempting too many changes at once invites failure. Success with one behaviour change encourages you to make other positive lifestyle changes.

- *Have reasonable expectations of yourself and your training program.* Many people become exercise dropouts because their expectations are too high. Be patient with yourself and your body. Give it sufficient time to reach your physical fitness goals.

- *Choose a specific time to be physically active and stick with it.* Learning to establish priorities and keeping to a schedule are vital steps toward improved physical fitness. Experiment by exercising at different times of the day to learn what time works and feels best for you.

- *Be physically active with a friend.* Reneging on an exercise commitment is more difficult if your plans include a friend. Enjoy the social aspects of exercising with a friend. Partners can motivate and encourage one another, provided they remember that progress will not be the same for each of them.

- *Make physical activity a positive habit.* Usually, if you are able to do a physical activity for three weeks, you will be able to incorporate it into your lifestyle. Be aware that for some individuals exercise can become a negative habit (addiction).

- *Keep a record of your progress.* A personal journal can be a good motivator. Your journal could include various facts about your physical activities (frequency, intensity, time, type) and chronicle your emotions and personal achievements as you progress in your training.

- *Take lapses in stride.* Physical deconditioning—a decline in fitness level—occurs at about the same rate as physical conditioning. If you have not exercised for three or more weeks after regular training, you will notice lower levels of cardiorespiratory and muscular fitness. First, renew your commitment, and then restart your exercise program.

CHECKLIST FOR CHANGE: MAKING COMMUNITY CHOICES

- Does your campus have facilities for physical activity and physical fitness training? Where are these facilities? Are they conveniently located? Is the use of facilities included in your student fees? What hours are those facilities available?

- What community facilities does your home town have available for physical activity? Where are these facilities? Are they conveniently located? Have you considered using these facilities? Why or why not?

- Does your community have walking and/or bicycling trails? Are the places you need to go regularly (for example, grocery store) within a walking distance? Is the scenery pleasant when you walk? These factors are associated with a higher level of walking.[57] Do they matter to you as well? Why or why not?

- What opportunities are available for you to volunteer at a local physical fitness or wellness facility? Have you considered volunteering to help low-income individuals or individuals with a physical or mental disability in physical activity or physical fitness programs? Why or why not?

CRITICAL THINKING

Your friend Silke catches everyone's eye: five years of intense bodybuilding have created a sleek, "jacked," hard body. She plans to enter bodybuilding contests within the next year. Silke started working out in high school after her father had a heart attack at age 38. Her family doctor pointed out that her family had a history of cardiovascular disease and that she should take steps to lower her own risk.

Although aerobic exercise was his suggestion, Silke works out 2 to 3 hours a day in the weight room, usually powerlifting to build bigger muscles for competition. When she had a higher-than-normal blood pressure reading last week, she was convinced that she had to train harder. From what you have learned, you want to suggest that she add aerobic exercise and flexibility training to her workout. However, because you do little more than walk 30 minutes a day, you are afraid she won't take your suggestion seriously.

Using the DECIDE model described in Chapter 1, decide how you could approach Silke to urge her to take a more balanced and perhaps more realistic approach to her workout regime.

SKILLS FOR BEHAVIOUR CHANGE

Better, Not Best

A popular, relatively new video game system (introduced in the fall of 2006) that promotes physical activity is the Nintendo Wii. Various games/activities are available (golf, bowling, baseball, tennis, and boxing, for instance), which are played in an interactive setting. The "player" holds a remote in one or both hands to perform the required actions of the game (that is, swing golf club, bowl, swing bat, etc.). The game can be played in the comfort of your own home and at a time that fits your personal schedule. Further simplifying the process and reducing common barriers to physical activity is the fact that you do not need someone to play with (though a number of players/gamers can be included at one time). Sound like a perfect way to build and/or maintain your physical fitness? Not quite. Research by Porcari, Schmidt, and Foster showed that the physical activities engaged in did burn significantly more calories than does the body at rest; however, not as many as the "real" physical activity in the "real" environment would. Specifically it was found that Wii golfing used approximately 3.1 calories per minute compared to 3.9 calories per minute for real golfing. Wii boxing was the most vigorous activity, using 7.2 calories per minute compared to 10.2 calories per minute of the real thing. The bottom line is that Wii provides another option for being physically active, *but* it may not provide the intensity of activity needed to build or maintain your physical fitness.

Source: Adapted from J. Porcari, K. Schmidt, and C. Foster. "As Good as the Real Thing?" *ACE Fitness Matters,* July/August (2008) 7–9.

condition resulting from abnormally low body core temperature—may result. Hypothermia can occur as a result of prolonged, vigorous exercise (for example, snowboarding or rugby) in 4°C to 10°C temperatures, particularly if there is rain, snow, or a strong wind.

As your body core temperature drops from the normal 37°C to 34°C, you will begin to shiver. Shivering— the involuntary contraction of nearly every muscle in your body—is designed to increase your body temperature by generating heat through muscle activity. During this first stage of hypothermia, you may also experience cold hands and feet, poor judgment, apathy, and amnesia.[56] Shivering ceases in most hypothermia victims as their core body temperature drops to between 32°C and 30°C, a sign that the body has lost its ability to generate heat. Death from hypothermia usually occurs at core body temperatures between 26.5°C and 24°C.

To prevent hypothermia, follow these guidelines: analyze weather conditions and your risk of hypothermia before engaging in your planned outdoor physical activity, remembering that wind and humidity are as significant as temperature; use the "buddy system"— that is, have a friend join you for your cold-weather outdoor activities; wear layers of appropriate clothing to prevent excessive heat loss (for example, polypropylene or woolen undergarments, a Gore-Tex windbreaker, and wool hat and gloves); and, finally, don't allow yourself to become dehydrated.

Go to MyHealthLab at **www.pearsoned.ca/myhealthlab**. Here you will find self-assessments, case studies, links to health on the net, and much more.

✱ DISCUSSION QUESTIONS

1. What is the difference between physical activity and physical fitness? How do each relate to health? What are the physiological and psychological benefits of engaging in regular physical activity and/or a higher level of physical fitness?

2. What are the key components of a physical fitness program? What should you consider when you begin a program?

3. When exercising to improve your cardiorespiratory endurance, how can you monitor the intensity of your exercise? How frequently do you need to exercise? For how long? What kind of physical activities would you do? Why should you consider cross training?

4. Compare and contrast strength training using your body as resistance versus weight training machines or free weights. Which would you prefer? Why?

5. How can you improve your flexibility? When is the most effective time to improve flexibility? Why?

6. Create a table with columns for the FITT prescription (Frequency, Intensity, Time and Type) and rows for cardiorespiratory endurance, muscular strength, muscular endurance, and flexibility.

7. How can you prevent fitness training–related injuries? How does footwear play a role in preventing injuries?

⟜◉ APPLICATION EXERCISE

Reread the "Consider This . . ." scenario at the beginning of the chapter and answer the following questions.

1. Assuming that Magda's workouts were about 45 to 60 minutes long and alternated each day between cardiorespiratory and muscular strength training, was she exercising in appropriately? What amount of exercise is too much? Too little? Just right? How can you tell?

2. Given that Magda is still tired and lonely even though she regularly works out, what advice would you give her? Is fatigue simply a part of university or college life, or can it be managed? How could you suggest she manage her loneliness?

MYSEARCHLAB EXERCISE

1. Log on to www.MySearchLab.com.

2. Find a recent article that examines physical activity and/or physical fitness and its relationship to health. Use various keywords and in various combination to see the number of articles available. Find one that interests you.

3. Read the article, and then respond to the following questions:

   a. What health benefit(s) from physical activity (or physical fitness) is/are described?

   b. How much physical activity is required to obtain the described health benefit? Are greater benefits obtained with higher levels of physical activity (fitness)?

   c. Is the amount of physical activity "doable"—that is, do you think the average Canadian can/will participate at this level? Why or why not?

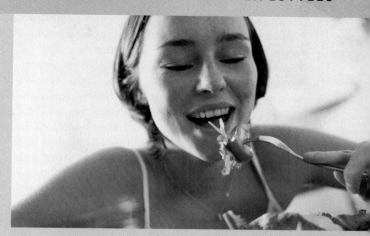

CHAPTER 5

NUTRITION

Eating for Optimum Health

CONSIDER THIS . . .

Ahmed is a first-year student living in residence and using the food services provided. At "food hall," the same sorts of choices are available to Ahmed each day (burgers and fries, pizza, stir fry, pasta and sauce, soup, sandwiches, and tossed salads), foods are often overcooked, there are few fresh vegetables or fruits, and beverages offered include soft drinks, iced tea, milk, and various watered-down juices. Although Ahmed eats daily at "food hall," he supplements his food intake with fast food, ice cream, and other salty and/or sweet snacks. Ahmed is gaining weight and not feeling very good about himself physically or emotionally. As a result, Ahmed wants to eat better, but when he goes to "food hall" or out to eat, he is not sure what to do differently.

What factors contribute to students' attitudes and behaviours toward their food choices? Why do some students find it difficult to eat well? Do you think Ahmed should change his eating habits? Why or why not? What would you suggest he do differently? Do you or your friends have similar problems? Where on your campus could you go for help?

CHAPTER OBJECTIVES

- Summarize the history of Eating Well with Canada's Food Guide and the objectives that guided each stage of its development.

- Describe how to ensure a healthy dietary intake by using the Food Guide.

- Review each major essential nutrient and the purpose each serves in maintaining overall health.

- Identify typical problems university or college students experience when trying to eat healthily.

- Identify current food safety concerns and what students can do to ensure their food is safe for consumption.

Today, we face dietary choices and nutritional challenges that our grandparents never dreamed of—exotic foreign foods; dietary supplements; artificial sweeteners; no-fat, low-fat, and artificial-fat alternatives; cholesterol-free, trans fat–free, sugar free, low sodium, high-protein, high-carbohydrate, and low-calorie products. Thousands of alternatives bombard us daily. Caught in the crossfire of advertised claims by the food industry and advice provided by health and nutrition experts, most of us find it challenging to make wise dietary choices. The ability to sift through the untruths, half-truths, and scientific realities and select a dietary plan that satisfies individual preferences and needs is an essential health-promoting skill—particularly when you are living away from home for the first time. Past patterns of eating influence current dietary attitudes and behaviours. Understanding the reasons behind your dietary attitudes and behaviours may help you make more positive dietary choices.

✳ HEALTHY EATING

We often take our ability to eat what we want, when we want, where we want for granted. We assume we will have sufficient food to get us through the day, and rarely are forced to eat foods we do not like for survival. Although we have undoubtedly experienced **hunger**, few of us have suffered the type of hunger that continues for days and threatens survival. We often eat because of **appetite**, a learned psychological desire to eat whether or not we are hungry. Our appetite can be triggered by smell, taste, time of day, special occasions, or proximity to favourite foods such as freshly baked bread, pizza, or chocolate chip cookies. Other factors also stimulate our desire to eat, including cultural and social meanings attached to food, convenience and advertising, habit or custom, emotional comfort, nutritional value, social interaction, and regional/seasonal trends. Finding the right balance between eating to maintain body functions (eating to live) and eating to satisfy our appetite and/ or cultural needs (living to eat) is a problem for many, as evidenced by the increased prevalence of overweight and obesity in our population.

Many factors influence what we eat, when we eat, why we eat, where we eat, and how much we eat. Social pressures, including family traditions, social events that involve food, and busy work schedules also influence the quality and quantity of our dietary intake. The Your Spiritual and Emotional Health box also discusses some of the cultural influences on our eating attitudes and behaviours.

Although our grandparents typically sat down to eat least three big meals per day, they also laboured heavily in the fields or at other physical work, effectively using the calories consumed. Today, eating three large meals combined with a physically inactive lifestyle—at work and at play—is the perfect recipe for weight and fat gain.

Nutrition is the science that investigates the relationship between physiological function and the elements of the foods we eat. With the abundance of food available in our society, the options available, and easy access to almost every **nutrient** (water, proteins, carbohydrates, fats, vitamins, and minerals) 24 hours a day, Canadians should have few nutritional problems. However, nutritionists believe that our "diet of affluence" is responsible for many diseases and disabilities. This country's history as a land of agricultural abundance accounts for the traditional Canadian diet: high in fats and calories with typically large servings of red meats, potatoes, and rich desserts. More recent trends indicate that Canadians are changing to a white-meat diet (that is, poultry and fish) with less fats and more vegetables and fruits.

Why do so many of us have nutritional problems? Much of our preoccupation with food and our tendency to eat too much of certain foods stems from our early eating habits.

Monitoring Calories

Canadians consume more calories per person per day than many other people in the world. A **calorie** is a unit of measure that indicates the amount of energy obtained from a particular food. Calories are eaten in the form of proteins, fats, and carbohydrates, three of the basic nutrients necessary for life. Three other nutrients also necessary for life—water, vitamins, and minerals—do not contribute calories to our dietary intake even though they provide vital functions.

Excess calorie consumption is a major factor in gaining weight. However, it is not just the quantity of food we eat that results in weight gain and associated diseases: it is also the relative proportion of nutrients consumed and, perhaps more importantly, low levels of physical activity. Canadian adults obtain their dietary energy from proteins (16–18 percent), carbohydrates (50–56 percent), and fats (29–31 percent), close to the recommended levels for their specific age/ sex groups.[1] It is the high concentration of fats in the Canadian diet—particularly saturated (largely animal fats) and trans fats (produced when polyunsaturated oils are hydrogenated)—that likely most increase risk

Cultural Practices and Healthy Eating

Many factors influence healthy eating, including culture. Culture permeates all aspects of life, including food preparation, food selection, and attitudes and behaviours toward eating. Some of the attitudes and behaviours relate to portion sizes, how, where, and when food is consumed as well as who with (or without). Food may also be consumed to sooth the spirit. This textbox focuses primarily on cultural eating of three ethnicities. Traditional dietary intakes such as Mediterranean, Asian, and Western are influenced by ethic and religious beliefs in addition to culture, climate, terrain, material resources, and technology. In regard to our nutrition and overall health, we can learn from other cultural eating practices.

MEDITERRANEAN

The traditional Mediterranean diet found in Spain, southern France and Italy, former Yugoslavia, Greece, Turkey, Cyprus, Crete, Lebanon, Israel, Palestine, Egypt, Libya, Algeria, Tunisia, and Morocco, typically includes a lot of bread and other cereal products (usually made of wheat), vegetables and fruits, fish, cheese, olive oil, tree nuts such as walnuts and almonds, and wine (in non-Islamic countries). Food is flavoured extensively with herbs and spices. Little meat is consumed, and when it is, it is most often included in everyday dishes. The traditional hot drink is coffee, which in modern times is sweetened with sugar. Desserts are also sweet, but consumption is relatively low such that overall sugar intake is low. This traditional Mediterranean diet has been associated with lower incidences of coronary heart disease. It is also thought that this dietary pattern may be protective against cancer.

ASIAN

Although Asian cuisines (including those of India, Sri Lanka, Thailand, Cambodia, Vietnam, China, and Korea) can be very diverse, the traditional Asian diet typically includes rice as its staple cereal and main source of energy. The consumption of vegetables, fruits, and fish varies based upon prosperity. Similar to the Mediterranean diet, herbs and spices are used extensively to flavour food. Tea is the traditional hot drink. Overall, the traditional Asian diet tends to be low in fat and sugar consumption. In addition to lower risks of coronary heart disease, individuals who consume a traditional Asian diet tend to have lower rates of obesity, type 2 diabetes, and some types of cancers.

WESTERN

"Traditional" dietary patterns considered Western are a result of an industrialized food system. The traditional Western diet is energy dense and includes increasingly more and more processed foods. Specifically, the traditional Western diet includes large amounts of meat, milk and milk products, fatty and/or sugary foods (that is, processed meats, pastries, baked goods, confectionery, etc.), and alcoholic drinks. Further, relatively low intakes of vegetables and fruits are common in traditional Western cuisine. As a result, this diet tends to be high in calories, fat, and sugar and low in fibre. Thus, the typical Western diet is associated with overweight and obesity as well as greater risk for type 2 diabetes, cardiovascular disease, stroke, some cancers, and other chronic diseases.

Source: Adapted from World Cancer Research Fund/American Institute for Cancer Research, 2007, *Food, Nutrition, Physical Activity, and the Prevention of Cancer: A Global Perspective*. Washington, DC: AICR.

for various chronic diseases, including heart disease. Elevated concentrations of highly processed sugars also increase risk for other diseases such as tooth decay.

what do you THINK?

Think about your eating habits. Why do you eat the way you do? What/who influences your food choices? How can you change your attitudes and behaviours to eat better?

Hunger: The feeling associated with the physiological need to eat.

Appetite: The desire to eat; often more psychologic than physiological.

Nutrition: The science that investigates the relationship between physiological function and the essential elements of foods we eat.

Nutrients: The constituents of food that sustain us physiologically: water, proteins, carbohydrates, fats, vitamins, and minerals.

Calorie: A unit of measure that indicates the amount of energy obtained from a particular food.

What's Your EQ (Eating Quotient)?

Keeping up with the latest on what to eat—or not eat—isn't easy. If you think a few facts might have slipped past you, this quiz should help. There's only one correct answer for each question.

1. Fresh fruits and vegetables contain more nutrients than canned or frozen varieties.

   True or False

2. While you are shopping, it makes a difference what area of the store you start in, in terms of keeping your foods safe.

   True or False

3. Fruit drinks count as a serving from the fruit group in the Food Guide.

   True or False

4. Baked potatoes have a higher glycemic index (carbohydrates' ability to raise blood sugar levels quickly) than sweet potatoes or apples.

   True or False

5. A late dinner is more likely to cause weight gain than eating the same meal earlier in the day.

   True or False

6. Nuts are okay to eat if you are trying to stick to a low-fat diet.

   True or False

7. Certain foods, such as grapefruit, celery or cabbage soup, can burn fat and make you lose weight.

   True or False

8. Which of the following has the most fibre?

   a. chuck roast

   b. dark-meat chicken with skin

   c. skinless chicken wing

   d. they are all about the same

9. Which of the following is the strongest predictor of obesity in Canada today?

   a. region of the country you live in

   b. ethnicity/culture

   c. lack of physical activity

   d. socioeconomic status

10. When you eat a meal, how long does it take for your brain to get the message that you are full?

    a. 10 minutes

    b. 20 minutes

    c. at least an hour

    d. 2 hours or more

11. Which of the following are at the top of the list in bacterial levels among domestically grown vegetables?

    a. green onions, cantaloupe, and cilantro

    b. beets, potatoes, and summer squash

    c. celery, leaf lettuce, and parsley

    d. strawberries, apples, and tomatoes

12. Which of the following foods contains the most grams of fibre per serving?

    a. 1/2 cup of strawberries

    b. 1/2 cup of kidney beans

    c. 1 cup popcorn

    d. 1 medium banana

13. To ensure that you are getting your antioxidants each day, which tip below would be most helpful?

    a. Eat several dark green vegetables and orange, red, and yellow fruits and vegetables.

    b. Eat at least 2 servings of lean red meat per day.

    c. Eat whole-grain foods with at least 2 grams of fibre per serving.

    d. Eat several servings of tuna and salmon per week.

14. Olive oil, one of the heart-healthy monounsaturated fats, is a great source for antioxidants. To reap the most benefits from olive oil, which recommendation should you follow?

    a. Buy it only in amounts that you will use relatively quickly. Nutrients are lost quickly after 12 months sitting on the shelf.

    b. If you buy larger bottles, separate it into smaller bottles and keep the lid on tightly to reduce oxidation from air contact. Refrigerate if possible. Refrigeration causes cloudiness but doesn't affect quality.

    c. Store it in opaque airtight glass bottles or metal tins away from heat and light.

    d. All of the above.

15. Which strategy will help you identify high-fibre breads to maximize your quality carbohydrate intake?

    a. Choose a whole-grain bread that lists a whole grain as the first ingredient.

    b. Try to purchase breads with 1 to 2 grams of fibre per slice.

    c. Look for bread that is dark coloured. The darker it is, the greater the chance that it has lots of good-quality fibre in its recipe.

    d. All of the above.

Answers

1. *False:* There is usually little difference, depending on how produce is handled and how quickly it reaches your supermarket. Canned and frozen produce is typically picked at its peak and may contain more nutrients than fresh produce that was picked overripe or too early, sat in a warehouse, spent days in transit, or sat at improper temperatures for prolonged periods. However, canned or frozen fruits and vegetables may have added salt or sugar, so check labels carefully. Whenever possible, buy local produce fresh from the fields or neighbouring areas.

2. *True:* As a general rule, milk, meat, and other perishables that have been left at room temperature for more than 2 hours have a significant risk of conveying a food-borne illness. Be sure to factor in the time that you spend driving home from the store or running other errands. Start your shopping in the canned and non-refrigerated sections of the store, and save your meat and dairy products and frozen foods until last. Run your other errands before you shop for food, and if you know it will take time to get home, bring a cooler with ice.

3. *False:* Even if fruit juice is an actual ingredient (often it is not), most fruit drinks consist primarily of water and high fructose corn syrup or other sweeteners, colourings, and fruit flavouring. It is always better to eat the whole fruit, because you will get added fibre, more nutrients, and other benefits. Next best are 100 percent fruit juices, preferably with added vitamin C. Lowest on the nutrient quality list are the sweetened, flavoured fruit drinks.

4. *True:* Unfortunately, we'd probably be better off with a sweet potato or apple instead of substituting baked potatoes for fries if we are trying to keep our blood sugar levels down or control diabetes. For more information, check the glycemic index reference books available at most bookstores, or use the handy guide found at www.diabetesnet.com/diabetes_food_diet/glycemic_index.php.

5. *False:* It's not when you eat but what you eat that makes a difference in weight gain. If you ate a 500-calorie salad at 10 PM and it was your only meal, you wouldn't gain weight. However, a 5000 calorie pizza for breakfast, followed by a big lunch and dinner would provide enough total calories to put more than muscle on the hips, buttocks, and waist.

6. *True:* Although they are high in fat, nuts contain mostly unsaturated (good) fat and are good sources of protein, magnesium, and the antioxidants vitamin E and selenium. Moderation is the key.

7. *False:* No foods can burn fat. Some foods with caffeine may speed up your metabolism for a short time, but they do not cause weight loss. One of the best ways to boost your metabolism is to increase your muscle mass through weight training and exercise—not by eating specific foods.

8. *d:* There is no fibre in animal foods. Fibre is found only in plants and plant-based foods such as fruits, beans, whole grains, and vegetables.

9. *d:* Although the other responses are all contributors to obesity, the greatest single predictor of obesity is low socioeconomic status. Although related factors such as education play a role, the poor nutritional quality of foods commonly eaten when people are forced to stretch their food budget—high-fat meats, hot dogs, inexpensive white breads and pastries, and other high-calorie, low-fibre foods—often increases the risk of obesity.

10. *b:* It takes about 20 minutes for your brain to get the message that you are full. To make sure you don't gorge yourself, eat slowly, talk with others, put your fork down after taking a bite, take a drink of water, or do other things to delay your meal. Let your brain catch up to your fork, and slow it down!

11. *a:* The bad news is that in a recent government study of bacterial levels found in domestic produce, green onions, cantaloupe, and cilantro scored the highest in positive tests for two common bacteria: *Salmonella* and *Shigella.* The good news is that out of nearly 1100 samples, only 2 to 3 percent were contaminated, but washing your produce (even the bagged and washed variety) is still a must; run a heavy stream of water over the produce while rubbing the outside under the water.

12. *b:* One-half cup of kidney beans provides 4.5 grams of fibre; the medium banana has 2 grams of fibre; strawberries and popcorn each have 1 gram of fibre per serving.

13. *a:* Antioxidants, particularly vitamins C and E, the mineral selenium, and plant pigments known as carotenoids (which include beta-carotene) are found in green leafy vegetables and orange, yellow, and red vegetables and fruit. Eating several servings of these per day may help avoid risks from selected health problems.

14. *d:* Olive oil does lose nutrients over time, with one year being the general guesstimate of "use by" time. Keeping it in the refrigerator helps prolong shelf life. If the oil smells rancid or if you note mould or other discolouration, discard the bottle.

15. *a:* A true whole-grain bread clearly says so on the label (for example, "100 percent whole wheat" or "100 percent stone-ground whole wheat"). If all the ingredients aren't whole grain, then it's not a true whole-grain bread. The more fibre in each slice, the better; look for a minimum of 3 grams per slice. Colour is not a good indicator of nutrient value. Dyes and colouring may make even the whitest white bread brown.

SCORING

If you answered all of the above correctly, congratulations! You clearly have a good sense of some of the current issues and facts surrounding dietary choices. If you missed one or more questions, read the corresponding section of this chapter to find out more. Don't despair. Nutrition information changes rapidly, and there is a wealth of information available. Check with your instructor for courses you can take to increase your nutritional knowledge. Review the resources that are recommended, and work hard to stay current.

* EATING WELL WITH CANADA'S FOOD GUIDE

In July 1942, the Official Food Rules, Canada's first food guide, was introduced.[2] The main objectives of the Official Food Rules were to promote healthy eating, prevent nutritional deficiencies, and improve the health of Canadians while recognizing the impact of wartime food rationing. Although the food guide has been transformed many times, it has never wavered from its original purpose of guiding food selection and promoting the health of Canadians. In addition to new looks and formats, the title of Canada's food guide has changed over time: from Canada's Official Food Rules (1942), to Canada's Food Rules (1944, 1949), to Canada's Food Guide (1961, 1977, 1982), to Canada's Food Guide to Healthy Eating (1992), and now to Eating Well with Canada's Food Guide (2007).

Canada's most recent Food Guide was created because it was important to ensure that it (1) promoted a pattern of eating to meet nutrient needs, (2) promoted health, and (3) minimized the risk of nutrition-related chronic disease. In revising this Food Guide, Health Canada worked closely with three advisory groups; (1) an external group called the Food Guide Advisory Committee, which included 12 individuals representing public health, health policy, nutrition education, disease prevention, industry, and communication; (2) an Interdepartmental Working Group of 13 representatives from several federal departments for which changes to the Food Guide would have an impact; and (3) an Expert Advisory Committee on Dietary Reference Intakes consisting of 11 appointed members.[3] Also part of the process was a stakeholders meeting held in January 2004, followed by a number of meetings throughout the country to update key stakeholders on proposed directions and to seek feedback on the planned approach, tools, and resources available. Finally, a national consultation was launched in Ottawa in November 2005, at which the proposed content and draft design of the new Food Guide were shared, with input sought using an online questionnaire (February to March 2006) and regional meetings in St. John's, Halifax, Montreal, Toronto, Winnipeg, Regina, Calgary, and Vancouver in April 2006.

The newest version of the Food Guide is intended to help a broader age range of Canadians, since it can be applied to anyone 2 years of age and older. Specifically, the objectives of the new Food Guide are to[4]

- describe a pattern of eating sufficient to meet nutrient needs;
- describe a pattern of eating that reduces risk of nutrition-related health problems;
- describe a pattern of eating that supports the achievement and maintenance of a healthy body weight;
- describe a pattern of eating that reflects the diversity of foods available to Canadians;
- support Canadians' awareness and understanding of what constitutes a pattern of healthy eating; and
- emphasize that healthy eating and regular physical activity are important for health.

Figure 5.1 shows Eating Well with Canada's Food Guide (2007), including recommended sex-specific servings for children, teens, and adults. Examples of one serving from each of the major food groups are also depicted.

The newest version of the Food Guide[5] continues to incorporate a rainbow approach in its presentation. This use of the "rainbow" is consistent with Canada's Physical Activity Guide (see Chapter 4) and visually depicts that we need some foods in amounts greater than others. New to the latest Food Guide are age- and sex-specific recommendations for children, teens, and adults for each of the four food groups (vegetables and fruit, grain products, milk and alternatives, meat and alternatives). Also new to the Food Guide is a specific recommendation to include a small amount of unsaturated fat each day (that is, 30–45 millilitres or 2–3 tablespoons.). The Food Guide continues to advocate for variety, balance, and moderation in your food intake. It is recommended that you eat as many different foods from each food group as possible to obtain variety. Generally, focusing on having lots of "colour" on your plate helps to achieve variety. In

It takes knowledge, resources, and planning to make healthy food choices, whether eating out, in the dining hall, or cooking meals at home.

terms of balance, it is recommended that you obtain the minimum number of servings from each food group *before* eating "extras" or "others" (that is, foods that do not fit into a food group, such as chips, soft drinks, chocolate bars, etc.). Finally, moderation refers to total calorie consumption as well as consumption of individual foods. In other words, moderate consumption meets your caloric needs and does not involve excessive consumption, nor does it involve an excessive consumption of one particular food (that is, a whole box of crackers or pint of ice cream). Something else to be remembered is that all foods can be part of healthy eating; some, like "extras" or "others" we simply need to eat less of.

---

what do you THINK?

Do you use the Food Guide? Why or why not? Examine the current version of the Food Guide (Figure 5.1). Of which food groups are you most likely to eat the recommended amounts? Which ones are you most likely to skimp on? Why? Do you meet the principles of variety, balance, and moderation? What are some simple changes that you could make right now to help you eat better?

THE DIGESTIVE PROCESS

Food provides the chemicals we need for physical activity and body maintenance. Because our bodies cannot synthesize or produce certain essential nutrients, we must get them from the foods we eat. Nutrients are the elements of food that physiologically sustain us, and, as mentioned, these include water, protein, carbohydrates, fats, vitamins, and minerals. Before foods can be utilized, the digestive system must break them down into smaller, more usable forms. The process by which foods are broken down and absorbed or excreted by the body is known as the **digestive process**.

Even before you take your first bite, your body has already begun a series of complex digestive responses. Your mouth prepares for the food by increasing saliva production. **Saliva** contains mostly water, which aids in chewing and swallowing, but it also contains important enzymes that begin the process of food breakdown. One such enzyme, amylase, initiates the digestive process for carbohydrates. From your mouth, food passes down your **esophagus**, a 23- to 25-centimetre tube that connects the mouth to the stomach. A series of contractions and relaxations by the muscles lining your esophagus gently moves food to the next digestive

organ, the **stomach**. Here, food mixes with enzymes and stomach acids. Hydrochloric acid works in combination with pepsin, another enzyme, to break down proteins. In most people, the stomach secretes enough mucus to protect the stomach lining from these harsh digestive juices. In others, there are problems with the lining that result in ulcers or other gastric problems.

Further digestive activity takes place in your **small intestine**, an 8-metre-long coiled tube containing three sections: the duodenum, the jejunum, and the ileum. Each section secretes digestive enzymes that, when combined with enzymes from the liver and the pancreas, contributes to the breakdown of proteins, fats, and carbohydrates. Once broken down, these nutrients are absorbed into the bloodstream and supply body cells with energy. The liver is the major organ that determines whether nutrients are stored, sent to cells or organs, or excreted. Solid wastes consisting of fibre, water, and salts are dumped into the large intestine, where most of the water and salts are reabsorbed into the system and the fibre is passed out through the anus. The entire digestive process takes approximately 24 hours (see Figure 5.2 on page 111).

Dietary Reference Intake vs. Recommended Nutrient Intake

Scientists in Canada and the United States collaborated to develop new, common recommendations for nutrient intake. Canada previously used Recommended Nutrient Intake (RNI) while the United States utilized the Recommended Dietary Allowance (RDA), with slight variations between the two. The new recommendations, called Dietary Reference Intakes (DRIs), are based on the amount of water, proteins, carbohydrates, fats, vitamins, and minerals we need to avoid deficiencies and reduce risk for chronic diseases while attempting to avoid overconsumption.[6] The RDA is now a reference standard within the DRIs and represents the average nutrient

Digestive process: The process by which foods are broken down and absorbed or excreted by the body.

Saliva: Fluid secreted by the salivary glands that contains enzymes that assist in the digestion of some foods.

Esophagus: Tube that transports food from the mouth to the stomach.

Stomach: Large muscular organ that temporarily stores, mixes, and digests foods.

Small intestine: Muscular, coiled digestive organ; consists of the duodenum, jejunum, and ileum.

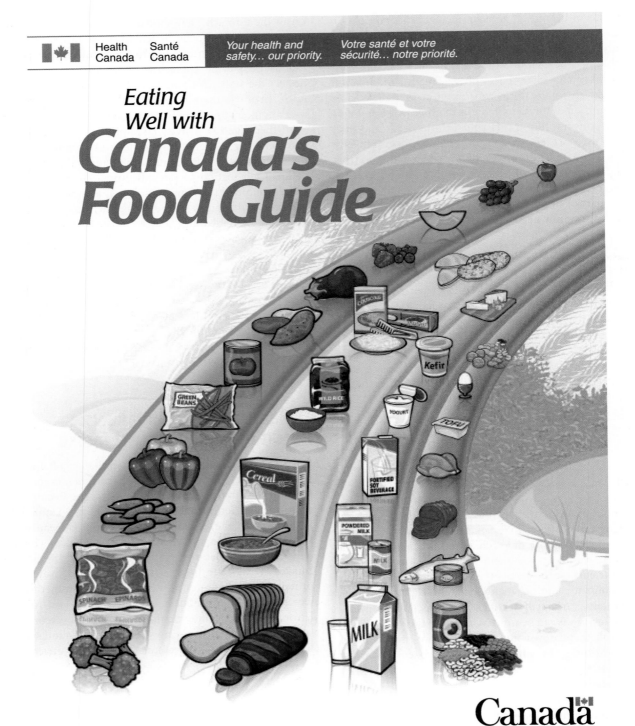

FIGURE 5.1

Eating Well with Canada's Food Guide

Source: Health Canada, 2009©. Adapted and Reproduced with the permission of the Minister of Public Works and Government Services Canada, 2009.

Recommended Number of Food Guide Servings per Day

	Children			Teens		Adults			
Age in Years	2-3	4-8	9-13	14-18		19-50		51+	
Sex	Girls and Boys			Females	Males	Females	Males	Females	Males
Vegetables and Fruit	4	5	6	7	8	7-8	8-10	7	7
Grain Products	3	4	6	6	7	6-7	8	6	7
Milk and Alternatives	2	2	3-4	3-4	3-4	2	2	3	3
Meat and Alternatives	1	1	1-2	2	3	2	3	2	3

The chart above shows how many Food Guide Servings you need from each of the four food groups every day.

Having the amount and type of food recommended and following the tips in *Canada's Food Guide* will help:

- Meet your needs for vitamins, minerals and other nutrients.
- Reduce your risk of obesity, type 2 diabetes, heart disease, certain types of cancer and osteoporosis.
- Contribute to your overall health and vitality.

Make each Food Guide Serving count...
wherever you are – at home, at school, at work or when eating out!

▶ **Eat at least one dark green and one orange vegetable each day.**
- Go for dark green vegetables such as broccoli, romaine lettuce and spinach.
- Go for orange vegetables such as carrots, sweet potatoes and winter squash.

▶ **Choose vegetables and fruit prepared with little or no added fat, sugar or salt.**
- Enjoy vegetables steamed, baked or stir-fried instead of deep-fried.

▶ **Have vegetables and fruit more often than juice.**

▶ **Make at least half of your grain products whole grain each day.**
- Eat a variety of whole grains such as barley, brown rice, oats, quinoa and wild rice.
- Enjoy whole grain breads, oatmeal or whole wheat pasta.

▶ **Choose grain products that are lower in fat, sugar or salt.**
- Compare the Nutrition Facts table on labels to make wise choices.
- Enjoy the true taste of grain products. When adding sauces or spreads, use small amounts.

▶ **Drink skim, 1%, or 2% milk each day.**
- Have 500 mL (2 cups) of milk every day for adequate vitamin D.
- Drink fortified soy beverages if you do not drink milk.

▶ **Select lower fat milk alternatives.**
- Compare the Nutrition Facts table on yogurts or cheeses to make wise choices.

▶ **Have meat alternatives such as beans, lentils and tofu often.**

▶ **Eat at least two Food Guide Servings of fish each week.***
- Choose fish such as char, herring, mackerel, salmon, sardines and trout.

▶ **Select lean meat and alternatives prepared with little or no added fat or salt.**
- Trim the visible fat from meats. Remove the skin on poultry.
- Use cooking methods such as roasting, baking or poaching that require little or no added fat.
- If you eat luncheon meats, sausages or prepackaged meats, choose those lower in salt (sodium) and fat.

Enjoy a variety of foods from the four food groups.

Satisfy your thirst with water!
Drink water regularly. It's a calorie-free way to quench your thirst. Drink more water in hot weather or when you are very active.

* Health Canada provides advice for limiting exposure to mercury from certain types of fish. Refer to www.healthcanada.gc.ca for the latest information.

What is One Food Guide Serving?
Look at the examples below.

Oils and Fats
- Include a small amount – 30 to 45 mL (2 to 3 Tbsp) – of unsaturated fat each day. This includes oil used for cooking, salad dressings, margarine and mayonnaise.
- Use vegetable oils such as canola, olive and soybean.
- Choose soft margarines that are low in saturated and trans fats.
- Limit butter, hard margarine, lard and shortening.

FIGURE 5.1 (continued)

Eating Well with Canada's Food Guide

Vitamin D: Many Canadians May Not Be Getting Enough

A May 25, 2006 news release from the Dietitians of Canada, the national professional association of dietitians, suggested many Canadians may not be getting enough vitamin D.

Why is there concern about vitamin D?

In addition to playing a vital role in bone health for people of all ages, vitamin D may have a positive effect on some types of cancers, in particular colorectal cancer, and other immune-related diseases.

We normally obtain vitamin D in one of two ways: (1) from the sun via UVB radiation absorbed through our skin, and (2) through our dietary intake, most often from fortified cows' milk.

Who is at greatest risk for inadequate vitamin D?

All Canadians—and anyone else who lives above 370° latitude—may be at risk in the winter months when there is insufficient UVB radiation from the sun, partly because of the reduced daylight hours and partly because of the level of the solstice. Other groups particularly at risk include:

- The elderly—because they produce less vitamin D in their bodies as a result of aging. Other contributing factors include an inadequate dietary intake, and limited exposure to the sunlight because the elderly are more likely to be housebound.

- Individuals with dark skin—because the darker one's skin, the lower the production of vitamin D.

- Exclusively breast-fed infants—because the vitamin D content of breast milk is not sufficient.

- Individuals who wear clothing covering the majority of their body when outside—because there is no exposed skin to absorb vitamin D from the sun and its UVB radiation.

- Individuals with low dietary intakes of vitamin D.

Can diet alone provide enough vitamin D?

As mentioned previously, most of the vitamin D obtained via dietary intake comes from fortified cows' milk. Other dietary sources include fatty fish, such as salmon and sardines, infant formulas, meal replacements, and nutritional supplements.

The dietary reference intakes (DRIs), the new dietary standard for Canada and the United States, recommend that adults up to the age of 50 obtain 200 IU each day, those between the ages of 51 and 70 require 400 IU per day, and individuals over the age of 71 need 600 IU per day. Further, the Osteoporosis Society of Canada recommends that adults over the age of 50 and at risk for osteoporosis obtain 800 IU of vitamin D or the equivalent of 750 mL of milk (around three glasses) per day.

Are vitamin D supplements recommended, and if so how much should one take?

Health Canada and the Canadian Paediatric Society currently recommend that exclusively breast-fed infants receive a daily supplement of 400 IU vitamin D per day.

If children and adults are able to have regular, brief, unprotected daily exposure to the sun and follow Eating Well with Canada's Food Guide, they should obtain sufficient vitamin D. However, adults over the age of 50 at risk of osteoporosis may need to supplement. These individuals should consult their physician and have their dietary intake evaluated by a registered dietitian. A blanket recommendation should not be made for everyone.

STUDY QUESTIONS

1. How much vitamin D do you need?
2. Where do you get your vitamin D from?
3. What can you do to ensure an adequate vitamin D intake?
4. Are vitamin D supplements an essential part of healthy living? Why or why not?

Source: Adapted from Dietitians of Canada News Releases, May 25, 2006, "Vitamin D—Many Canadians May Not Be Getting Enough." Retrieved on May 25, 2006, from www.dietitians.ca/news/media.

intake that meets the requirements of 97 to 98 percent of healthy males and females at a particular age.[7] Another term to become familiar with in regard to nutrient consumption is *adequate intake* (AI). AI refers to the recommended average daily nutrient intake based on observed or experimentally determined estimates of nutrient intake for a group of healthy people.

These estimates are used when an RDA cannot be established and are assumed to be adequate.[8]

OBTAINING ESSENTIAL NUTRIENTS

Water

Most of us are aware that we could survive much longer without food than without water. Even in severe conditions, the average person can go for weeks without certain vitamins and minerals before experiencing

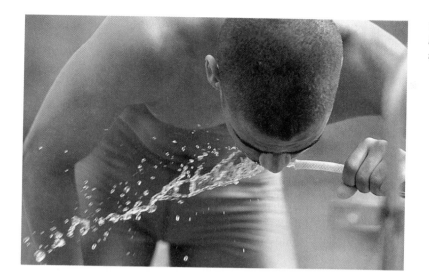

serious deficiency symptoms. However, **dehydration** (abnormal depletion of body fluids) can cause serious health-related issues within hours, and death after a few days.

Just what function does water serve in the body? Between 50 and 60 percent of our total body weight is water. The water in our system bathes cells, aids in fluid and electrolyte balance, maintains pH balance, and transports molecules and cells throughout the body. Water is the major component of blood, which carries oxygen and nutrients to the tissues and is responsible for maintaining cells in working order.

How much water do you need? Most experts believe that six to eight glasses of water per day are necessary. Because of high concentrations of water in most foods we consume, the actual number of glasses needed each day is somewhat less than this for the average person. The DRIs are somewhat greater than this recommendation, at approximately 13 cups of beverages for men and nine for women. More specifically, the DRI for men between the ages of 19 and 50 years is 3.7 litres of total water per day (includes 3.0 litres of beverages) while the recommendation for women (ages 19 to 50 years) is 2.7 litres (includes 2.2 litres of beverages). Individual needs vary according to dietary factors, age, size, environmental temperature and humidity levels, physical activity, and the effectiveness of the individual's system. It is not unusual for athletes to lose 1 to 2 litres of fluid per hour in hot, humid weather when exercising. To maintain hydration levels, athletes should weigh themselves before and after their workouts and drink one litre of fluid for every kilogram of weight lost. Thirst is not a good indicator of your need for fluids. In fact, if you wait until you are thirsty to replenish your fluids, you have waited too long. The best method of ensuring that your body is adequately hydrated is to monitor the colour of your urine. If it is a pale yellow, your body is sufficiently hydrated; if it is a darker yellow, your body needs fluids.

Are sports drinks necessary? Not likely as often as they are consumed. Most sport drinks are absorbed as effectively as water, and some are absorbed better than juice. In terms of hydration, it is important to note that people are likely to drink more fluid when it is flavoured. The intent of sport drinks is to replenish electrolytes lost through perspiration. They are also

Parotid gland (salivary)

Esophagus

Liver

Duodenum
Gall bladder
Jejunum
Ascending colon

Cecum

Rectum

Teeth
Tongue
Oral cavity

Sublingual and submaxillary (salivary) glands

Stomach
Pancreas
Transverse colon
Descending colon

Ileum
Sigmoid colon

FIGURE 5.2

The Digestive System

Dehydration: Abnormal depletion of body fluids.

used to replenish glycogen or energy stores. Thus, when your perspiration is profuse for 60 minutes or longer, a sports drink may be necessary. However, for physical activity of shorter duration or that is not accompanied by heavy sweating, a sports drink is not needed; water can adequately meet your needs.

Recently, interest has been given to milk and its potential to hydrate the body and replenish nutrients.[9] Milk is a liquid that not only hydrates but also is a rich source of carbohydrates for energy as well as a rich source of protein, which is vital for muscle repair. Milk also contains the electrolytes sodium and potassium, which are involved in the body's hydration process—and with which sports drinks are often fortified.

Proteins

Next to water, proteins are the most abundant substances in the human body. **Proteins** are major components of nearly every cell and are often referred to as "building blocks" because of their role in the development and repair of bone, muscle, skin, and blood cells. Proteins are also the key elements of the antibodies that protect us from disease, of enzymes that control chemical activities in the body, and of hormones that regulate bodily functions. Moreover, proteins aid in the transport of iron, oxygen, and nutrients to the body's cells. Finally, proteins are also involved in fluid, electrolyte, and acid–base balance (pH). Normally proteins are not a source of energy, but can be broken down to supply energy if carbohydrates and fat are not available. Proteins provide 4 calories of energy per gram of intake.

Most Canadians consume more protein than needed. In particular, they consume too much protein in the form of meat and high-fat dairy products, which are associated with higher blood cholesterol levels.[10] The recommended protein intake for the average person is 0.8 gram per kilogram of body weight per day, equivalent to about 12 to 20 percent of total energy intake.[11] The excess is stored, like other extra calories, as fat.

Proteins are made up of smaller molecules known as **amino acids**. Amino acids are composed of chains that link together like beads on a necklace in differing combinations. More than 22 different amino acids are found in animal tissue, and humans cannot synthesize all of them. The eight amino acids that the adult body cannot make adequately are referred to as **essential amino acids**. They must be obtained from the foods we eat.

Complete (high-quality) proteins are found in foods that naturally contain the eight essential amino acids together. If we consume a food deficient in an essential amino acid, the total amount of protein that can be synthesized by the other amino acids is limited by the missing amino acid(s). It is important to remember that the fact that essential amino acids are present in a food does not guarantee that they will be synthesized. The quality of protein depends on the presence of amino acids in digestible form and in amounts proportional to body requirements.

The most common sources of dietary protein in Canada are meats, poultry, seafood, dairy products, eggs, soy products, legumes, whole grains, and nuts. In addition to providing high-quality proteins, some of these foods (that is, meats, poultry, high-fat dairy products, and eggs) also contain high levels of saturated fat. Selecting leaner cuts of meat, removing the fat and skin from poultry, and choosing low-fat dairy products enables you to get high-quality proteins with less fat.

What about plant sources of protein? Proteins from plant sources are **incomplete proteins** in that they are missing one or two essential amino acids. It is relatively easy for the non–meat eater to combine plant foods effectively and eat complementary sources of plant protein. An excellent example is eating peanut butter on whole-grain bread. Although separately peanut butter and whole wheat bread are deficient in essential amino acids, eating them together provides high-quality protein because all amino acids are eaten at the same time.

As illustrated in Figure 5.3, plant sources of protein fall into four general categories: legumes (beans, peas, peanuts, and soy products), grains (whole grains, corn, and pasta products), nuts and seeds, and other vegetables, such as leafy greens and broccoli. Mixing two or

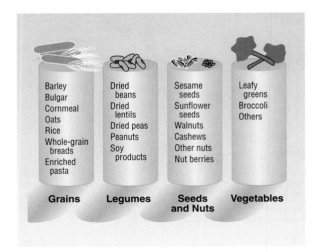

FIGURE 5.3

Complementary Proteins

Source: Adapted by permission from page 205 of *Nutrition Concepts and Controversies*, 6th ed., by Eva Hamilton, Eleanor Whitney, and Frances Sizer. Copyright 1994 by West Publishing Company. All rights reserved.

more foods from each of these categories at the same meal provides all the essential amino acids necessary to ensure adequate protein absorption. People not interested in obtaining all their protein from plants can combine incomplete plant proteins with complete low-fat animal proteins such as poultry, seafood, and lean cuts of pork or beef. Further, low-fat cottage cheese, skim milk, egg whites, and nonfat dry milk provide high-quality proteins, few calories, and little dietary fat.

Carbohydrates

Carbohydrates supply us with the energy (4 calories per gram) needed to sustain normal daily activity. Long maligned by weight-conscious people, carbohydrates are often metabolized more quickly and efficiently than proteins. Carbohydrates are a quick source of energy for the body, easily converted to glucose, a fuel for the body's cells. Carbohydrates are actually the preferred fuel for red blood and nerve cells—including those in the brain.[12] Carbohydrates also play an important role in the functioning of the internal organs, the nervous system, and the muscles. They are the best source of energy for endurance athletes because they provide an immediate and a time-released energy source as they are digested easily and continuously metabolized in the bloodstream.

There are two major types of carbohydrates: **simple carbohydrates**, found primarily in fruits, and **complex carbohydrates**, found mostly in grains, cereals, dark green leafy vegetables, yellow fruits and vegetables (carrots, yams), cruciferous vegetables (such as broccoli, cabbage, and cauliflower), and root vegetables, such as potatoes. Most Canadians do not eat enough complex carbohydrates and, in particular, not enough fibre (this will be discussed in greater detail later).

Canadians typically consume a lot of simple sugars. A high intake of simple sugars is linked to consumption of soft drinks (also high in children and youth). The most common form is glucose. The human body converts all simple sugars to glucose to provide energy to cells. In its natural form, glucose is sweet and obtained from foods such as corn syrup, honey, molasses, vegetables, and fruits. Fructose is another simple sugar found in fruits and berries. Glucose and fructose are classified as **monosaccharides** because they contain only one molecule of sugar.

Disaccharides are combinations of two monosaccharides or two molecules of simple sugar. Perhaps the best-known disaccharide is table sugar (known as sucrose), which is made of fructose and glucose. Lactose, found in milk and milk products, is also a disaccharide, formed by the combination of glucose and galactose. Disaccharides must be broken down into simple sugars before they can be used by the body.

Polysaccharides are complex carbohydrates formed from the combination of long chains of saccharides. Like disaccharides, they must be broken down into simple sugars before they can be utilized by the body.

The World Health Organization (WHO) recommends an intake of free sugars of less than 10 percent of total caloric intake.[13] Free sugars refer to the monosaccharides and disaccharides added to foods by the manufacturer, food preparer, or consumer as well as sugar naturally occurring in honey, syrups, and fruit juices. A limit of free sugars is recommended because they (1) contribute to the overall density of dietary intake, (2) promote a positive energy balance, and (3) reduce appetite control. Of particular interest regarding the last point is the reduced compensatory decrease in food intake that follows the consumption of high-sugar drinks, like soft drinks, compared to when the equivalent number of calories are consumed in food.

There are two major forms of complex carbohydrates: starches and **fibre**. Starches make up the majority of the complex carbohydrates. We obtain dietary starches from flours, breads, pasta, potatoes, and related foods. Starches are stored in the muscles and liver in a polysaccharide form called **glycogen**. When the body requires a sudden burst of energy, it breaks down glycogen into glucose.

Proteins: An essential constituent of nearly all body cells, necessary for the development and repair of bone, muscle, skin, and blood, and key elements of antibodies, enzymes, and hormones.

Amino acids: The building blocks of protein.

Essential amino acids: Eight of the basic nitrogen-containing building blocks of protein.

Complete (high-quality) proteins: Proteins that contain all eight essential amino acids.

Incomplete proteins: Proteins lacking in one or more essential amino acids.

Carbohydrates: Basic nutrients that supply the body with energy (4 kcal/gram).

Simple carbohydrates: Found primarily in fruits; are quickly digested.

Complex carbohydrates: Found in grains, cereals, and vegetables; require more time to be digested.

Monosaccharide: A simple carbohydrate that contains only one molecule of sugar.

Disaccharide: A combination of two monosaccharides.

Polysaccharide: A complex carbohydrate formed by the combination of long chains of saccharides.

Fibre: Refers to the non-digestible part of plants.

Glycogen: The polysaccharide form in which glucose is stored in the liver.

Carbohydrates and Athletic Performance

Many athletes and/or fitness enthusiasts view carbohydrates as their "health foods." Some of these individuals consume concentrated sugary foods or drinks before or during athletic activity, thinking that the sugars will provide extra energy. However, this practice may actually be counterproductive.[14] One possible problem involves the gastrointestinal tract. If your intestines react to physical activity (or the nervousness before competition) by moving material through the small intestine more rapidly than usual, undigested disaccharides or unabsorbed monosaccharides will reach the colon, which can result in an inopportune bout of diarrhea.[15]

In an attempt to improve performance, endurance athletes often attempt to increase stores of glycogen in their body through a process known as carbohydrate loading, glycogen loading, or glycogen supercompensation.[16] Although a variety of strategies— which vary in duration, dietary manipulation, and the amount and intensity of training—can be used to effectively increase muscle glycogen stores, a common process involves modifying these variables, usually a week or so before competition. Athletes train very hard several days before the competition while eating only a small amount of carbohydrates. Then, the day before competition, they dramatically increase their intake of carbohydrates. This depletion and repletion of carbohydrates forces the body to store increased levels of glycogen, which are presumably then used in the later stages of endurance activities (such as the last kilometre or so of a marathon). There are a variety of techniques to carbohydrate load, with most research on its effectiveness done on men. Canadian researcher, Mark Tarnopolsky and associates[17] reported no significant increase in glycogen stores or performance in women, however. This team of researchers suggested that women's lower total energy requirements (compared to men) may limit their ability to carbohydrate load effectively.[18] Further speculation indicates that the menstrual cycle may also play a role. More research is needed on this topic with women.

Carbohydrates and Weight Loss

As previously mentioned, carbohydrates have often been given a bad "rap" when it comes to weight control. As a result, many individuals interested in weight loss often reduce the amount of carbohydrates they consume. Examples of low-carbohydrate diets include (but are not limited to) the Atkins Diet, Protein Power, The Zone, and the South Beach Diet. Although it may seem that a low-carbohydrate dietary intake reduces body weight (at least in the short term), the long-term negative health effects have serious implications. See Chapter 6 for more details.

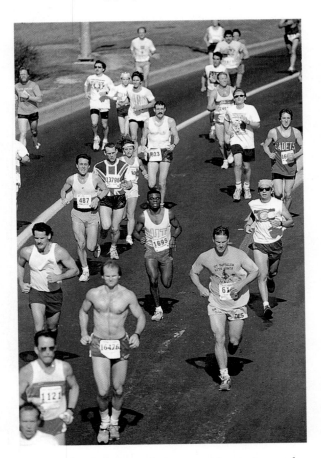

Carbo-loading before an endurance event is a strategy used by many athletes to build energy reserves for the last few kilometres.

> ## what do you THINK?
> Do you eat enough carbohydrates? Do you eat sufficient complex carbohydrates? What easy changes could you make now to eat better?

Fibre

Fibre is often referred to as "bulk" or "roughage." It is the indigestible portion of plant foods that helps move foods through the digestive system and softens stools by absorbing water. Fibre has a number of definitions: dietary, functional, and total.[19] Dietary fibre refers to the nondigestible parts of plants, such as leaves, stems, and seeds. Functional fibre refers to the nondigestible forms of carbohydrates with health benefits that are extracted from plants or manufactured.

Total fibre refers to the combination of dietary and functional fibre. Although the terms *dietary fibre*, *functional fibre*, and *total fibre* provide the most recent scientific definitions and distinctions for fibre, most people prefer to describe it according to its physical properties—that is, solubility.[20] Insoluble fibres are associated with gastrointestinal benefits and reduce the risk of several forms of cancer. Specifically, insoluble fibres attract water by clinging to it, thus facilitating passage of the contents of the large intestine for excretion. The main insoluble fibres are lignin (found in vegetables), cellulose (found in wheat), and hemicellulose (found in cereals and vegetables).[21] Soluble fibres absorb water and swell to form gels that trap nutrients such as glucose and slow their absorption in the blood. Food then stays longer in the small intestine, providing a feeling of "fullness," which may assist in the regulation of blood sugars and weight control. Sources of soluble fibre include oat bran, oatmeal, barley, and legumes, as well as naturally occurring pectins in some fruits (apples, bananas, grapefruits, oranges, and strawberries).

The best way to increase your intake of dietary fibre is to eat more complex carbohydrates, such as whole grains, fruits, vegetables, dried peas and beans, nuts, and seeds. A few years ago, fibre was thought to be the remedy for just about everything. Current research supports its function in the following:[22]

- protection against colorectal cancer
- protection against breast cancer
- protection against constipation
- protection against diverticulosis
- protection against heart disease
- protection against diabetes
- enhanced weight control

The AI for fibre is 25 grams per day for women and 38 grams per day for men—or an amount equivalent to 14 grams of fibre for every 1000 calories consumed.[23] Most Canadians do not eat sufficient fibre; thus, to increase your dietary intake of fibre, the following steps are recommended:

- Select breads and cereals made with whole grains such as wheat, oats, barley, and rye.
- Choose foods with at least 2 to 3 grams of fibre per serving.
- Choose fresh fruits and vegetables whenever possible. When appropriate, eat the peel or skin of fresh fruits and vegetables (potatoes, pears, apples, mangoes, and kiwi fruit).
- Eat legumes frequently—every day, if possible.
- Drink plenty of fluids.

Fats

Fats (or lipids), another basic nutrient, are perhaps the most misunderstood of the body's required energy sources. Most of us do not realize that fat is a source of essential fatty acids (omega-3 and omega-6) and plays a vital role in the maintenance of healthy skin and hair, insulation of the body organs against shock, maintenance of body temperature, and the proper functioning of the cells themselves. Fats help our food taste better, provide texture to food, and carry the fat-soluble vitamins A, D, E, and K to the cells. They also provide a concentrated form of energy at 9 calories per gram. If fats perform all these functions, why are we frequently reminded to reduce our intake?

Although a moderate consumption of fats is essential to health, overconsumption can be dangerous. The most common form of fat circulating in the blood is the **triglyceride**, which makes up about 95 percent of total body fat. When we consume too many calories, the excess is converted into triglycerides in the liver, which are stored in obvious places on our bodies. The remaining five percent of body fat is composed of substances such as **cholesterol**, which can accumulate on the inner walls of arteries, causing a narrowing of the channel through which blood flows. This buildup, "plaque," is a major cause of arteriosclerosis (discussed in detail in Chapter 11).

Fat cells consist of chains of carbon and hydrogen atoms. Those not able to hold any more hydrogen in their chemical structure are labelled **saturated fats**. These generally come from animal sources, such as meats and dairy products, and are solid at room temperature. **Unsaturated fats**, which come from plants and most vegetable oils, are generally liquid at room temperature and have room for additional hydrogen atoms in their chemical structure. The terms *monounsaturated fat* and *polyunsaturated fat* refer to the relative number of hydrogen atoms missing. Peanut and olive oils are high in monounsaturated fats, whereas corn, sunflower, and safflower oils are high in polyunsaturated fats.

Fats: Basic nutrients that provide taste and texture to food, absorb vitamins A, D, E, and K, and are needed for the proper functioning of cells, insulation of body organs against shock, maintenance of body temperature, and healthy skin and hair.

Triglyceride: The most common form of fat in the body.

Cholesterol: A form of fat circulating in the blood that can accumulate on the inner walls of arteries.

Saturated fats: Fats that are unable to hold any more hydrogen in their chemical structure; derived mostly from animal sources; solid at room temperature.

Unsaturated fats: Fats that have room for more hydrogen in their chemical structure; derived mostly from plants; liquid at room temperature.

Reducing Fat in Your Daily Dietary Intake

The small choices you make daily add up to make a tremendous difference in the amount of fat you eat over time. Trimming just 5 mL (1 tsp.) of fat each day can cut more than 2 kg from your dietary intake in one year—without removing great-tasting foods or causing noticeable changes. Consider the following:

1. "Butter" your toast, muffins, or bagels with "fruit-only" jams instead of butter, margarine, cream cheese, or other high-fat spreads.
   - 15 mL butter or margarine   108 calories   12 g fat
   - 15 mL sugarless jam   8 calories   0 g fat
   - Savings   90 calories   12 g fat

2. Sauté or stir fry meat and vegetables in chicken broth or wine (most of which burns off during cooking) rather than oil.
   - 15 mL oil   240 calories   27 g fat
   - wine or broth   0 calories   0 g fat
   - Savings   240 calories   27 g fat

3. Remove the skin from chicken before cooking.
   - 100 g breast   193 calories   8 g fat
   - 100 g skinless breast   142 calories   3 g fat
   - Savings   51 calories   5 g fat

4. Use low-fat or no-fat salad dressings on your sandwiches and salads.
   - 15 mL mayonnaise   100 calories   11 g fat
   - 15 mL low-fat dressing   7 calories   0 g fat
   - Savings   93 calories   11 g fat

5. Choose nonfat frozen yogurt instead of ice cream.
   - 125 mL ice cream   400 calories   25 g fat
   - 125 mL nonfat yogurt   120 calories   0 g fat
   - Savings   280 calories   25 g fat

6. Mix in a blender three parts low-fat cottage cheese with one part nonfat yogurt and use as a delicious dip, spread, or topping.
   - 30 mL cream cheese   99 calories   10 g fat
   - 30 mL mock cream cheese   20 calories   0 g fat
   - Savings   79 calories   10 g fat

7. Eat broth-based rather than cream-based soups.
   - 250 mL cream of chicken soup   191 calories   15 g fat
   - 250 mL chicken noodle soup   75 calories   2 g fat
   - Savings   116 calories   13 g fat

8. Eat seafood at least twice per week.
   - 85 g top round beef   162 calories   5 g fat
   - 100 g skinless chicken breast   142 calories   3 g fat
   - 85 g cod   70 calories   0.5 g fat
   - Savings   164 calories   7.0 g fat

9. Substitute two egg whites for one whole egg in recipes or omelettes.
   - 1 whole egg   79 calories   6 g fat
   - 2 egg whites   32 calories   0 g fat
   - Savings   47 calories   6 g fat

10. Choose meatless entrées such as lentil soup or vegetarian chili.
    - 270 g beef chili   256 calories   6 g fat
    - 270 g lentil soup   164 calories   1 g fat
    - Savings   92 calories   5 g fat

GENERAL ADVICE

Read food labels carefully and select products that contain no more than 3 grams of fat for every 100 calories,

List the small changes that you can make this week to reduce fat from your dietary intake:

1.

2.

3.

4.

5.

What other things can you do to help reduce your overall fat consumption?

Source: www.EvelynTribole.com

Healthier fats contain polyunsaturated and monounsaturated fatty acids (found in vegetable oils—canola, soybean, olive—soft non-hydrogenated margarines, nuts, seeds, avocados, olives, and fatty fish;[24] it is recommended that we include approximately 45 millilitres (2–3 tablespoons) in our daily dietary intake of these fats).[25] Part of our fat intake should include omega-3 and omega-6, which are polyunsaturated fatty acids. Canadians typically ingest sufficient omega-6 fats in the form of polyunsaturated margarines and sunflower, corn, and sesame oil. However, our intake of omega-3 fatty acids tends to be low. As such, we need to increase our intake of fish, flaxseed, walnuts, canola, and soybean oil.[26]

Another group of fats we need to be aware of are **trans fatty acids** or trans fat. Trans fats are fatty acids produced by adding hydrogen molecules to liquid oil to make the oil solid. Unlike regular fats and oils, these "partially hydrogenated" fats stay solid or semisolid at room temperature. They change into irregular shapes at the molecular level, priming them to clog arteries. Trans fats are used in margarines, commercially baked goods, and many restaurant deep fryers. Trans fats are more harmful than saturated fats because they increase LDL levels and decrease HDL levels in the bloodstream. In other words, they increase our "bad" cholesterol and decrease our "good" cholesterol.[27] Canada was the first country in the world to include trans fat on food labels: starting in December 2005 all prepackaged food sold in Canada had to include the trans fat content. In regard to food labelling, "trans fat free" or "0 trans fat" can be used only if the stated serving amount contains less than 0.2 grams of trans fat or if the total amount of saturated and trans fat in a stated serving is 2 grams or less.[28]

Reducing Fat in Your Diet

Finding the best ways to reduce fat in your dietary intake is largely dependent on your determining what does and does not work for you and your lifestyle. The following basic guidelines are a place to start:

- Know what you are putting in your mouth. Read food labels. No more than 10 percent of your total calories should come from saturated and/or trans fat, and no more than 30 percent should come from all forms of fat combined.

- Choose fat-free or low-fat versions of foods whenever possible.

- Use olive oil for baking, stir frying, and sautéing.

- Whenever possible, use liquid, diet, or whipped margarine: these forms have far less trans fat than solid fat.

- Choose lean meats, seafood, or poultry. Remove skin and visible fat. Broil or bake whenever possible. In general, the more well-done the meat, the fewer the calories from fat. Drain fat after cooking.

- Limit intake of cold cuts, bacon, sausage, hot dogs, and organ meats.

- Select nonfat or low-fat dairy products whenever possible.

- When cooking, substitute chicken broth, wine, vinegar, low-fat/no-fat dressings and low-fat/no-fat sour cream for butter, margarine, oils, regular fat sour cream, mayonnaise, and salad dressings.

- Remember to think of your food intake as an average over a day or several days. If you have a high-fat breakfast or lunch, have a low-fat dinner to balance it out.

For more specific ways to reduce fat in your dietary intake, see the Skills for Behaviour Change box.

Vitamins

Although they do not provide energy (that is, calories), **vitamins** are potent, essential, organic compounds that promote growth and help maintain life and health. Every minute of every day, vitamins help maintain your nerves and skin, produce blood cells, build bones and teeth, heal wounds, and convert food energy to body energy.

Age, heat, and other environmental conditions can destroy vitamins in food. Vitamins are classified as either fat-soluble, meaning that they are absorbed through the intestinal tract with the help of fats, or water-soluble, meaning that they are easily dissolved in water. Vitamins A, D, E, and K are fat-soluble; B-complex vitamins and vitamin C are water-soluble. Fat-soluble vitamins tend to be stored in the body, and toxicity can occur if too much is consumed. Water-soluble vitamins are generally excreted and cause few toxicity problems. Table 5.1 provides a list of vitamins, the recommended dietary intake, best sources, and major functions in the body, as well as the symptoms of deficiency and toxicity.

Despite all media suggestions to the contrary, few Canadians suffer from vitamin deficiencies if they consume the recommended number of servings from each of the food groups most days of the week.

Nevertheless, Canadians continue to purchase and consume large quantities of vitamin supplements. For the most part, vitamin supplements are unnecessary and in certain instances may even be harmful. See also the Health in the Media box.

---

what do you THINK?

Of all of the nutrients discussed in this chapter, which one do you worry most about not getting enough of? Why? Are there any nutrients you consume too much of? What actions do you plan to make sure your daily dietary intake is adequate?

Trans-fatty acids: Fatty acids produced when polyunsaturated oils are hydrogenated to make them more solid.

Vitamins: Essential organic compounds that promote growth and reproduction and maintain life and health.

TABLE 5.1
A Guide to Vitamins

Vitamin	Best Sources	Chief Functions in the Body	Deficiency Symptoms	Toxicity Symptoms
Water-Soluble Vitamins				
Vitamin B1 (thiamine) 1.5 mg (RDA & RDI)	Meat, pork, liver, fish, poultry, whole-grain and enriched breads, cereals, pasta, nuts, legumes, wheat germ, oats	Helps carbohydrate convert to energy; supports normal appetite and nervous system function	Beriberi, edema, heart irregularity, mental confusion, muscle weakness, low morale, impaired growth	Rapid pulse, weakness, headaches, insomnia, irritability
Vitamin B2 (riboflavin) 1.7 mg (RDA & RDI)	Milk, dark green vegetables, yogurt, cottage cheese, liver, meat, whole-grain or enriched breads and cereals	Helps carbohydrates, fat, and protein convert to energy; promotes healthy skin and normal vision	Eye problems, skin disorders around nose and mouth	None reported, but an excess of any of the B vitamins can cause a deficiency of the others
Niacin 20 mg NE (RDA & RDI)	Meat, eggs, poultry, fish, milk, whole-grain and enriched breads and cereals, nuts, legumes, peanuts, nutritional yeast, all protein foods	Helps convert nutrients to energy; promotes health of skin, nerves, and digestive system	Pellagra: skin rash on parts exposed to sun, loss of appetite, dizziness, weakness, irritability, fatigue, mental confusion, indigestion	Flushing, nausea, headaches, cramps, ulcer irritation, heartburn, abnormal liver function, low blood pressure
Vitamin B6 (pyridoxine) 2.0 mg (RDA & RDI)	Meat, poultry, fish, shellfish, legumes, whole-grain products, green leafy vegetables, bananas	Protein and fat metabolism; formation of antibodies and red blood cells; helps convert tryptophan to niacin	Nervous disorders, skin rash, muscle weakness, anemia, convulsions, kidney stones	Depression, fatigue, irritability, headaches, numbness, damage to nerves, difficulty walking
Folate 400 µg (DFE & RDA)	Green leafy vegetables, liver, legumes, seeds	Red blood cell formation; protein metabolism; new cell division; prevents neural tube birth defects	Anemia, heartburn, diarrhea, smooth tongue, depression, poor growth	Diarrhea, insomnia, irritability, may mask a vitamin B12 deficiency
Vitamin B12 (cobalamin) 2.4 mg (RDA)	Meat, fish, poultry, shellfish, milk, cheese, eggs, nutritional yeast	Maintenance of nerve cells; red blood cell formation; synthesis of genetic material	Anemia, smooth tongue, fatigue, nerve degeneration progressing to paralysis	None reported
Pantothenic acid 5–7 mg (AI)	Widespread in foods	Coenzyme in energy metabolism	Rare; sleep disturbances, nausea, fatigue	Occasional diarrhea
Biotin 30 µg (AI)	Widespread in foods	Coenzyme in energy metabolism; fat synthesis; glycogen formation	Loss of appetite, nausea, depression, muscle pain, weakness, fatigue, rash	None reported
Vitamin C (ascorbic acid) 60 mg (RDI & RDA)	Citrus fruits, cabbage-type vegetables, tomatoes, potatoes, dark green vegetables, peppers, lettuce, cantaloupe, strawberries	Heals wounds, maintains bones and teeth, strengthens blood vessels; antioxidant; strengthens resistance to infection; aids iron absorption	Scurvy, anemia, depression, frequent infections, bleeding gums, loosened teeth, muscle degeneration, rough skin, bone fragility, poor wound healing	Nausea, abdominal cramps, diarrhea, breakdown of red blood cells in persons with certain genetic disorders; deficiency symptoms may appear at first on withdrawal of high doses

TABLE 5.1 (Continued)
A Guide to Vitamins

Vitamin	Best Sources	Chief Functions in the Body	Deficiency Symptoms	Toxicity Symptoms
Fat-Soluble Vitamins				
Vitamin A 5000 IU	Fortified milk and margarine, cream, cheese, butter, eggs, liver, spinach, and other dark leafy greens, broccoli, deep orange fruits and vegetables (carrots, sweet potatoes, peaches)	Vision; growth and repair of body tissues; reproduction; bone and tooth formation; immunity; cancer protection; hormone synthesis	Night blindness, rough skin, susceptibility to infection, impaired bone growth, vision problems	Nosebleeds, abdominal cramps, nausea, diarrhea, weight loss, blurred vision, irritability, bone pain, rashes, cessation of menstruation, growth retardation
Vitamin D 400–600 IU (RDA & RDI)	Self-synthesis with sunlight; fortified milk, fortified margarine, eggs, liver, fish	Calcium and phosphorus metabolism (bone and tooth formation); aids body's absorption of calcium	Rickets in children; osteomalacia in adults; abnormal growth, joint pain, soft bones	Raised blood calcium, constipation, weight loss, irritability, weakness, nausea, kidney stones, mental and physical retardation
Vitamin E 30 IU (RDA & RDI)	Vegetable oils, green leafy vegetables, wheat germ, whole-grain products, butter, liver, egg yolk, milk fat, nuts, seeds	Protects red blood cells; antioxidant; stabilization of cell membranes	Muscle wasting, weakness, red blood cell breakage, anemia, hemorrhaging, fibrocystic breast disease	Interference with anticlotting medication, general discomfort
Vitamin K 70–140 μg	Liver, green leafy and cabbage-type vegetables; milk	Bacterial synthesis in digestive tract; synthesis of blood-clotting proteins and a blood protein that regulates blood calcium	Hemorrhaging	Interference with anticlotting medication; may cause jaundice

Source: From J. Thompson and M. Manore, *Nutrition: An Applied Approach*. Copyright © 2005. Reprinted by permission of Pearson Education, Inc.

Minerals

Minerals are the inorganic, indestructible elements that aid physiological processes in the body. Without minerals, vitamins could not be absorbed. Minerals are readily excreted and usually not toxic. Macrominerals are minerals that the body needs in fairly large amounts: sodium, calcium, phosphorus, magnesium, potassium, sulphur, and chloride. Trace minerals include iron, zinc, manganese, copper, iodine, and cobalt, so-called because only trace amounts of these minerals are needed. Serious problems may result if excesses or deficiencies occur. Specific types of minerals, the recommended dietary intake, best sources, and their major functions in the body, as well as symptoms of deficiency and toxicity are listed in Table 5.2. Although minerals are necessary for body function, there are limits on how much of them we should consume.

Sodium

Sodium is necessary for the regulation of blood and body fluids, for the transmission of nerve impulses, for heart activity, for muscle contraction, and for other metabolic functions. Sodium also enhances flavour, balances the bitterness of some foods, acts as a preservative, and tenderizes meat. Although vital to our survival—and to the good taste of food—we tend to consume much more sodium than we need. The AI for sodium is 1500 mg per day for the average adult,[29] yet the average Canadian consumes at least 12 times this amount. The most common source of sodium for Canadians is table salt (that is, sodium chloride, which is about 40 percent sodium and 60 percent chloride by weight).[30] The remainder of dietary sodium comes from the water we drink and highly processed foods such as pickles, salty snack foods, processed cheeses, many breads and bakery products, smoked meats and sausages, many fast-food entrées, and soft drinks.

Many experts believe there is a link between excessive sodium intake and hypertension (high blood pressure). As a result, many organizations recommend

Minerals: Inorganic, indestructible elements that aid physiological processes.

TABLE 5.2

A Guide to Minerals

Mineral	Significant Sources	Chief Functions in the Body	Deficiency Symptoms	Toxicity Symptoms
Calcium AI: 1000 mg/day (men and women aged 19 to 50); 1200 mg/day (men and women over 50)	Milk and milk products, small fish (with bones), tofu, greens, legumes	Principal mineral of bones and teeth; involved in muscle contraction and relaxation, nerve function, blood clotting, blood pressure	Stunted growth in children; bone loss (osteoporosis) in adults	Excess calcium is excreted except in hormonal imbalance states
Phosphorus RDA = 700 mg/day	All animal tissues	Part of every cell; involved in acid-base balance	Unknown	Can create relative deficiency of calcium
Magnesium RDA = 400 mg/day (men); 310 mg/day (women)	Nuts, legumes, whole grains, dark green vegetables, seafood, chocolate, cocoa	Involved in bone mineralization, protein synthesis, enzyme action, normal muscular contraction, nerve transmission	Weakness, confusion, depressed pancreatic hormone secretion, growth failure, behavioural disturbances, muscle spasms	Pharmacological overuse can cause nausea, cramps, dehydration
Sodium AI: 1.5 g/day	Salt, soy sauce; processed foods; cured, canned, and pickled foods	Helps maintain normal fluid and acid-base balance	Muscle cramps, mental apathy, loss of appetite	Hypertension (in salt-sensitive persons)
Chloride AI: 2.3 g/day	Salt, soy sauce; processed foods	Part of stomach acid, necessary for proper digestion, fluid balance	Growth failure in children, muscle cramps, mental apathy, loss of appetite	Normally harmless (different from poisonous chlorine gas); disturbed acid-base balance; vomiting
Potassium AI: 4.7 g/day	All whole foods: meats, milk, fruits, vegetables, grains, legumes	Facilitates many reactions including protein synthesis, fluid balance, nerve transmission, and contraction of muscles	Muscle weakness, paralysis, confusion; can cause death, accompanies dehydration	Causes muscular weakness; triggers vomiting; if given into a vein, can stop the heart
Iodine RDA = 150 μg	Iodized salt, seafood	Part of thyroxine, which regulates metabolism	Goitre, cretinism	Very high intakes depress thyroid activity
Iron RDA = 8 mg/day (men; women over 51); 18 mg/day (women aged 19 to 50)	Beef, fish, poultry, shellfish, eggs, legumes, dried fruits	Hemoglobin formation; part of myoglobin; energy use	Anemia: weakness, pallor, headaches, reduced resistance to infection, inability to concentrate	Nausea, vomiting, dizziness, damage to organs, death
Zinc RDA = 11 mg/day (men); 8 mg/day (women)	Protein-containing foods: meats, fish, poultry, grains, vegetables	Part of many enzymes; present in insulin; involved in making genetic material and proteins, immunity, vitamin A transport, taste, wound healing, sperm creation, normal fetal development	Growth failure in children, delayed development of sexual organs, loss of taste, poor wound healing	Fever, nausea, vomiting, diarrhea
Fluoride AI: 3 to 4 mg/day	Drinking water (if naturally fluoride-containing or fluoridated), tea, seafood	Formation of bones and teeth; helps make teeth resistant to decay and bones resistant to mineral loss	Susceptibility to tooth decay and bone loss	Fluorosis (discolouration of teeth)
Selenium RDA = 55 μg	Seafood, meats, grains	Helps protect body compounds from oxidation	Impaired immune function, depression, muscle pain	Vomiting, nausea, rash, brittle hair and nails

Source: From J. Thompson and M. Manore, *Nutrition: An Applied Approach*. Copyright © 2005. Reprinted by permission of Pearson Education, Inc.

The Continuing Debate on the Benefits and Risks of Supplemental Vitamins and Minerals

In August 2008, Dietitians of Canada released a report on the benefits and risks of vitamin and mineral supplements.

Given the controversial media attention given to nutritional intake, it is often difficult for consumers to decide what is good or not good for them. Specific to vitamin and mineral supplementation, the difficulty in understanding their importance and relationship to health increased with a flurry of media attention paid to the issue in April 2008. Three articles surfaced around the same time:

1. A Cochrane review (a database that compiles and reviews large numbers of existing research studies) of the use of antioxidants,

2. the Maclean's cover story titled "Vitamins Are Hazardous to Your Health", and

3. a news item that appeared on internet health sites regarding a Harvard newsletter story titled "No One Needs to Take a Multivitamin".

What is a safe dose of vitamins and minerals and is supplementation—general and specific—recommended? Canadian researchers Whiting and Adolphe considered these questions in their recent report published by Dietitians of Canada.

When the DRIs were set, the benefits of vitamins and minerals beyond preventing deficiency diseases were not clearly established. Thus, Whiting and Adolphe conducted a review of recent research to clarify the risks and benefits of high supplemental doses of vitamins and minerals. These authors concluded that both too little and too much of a single nutrient can potentially cause harm. Further, it is important to take into account an individual's dietary habits and lifestyle when making decisions about the appropriateness of recommending vitamin and/or mineral supplements. It was also suggested as a Dietitian Practice Point that "until further research confirms a benefit of high intakes, it is best to keep intake from supplements within the boundaries set by the RDA/AI and the UL. However, risks and benefits of vitamin and mineral intakes with respect to chronic disease risk reduction should be communicated to clients."

Readers may be interested to learn more about Canada's Natural Health Products and their Regulations at: www.hc-sc.gc.ca/dhp-mps/prodnatur/about-apropos/index-eng.php.

Source: Adapted from S.J. Whiting and J. Adolphe. "The Continuing Debate on the Benefits and Risks of Supplemental Vitamins and Minerals." *Current Issues: The Inside Story* August (2008). Retrieved on September 11, 2008 from www.dietitians.ca/news/media/asp.

that Canadians cut back on sodium consumption to reduce their risk for cardiovascular diseases, debilitating bone fractures, and other health problems.[31]

Canadians between ages 19 and 50 do not consume the recommended 1000 milligrams of calcium per day, with particularly inadequate intakes in older

what do you THINK?

Do you use salt frequently? Pay attention to how often you use a salt shaker over the next few days. Do you "salt" your food prior to tasting? Why? Can you get by without salting your food? Have you tried salt-free herbs and spices? Why or why not?

Calcium

The issue of calcium consumption has gained national attention with the rising incidence of osteoporosis (see Chapter 16) among the elderly, particularly among older women. Although calcium plays a vital role in building strong bones and teeth, contracting muscles, clotting blood, transmitting nerve impulses, regulating heartbeat, and balancing fluid within cells, most adult

try it NOW!

Shake your salt habit! Did you know that the average Canadian consumes 1150 mg per 1000 calories eaten (or 2900 mg for 2500 calories)?[32] Extra salt can be found in almost everything from cereal to snack foods. Take simple steps today to reduce your overall sodium intake: read food labels and choose products labelled as low sodium (containing fewer than 500 mg per serving) or sodium/salt-free. Order your popcorn without salt, and, when dining out, ask the chef to cook with low-sodium products. Switch to kosher salt, it contains 25 percent less sodium than regular table salt. Instead of adding salt to food you prepare, use fresh or dried herbs for seasonings. Train yourself to taste the natural flavours of food. Once you reduce your sodium intake, you will taste the difference the next time you eat a sodium-laden product. Check out the following website for more information: www.sodium101.ca.

Canadians (>50 years), who are advised to consume 1200 milligrams of calcium per day.[33] Another reason to ensure adequate calcium intake relates to obesity prevention. Recent research suggests a positive relationship between calcium intake and healthy weight maintenance (or in other words, people who do not consume sufficient calcium are more likely to be overweight or obese).[34] Of equal importance is to evaluate the trend toward choosing soft drinks instead of milk. Soft drinks not only contain a high percentage of free sugars but also do not provide the necessary nutrients found in milk.

Increasing Your Dietary Calcium Intake

Because calcium intake is so important throughout your life, it is critical that you consume the minimum required each day. More than half our calcium intake usually comes from milk, one of the best sources of dietary calcium. Although many green, leafy vegetables are sources of calcium, some contain oxalic acid, which makes their calcium harder to absorb. Spinach, chard, and beet greens are not particularly valuable sources of calcium, whereas broccoli, cauliflower, and many peas and beans (pinto beans and soybeans) are a source of calcium. Many nuts, particularly almonds, Brazil nuts, and hazelnuts, and seeds such as sunflower and sesame contain calcium as well. Molasses is a source of calcium, as are canned salmon (if you eat the bones) and sardines. Some fruits—such as citrus, figs, raisins, and dried apricots—have moderate amounts.

Of interest to those who drink carbonated soft drinks is that the added phosphoric acid (phosphate) in these drinks can cause you to excrete calcium. Calcium and phosphorus imbalances may lead to kidney stones and other calcification problems, as well as to increased arteriosclerotic plaque.[35]

Vitamin D improves absorption of calcium; thus, exposure to sunlight is like having an extra calcium source. (See also the Focus on Canada box earlier in this chapter.) Stress, on the other hand, contributes to calcium depletion. Although calcium supplements are available, the best way to meet your needs is to consume calcium as part of a balanced, varied dietary intake throughout the day in foods containing protein, vitamin D, and vitamin C for optimum absorption.

Iron

Iron deficiency is the most common nutrient deficiency worldwide, affecting more than 2 billion people or about one third of the population. Although less prevalent an issue in Canada, it is still the most common nutrient deficiency. Females aged 19 to 50 require 18 milligrams of iron per day, and males aged 19 to 50 about 8 milligrams per day.[36] After the age of 50 (postmenopausal for women), men and women each require about 8 milligrams of iron per day.[37] Pregnant women require 27 milligrams of iron per day.[38] Iron deficiencies can lead to **anemia**, a problem resulting from the body's inability to produce hemoglobin, the bright red, oxygen-carrying component of the blood. When this occurs, body cells receive less oxygen, and carbon dioxide wastes are removed less efficiently, resulting in a person feeling tired and run down. Another problem with iron deficiency is that the immune system becomes less effective, which can lead to increased risk of illness. A less common problem, iron toxicity, is caused by too much iron in the blood. Women are more likely than men to suffer from iron deficiency problems, partly because they typically eat less than men and because of blood loss from menstrual flows.

Sex Differences in Nutritional Needs

Men and women differ in body size, body composition, and overall metabolic rates. These differences result in distinctive requirements for most nutrients throughout the life cycle and mean that men and women face unique challenges in meeting their dietary goals. Some of these differences have already been discussed. However, there are some dietary factors that need further consideration. One factor is that women have a lower ratio of lean body mass to adipose (fatty) tissue at all ages, particularly after puberty. Also, after puberty, metabolism is higher in men, meaning that they require more calories than women to do the same things.

Different Cycles, Different Needs

Women also have many more "landmark" times in their lives when their nutritional needs vary significantly. From menarche to menopause, women undergo cyclical physiological changes that can have dramatic effects on metabolism, nutrition needs, and efforts to maintain a nutrition plan. For example, during pregnancy and lactation, nutrition requirements increase substantially for women. Those unable to follow the dietary recommendations may gain more weight during pregnancy and retain it afterward. During the menstrual cycle, many women report significant food cravings that result in overeating. At menopause, nutrition needs change again rather dramatically. With the hormone estrogen reduced, the body needs more calcium to combat losses in bone mineral density.

Eating Too Much Meat!

Although men do not have the same cyclical patterns and dietary needs as women, they often have dietary excesses or habits resistant to change. Consider the following:

- Men who eat red meat as a main dish five or more times a week are four times more at risk of colorectal cancer than men who eat red meat less than once a month.

- Heavy-red-meat-eaters are more than twice as likely to get prostate cancer.

- For every three servings of vegetables or fruits consumed per day, men can expect a 22 percent lower risk of stroke.

- High vegetable and fruit dietary intakes may lower the risk of lung cancer in smokers, from 20 times the risk of nonsmokers to "only" 10 times the risk. They may also protect against oral, throat, pancreas, and bladder cancers, all of which are more common in smokers.

- While obesity seems to be a factor in cancer of the esophagus, an increasingly common malignancy among men, consumption of vegetables and fruits can help protect against it.

Meals like this vegetable and tofu stir-fry provide a vegan with essential vitamins, minerals, and protein. Adding a whole grain, such as brown rice or whole wheat bread/rolls would further enhance this meal by making use of complementary plant proteins.

what do you THINK?

Think about women you know who have difficulty maintaining their weight. What are their ages? What factors may influence them to have more (or less) difficulty than you have? What advantages, if any, do men have in managing their eating behaviours and their weight? How can you help these men and women in their efforts to maintain their weight?

VEGETARIANISM

For a variety of reasons, some people choose not to eat meat; approximately 4 percent of Canadians are identified as **vegetarian**.[39] Vegetarianism can provide a positive alternative to the typical high-fat, high-calorie, meat-based cuisine of most Canadians. However, without knowledge and careful food selection, vegetarians can have several dietary problems.

The term *vegetarian* means different things to different people. Strict vegetarians, or vegans, avoid all foods of animal origin, including dairy products and eggs. The people who fall into this category must carefully plan their dietary intake to ensure they obtain the necessary nutrients. Far more common are people who are lacto-vegetarians. These people eat dairy products but avoid flesh foods; as a result, their diet is often low in fat and cholesterol, but only if they consume skim milk and other low-fat or nonfat dairy products. Ovo-vegetarians add eggs to their diet, while lacto-ovo-vegetarians eat dairy products and eggs. Pesco-vegetarians eat seafood, dairy products, and eggs, while semi-vegetarians eat poultry, seafood, dairy products, and eggs. Some people in the semi-vegetarian category prefer to call themselves non–red meat eaters.

Anemia: Iron-deficiency disease that results from the body's inability to produce hemoglobin.

Vegetarian: A term with a variety of meanings: vegans avoid all foods of animal origin; lacto-vegetarians avoid flesh foods and eat dairy products; ovo-vegetarians avoid flesh foods and eat eggs; lacto-ovo-vegetarians avoid flesh foods and eat dairy products and eggs; pesco-vegetarians avoid meat but eat seafood, dairy products, and eggs; semi-vegetarians eat chicken, seafood, dairy products, and eggs.

Maintaining a healthy dietary intake can be a challenge for post-secondary students, particularly with fast-food chains on most campuses.

what do you THINK?

Have you ever considered becoming or are you currently a vegetarian? What would be (or is) your reason for making this choice? Do you find it difficult to select vegetarian foods in restaurants or other eating places on your campus? What actions can you take to obtain more vegetarian choices?

Generally, people who follow a vegetarian diet weigh less, have better cholesterol levels, fewer problems with irregular bowel movements (constipation and diarrhea), and a lower risk of heart disease than nonvegetarians. Preliminary evidence suggests that vegetarians may also have a reduced risk for colorectal and breast cancer. Whether these lower risks are due to the vegetarian diet per se or to a combination of lifestyle variables remains unclear.

The modern vegetarian is usually adept at combining the right types of foods to ensure proper nutrient intake. People who eat dairy products and small amounts of poultry or seafood are seldom nutrient-deficient; in fact, while vegans typically get 50 to 60 grams of protein per day, lacto-ovo-vegetarians normally consume between 70 and 90 grams per day, well beyond the DRIs. Vegan diets may be deficient in vitamins B2 (riboflavin), B12, and D. See Table 5.1 for "best sources" of these vitamins. Vegans are also at risk for calcium, iron, zinc, and other mineral deficiencies, but these nutrients can be obtained from supplements. Strict vegans have to pay much more attention to what they eat than the average person, but by eating complementary combinations of plant products (as shown previously in Figure 5.3) they can obtain an adequate amount of essential amino acids.

✳ EATING WELL AS A STUDENT

Post-secondary students face unique challenges when trying to maintain a healthy dietary intake. Some students live in residence and eat at university or college food services where food choices may be limited. Further, most students who live in residences do not have their own—or have limited—cooking or refrigeration equipment. Others live in crowded apartments where roommates forage in the refrigerator for everyone else's food. Most students also have time constraints that make buying and preparing food a difficult task. In addition, many lack the financial resources needed to buy some of the foods that their parents purchased while they lived at home. What's a student to do? We offer suggestions that may help to make healthy eating the easier and more frequent choice.

Fast Foods: Eating on the Run

Most campuses include an array of fast-food options that fit students' desires for a quick bite of food at a relatively reasonable price. Most of us know that many fast foods are high in fat and sodium—so is it possible to eat well and consume them? Yes. Not all fast foods are created equal and not all of them are "bad" for you. Keep in mind, as well, that all foods can be part of a healthy dietary intake; some simply in lesser quantities and less often than others. Many fast-food places offer "healthy eating" options for the discriminating consumer. The key word is *discriminating*. It is possible to eat well at fast-food chains if you follow the suggestions

Tips for Choosing Fast Foods Wisely

While some restaurants offer hints for health-conscious diners, you are on your own most of the time. To help you order wisely, this box includes lower-fat options and high-fat pitfalls. "Best" options contain fewer than 30 grams of fat. "Worst" options have up to 100 grams of fat. Keep in mind the portions often served; adjust your daily intake accordingly.

FAST FOOD

Best   Grilled chicken sandwich; roast beef sandwich; single hamburger; salad with light vinaigrette

Worst   Bacon burger; double cheeseburger; french fries; onion rings

Tips   Order sandwiches without mayo or special sauce. Limit deep-fried items like fish fillets, chicken nuggets, and french fries.

ITALIAN

Best   Pasta with red or white clam sauce; spaghetti with marinara or tomato-and-meat sauce

Worst   Eggplant parmigiana; fettuccine alfredo; fried calamari; lasagna

Tips   Stick with plain bread instead of garlic bread made with butter or oil. Ask for the server's help in avoiding cream- or egg-based sauces. Try vegetarian pizza—without extra cheese.

MEXICAN

Best   Bean burrito (no cheese); chicken fajitas

Worst   Beef chimichanga; chile relleno; quesadilla; refried beans

Tips   Choose soft tortillas (not fried) with fresh salsa, not guacamole. Special-order grilled shrimp, fish, or chicken. Ask for beans made without lard or fat and for cheeses and sour cream provided on the side. Ask for low-fat or no-fat varieties.

CHINESE

Best   Hot-and-sour soup; stir-fried vegetables; shrimp with garlic sauce; Szechuan shrimp; wonton soup

Worst   Crispy chicken; kung pao chicken; moo shu pork; sweet-and-sour pork

Tips   Share a stir-fry; help yourself to steamed rice. Ask for vegetables steamed or stirfried with less oil. Order moo shu vegetables instead of pork. Limit fried rice, breaded dishes, egg rolls, spring rolls, and items loaded with nuts. Limit high-sodium sauces.

JAPANESE

Best   Steamed rice and vegetables; tofu as a substitute for meat; broiled or steamed chicken and fish

Worst   Fried rice dishes; miso (very high in sodium); tempura

Tips   Limit soy sauces. Use caution in eating sashimi and sushi (raw fish) dishes to reduce risk of bacteria or parasites.

THAI

Best   Clear broth soups; stir-fried chicken and vegetables; grilled meats

Worst   Coconut milk; peanut sauces; deep-fried dishes

Tips   Limit coconut-based curries. Ask for steamed, not fried, rice.

BREAKFAST

Best   Hot or cold cereal with 1 percent or skim milk; pancakes or French toast with syrup; scrambled eggs with whole wheat toast

Worst   Belgian waffle with sausage; sausage and eggs with biscuits and gravy; ham-and-cheese omelette with hash browns and toast

Tips   Ask for whole-grain cereal or shredded wheat with 1 percent or skim milk or whole wheat toast without butter or margarine. Order omelettes without cheese, and fried eggs without bacon or sausage.

SANDWICHES

Best   Ham and Swiss cheese; roast beef; turkey; vegetarian

Worst   Tuna salad; Reuben; salami, pepperoni

Tips   Ask for mustard; hold the mayo, cheese, and salt. See if turkey-ham is available, and load up on the veggies.

SEAFOOD

Best   Broiled bass, halibut, or snapper; grilled scallops; steamed crab or lobster

Worst   Fried fish, fried seafood platter; blackened catfish

Tips   Order fish broiled, baked, grilled, or steamed—not pan-fried, sautéed, or breaded and deep fried. Ask for fresh lemon instead of tartar sauce. Limit creamy and buttery sauces.

Sources: American Dietetic Association, 2002, www.eatright.org; *Health* 10 (November/December 1996): 79.

below and those found in the Skills for Behaviour Change box:

- Ask for nutritional analyses of items on the menu.
- Order it "your way"—limit mayonnaise or sauces and other add-ons. Some places have fat-free or reduced fat mayonnaise, so ask.
- Order single, small burgers. Put on your own ketchup in moderation.
- Order salads, and use the dressing with moderation. Try vinegar and oil or low-fat/no-fat alternative dressings. Limit high-fat add-ons such as bacon bits, croutons, and parmesan cheese.
- Check to see what type of oil is used to cook fries if you have them. Avoid lard-based or other saturated-fat products.
- Order whole-wheat buns and bread and ask them to hold/reduce the butter or margarine.
- Limit fried foods in general, including hot apple pies and other crust-based fried foods.
- Choose broiled rather than fried.
- Choose low-fat skim milk or water instead of soft drinks.

When Funds Are Short

Balancing the need for adequate nutrition with the many other activities that are part of college or university life can become a difficult task. However, if you take the time to plan a healthy dietary intake, you may find that you are eating better, enjoying eating more, and saving money. Understanding the terminology used by the food industry may also help you eat more healthily. The Building Communication Skills box reviews some of these pertinent terms. Figure 5.4 shows an example of a Nutrition Facts label.

In addition, you can take these steps to help ensure a quality diet:

- Do not shop when hungry; hunger influences the quantity and quality of what you buy.
- Buy fruits and vegetables in season for lower cost and higher nutrient quality. Out-of-season, flash-frozen varieties are available at a reasonable price and are a high-nutrient-quality choice, if you have the capacity to store frozen foods.
- Check out the flyers before shopping. Use coupons and specials for price reductions.
- Shop whenever possible at discount warehouse food chains; capitalize on volume discounts and no-frills products.
- Plan ahead to get the most for your dollar and limit extra trips to the store. Make a menu and grocery list and then stick to it.
- Purchase meats and other products in volume, freezing portions for future needs (again if you have the capacity to do so). Or purchase small amounts of meats and other expensive proteins and combine them with beans and plant proteins for reduced total cost, calories, and fat.
- Cook large meals and freeze smaller portions for later use, if you have the capacity to do so.
- If you find that you have no/limited money for food, check with the local food bank or social service department. Assistance may also be available on your campus.

Healthy Eating in Residence

Some university or college food services have responded positively to new guidelines for low-fat,

FIGURE 5.4

The Nutrition Facts Label

Source: Health Canada, 2009©. Adapted and Reproduced with the permission of the Minister of Public Works and Government Services Canada, 2009.

Information in the Nutrition Facts table is based on a specified amount of food. Compare this to the amount you eat.

This number is the amount of the nutrient in the specified quantity of food.

The Nutrition Facts table will include this list of calories and 13 nutrients.

Per 125 mL (87 g))

Amount	% Daily Value
Calories 80	
Fat 0.5 g	
Saturated 0 g	0%
+Trans 0 g	
Cholesterol 0 mg	
Sodium 0 mg	0%
Carbohydrates 18 g	6%
Fibre 2 g	
Sugars 2 g	8%
Protein 3 g	

Use % Daily Value to see if a food has a little or a lot of a nutrient.

Understanding Nutrition and Health Claims

Nutritional labelling regulations became mandatory for packaged foods distributed from larger businesses on December 12, 2005 and for smaller businesses on December 12, 2007. These regulations require pre-packaged food labels to carry a Nutrition Facts table that lists calories and 13 key nutrients in a specified amount of food (that is, a usual serving). The regulations were introduced in 2003, with many food distributors adapting their food labels to meet the regulations prior to the mandatory dates.

In addition to the labelling regulations, Health Canada updated the requirements of more than 40 nutrient content claims and decided to allow only certain health claims (re: the diet–health relationships) on food labels or in advertisements. It is up to the manufacturer whether to include a nutrition content or diet–health claim on the label or in the advertisement of the food. Often the claims are made—and done so attractively—because they positively influence consumers purchasing habits.

EXAMPLES OF NUTRIENT CONTENT CLAIMS:

Source of fibre–the food must contain at least 2 grams of dietary fibre in the amount of food specified as a serving in the Nutrition Facts table.

Low fat–the food contains no more than 3 grams of fat in the amount of food specified as a serving in the Nutrition Facts table.

Trans fat free – the food contains less than 0.2 grams of trans fat in the amount of food specified or the total amount of saturated and trans fat add up to 2 grams or less per specified serving in the Nutrition Facts table.

Cholesterol-free–the food has a negligible amount of cholesterol (less than 2 mg) in the amount of food specified as a serving in the Nutrition Facts table. The food must also be low in saturated and trans fat.

Sodium-free–the food contains less than 5 mg of sodium in the amount of food specified as a serving in the Nutrition Facts table.

Reduced in calories–the food has at least 25 percent fewer calories than the food it is compared to.

Light–in regard to the nutritional characteristics of a product, "light" is allowed on foods reduced in fat or reduced in calories. "Light" may also be used to describe sensory characteristics associated with a particular food—so long as that characteristic is clearly identified with the claim (for example, light tasting, light coloured).

WHAT DO THE WORDS IN NUTRIENT CONTENT CLAIMS MEAN?

Free–none or hardly any

Low–a small amount

Reduced–at least 25 percent less than in a similar product

Light–allowed only on labels reduced in fat or reduced in calories. If used in reference to the characteristic of the food, the characteristic must accompany the claim.

Source–contains a useful amount

High or good source–contains a high amount

Very high or excellent source–contains a very high amount

WHAT ARE HEALTH CLAIMS?

Only the following diet–health claims can be made:

1. A healthy diet low in saturated and trans fat may reduce the risk of heart disease.

2. A healthy diet with adequate calcium and vitamin D, and regular physical activity, helps to achieve strong bones and may reduce the risk of osteoporosis.

3. A healthy diet rich in a variety of vegetables and fruit may help reduce the risk of some types of cancer.

4. A healthy diet containing foods high in potassium and low in sodium may reduce the risk of high blood pressure, a risk factor for stroke and heart disease.

Source: Adapted from Health Canada: Food and Nutrition, "Interactive Nutrition Label: Get the Facts," retrieved on May 25, 2006, from www.hc-sc.gc.ca and S. Conrad"s. "Current Perspectives on Understanding Fat," retrieved on September 11, 2008 from www.cfcn.ca/in_action/fact_sheets.asp.

high-carbohydrate eating. Many offer vegetarian entrées, choices among broiled, baked, or fried foods, skim and other reduced-fat milks, nonfat yogurts, and full-service salad and pasta bars. Unfortunately, others have not changed and offer only limited choices for students, providing a limited selection of foods with primarily high- and higher-fat choices. If you find that your institution provides health-conscious food services, the guidelines and tips provided throughout this chapter should be helpful (see also Table 5.3). If not, the following are some actions you might take to help them change their food offerings and cooking practices:

- Ask if anyone has ever done a nutrient analysis of menu items at the food service or residence. If they have, find out what happened to the information obtained. If not, find out what you can do to get one done. Your student health service, health class, nutrition department, or local hospital may be a good resource.

TABLE 5.3

Eating Well in the Dining Hall

Choose lean meats, grilled chicken, seafood, or vegetable dishes. Limit fried chicken, fatty cuts of red meat, and dishes smothered in creamy or oily sauce.

Hit the salad bar and load up on leafy greens, beans, tuna, or tofu. Choose items such as avocado or nuts for a little "good" fat, and go easy on the dressing.

Get creative: Choose items such as a baked potato with salsa, or add a grilled chicken breast to your salad. Toast some bread, and top it with veggies, hummus, or grilled chicken or tuna.

When choosing foods from a made-to-order food station, ask the preparer to hold the butter or oil, mayonnaise, sour cream, or cheese or cream-based sauce. Ask for extra servings of veggies and lean meats.

Limit going back for seconds and consuming large portions. Many colleges and universities limit the number of visits you make each day to the dining hall; do not view this as a reason to overeat.

If there is something you would like but you do not see it in your dining hall, or you are vegetarian and feel like your food options are limited, speak to your food services manager and provide suggestions.

Limit high-calorie, low-nutrient rich foods such as sugary cereals, soft-serve ice cream, waffles, and other sweet treats. Choose fruit or low-fat yogurt to satisfy your sweet tooth.

- Once you've identified the nutrient content of these meals, take your findings to the food service provider so that changes can be made. If action does not result, contact your student newspaper and the student government to find someone willing to push for food service reform.

- If you are dissatisfied with cafeteria foods, make your complaints known in writing to the director of student services or the food service administrator. Be sure to include practical recommendations for improvements.

- Find out what is being done on other campuses in your province and throughout the country. Competition among universities and colleges often goes beyond the sports field. You may spur someone to action.

- Use the suggestion box provided in the cafeteria. If there isn't one, try to get one.

- Be positive in your approach. More support is gained by providing suggestions for change than by simply criticizing current practice.

what do you THINK?

What causes you the most difficulty when you try to eat better? Are these problems in your family, too, or are they unique to your current situation as a student? What actions can you take that would help improve your current eating attitudes and behaviours?

FOOD SAFETY CONCERNS

Food-Borne Illness

Most of us have experienced the characteristic symptoms of diarrhea, nausea, cramping, and vomiting that prompted us to say, "It must be something I ate." The number of cases of food poisoning in Canada has been growing (there are 10 000 reported cases per year; for every reported case, there are many more unreported cases). Symptoms of food-borne illness vary according to the type of organism and the amount of contaminant eaten. These symptoms may appear as early as a half hour after eating, or take several days or weeks to develop. In most people, they come on five to eight hours after eating and last only a day or two. In others, such as the very old, the very young, and those with a compromised immune system, food-borne illness can be life-threatening.

Several factors may be contributing to the increase in food-borne illnesses. One factor is the move away from a traditional meat-and-potato dietary intake to "heart-healthy" eating—increased consumption of fruits, vegetables, and grains—because it has spurred demand for fresh foods not in season most of the year.[40] This results in greater imports of fresh vegetables and fruits, thus putting ourselves at risk for ingesting exotic pathogens. Although we are told when we travel to developing countries to "boil it, peel it, or don't eat it," we bring these foods into our kitchens and eat them, often without washing them.[41] Food can also become contaminated by being watered with contaminated water, fertilized with "organic" fertilizers (animal

Learning to shop carefully for fresh, high-quality foods can help ensure that your food is safe and help you to attain nutritional health.

manure), or not subjected to the same rigorous pesticide regulations as Canadian-raised produce. To give you an idea of the implications, studies have shown that *Escherichia coli* (a lethal bacterial pathogen) can survive in cow manure for up to 70 days and multiply in foods grown with manure unless heat or additives such as salt or preservatives are used to kill them.[42] There are essentially no regulations that prohibit farmers from using animal manure to fertilize crops.

Other key factors associated with the increasing spread of food-borne diseases include inadvertent introduction of pathogens into new geographic regions and insufficient education about food safety.[43]

Part of the responsibility for preventing food-borne illness lies with consumers: more than 30 percent of such illnesses result from unsafe handling of food at home. The following are actions you can take to minimize your risk:[44]

- When shopping, pick up your packaged and canned foods first and frozen foods and perishables such as dairy products, meat, poultry, and seafood at the end.

- Check for cleanliness and food safety at the salad bar, meat, and seafood counters. Cooked shrimp, crab, or lobster lying on the same bed of ice as raw seafood can become contaminated.

- When shopping for seafood, buy from markets that get their supplies from approved sources.

- Most fresh meat, seafood, and poultry should be kept in the refrigerator no more than one or two days. Check the shelf life of all products before buying.

- Leftovers should be eaten within three days.

- Use a thermometer to ensure that meats are completely cooked. Beef and lamb steaks and roasts should be cooked to at least 63°C, ground meat, pork chops, ribs, and egg dishes to 71°C, chicken and poultry breasts to 77°C, and chicken and turkey legs, thighs, and whole birds to 82°C.

- Fish is done when the thickest part becomes opaque and the fish flakes easily.

- Cooked food should never be left standing on the stove or table for more than two hours. Keep hot foods hot and cold foods cold.

- Never thaw frozen foods at room temperature. Put in the refrigerator for a day to thaw, or thaw in cold water, changing the water every 30 minutes.

- Wash your hands with soap and water before, during, and after food preparations, particularly after handling meat, seafood, or poultry. Wash the countertop and all utensils thoroughly and with a bacteria-killing cleanser before using them for other foods.

- When freezing raw foods, in particular meat, make sure juices cannot spill into ice cubes or other areas of the refrigerator.

- When packing lunch for school, ensure appropriate temperatures are maintained.

Food Additives

Additives are substances added to food to reduce the risk of food-borne illness, prevent spoilage, and enhance the look and taste. Additives can also enhance the nutrient value; for example, the fortification of milk with Vitamin D and of grain products with folate. Although Health Canada regulates additives according to effectiveness, safety and ability to detect them in foods, questions are often raised about their safety—in particular because some additives interact with medications. Generally, the fewer the chemicals, colorants, and preservatives, the better.

Examples of common additives include

- antimicrobial agents: substances such as salt, sugar, nitrites, and others that tend to make foods less hospitable for microbes
- antioxidants: substances that preserve colour and flavour by reducing loss due to oxygen exposure. Vitamins C and E as well as the additives BHA and HHT are common antioxidants.
- artificial colours, nutrient additions, and flavour enhancers such as MSG (monosodium glutamate)
- sulfites: used to preserve vegetable colour
- dioxins: found in coffee filters, milk containers, and frozen foods
- methylene chloride: found in decaffeinated coffee
- hormones: bovine growth hormone found in animal meat and milk

Food Allergies

Up to 8 percent of children, and a smaller proportion of adults, are allergic to at least one food. True **food allergies** occur when the body overreacts to normally harmless proteins, perceiving them as allergens. The body then produces antibodies that activate immune cells known as histamines, triggering a variety of allergic symptoms. Such allergic reactions vary tremendously and range from a case of hives or a body rash to swelling of certain body parts (especially the lips), to pain, itchiness, diarrhea, nausea, or vomiting. In more severe cases, irregularities in breathing and heartbeat are experienced, along with blood pressure fluctuations, shock, and, if untreated, death. Symptoms may occur within minutes or over a two- to three-hour period.

The most common culprits are soybeans, legumes (including peanuts), nuts, shellfish, eggs, wheat, and milk. People are often allergic to a whole family of foods; this is called "cross-reactivity." Unlike many other allergies, food allergies do not appear to be inherited. Individuals breast-fed as infants seem to have fewer food allergies. If you think you have a food allergy, get tested by a trained allergist.

Some common reactions to food that may imitate allergies but do not involve the immune system are listed below.[45]

- **Food intolerance** occurs in people who lack certain digestive enzymes and suffer adverse effects when they consume substances they are intolerant to. One of the most common examples is lactose intolerance, experienced by people without the digestive enzymes needed to digest the lactose in milk.
- Reactions to food additives, such as sulphites and MSG.
- Reactions to substances occurring naturally in some foods, such as tyramine in cheese, phenylethylamine in chocolate, caffeine in coffee, and some compounds in alcohol.
- Unknown reactions in people who have adverse symptoms that they attribute to foods and that may actually go away when treated as allergies but for which there is no physiological basis.

Organic Foods

Due to mounting concerns about food safety, many people refuse to buy processed foods and mass-produced agricultural products. Instead, they purchase foods **organically grown**—foods reported to be pesticide- and chemical-free. Not that long ago, buying organic foods meant going to a specialty store and paying premium prices for produce that was likely wilted, wormy, and smaller than its nonorganic alternative. Further, there was no guarantee that these products were really grown in an organic environment. People who bought these foods did so out of the desire to eat healthier produce and to avoid potentially harmful chemicals, and to support the environment.

Enter the organics of the twenty-first century— larger, more attractive, and fresher looking but still often carrying a heavier price tag. Another difficulty is in ensuring that what you buy as organic does not have "second-hand" pesticides or chemicals on it. Currently, Canadian farms can be certified as organic so long as they do not use chemicals themselves regardless of the chemicals used on neighbouring farms.

Is buying organic really better for you? Perhaps if we could put a group of people in a pristine environment and ensure that they never ate, drank, or were exposed to chemicals, we could test this hypothesis. In real life, however, it is almost impossible to assess the health impact of organic versus non-organic produce. Nevertheless, the market for organic products continues to increase each year, particularly as people's concern for the environment increases. In addition to purchasing organically grown produce, people are interested in purchasing locally grown produce— produce that does not have to travel a great distance to get to them—which is an environmentally sound approach as well.

Food allergies: Overreaction by the body to normally harmless proteins perceived as allergens. In response, the body produces antibodies, triggering allergic symptoms.

Food intolerance: Adverse effects resulting when people who lack the digestive chemicals needed to break down certain substances eat those substances.

Organically grown: Foods grown without pesticides or chemicals.

Managing Your Nutrition

Let's face it, eating well is not easy. It takes knowledge, careful thought and analysis, and the ability to put it all together to make the best decisions for your lifestyle and personal goals within your budgetary limits. By focusing on the issue, reading, seeking help from reputable, trained professionals, and planning ahead, you can improve your nutrition health. The following recommendations may also help.

MAKING DECISIONS FOR YOU

1. List the four biggest improvements to your current dietary intake you want to make. Be specific.

2. Prioritize the items in the above list. Determine when you want to accomplish each item and outline a plan of action for accomplishing each goal.

3. List the little actions that you can take that may make a difference in your overall plan. List the big changes that you can make to accomplish your overall goals.

4. On the basis of your past history of trying to change these behaviours, what techniques do you think may most likely work for you? Indicate what you will use from these past attempts and what you will do differently.

CHECKLIST FOR CHANGE: MAKING PERSONAL CHOICES

- *Eat lower on the food chain.* Try to substitute vegetables, fruits, nuts, or grains for animal products at least once a day.

- *Eat seasonal foods whenever possible.* By eating foods at the peak of harvest, you are most apt to avoid nutrient losses incurred by storage, freezing, canning, and so on—and are likely to obtain a lower-cost option.

- *Eat lean.* The evidence against high-fat foods mounts daily. Pay attention to labels, assess your food intake, and balance high-fat with low-fat choices. Choose leaner cuts of meat and bake, grill, boil, or broil whenever possible.

- *Eat more colour.* Generally, the more vibrant the colours in the vegetable or fruit, the more nutrients available. In particular, eat more dark greens and oranges. Try a new vegetable or fruit each week.

- *Increase your consumption of vegetables and fruits.* Use the real thing instead of juices and get more for your money.

- *Practise responsible consumer safety.* Avoid unnecessary chemicals and buy, prepare, and store foods prudently to avoid food-borne illness.

- *Eat in moderation.* Learn to separate true hunger feelings from the food cravings that come from boredom. Recognize when your body is signalling that it is getting full, and stop eating. Moderate your caloric consumption and reduce your consumption of sugars and other dietary "extras."

- *Keep your systems functioning well.* Even the best plans are doomed to fail if life problems are dragging your systems down, particularly your digestive system.

- *Balance your dietary intake.* Consume appropriate amounts of water, proteins, carbohydrates, fats, vitamins, and minerals.

- *Pay attention to changing nutrient needs.* Various factors in your life, such as pregnancy or illness, may require adjustments to your nutrition intake. Prepare for these changes and remain informed about reputable sources of information concerning nutrient benefits and risks.

CHECKLIST FOR CHANGE: MAKING COMMUNITY CHOICES

- Evaluate the types of eating establishments available on your campus. If you don't have the options you think you should, take action. Involve your student newspaper and student organizations, talk with food service representatives, involve your student health service, and solicit the support of key campus representatives.

- Assess your elected officials' priorities regarding nutrition as it pertains to the elderly, pregnant women, and the homeless. Are they supporting actions to ensure adequate nutrition for high-risk groups? If not, why not? Write letters asking for clarification of their positions. Seek alternative candidates if these individuals do not represent your views.

- If you patronize certain food establishments, review the food options. Tell them when they are doing a good job and request other options when they are not.

- Find out about government-subsidized foods. Who is eligible for these programs? What is their purpose? What are their limitations? Strengths? Be informed about these programs. Support or refute them on the basis of sound information rather than on emotional reactions.

- Be informed about key nutritional concepts. Speak up when you see information that is false or misleading. Demand accuracy in reported claims. Give advice only when you have taken the time to read and study the issues. Read reliable nutrition sources. When in doubt, seek help from professors or experts in the community.

CRITICAL THINKING

You and your best friend chose to move into an apartment off campus this year and you have decided to make your meals together. You were raised on meals where meat was the focal point; your best friend/roommate is a lacto-ovo vegetarian. Using the DECIDE model described in Chapter 1, decide how you two will come up with a menu that works for you both.

Go to MyHealthLab at **www.pearsoned.ca/myhealthlab.** Here you will find self-assessments, case studies, links to health on the net, and much more.

DISCUSSION QUESTIONS

1. What factors influence the dietary patterns, attitudes, and behaviours of the typical university or college student? Which of these factors has the greatest influence on your eating attitudes and behaviours? Why is it important that you know about your dietary influences as you think about changing your eating patterns, attitudes, and behaviours?

2. What are the four food groups in Eating Well with Canada's Food Guide? How many servings do you need of each? What groups might you find it difficult to get enough servings from? What food group do you get too many servings from? What can you do to increase or decrease your intake of selected food groups? How can you remember the four food groups?

3. What other recommendations are made in Eating Well with Canada's Food Guide (other than servings from each food group)? Are these recommendations difficult to follow, particularly as a university or college student? Why or why not?

4. What are the major types of nutrients that you should be getting from the foods you eat? What happens if you do not get enough of one or more of these nutrients? Are vitamin and mineral supplements necessary for you individually? Why or why not?

5. Distinguish between the different types of vegetarianism. Which types are most likely to lead to nutrient deficiencies? What can be done to ensure that even the strictest vegetarian gets sufficient nutrients?

6. What are the problems many post-secondary students face when trying to eat well? List five ways you could improve your dietary intake now.

7. What are the major risks for food-borne illnesses and what can you do to protect yourself at school? At home? Why are additives added to food? What are the potential risks of these additives? How are food illnesses and food allergies different?

APPLICATION EXERCISE

Reread the "Consider This . . ." scenario at the beginning of the chapter and respond to the following:

1. Critique Ahmed's eating habits. What suggestions could you make to help him? How can you make these suggestions in a way that does not offend him?

2. Is there anything Ahmed can do to improve his eating situation? Imagine Ahmed attends your university or college; is the food available really that unhealthy or does he need more knowledge and motivation to make better choices? What specific suggestions would you make?

MYSEARCHLAB EXERCISE

1. Log on to www.MySearchLab.com.
2. Retrieve article AN 31384794, "You're Not Sick, You're Thirsty: Drink Up!" by Joey Shulman.
3. Read the article, then respond to the following questions:
   a. What health conditions may result when chronically dehydrated?
   b. How much water should you drink?
   c. Why do older people need more water?
   d. What other suggestions would you make to assist in consuming sufficient water/fluids on a daily basis?

CHAPTER 6

MANAGING YOUR WEIGHT

Finding a Healthy Balance

CONSIDER THIS . . .

Denzel, aged 20, desperately wants to lose the "frosh 15"–that is, the 7 kilograms (or 15 pounds) he put on during his first year at university. In his first year, he spent much of his time in sedentary activities and made little time for physical activity. He also often rewarded his study efforts with food-related breaks with his friends. Because he wants to lose the "frosh 15" quickly so he can be buff for spring break, Denzel goes on a crash diet and begins an intense running and weightlifting program. After three weeks following this regimen, his friends tell him how great he looks. Bolstered by their support, Denzel decides to cut his already low food intake even more, increase his running and weightlifting workouts, and take a fat-loss supplement.

What risks are associated with Denzel's rapid weight loss? Is his thinking typical of others on similar weight loss plans? What are his motivations for losing weight? How do the opinions of others appear to influence him? As a friend, what could you do to help Denzel without compromising his health?

CHAPTER OBJECTIVES

- Distinguish between overweight and obesity, including how they are measured.

- Summarize the factors that result in obesity.

- Explain the roles of physical activity, dietary intake, and other factors in weight maintenance.

- Identify the common factors that lead to dieting, body image disturbances, and the development of eating disorders.

Canadians are concerned about their body weight and shape—and should be, since more than half are classified as overweight or obese according to body mass index (BMI) calculations derived from measured height and weight in the most recent Canadian Community Health Survey.[1] Equally alarming is the high percentage of Canadian children and youth considered at risk of overweight or overweight. In addition to a greater number of Canadian adults, children, and youth classified as overweight or obese, their average BMI and fat levels have increased too. Specifically, the average BMI of adults increased from 25.1 in 1978–79 to 27.0 in 2004[2] and the average level of fat as measured by skinfolds was greater in children and adolescents measured in the 1990s than in those measured in the 1960s.[3] Given the attention to overweight and obesity in the media, you are likely aware of the health risks associated with these conditions. Briefly, these include increased risk of heart disease, stroke, high blood pressure, some types of cancer, type 2 diabetes, gall bladder disease, and osteoarthritis.[4] Of equal concern are the emotional, spiritual, and social health risks associated with obesity partly due to the stigma surrounding it. You are also likely aware of the "simple" solution to obesity often depicted in the media: eat less, do more. However, it is not that simple—if it was, our population would not be experiencing the current levels of overweight and obesity.

This chapter is designed to help you better understand what overweight and obesity really mean, what factors lead to their development, and why weight maintenance is essential to overall health. This chapter also includes practical and realistic strategies for maintaining your weight and learning to appreciate your body size and shape as it is.

OVERWEIGHT AND OBESITY

Confusion exists in the understanding of the terms *overweight* and *obesity*. Part of the confusion relates to measurement and another part is the inconsistent and inappropriate use of each term. **Overweight** refers to a weight greater than expected for a specific height (and is usually determined from height–weight charts or calculating BMI). **Obesity** refers to an excessive accumulation of body fat such that the individual is at increased risk for developing health problems (see Figure 6.1). Interestingly, a person can be overweight and not obese. For example, a male weightlifter or football athlete may be

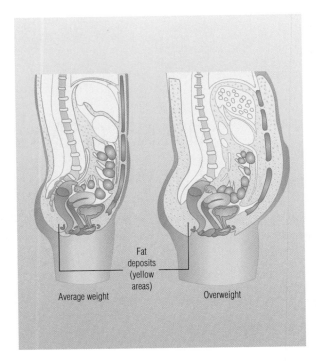

FIGURE 6.1

The figure compares a person with an average level of body fat to a person with excess body fat. Note the fat deposits directly under the skin (subcutaneous fat) and around the internal organs (visceral fat).

overweight according to a height–weight chart and BMI classification because of his high level of lean body or muscle mass but clearly not be obese. Similarly, a person can be obese without being overweight. A female student, 20 years of age, who weighs 54 kilograms and is 160 centimetres tall can have more than 30 percent of her weight coming from fat if she does not exercise, engages in little physical activity, spends lots of time on the computer and studying, and eats a high-fat diet. Thus, weight by itself or in combination with height is not a valid indicator of obesity or fatness.

As previously mentioned, physical health risks associated with obesity or an excessive accumulation of fat include, but should not be limited to, an increased chance of developing atherosclerosis, coronary artery disease, hypertension, colon cancer, postmenopausal breast cancer, type 2 diabetes, gallbladder disease, and osteoarthritis.[5] Excessive fatness may also contribute to a poor body image and reduced self-esteem. Most health professionals agree that a level of total body fat that exceeds 20 percent in men and 30 percent in women puts them at risk for health problems. Table 6.1 provides general ratings for adults aged 18 to 30 in terms of overall percentages of body fat.

✳ Determining the Right Weight for You

The answer to whether you are at a healthy weight depends on your body structure and how your weight is distributed. Traditionally, people compared their weight to the range given on height-and-weight charts. These charts usually give the "ideal" weight for males and females of a given height and frame size. If you were above your ideal weight, you would then be classified as overweight.

More common today is to determine your weight status based on calculating your **BMI**. BMI is obtained by dividing your weight (in kilograms) by your height (in metres) squared. Weight should be taken without shoes or clothing, and height should be measured without shoes. Table 6.2 and Figure 6.2 depict classifications for health risk according to BMI for men and women.[6] In general, a BMI range of 18.5 to 24.9 is considered a healthy weight. BMI values above 25.0 are referred to as overweight and are associated with increased health risk. Although not a measure of fatness per se, a BMI greater than 30 results in an "obese" classification because of the associated health risks found in the population at this level of BMI and greater. As noted in Table 6.2, obesity is further broken into classes with associated health risks. Specifically, a BMI between 30.0 and 34.9 refers to Obese Class I with high health risk, a BMI between 35.0 and 39.9 refers to Obese Class II and very high health risk, and a BMI greater than 40.0 is classified as Obese Class III with extremely high health risk.

Why the difference in acceptable fat levels between men and women? Much of it can be attributed to genetics and, more specifically, related to the structure of the female body and to sex hormones. Body composition is most often broken down into two main components: fat-free mass and fat mass. Fat-free mass is made up of all the body's components other than fat—that is, the structural and functional elements in cells, body water, muscle, bones, and other body organs such as the heart, liver, and kidneys. Compared with men, women have a lower ratio of fat-free mass to fat mass, in part due to the genetic differences in bone size and mass, muscle size, and other variables. Women also experience greater weight and fat fluctuation due to hormonal changes, pregnancy, and menopause.

Body fat is composed of two types: essential fat and storage fat. Essential fat is necessary for normal physiological functioning, such as nerve conduction. Essential fat makes up approximately three to seven percent of total body weight in men and approximately 10 to 15 percent in women. Storage fat, which serves to insulate, pad, and protect the body from cold and trauma, makes up the remainder of our fat. It accounts for only a small percentage of total body weight for very lean people and between 5 and 25 percent of body weight for most healthy Canadian adults. Female bodybuilders, who are among the leanest of female athletes, may have a healthy body fat percentage in the range of 8 to 13 percent, nearly all of which is essential fat.

Similar to too much fat putting one's health at risk, too little fat also can relate to poor health. A minimal amount of fat is necessary for insulating the body, for cushioning between parts of the body and vital organs, and for maintaining several body functions. Although tremendous variation exists, it is generally suggested that in men this lower limit is approximately 3 to 4 percent and for women, 8 percent. Excessively low

TABLE 6.1

General Ratings of Body Fat Percentages by Age and Sex

Rating	Males (ages 18–30) (%)	Females (ages 18–30) (%)
Athletic*	6–10	10–15
Good	11–14	16–19
Acceptable	15–17	20–24
Overfat	18–19	25–29
Obese	20 or over	30 or over

* The ratings in the Athletic category are general guidelines for athletes involved in aesthetic or lean-weight sports such as gymnastics, diving, distance running, etc. where a low level of body fat and/or weight often confers a competitive advantage.

TABLE 6.2

Health Risk Classification for Adults* According to BMI

BMI	Weight Classification	Risk of Developing a Health Problem
30.0	Obese	High
30.1–34.9	Obese Class I	High
35.0–39.9	Obese Class II	Very high
> 40.0	Obese Class III	Extremely high

* These cut-off values and weight and health classifications are not applicable to growing children and adolescents.

Overweight: A weight greater than expected for a specific height.

Obesity: An excessive accumulation of body fat at which level the risk for health problems is increased.

Body mass index (BMI): A technique of weight assessment based on the relationship of weight to height.

Body Mass Index

Height (feet / inches)

Weight (lb)	5'0"	5'1"	5'2"	5'3"	5'4"	5'5"	5'6"	5'7"	5'8"	5'9"	5'10"	5'11"	6'0"	6'1"	6'2"	6'3"	6'4"	Weight (kg)
100	20	19	18	18	17	17	16	16	15	15	14	14	14	13	13	12	12	45
105	21	20	19	19	18	17	17	16	16	16	15	15	14	14	13	13	13	47
110	21	21	20	19	19	18	18	17	17	16	16	15	15	15	14	14	13	50
115	22	22	21	20	20	19	19	18	17	17	17	16	16	15	15	14	14	52
120	23	23	22	21	21	20	19	19	18	18	17	17	16	16	15	15	15	54
125	24	24	23	22	21	21	20	20	19	18	18	17	17	16	16	16	15	57
130	25	25	24	23	22	22	21	20	20	19	19	18	18	17	17	16	16	59
135	26	26	25	24	23	22	22	21	21	20	20	19	18	18	17	17	16	61
140	27	26	26	25	24	23	23	22	21	21	20	20	19	18	18	17	17	63
145	28	27	27	26	25	24	23	23	22	21	21	20	20	19	19	18	18	66
150	29	28	27	27	26	25	24	23	23	22	22	21	20	20	19	19	18	68
155	30	29	28	27	27	26	25	24	24	23	22	22	21	20	20	19	19	70
160	31	30	29	28	27	27	26	25	24	24	23	22	22	21	21	20	19	72
165	32	31	30	29	28	27	27	26	25	24	24	23	22	22	21	21	20	75
170	33	32	31	30	29	28	27	27	26	25	24	24	23	22	22	21	21	77
175	34	33	32	31	30	29	28	27	27	26	25	24	24	23	23	22	21	79
180	35	34	33	32	31	30	29	28	27	27	26	25	24	24	23	22	22	82
185	36	35	34	33	32	31	30	29	28	27	27	26	25	24	24	23	23	84
190	37	36	35	34	33	32	31	30	29	28	27	26	26	25	25	24	23	86
195	38	37	36	35	33	32	31	31	30	29	28	27	26	26	25	24	24	88
200	39	38	37	35	34	33	32	31	30	30	29	28	27	26	26	25	24	91
205	40	39	37	36	35	34	33	32	31	30	29	29	28	27	26	26	25	93
210	41	40	38	37	36	35	34	33	32	31	30	29	28	28	27	26	26	95
215	42	41	39	38	37	36	35	34	33	32	31	30	29	28	28	27	26	98
220	43	42	40	39	38	37	36	34	33	32	32	31	30	29	28	27	27	100
225	44	43	41	40	39	37	36	35	34	33	32	31	31	30	29	28	27	102
230	45	43	42	41	39	38	37	36	35	34	33	32	31	30	30	29	28	104
235	46	44	43	42	40	39	38	37	36	35	34	33	32	31	30	29	29	107
240	47	45	44	43	41	40	39	38	36	35	34	33	33	32	31	30	29	109
245	48	46	45	43	42	41	40	38	37	36	35	34	33	32	31	31	30	111
250	49	47	46	44	43	42	40	39	38	37	36	35	34	33	32	31	30	114
Height (centimetres)	150.0	152.5	155.0	157.5	160.0	162.5	165.0	167.5	170.0	172.5	175.0	177.5	180.0	182.5	185.0	187.5	190.0	

Legend:
- Underweight
- Weight appropriate
- Overweight
- Obese

FIGURE 6.2

What is your weight status? To find out, find your height (either at the top [in feet and inches] or bottom [in centimetres]) and your weight (at the right [in kilograms] or left [in pounds]) and find where these two intersect.

Nutrition: Findings from the Canadian Community Health Survey—Measured Obesity

Information on the prevalence of obesity (based on BMI) in adults gathered from the 2004 Canadian Community Health Survey (CCHS) was released in July 2005. Unique to this survey was that body mass index (BMI) was calculated from measured rather than self-reported height and weight. This is significant because, typically, people overestimate their height and underestimate their weight in measures of self-report, resulting in an underestimation of BMI. Thus, it is important to keep in mind that it is likely that the data reported in previous surveys underestimated the prevalence of overweight and obesity in the Canadian population.

Results from the CCHS indicate that 23.1 percent of adult Canadians (aged 18 or older) were classified as obese (BMI ≥ 30). Further, 36.1 percent of Canadian adults were considered overweight (BMI > 25 < 30). All together, more than half (59.1 percent) of the Canadian population is overweight or obese. Of significant concern is the percentage of the population that meet the criteria for Class II (BMI 35–39.99) and Class III (BMI ≥ 40) obesity; that is, 5.1 percent and 2.7 percent, respectively.

The percentage of males classified as overweight (42.0 percent) was significantly greater than that of females (30.2 percent). Although, there were no significant differences in the estimates of males (22.9 percent) and females for obesity (23.2 percent), when the three classes of obesity (that is, a BMI 30–34.9, BMI 35.–39.9, and BMI ≥ 40.) were combined, there were a greater percentage of females (3.8 versus 1.6 percent) in the Class III category (that is, BMI ≥ 40.0).

Obesity rates were greatest among the 45- to 54-year-olds and lowest in the 18- to 24-year-olds (29.9 vs. 10.7 percent). Overweight was greatest in the 65- to 74-year-olds and lowest in the 18- to 24-year-olds (52.7 vs. 27.0 percent).

In regard to provincial data, the highest rates of obesity were found in Newfoundland and Labrador (33.3 percent), New Brunswick (30.8 percent), and Saskatchewan (30.4 percent), with the lowest prevalence in British Columbia (18.2 percent).

STUDY QUESTIONS:

1. Why do think the rate of overweight and obesity increased in the Canadian population? Is this a real change or simply an issue of more accurate measurement?

2. What effect will this rise in overweight and obesity have on Canada's Health System? On individual health and wellness?

Source: Statistics Canada, 2005, "Nutrition: Findings from the Canadian Community Health Survey, Measured Obesity, Adult Obesity in Canada: Measured Height and Weight," Catalogue No. 82-620-MWE2005001. Retrieved on December 9, 2005, from www.statcan.ca/english/research/82-620-MIE/2005001/articles/adults/aobesity.htm. Adapted and reproduced with permission of the Minister of Public Works and Government Services of Canada, 2007.

---

body fat in females may lead to amenorrhea or oligomenorrhea, a cessation or disruption of the menstrual cycle respectively. The critical level of body fat necessary to maintain normal menstrual flow is believed to be between 8 and 13 percent, with exceptions to this rule and many additional factors that affect the menstrual cycle. Under extreme circumstances, such as starvation diets and certain diseases, the body exhausts available fat reserves and begins breaking down muscle tissue in a last-ditch effort to obtain sufficient nourishment.

Assessing Your Body Fat Content

Since both too little and too much body fat may pose a health risk, it can be important to know your actual level of body fat. But how is fat measured? Many options are available and an accurate assessment of body fat requires a different type of measurement than

what can be obtained using traditional height–weight charts or calculations of BMI. How do you decide which of the techniques available are the best for you? Several factors should be considered before you make this decision. Cost and access may be two of those factors, since some techniques are relatively expensive and inaccessible. Another factor to consider is your reason for wanting to know your body fat content and whether or not it is essential for you to have a precise measure. At the most basic level, if your previously well-fitting jeans are now too tight, you know you have gained weight/fat and ought to take action to prevent further weight gain. Similarly, if your well-fitting jeans continue to fit well, you have maintained your weight.

Although assessments of body composition generally quantify body weight into its basic components—that is, fat-free mass and fat mass[7]—estimates of body fat are considered most important for the health-related components of physical fitness. Further, although the various methods used to measure body fat can be useful, there are limits to the accuracy of measurement, even when the testers are skilful and well trained. Before agreeing to any procedure, be aware of the expense, risks, measurement error, and training of the tester. Further, consider what you will do with the value, once known.

Dual-Energy X-Ray Absorptiometry

Dual-energy X-ray absorptiometry (DXA) measures bone mineral content and lean and fat tissue.[8] This technique requires a low radiation exposure from a low-energy and high-energy photon beam. Based on appropriate computer algorithms and the amount of absorption of the photon beams by the atoms in bone mineral and soft tissues, an estimate of bone mineral, fat-free soft tissue, and fat tissue is made. A strength of the DXA method is that total body fat can be determined as well as regional body fat distribution. Further, some consider DXA to be the most accurate or "gold standard" assessment of body composition.

Hydrostatic Weighing

Hydrostatic weighing was previously considered the gold standard for measuring body composition. This method measures the amount of water a person displaces when completely submerged. Because fat tissue has a lower density than muscle or bone tissue, body fat can be computed using a person's underwater and out-of-water weights.

Air Displacement Plethysmography

Air displacement plethysmography (ADP) has become popular in recent years to measure body composition. Based on the same premises as

The Bod Pod is an example of air displacement plethysmography.

hydrostatic weighing, total body volume is measured—this time from air displacement—from which an estimate of body fat can be made. Estimates of total body volume (either in water or air) use the formula density = mass ÷ volume.[9] The major assumption and limitation of these two methods is that the density of fat and fat-free mass (fat-free mass being all components of the body except fat) is considered constant. The limitation, then, relates to bone mineral content and density, which is known to vary throughout the life cycle.

Skinfold Measurements

Perhaps the most commonly used method to estimate body fat is **skinfold measurements**. In this procedure, a person grasps folds of skin and the underlying tissue with the thumb and index finger and then a specially calibrated instrument called a "skinfold" caliper is applied to take the measurement. The eight sites most commonly measured on the right side of the body include the triceps (back of the arm), biceps (front of the arm), subscapular (on the back), iliac crest (on the side of the body—near the "love handles"), supraspinale (along the front of the body over the hip), abdominal (next to the umbilicus—belly button), front thigh (middle of the upper leg), and medial calf (middle, inside of the lower leg). Once these sites

Hydrostatic weighing is one technique used to estimate body fat.

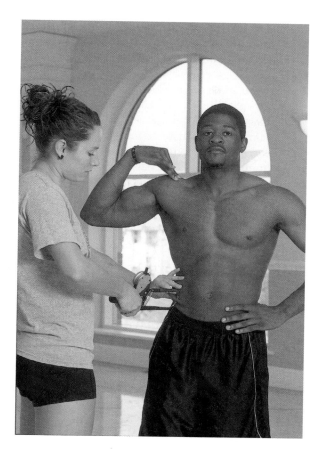

In the hands of a trained professional, skinfold calipers can be used to provide an accurate measure of body fat for people who are not overly fat.

what do you THINK?

Is it important to you to know your current level of body fat? Why or why not? Which of the tests would you feel comfortable taking? Would any make you feel uncomfortable? Why or why not?

Waist Circumference

A common method of assessing abdominal body fat is **waist circumference**. A simple measuring tape is used to take the girth, or circumference, measurement at the superior border or top of the iliac crest or hip bones. Regardless of where measured (for example, at the smallest point of the torso, at the level of the umbilicus [that is, belly button], or the top of the hip bones), a larger waist circumference is associated with greater health risk.[11] Specifically, a waist circumference greater than 102 centimetres in men and 88 centimetres in women indicates increased risk of heart disease, type 2 diabetes, metabolic syndrome, hypertension, and hyperlipidemia.[12]

Bioelectrical Impedance Analysis

Another method of determining body fat levels, **bioelectrical impedance analysis (BIA)**, involves sending a weak electric current through the body. The rationale for this technique is based on the greater electrolyte and water content of fat free versus fat tissue.[13] The amount of resistance to the current, along with the person's age, sex, and other physical characteristics, is then fed into a computer that uses a special formula to determine the total amount of fat-free and

are measured, formulas can be used to predict total body fat.[10] In the hands of trained technicians, this procedure can be fairly accurate. However, the fatter a person is, the more prone this technique is to error. For people who are obese, difficulties in assessment are magnified because of problems distinguishing between flaccid muscles and fat. Also, most skinfold calipers do not expand far enough to obtain measurements from the moderately obese (20 to 40 percent fat) or morbidly obese (more than 40 percent fat). Additional errors in estimating percentage of body fat from skinfold assessments may occur as a result of failure to account for certain age, sex, and ethnic differences in the calculations.

An alternative to predicting percentage of body fat from skinfold measurements is to simply total them. A "sum of skinfolds" also allows for comparison of "before" and "after" measurements. Since approximately 50 percent of body fat lies below the skin (that is, as subcutaneous fat), a loss in total sum of skinfolds indicates a loss of total body fat. Similarly, a gain in sum of skinfolds indicates a gain in total body fat.

Dual-energy X-ray absorptiometry (DXA): A method of body composition assessment in which estimates are made of bone mineral content and lean and fat mass.

Hydrostatic weighing: A method of determining body fat by measuring the amount of water displaced when a person is completely submerged.

Air displacement plethysmography (ADP): A method used to determine body fat from estimates of total body volume.

Skinfold measurements: A method of assessing body fat where double folds of skin and the underlying tissue are measured with skinfold calipers.

Waist circumference: A method of assessing abdominal fat where a measuring tape is used to assess the girth at the top of the iliac crest.

Bioelectrical impedance analysis (BIA): A technique of body fat assessment in which the resistance to a weak electrical current is measured.

fat tissue. This technique has increased in use in recent years, likely because of its convenience, low cost, non-invasiveness, and quick estimate of body fat. Keep in mind however that it is important for the body to be normally hydrated when using BIA because even small fluctuations in body water content alter the assessment. Even with adequate hydration and nutritional status, significant error can result in body composition estimates from BIA.

MANAGING YOUR WEIGHT

At some point in our lives, almost all of us will decide we need to do something about our weight. Many will choose to go on a diet, with initially successful results, but few of us will achieve long-term weight loss. The problem is that we think about losing weight via dieting, or lowering our calorie intake for the short term. Even if combined with increased exercise or physical activity, the change is viewed as temporary. What is needed instead is a lifetime approach to eating well, being physically active, and managing our behaviours around food, physical activity, and sedentary activities.

Keeping Weight Loss in Perspective

Long-term weight loss is difficult for many people and requires support from friends, family, and the community. As mentioned previously, it is often believed that losing weight is simple: we just need to burn more calories than we consume. Putting this principle into practice, however, is far from simple given our cultural attitudes and behaviours toward food and habitual levels of physical activity and sedentary activities. Other factors are involved, too—factors such as stress, food availability and accessibility, and depression. To reach and maintain the weight that is right for you— the weight at which you will be most healthy—you need to develop a lifelong approach to healthy eating, physical activity, and sedentary behaviours. Your eating habits cannot simply be a "diet" that you go on, because then it will be a diet that you can go off of as well. Similarly, your approach to being physically active must also be for your lifetime—while recognizing that there will be times when you will be more or less physically active.

What Is a Calorie?

A calorie is a unit of measurement that indicates the amount of energy obtained from a particular food. A kilogram of body fat contains approximately 7500 calories. So each time you consume 7500 calories more than your body needs, you gain a kilogram (or, roughly, two pounds). Conversely, each time your body expends an extra 7500 calories, you lose a kilogram. If you add a can of Coca-Cola (140 calories) to your daily caloric intake and make no other changes in your dietary intake or physical activity, you would gain a kilogram in approximately 54 days (7500 calories ÷ 140 calories/day = 53.6 days). Conversely, if you walked for half an hour each day at a pace of 9 minutes per kilometre (172 calories burned), you would lose a kilogram in 44 days (7500 calories ÷ 172 calories/ day = 43.6 days), assuming you make no other changes to dietary intake or physical activity habits.

✳ Physical Activity

Approximately 90 percent of the daily calorie expenditures of most people occurs as a result of their **resting metabolic rate (RMR)**. RMR is greater than BMR (or **basal metabolic rate**, which is the amount of energy our bodies burn at complete rest; this will be discussed at greater length later in the chapter); RMR includes BMR plus any additional energy expended through daily sedentary activities, such as food digestion, sitting, studying, or standing.

Exercise metabolic rate (EMR) accounts for the remaining 10 percent and specifically refers to the energy expenditure as a result of physical activity. For most of us, this caloric expenditure comes in the form of light daily activities, such as walking, climbing stairs, doing the dishes, running the vacuum, and mowing the lawn. If we increase the level and intensity of our physical activity to moderate or heavy, our EMR may be 10 to 20 times greater and contribute more substantially to our energy needs.

Increasing BMR (which is the energy expenditure of the body under resting conditions at normal room temperature), RMR, or EMR levels will require more

try it NOW!

Set SuPeRSMART goals for weight maintenance or even weight loss. Give your goals a reality check: are they Self-controllable, Public, Rewarded, Specific, Measurable, Achievable, Relevant, and Time Specific? For example, rather than aiming to lose 10 kilograms this month (which is *not* healthy—nor realistic or achievable), set a comfortable goal of not *gaining* any weight and/or losing 1 to 2 kilograms. Realistic goals encourage success by boosting confidence in your ability to make lifelong healthy changes.

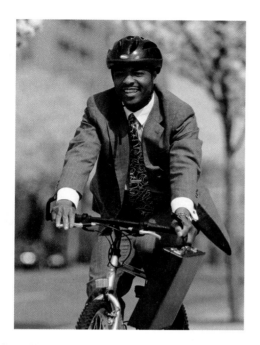

A physically active lifestyle is the key to balancing caloric intake with caloric output for weight maintenance.

calories for weight maintenance. An increase in the intensity, frequency, and time or duration of your daily physical activities will have a significant impact on your total calorie expenditure and ability to manage your weight. Current recommendations are that at least 60 minutes of moderate-intensity physical activity each day are required for weight management. Further, emphasis should be placed on cardiorespiratory and strength-related physical activities.

Physical activity makes a greater contribution to EMR when large muscle groups are used. The energy spent on physical activity includes the energy used to move the body's muscles—the muscles of the arms, back, abdomen, legs, and so on—and the extra energy required to increase heartbeat, respiration rate, blood pressure, body cooling, etc. The number of calories expended depends on three factors:

1. the amount of muscle mass being moved
2. the amount of weight being moved
3. the amount of time the activity takes

For example, an activity involving the arms and the legs burns more calories than one involving only the legs, an activity performed by a heavy person burns more calories than one performed by a lighter person, and an activity performed for 40 minutes requires twice as much energy as the same activity performed for 20 minutes. Thus, persons who are obese who walk 1 kilometre burn more calories than people who are slim and walk the same distance. It may also take a person who is obese longer to walk a specified dis-

tance, which means they burn energy for a longer time and therefore expend more overall calories than walkers who are thin and complete the walk in a shorter time.[14]

Determining the Caloric Output of Your Physical Activity

The number of calories required to do a physical activity depends on a number of factors, one of which is how much you weigh. The more you weigh, the greater the caloric cost of the physical activity. In other words, you use more calories when you weigh more. Another factor is how intensely—or how hard—you participate in that physical activity. More intense physical activities require more energy to perform. The third factor that influences the number of calories required to do a particular physical activity is time. Obviously, the longer you do the physical activity, the more energy it requires. The latter two factors, intensity of activity and length of time, interact. Most often, more intense physical activities (for instance, running) can only be done for shorter periods of time, and less intense physical activities (for instance, walking) can be done for longer periods of time.

The following physical activities each require about 150 calories of energy to perform (with an average body weight of around 68 kilograms):[15]

- gardening for 30 to 45 minutes
- raking leaves for 30 minutes
- shovelling snow for 15 minutes
- walking 3 kilometres in approximately 30 minutes
- pushing a stroller when walking for 30 minutes
- running 2.25 kilometres in 15 minutes
- climbing the stairs for 15 minutes
- playing touch football for 30 to 45 minutes
- playing basketball (that is, shooting baskets) for 30 minutes
- playing basketball (that is, a game) for 15 to 20 minutes
- playing wheelchair basketball for 20 minutes

Resting metabolic rate (RMR): The energy expenditure of the body while at rest, which includes basal metabolic rate (the metabolic rate of the body at complete rest) plus the energy required by sedentary activities, such as food digestion, sitting, studying, or standing.

Basal metabolic rate (BMR): The energy expenditure of the body under resting conditions at normal room temperature.

Exercise metabolic rate (EMR): The energy expenditure of physical activity.

- bicycling 7.5 kilometres in 30 minutes
- dancing (social) for 30 minutes
- swimming laps for 20 minutes
- water fitness classes for 30 minutes
- jumping rope for 30 minutes

Another way to determine the number of calories required by a particular physical activity is to use established energy costs for that physical activity, along with your body weight (in kilograms) and the time you engaged in that physical activity, to calculate your energy costs. This method takes into account the three factors that are involved in determining the energy costs of physical activity: body weight, intensity, and time.

Table 6.3 provides a sample of the energy costs of selected physical activities per minute per kilogram. Thus, if you weigh 65 kilograms and go for a 30-minute run at a pace of 5 minutes per kilometre, you will use 362 calories (65 kg × 0.1856 cal/min/kg × 30 minutes = 362 calories). You would need to run for only 24 minutes at a pace of 3.7 minutes per kilometre to use the same approximate number of calories (that is, 65 kg × 0.2350 cal/min/kg × 24 minutes = 367 calories).

✱ Is Dieting Healthy?

Most experts agree that the ultimate goal of a weight-loss program should be improved quality of life and lifetime weight maintenance.[16] Weight goals should be set to reduce health risks and address medical problems and to help people improve their ability to perform daily tasks without undue stress and strain—rather than to achieve an "ideal" weight or shape. In addition, experts agree that weight-loss programs that promote qualitative rather than quantitative changes

in food intake improve health and long-term weight maintenance and are more easily sustained than those that force people to severely restrict intake of calories or specific foods.[17] But while the experts seem to agree on these points, many weight-loss programs fail to follow these basic premises. What happens to people who get caught up in "lose weight fast and furiously" campaigns? Researchers are increasingly concerned that:

- dieting to lose weight may be more harmful than helpful in promoting physiological health and psychological well-being[18]
- because dieting only rarely produces successful long-term weight loss, the physiological and psychological stress, damage to self-esteem, and other emotional disturbances are without purpose[19]
- dieting causes repeated cycles of weight loss and regain, changes in metabolic rates, increased risk for cardiovascular problems, and other conditions adverse to health[20]
- dieting contributes to the development of eating disorders such as anorexia and bulimia nervosa, and compulsive eating or binge eating disorder[21]

Most health authorities recommend that, rather than going on a diet, a person should adopt a lifetime approach to healthy eating, physical activity, and sedentary activities aimed at enhancing metabolic rates and maintaining muscle mass.

what do you THINK?

Consider your approach to eating; Do you think about your food choices (including quantity) as part of your overall approach to being healthy in the long-term? Or do you make decisions related to short-term gain (that is, dieting)? How can you develop a lifetime approach to healthy eating?

TABLE 6.3

Energy Costs of Selected Physical Activities (min/kg)

Physical Activity	Time	Cal/min/kg
Walking (on a grassy surface)	10.5 min/km	0.0794
Cycling	4 min/km	0.0985
Cycling	3.1 min/km	0.1559
Swimming	55 min/km	0.1333
Running	3.7 min/km	0.2350
Running	5 min/km	0.1856

Source: Adapted from B. Getchell, *Physical Fitness: A Way of Life* (Benjamin Cummings, 1992).

✱ Improving Your Eating Habits

Before you can change a given behaviour, you must first determine what causes and relates to that behaviour. Why do you suddenly find yourself at the refrigerator door eating? Why do you take a second and third helping of potatoes or dessert when you know that you have had enough to eat and your body does not need more? Our eating is influenced by a number of things including individual and environmental determinants.[22] Individual determinants include our physiological state (that is, whether or not we are hungry), food preferences, nutritional knowledge, perceptions of healthy eating, and psychological factors. Environmental factors include the interpersonal environment created by our family and peers, the physical environment, which determines food accessibility and availability, the economic and social environment, and the cultural milieu surrounding food choices. Further, food policy has an overarching influence on the individual and environmental factors influencing our eating behaviours.

Many people discovered that one of the best ways of assessing their eating behaviours is to chart exactly when they feel like eating, where they are when they eat, the amount of time they spend eating, other activities they engage in while eating (watching television, reading, or something else), whether they eat alone or with others, what and how much they eat, and how they feel before they take their first bite. If you keep a detailed log each day for a week, you will discover useful clues about what in your environment or in your emotional makeup relates to your eating habits. Typically, these "triggers" centre on issues related to everyday living rather than on real hunger/need to eat. As you record this information, your reasons for eating will often become apparent. Many people discover that they eat compulsively when stressed or when they have problems in their relationships. For others, it is the smell of a particular food (for example, popcorn) or a routine (for example, eating while studying) that causes them to eat, rather than hunger itself.

Once you recognize the factors that relate to your eating, remove the triggers or substitute other activities so that you develop more sensible eating behaviours. Here are some examples (see also Skills for Behaviour Change):

1. When eating dinner, turn off all distractions, including the television, radio, and your computer.
2. Include physical activity in your coffee breaks.
3. Instead of gulping your food, chew slowly, putting your fork down between each bite.
4. Instead of eating by the clock, eat when you are hungry.
5. Eat frequently throughout the day—three smaller meals per day plus snacks—rather than loading up at one meal and skipping others.
6. If you find that you generally eat all that is on a plate, use smaller plates, or serve smaller portions. Serve your plate at the counter/stove rather than having pots/bowls on the table where you are eating.
7. If you find that you are continually seeking your favourite foods, buy them in smaller quantities, serve them in smaller portions, and store them in an inconvenient spot.
8. Eat breakfast every day.
9. Replace soft drinks with water.

what do you THINK?

Based on what you have read so far, what triggers your eating? Is it certain people? Places? Situations? What can you do to manage these triggers?

Selecting a Nutritional Plan

Once you discover what factors influence your eating, you will be on your way to successful weight maintenance. To be successful, however, you must plan for success.

Seek help from reputable sources in choosing a dietary plan that is easy to follow and includes adequate nutrients. Registered dietitians, holistic physicians (only holistic physicians have strong backgrounds in nutrition, which includes some MDs), health educators, exercise physiologists with nutritional backgrounds, and other health professionals can provide reliable information. Avoid quick weight-loss programs that promise miracle results. The majority of these programs are expensive, and most people regain the weight soon after completing them. Ask questions about the credentials of the adviser in any weight-loss program/centre, assess the nutrient value of the prescribed diet, verify that dietary guidelines are consistent with information from reliable dietary research, and analyze how suitable the dietary plan is for your tastes, budget, and lifestyle to avoid putting yourself in a risky, expensive, or unhealthy dietary situation. Any diet that requires radical behaviour changes or cannot be followed for a lifetime is doomed to fail. Dietary plans that do not ask you to sacrifice what you enjoy and that allow you to make choices are usually the most successful.

"Miracle" Diets

Fasting, starvation diets, and other forms of **very low-calorie diets (VLCDs)** are related to significant health risks. Typically, when you deprive your body of food for prolonged periods, it makes adjustments to save you from inevitable organ shutdown. First, it depletes its energy reserves to maintain its supply of glucose. One of the first reserves to which the body turns is lean protein tissue. When this occurs you lose weight rapidly because significant water is lost as well. Over time, the body begins to run out of liver tissue, heart muscle, blood, and so on, as these readily available substances are used to supply energy. Only after

Very-low-calorie diets (VLCDs): Diets with caloric value of 400 to 700 calories per day.

General Tips for Managing Your Weight

WHEN EATING AT HOME

- Eat only in the kitchen or dining room. Keep food out of the living room, bedroom, and study spaces.
- Spread your caloric intake throughout the day by eating smaller meals four to five times a day (this enhances RMR).
- Use a smaller plate and fill it with low-calorie, nutrient-dense foods such as salad without dressing or with a small amount of dressing on the side, and pasta with a low-fat sauce.
- Take more time to eat; at least 20 minutes per meal is recommended. Chew your food carefully, setting your fork down between bites and enjoying the taste.
- Drink a glass of water before your meal.
- Drink a glass of water when you think you are hungry; you may actually be thirsty; hunger is often mistaken for thirst.
- Brush your teeth after eating to signify the end of your meal.
- Limit your purchases of high-calorie, high-fat, low-nutrient foods, even for guests or even on holidays.
- When having desserts, limit yourself to a small taste, or choose lower-calorie, lower-fat options.
- Get in tune with your true feelings of hunger. Eat when you are really hungry, not by the clock.
- Develop stress-management skills that do not involve eating.
- Get enough sleep; individuals with a "sleep debt" are at greater risk for obesity.
- Try not to allow yourself to get too hungry before eating.

- Limit the amount you eat immediately before going to bed.
- Put serving dishes on the counter or stove while you are eating. Leaving them on the table encourages second helpings even when you are no longer hungry.

WHEN EATING OUT

- Ask for it "your way." Request that the cheese be left off, the sauce cut in half, salad dressing on the side, and so on.
- Ask that entrées be broiled, steamed, baked, grilled, poached, or roasted, with only a small amount of fat used for the cooking process.
- When ordering omelettes, ask for a one- or two-egg-yolk version containing only the whites of the other eggs. Limit meat and cheese fillings. Choose vegetable fillings whenever possible.
- Reduce portion size. Order à la carte if possible, with a salad or fresh vegetable on the side.
- Limit how frequently you eat at an all-you-can-eat restaurant.
- Drink at least one glass of water before starting your meal. Try to relax while eating and make your mealtime last. Talk more, put your fork down more frequently, chew more, and generally slow down.
- Order fresh fruits and low- or no-fat yoghurts in place of heavy desserts.
- Frequent restaurants that offer low-fat, high-complex-carbohydrate meals.
- Choose water or low-fat milk as your beverage.

---

the readily available proteins from these sources are depleted will your body begin to use fat reserves. In this process, known as **ketosis**, the body adapts to prolonged fasting or carbohydrate deprivation by converting body fat to ketones, which can be used as fuel for

try it NOW!

Make healthy substitutions at meal time—a successful key to weight maintenance! The next time you make dinner, take a look at the portions on your plate. Vegetables and whole grains should take up most of the space; if not, substitute a portion of meat, pasta, or cheese for an equal portion of legumes, salad greens, or a favourite vegetable. This will reduce the calorie content of your meal without sacrificing quantity.

some brain cells. About 10 days after the typical adult begins a complete fast, the body has used many of its energy stores and death may occur.

In very-low-calorie diets, powdered formulas are usually given to patients under medical supervision. These formulas range from 400 to 700 calories plus vitamin and mineral supplements. Although these diets may be beneficial for people who have failed at all conventional weight-loss methods and who face severe threats to their health complicated by their obesity, they should never be undertaken without close medical supervision. Problems associated with fasting, VLCDs, and other forms of severe calorie deprivation include blood sugar imbalances, cold intolerance, constipation, decreased BMR, dehydration, diarrhea, emotional problems, fatigue, headaches, heart irregularity, ketosis, kidney infections and failure, loss of lean body tissue, weakness, and weight gain due to the yo-yo effect and other problems.

Trying to Gain Weight

Although trying to lose weight poses a major challenge for many, there is a another group of people who, for a variety of metabolic, hereditary, psychological, and other reasons, cannot seem to gain weight no matter how hard they try. If you are one of these individuals, you must determine why you have difficulty in gaining weight—just like someone who has difficulty keeping his or her weight down. Once you have answered this question, there are several things you can do to help yourself:

- Monitor your physical activity. Keep a careful record of calories burned; perhaps you are not eating enough to compensate. In addition to your exercise, monitor your incidental movements (that is, active transportation, fidgeting behaviours, etc.). These contribute to caloric needs as well.

- Eat more. Eat more often. It is possible that you are not eating enough calories to support your body's needs. Eat more frequently, spend more time eating, and eat high-calorie, nutrient-dense foods first if you tend to fill up fast. Take time to shop and to cook, and eat slowly. Make your sandwiches with extra-thick slices of bread and add more filling such as peanut butter, cream cheese, or cheese. Eat second helpings whenever possible and eat high-calorie, nutrient-dense snacks during the day.

- Drink more of your calories; instead of water, choose milk or juice.

- Try to relax. Many people who are underweight also suffer from anxiety and the "hurry syndrome." Slow down and try to manage your reactions to stress.

RISK FACTORS FOR OBESITY

It would seem that the cause of obesity is quite simple: when you take in more calories than you burn, you gain weight—most often in the form of fat. If you do this frequently enough, you will become obese. If we know what the cause is, we should be able to offer a simple solution for prevention, right?

Wrong. Although the calorie balance equation (that is, if calories in equals calories out there is no weight gain) explanation of weight management is valid, it offers only two simple reasons for a person's weight gain: we eat too much and do too little. It does not include the many other sociocultural factors surrounding dietary intake and our physical activity behaviours that contribute to excessive food consumption or low levels of physical activity. It also fails to answer many other critical questions. If we know that eating too much will cause us to gain weight, why do we continue to eat so much? If we know we should be more physically active, why don't we simply get out there and "do it"? Is there a metabolic explanation for obesity? Why is there limited success for permanent weight loss from dieting?

✔• Heredity and Genetic Factors

Are some people born to be fat? Many factors influence why one person becomes obese and another remains thin; genes seem to interact with many of these factors. More than 250 gene markers have been identified as related to obesity in more than 400 studies.[23]

Body Type and Genes

In some animal species, the shape and size of the individual's body is largely determined by the shape and size of its parents' bodies. Many scientists have explored the role of heredity in determining human body shapes or physiques. As early as 1940, Harvard psychologist William Sheldon analyzed weight problems in terms of somatotypes.[24] A somatotype provides a classification of an individual's physique or body as a whole and is comprised of three components: endomorphy, mesomorphy, and ectomorphy.[25] Endomorphy describes the relative fatness of the body, specifically referring to roundness and soft appearance. In Sheldon's work, individuals with a high endomorphic rating often had a large abdomen and typically reported a history of weight problems beginning in childhood. Mesomorphy refers to the relative muscularity of the body; individuals with a high mesomorphic rating have a tendency to gain weight later in life. Ectomorphy describes the relative linearity of the body, with individuals rating high in this component characterized as tall with slender frames and generally experiencing few difficulties with weight control.

Although somatotype may play a role in the development of obesity, most researchers contend that heredity plays a more subtle role. These researchers argue that obesity has a strong genetic determinant (it tends to run in families) and cite statistics suggesting that 40 percent of children with one obese parent and 80 percent of children with two obese parents are also likely to be obese.[26] Studies of identical twins separated at birth and raised in different environments have provided some of the most compelling evidence to date that obesity may be genetically determined.

Ketosis: A condition in which the body adapts to prolonged fasting or carbohydrate deprivation by converting body fat to ketones, which can be used as fuel for some brain activity.

Whether raised in environments with fat or thin family members, twins with obese birth parents tended to be obese in later life.[27] According to another study, identical twins separated and raised in different families who ate widely different diets still grew up to weigh about the same.[28]

Obesity Genes?

Recent research points to the existence of a "fat gene." Rather than inheriting a particular body type that predisposes us to become overweight or obese, it may be that our genes predispose us toward certain satiety and feeding behaviours. This "I need to eat" gene may account for up to one-third of our risk for obesity.[29] The most promising candidate is the GAD2 gene. For some individuals, a variation in this gene increases the production of a chemical that boosts appetite and signals a person to eat.[30]

Another gene getting a lot of attention is an Ob gene (for obesity) which is believed to disrupt the body's "I've had enough to eat" signalling system and may prompt individuals to keep eating past the point of being comfortably full. Research on Pima Indians, a group with an estimated 75 percent obesity rate and 90 percent rate of overweight, points to an Ob gene that is a "thrifty gene." It is theorized that because their ancestors struggled through centuries of famine, during which the Ob gene prompted them to eat as much as possible when food was available and to conserve when not, their basal metabolic rates slowed, which allowed them to store precious fat. Survivors may have passed their genes on to their descendants, which may explain their lower metabolic rates and tendency toward obesity today.[31]

Endocrine Influences: The Hungry Hormones

Over the years, many people attributed obesity to problems with their thyroid gland and resultant hormonal imbalances. They believed that an underactive thyroid impeded their ability to burn calories. Research indicates that less than 2 percent of the population that is obese can trace their weight and/or fat problems to their thyroid, or metabolic or hormonal imbalances.[32] Researchers continue to investigate the influence of various hormones on a person's ability to attain and maintain weight loss, and control appetite and satiety or sense of fullness.

One such hormone that researchers suspect may play a role in our ability to maintain weight loss, based on its role in appetite stimulation, is ghrelin. Specifically, it was noted in a small group of people who were obese and lost weight over six months that

their ghrelin levels—which are produced in the stomach—rose before every meal and fell drastically shortly after. Another hormone believed to be involved in the satiety signal from the brain, which tells us to stop eating because we are full, is leptin. Leptin and ghrelin are both believed to be influenced by lack of sleep. More specifically, fewer hours of sleep in standardized experimental sleeping conditions resulted in an increase in hunger accompanied by a decrease in leptin and an increase in ghrelin.[33] Yet another hormone involved in slowing the passage of food through the intestines is called GLP-1. It is believed that GLP-1 may stimulate insulin production and be a key factor in preventing and controlling type 2 diabetes and obesity.[34] It is further speculated that leptin and GLP-1 play complementary roles in weight control, where leptin regulates body weight and fat levels over the long term, calling on the fast-acting appetite suppressants GLP-1 when needed.

✳ Hunger, Appetite, and Satiety

Scientists distinguish between **hunger**, an inborn physiological response to nutritional needs, and **appetite**, a learned response to food tied to an emotional or psychological craving for food often unrelated to nutritional need. Obese people may be more likely than people at a healthy weight to satisfy their appetite and eat for reasons other than nutrition.

In some instances, the problem with overconsumption may be more related to **satiety** than to appetite or hunger. People generally feel satiated, or full, when they have satisfied their nutritional needs and their stomach signals "no more." For undetermined reasons, people who are obese may not feel full until much later than people who are at a healthy weight.

Theories abound concerning the mechanisms that regulate food intake. Some sources indicate that the hypothalamus (the part of the brain that regulates appetite) closely monitors levels of certain nutrients in the blood. When these levels begin to fall, the brain signals us to eat. In persons who are obese, it is possible that the monitoring system does not work properly and that the cues to eat are more frequent and intense than in people of a healthy weight.

Other sources indicate that people who are at a healthy weight may send more effective messages to the hypothalamus. This concept, known as **adaptive thermogenesis**, states that some people can consume lots of food without gaining weight because the appetite centre of their brains speeds up metabolic activity to compensate for the increased consumption. Still other studies indicate the possibility that specialized types of fat cells, called **brown fat cells**, may send signals to the brain, which controls the thermogenesis response.

Developmental Factors

Some people who are obese may have an excessive number of fat cells. **Hyperplasia**, which refers to an increase in the number of cells, normally occurs during specific periods of the growth process.[35] The only periods during which fat cells normally increase in number is during infancy and the rapid growth period of puberty. However, fat cells can also increase in number when an individual is under chronic positive energy balance (that is, they continuously consume more calories than they burn) and their current fat cells are "full." Fat cells also have the ability to increase in size. This process is called **hypertrophy**, and can occur at any time in childhood, adolescence, and adulthood—if calorie intake exceeds calorie output. Thus, fat gain is tied to the number of fat cells in the body (during infancy and puberty) and the capacity of the fat cells to increase in size (childhood, adolescence, and adulthood).

An adult of average weight and fat levels has approximately 30 to 50 billion fat cells,[36] an adult who is moderately obese has about 60 billion to 100 billion, and an adult who is extremely obese may have as many as 200 billion. The size of fat cells in a young adult of a healthy weight is about 80 to 100 micrometres (μm). (See Figure 6.3.)

People who are obese and have a large number of fat cells may have difficulty attaining long-term fat loss because there may be a trigger released once they have substantially decreased the size of each fat cell, resulting in an increase in appetite.

Metabolic Rates and Weight

Even at rest, our bodies need a certain amount of energy. As previously noted, the amount of energy the body requires at complete rest is called basal metabolic rate (BMR). In physically active individuals, about 60 to 70 percent of all the calories consumed support basal metabolism, which provides the energy (that is, calories) needed for bodily functions such as heartbeat, breathing, maintaining body temperature, and so on. So if you consume 2000 calories per day, between 1200 and 1400 of those calories are required for regular body maintenance. The remaining 600 to 800 calories supply the energy required for your physical activities. The key factor here is the amount of physical activity you do.

BMR fluctuates considerably. In general, the younger you are, the higher your BMR. BMR is greatest when we are younger partly because cells undergo rapid subdivision in young people, which requires a good deal of energy. Thus, BMR is highest during infancy, puberty, and pregnancy, when bodily changes are most rapid.

BMR is also influenced by body composition. Muscle tissue is highly active—even at rest—compared to fat tissue. In essence, the more muscle tissue you have, the greater your BMR. Thus, men usually have a higher BMR than women, because they have a greater muscle mass.

Age is another factor that affects BMR. After the age of 30, BMR slows down by about 1 to 2 percent per year. Therefore, people over 30 commonly find that they either have to eat less or do more physical activity to maintain their body weight. "Middle-aged spread," a reference to the tendency to gain weight or fat after the age of 30, is partly related to this change. A slower BMR, coupled with an inclination to be less physically

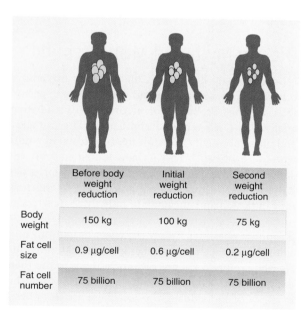

	Before body weight reduction	Initial weight reduction	Second weight reduction
Body weight	150 kg	100 kg	75 kg
Fat cell size	0.9 μg/cell	0.6 μg/cell	0.2 μg/cell
Fat cell number	75 billion	75 billion	75 billion

FIGURE 6.3

The figure depicts one person at various stages of fat loss. Note that the number of fat cells remains constant but the cells' size decreases.

Hunger: An inborn physiological response to nutritional needs.

Appetite: A learned response tied to an emotional or psychological craving for food often unrelated to nutritional need.

Satiety: The feeling of fullness or satisfaction after eating.

Adaptive thermogenesis: Theoretical mechanism by which the brain regulates metabolic activity according to caloric intake.

Brown fat cells: Specialized type of fat cell that affects the ability to regulate fat metabolism.

Hyperplasia: An increase in the number of cells.

Hypertrophy: An increase in the size of cells.

active, puts many middle-aged people's weight over healthy limits.

In addition, the body has a number of self-protective mechanisms that signal BMR to speed up or slow down. For example, when you have a fever, the energy needs of your cells increase, and this increased activity generates heat and increases your BMR. In starvation situations, the body protects itself by slowing the BMR to conserve energy. Thus, when people repeatedly resort to low-calorie diets, their bodies "reset" their BMRs to lower rates. **Yo-yo diets**, which involve people repeatedly gaining and losing weight, lower BMR in the process, and as a result are doomed to failure. When the dieters begin to eat again after the weight loss, their BMR is set lower, making it almost certain that they will regain the weight lost—and more. After repeated cycles of such dieting/regaining, these people find it increasingly hard to lose weight and increasingly easy to regain it, and so they become fatter. Besides an increase in fat, weight-cycling may also have a negative effect on an individual's risk for heart disease. Specifically, other health risks research indicated that middle-aged men who maintained a steady weight (even if overweight) had a lower risk of heart attack than men whose weight cycled in a yo-yo pattern.[37] Furthermore, it was noted that smaller, maintained weight losses were more beneficial for reducing cardiovascular risk than larger, poorly maintained weight losses.

Related to metabolic rate is a highly controversial theory called the **setpoint theory**. It states that a person's body has a setpoint of weight at which it is programmed to be comfortable. If your setpoint is 70 kilograms, you will gain and lose weight fairly easily within a given range around that setpoint. Can a person change this predetermined setpoint? Proponents of this theory argue that it is possible to raise one's setpoint over time by continually gaining weight and failing to engage in regular physical activity. Conversely, reducing caloric intake and being physically active over a long period of time may slowly decrease one's setpoint.

Psychosocial Factors

The relationship of weight problems to deeply rooted emotional insecurities, needs, and wants remains uncertain. Food is often used inappropriately as a reward for good behaviour in childhood. As adults face various stresses in their lives, food is often also used as a comforting mechanism. Again, the research underlying this theory is controversial. What is certain is that in mainstream Canada, eating tends to be a focal point of people's lives—a major part of our socialization; a social ritual associated with companionship, celebration, and enjoyment.

✳ Eating Cues

At least one major factor in our preoccupation with food is the pressure placed on us by the highly sophisticated, heavily advertised "eating" campaigns launched by the food industry. Although salads and other lower-fat, lower-calorie options are available at most, if not all, fast-food restaurants, we still have the gauntlet of starchy, meaty delights and tasty high-fat fries to choose from. Food-related messages permeate the media, particularly for children and youth.[38] Compared to the foods recommended in Eating Well with Canada's Food Guide, most advertised foods are lower in nutrient density, fibre, and complex carbohydrates and higher in fat, sodium, simple carbohydrates, caffeine, and alcohol.

Increasingly, a large percentage of the foods we eat come from fast-food restaurants. We eat at fast-food restaurants for a number of reasons, including the relatively low cost and the perceived time saved. It should be kept in mind however that: (1) fast food is typically high in calories, fat, sodium, and simple carbohydrates; (2) it tends to all be eaten, even though portions are often much bigger than needed; and (3) it tends to be eaten quickly, so there is not enough time for the "I am full" signal to get to your mouth before the last bite of food is consumed.[39] This is a particular problem for post-secondary students, who encounter fast-food restaurants on campus, in addition to the all-you-can-eat buffets at food hall, combined with a perceived time shortage to focus on a sit-down, healthy, family meal.

Dietary Myth and Misperception

Most of us have heard someone say "I eat like a bird, but I can't lose weight." Should you believe the person who says this? Probably not, according to a study that analyzed the self-reported and actual caloric intakes and physical activity expenditures of a group of adults who were obese.[40] Though the individuals in this study claimed to consume fewer than 1200 calories per day, they were actually eating nearly twice as much as they indicated and engaging in only three-quarters as much physical activity as they reported. Does this mean that obesity is simply the result of gluttony and sloth? No. In fact, many studies indicate that individuals who are obese do not eat much, if any, more than their counterparts at a healthy weight. However, the majority of individuals who are obese are less physically active than people at a healthy weight.

Lifestyle

Of all the factors affecting obesity, perhaps the most critical one relates to lifestyle. As noted in Chapter 4, about 50 percent of the Canadian population aged 12 and over were classified as sedentary or inactive in their leisure time.[41] One of the reasons for low levels of physical activity participation may relate to poor or inadequate experiences in physical education classes. Currently, physical education is optional in most high schools (although recently the provinces of Alberta and Nova Scotia have added a physical education requirement to graduate from high school) and is seldom offered daily in elementary and junior schools. Furthermore, many children and youth are transported to and from school on a daily basis. This may limit the desire for active transportation later in life as well as leading to the attitude that one must be transported to one's activities.

You probably know someone who seems to be able to eat a lot and does not appear to do any more physical activity than you, yet never seems to gain weight. It is hard to understand how this person maintains his or her weight. With few exceptions, if you were to follow this person around for a typical day and monitor their level and intensity of physical activity, you would discover the answer to your question. Although the person's day may not include scheduled exercise, it probably includes a high level of physical activity. Walking up a flight of stairs rather than taking the elevator, speeding up the pace while mowing the lawn, getting up to change the TV channel rather than using the remote, and doing housework vigorously all burn extra calories. A major cause of low physical activity levels is the abundance of labour-saving devices in the modern household. Using a blender instead of chopping vegetables or pushing remote-control buttons on the television and stereo equipment as well as on garage doors results in a reduced caloric expenditure compared to previous generations. The automobile is also a great convenience, but using it has significantly reduced our daily physical activity.

what do you THINK?
Based on the risk factors for obesity discussed thus far, which ones do you think pose the greatest risk for you? Why? What can you do about it? What will motivate you to do something about it now?

SOCIAL BIAS AGAINST THE OVERWEIGHT

Although much has been written about the potentially devastating physical consequences of being overweight and obese, the social consequences of excessive weight and/or fat are rarely discussed. Difficulty in finding a suitable job, workplace discrimination, and problems in most every aspect of their social life have been noted for people who are obese.

Research increasingly points to a nation of weight bias. **Weight bias** refers to negative attitudes that have a detrimental effect on interpersonal interactions and activities with individuals who are obese. The stigma against fat people may come in several forms, including verbal types of bias (such as ridicule, teasing, insults, stereotypes, derogatory names, or pejorative language), physical stigma (such as touching, grabbing, or other aggressive behaviours), or other barriers and obstacles for people who are obese, such as the inadequate size of the seats in movie theatres, stadiums, and airplanes. In an extreme form, this stigma results in subtle and overt forms of discrimination, such as the denial of a promotion or a raise.[42]

Bias and stigmatization can lead to social isolation and a host of other problems for individuals who are obese. People who experience bias and stigma have higher rates of depression, poorer psychological adjustment, and higher rates of suicide. They may feel that they are "unlovable" and have difficulties in relationships. They also may have higher rates of disordered eating (discussed in the next section), issues with self-esteem, more difficulties in obtaining health care, and host of other problems.[43]

what do you THINK?
Are you biased against people who are overweight or obese? When you see a person who is fat, do you make judgments about him or her? His or her level of physical activity? Dietary intake? Personal lifestyle? Would you date someone who was obese? Why or why not? Should certain jobs have weight or fat restrictions? Why or why not?

Yo-yo diet: Cycles in which people repeatedly gain and lose weight. This lowers their BMR, which favours the weight gain process.

Setpoint theory: A theory that suggests fat storage is determined by a thermostatic mechanism in the body that acts to maintain a specific amount of body fat.

Weight bias: Negative attitudes that have a harmful effect on a person's interpersonal interactions and activities with persons who are obese.

✳ THINKING THIN: BODY IMAGE DISORDERS

Most of us think of the obsession with thinness as a phenomenon of recent years. Beginning with super-model Twiggy in the 1960s and continuing with super-model Kate Moss in the 1990s, the thin look has dominated fashion ads. And not only that: television, movies, the internet, and magazines constantly project images of lean, fit bodies. We have been led to believe that if we are thin, with shapely curves or well-defined muscles, we will be more desirable. But variations of this thin look have been around for a long time. During the Victorian era, corsets were used to achieve unrealistically tiny waists. And by the 1920s, it was common knowledge that obesity was linked to poor health. Today, beautiful female models and under-weight beauty pageant contestants in size 0 or 2 clothes exemplify desirability and success, delivering the subtle message that thin is in.

EATING DISORDERS

Obesity itself is neither a psychiatric disorder nor an **eating disorder**. Eating disorders involve severe disturbances in eating behaviours, unhealthy efforts to control body fat and weight, as well as abnormal and unrealistic attitudes about one's body weight and shape. In general, individuals who develop eating disorders have low self-esteem and excessive concern about their body weight and shape.

Eating disorders, regardless of type, occur more frequently in females with 90 to 95 percent of all diagnosed cases occurring in women. Further, it tends to be younger women who are most often diagnosed, with the majority of diagnoses occurring between the ages of 15 and 24 years.[44] Eating disorders are not restricted to middle-class white females with overprotective or over-perfectionist parents. Eating disorders span social classes and ethnic groups. They occur with similar frequencies in most industrialized countries, including Canada, the United States, Europe, Australia, Japan, New Zealand, and South Africa. Emigrants from cultures where eating disorders are rare and who come to cultures where they are more prevalent may develop eating disorders as they assimilate to the sociocultural pressures surrounding body weight and shape in their adopted culture.

Anorexia Nervosa

Anorexia nervosa is characterized by an obsession with controlling eating. It is often believed that if eating can be controlled, the rest of one's life can be controlled too.[45] This obsession usually leads to self-starvation motivated by an intense fear of gaining weight, along with an inability to see one's body the way it really is. When anorexia nervosa develops in childhood or early adolescence, one of the first signs can be the failure to gain weight associated with normal growth rather than actual weight loss. About 0.5 to 1 percent of females in late adolescence or early adulthood meet the diagnostic criteria of anorexia nervosa.

The following characteristics can often be recognized in an individual with anorexia nervosa: [46]

- significant weight loss (approximately 15 to 25 percent of body weight) without any logical reason
- an inability to maintain a weight considered healthy for age and height
- an obsessive desire to be thinner
- an intense fear of becoming fat
- distorted body image (that is, the inability to see one's body the way it really is; generally the perception is that the body is fat, even though emaciated)
- weight and shape (and/or number on the bathroom scale) dictates how one feels about oneself
- strong desire to control life; believed to be done through dietary (and exercise) manipulation
- significant reduction in eating, along with repeated denials of hunger

The medical problems associated with anorexia nervosa are many. Starvation damages the bones, the muscles, and the organs as well as the immune, nervous, and digestive systems. People with anorexia nervosa often lose their hair or develop excessive fine facial and body hair. A woman's menstrual cycle usually stops as well (that is, amenorrhea occurs). Further, between 10 and 15 percent of individuals with anorexia nervosa die as a result of the disorder.[47]

✳ Bulimia Nervosa

Bulimia nervosa involves cycles of binge eating and purging. Purging behaviours include self-induced vomiting, using laxatives, enemas, or diuretics, excessive exercising, or fasting.[48] As with anorexia nervosa, the eating behaviours of individuals with bulimia nervosa are strongly influenced by a desire to be in control of their body weight and shape. The cycle begins with a binge—or the rapid ingestion of a large amount of food at one time—then continues with some sort of purging behaviour. Usually the eating feels automatic and the person feels helpless since their eating may initially placate feelings of anger or sadness. Due to the ingestion of a large number of calories, the binge

The self-starvation associated with eating disorders like anorexia nervosa can damage bones, muscles, and organs and create a host of other serious and, in some cases, life-threatening medical problems.

causes considerable physical discomfort and a worry about weight gain. The cycle then continues with efforts to prevent calorie absorption with some form of purging.

Binge eating usually occurs in secrecy and is accompanied by a lack of control; it is difficult for a person to stop a binge once it has started. About 1 to 3 percent of adolescent and young adult females have bulimia nervosa; the rate among men is about 10 percent of that among females. Unlike individuals with anorexia nervosa, the body weight of individuals with bulimia nervosa is typically within the healthy weight range. One frequent health issue often experienced by individuals with bulimia nervosa relates to the acid in vomit, which causes tooth enamel to dissolve. Calluses may also appear on the outer fingers/knuckles from frequent scraping along the teeth when inducing vomiting by putting one or more fingers down the throat.

Binge Eating Disorder

People with a **binge eating disorder (BED)** engage in recurrent binge eating but, unlike those with bulimia nervosa, do not purge. Most people with a BED binge because they are very hungry as a result of restrictive eating or dieting or to comfort themselves, avoid uncomfortable situations, or numb their feelings. Generally, individuals with BED do not have abnormal attitudes about dieting or body weight and shape. Rather, BED occurs predominantly in individuals who are obese, with

estimates of one in five being diagnosed.[49] BED is often referred to as "compulsive overeating."

Eating Disorder Not Otherwise Specified

When individuals cannot be clearly diagnosed with one of the eating disorders described above yet still have obvious problems with their eating and body image, they are said to have an Eating Disorder Not Otherwise Specified (ED-NOS). For example, women who meet some of the criteria for anorexia nervosa but continue to menstruate would fit in this category, as do men and women who lose a lot of weight but remain within a healthy weight range despite their abnormal eating behaviours. Common behaviours of individuals with ED-NOS include[50]

- purging after normal eating
- chewing food repeatedly and then spitting it out (rather than swallowing)
- binge eating and purging (but not with the regularity required for a bulimia nervosa diagnosis)

Disordered Eating

Although not clinically diagnosed, disordered eating refers to a wide range of abnormal eating behaviours including various actions seen in individuals with anorexia nervosa, bulimia nervosa, and BED. These behaviours include chronic restrained eating, compulsive eating, habitual dieting, and irregular chaotic eating patterns where hunger and satiety are ignored. Similar to other eating disorders, disordered eating has negative health implications for overall and emotional, spiritual, social, and physical health. Further, disordered eating is highly prevalent in our culture, with most young women exhibiting one or more of these behaviours at one or more times in their lives. For example, in a recent study, 27 percent of Ontario girls aged 12 to 18 reported severely problematic food and weight behaviour.[51]

Eating disorder: A term used to describe a collection of psychiatric diseases that involve severe disturbances in eating behaviours, unhealthy efforts to control body fat and weight, and abnormal attitudes toward one's body weight and shape.

Anorexia nervosa: Eating disorder characterized by excessive preoccupation with food, self-starvation, and/or extreme exercising to achieve weight loss.

Bulimia nervosa: Eating disorder characterized by cycles of binge eating and purging (that is, various methods taken to prevent calorie absorption).

Binge eating disorder (BED): Eating disorder characterized by recurrent binge eating without any purging behaviours.

Anorexia Athletica

Similar to disordered eating, anorexia athletica is not a recognized diagnosis. Many people preoccupied with food and weight exercise compulsively to control their weight in misguided attempts to gain a sense of power, control, and self-respect.

Symptoms of anorexia athletica include[52]

- exercising beyond the requirements for good health
- being fanatical about weight and dietary intake
- stealing time from work, school, and relationships to exercise
- focusing on calorie burning and forgetting that physical activity and/or exercise can be fun
- defining self-worth in terms of performance
- rarely or never being satisfied with athletic achievements
- always pushing on to the next physical challenge
- justifying excessive behaviours by defining self as an athlete or insisting that current exercising behaviours are healthy

Who's at Risk?

Disordered eating patterns are the result of many factors and there is no simple explanation for why intelligent, often highly accomplished individuals spiral downwards into the destructive behaviours that lead to eating disorders. One potential factor is the desperate need to win social approval or gain control of their lives with food.

Many persons with disordered eating patterns also suffer from other problems such as clinical depression, alcohol abuse, compulsive stealing, gambling, or other addictions.[53] Some studies using identical twins have shown a possible association between heredity and eating disorders, as have others that point to the proportionally large number of persons with an eating disorder who have a mother or sister with a similar disease.

Treating Eating Disorders

As noted in the Building Communication Skills textbox, people can and do recover from eating disorders, the likelihood of success being greatest when the diagnosis is early and the individual acknowledges the need for treatment. The most effective treatments combine different approaches into a package that involves the patient and his or her family and friends. People with eating disorders usually come to the attention of medical personnel because someone else shows concern.

Treatment options for people with eating disorders vary and often need to be individualized. Often the individual requires hospitalization, with the first goal of treatment being to restore near-normal body weight. Concurrently, individual and group psychotherapy provide an opportunity to enhance self-confidence, self-esteem, and feelings of power and control. At this time, the person learns new, more effective ways to handle stress and gain a measure of control over her or his life, so that it is no longer necessary to turn to or away from food as the solution.

> ## what do you THINK?
>
> Why are young women in particular at risk of developing disordered eating and/or eating disorders? What programs or services on your campus are available to assist someone with an eating disorder?

Helping Someone with an Eating Disorder

Although people can, and do, recover from eating disorders, professional help is almost always required. However, recovery is more difficult the longer symptoms are denied or ignored. It is not easy to approach someone who you think has an eating disorder. What should you say? What should you do? The following are suggestions to help someone you think may be at risk.

Be patient: When you first approach the individual, do not be surprised if your expression of concern is rejected and treated with anger and denial. Shame and pain tend to go along with an eating disorder. It is also important not to rush and to accept that it will take time for the person to recognize that he or she has an eating disorder and needs to change.

Be knowledgeable: It is important to understand that an eating disorder results from a misguided coping strategy to deal with deeper issues around control. In other words, eating disorders are about more than just not eating or being thin! Learn more about eating disorders and in particular the eating disorder you think this individual has.

Be compassionate: Eating disorders are complex problems where issues with food, body weight and shape result. It is important to understand that the person might prefer to use healthier coping mechanisms, but simply does not know how.

Be encouraging: Encourage the person to define him or herself in ways that do not involve the eating disorder. Do this by talking about other aspects of his or her life, and of life more generally. Affirm strengths and interests unrelated to food or physical appearance.

Be non-judgmental: It is important to express your needs in the relationship, without blaming or shaming the other person. Remember that the individual with the eating disorder will have to decide on when and how to get help, and what kind. Provide support by validating healthy changes made, no matter how small they may be.

Take care of yourself: Seeing someone you care about struggling with an eating disorder might make you scared, angry, frustrated, and helpless. Still, be careful not to blame this person for his or her condition. Try to understand that eating disorders result from the behaviours used to deal with painful emotions or experiences and are a result of an attempt to gain control. The person with an eating disorder may know that his or her condition is upsetting other people, but may not be ready for or capable of change.

Do not take on the role of a therapist: Do only what you feel capable of. Get support for yourself. You need to take care of yourself while dealing with your friend or family member. Remember, you need to put on your own oxygen mask before helping others with theirs. Also remember that this person can only get better at his or her own pace. You can be supportive and gently share information. You can help this person to see and consider alternatives to their current behaviours. You cannot make them get better; you cannot even force them to seek treatment.

CONVERSATION GUIDE
Focus on feelings and relationships:

- Express concern about this person's health, yet respect his or her privacy.
- Do not comment on how this person or any others look, how fat or thin they are, how much they eat, etc. This person is already aware of his or her body, eating habits, and likely has a distorted view of his or her body, exercise, and eating behaviours. Even if you use compliments, comments about weight or appearance reinforce the obsession with body image and weight.
- Be positive. Find neutral, comfortable places and times to talk. For example:
  Instead of saying, "You could control/stop this if you wanted to," say, "I know how hard it is for you. Let's talk about how we can find ways to make things better."
- Keep calm, focused, and respectful during difficult conversations. Set caring and reasonable limits. Be firm and consistent. For example, know how you will respond when the person wants to skip meals or eat alone, or when they get angry if someone eats their "special" food.
- Avoid power struggles about eating. Do not demand change. Do not criticize eating habits. People with eating disorders are trying to gain control because they do not feel in control of other aspects of their life. Trying to trick or force them to eat can make things worse.
- Examine your attitudes about food, weight, body image, and body size. Think about the way you personally are affected by body-image pressures, and how it is that you speak about your body, your eating, and the pressures you experience.
- Do not convey any fat prejudice, or reinforce the desire to be thin. If this person says he or she feels fat or wants to lose weight, do not say, "You are not fat." Instead, suggest that they explore their reasons for dieting, and what they think they can achieve by weight loss. Encourage them to reflect on the pressure to look a certain way in society, and how this makes us feel about ourselves.

Source: Adapted from "Help for Family and Friends," National Eating Disorder Information Centre (NEDIC).

Managing Your Weight

Managing your weight is not an easy task. To ensure success, consider it a lifelong commitment rather than a temporary diet—that is, something you follow for a lifetime rather than sticking with for a few weeks and then returning to previous dietary behaviours.

MAKING DECISIONS FOR YOU

The first step in managing your weight is an honest self-assessment of where you are. You don't need sophisticated fat-measurement techniques. What you need is a scale and/or a mirror. You also know if your favourite jeans are too tight! Next, you need to set a realistic goal. Ask yourself, why do I want to meet this goal? What will I do when I reach this goal? Then set out a plan to reach your goal. Keep in mind what you enjoy doing. If you like taking walks, you might make walking part of your program. If you absolutely love chocolate chip cookies, you might consider limiting yourself to two cookies per day or every other day.

CHECKLIST FOR CHANGE: MAKING PERSONAL CHOICES

- Design your plan to meet your needs. Your plan must fit your personality, your priorities, and your study, work, and recreation schedules. It should also allow for sufficient rest and relaxation.
- Plan for nutrient-dense foods. Attempt to get the most from the foods you eat by selecting foods with high nutritional value.
- Spread caloric intake throughout the day. Most research indicates that the body burns calories more efficiently when they are consumed in small amounts spread throughout the day.
- Chart your progress. For many people, the daily "weigh-in" is a critical factor in maintaining their program. However, for others, the daily monitoring of weight negatively influences self-esteem. If you choose to weigh yourself daily, keep in mind that body weight normally fluctuates throughout the week and a once per week "weigh-in" may be more appropriate.
- Chart your eating setbacks. Rather than thinking in terms of failure and punishment, think in terms of temporary setbacks and how to accommodate them. By carefully recording your emotional states when eating, eating habits, environmental cues, and feelings, you may determine why you needed that particular food in that quantity. Successful weight maintenance accommodates hormonal fluctuations and their potential influence on dietary habits.
- Chart your exercise setbacks. Similar to monitoring your setbacks in dietary intake, you should keep track of your challenges in regard to your physical activity behaviours. Once again, carefully recording how you felt prior to missing your physical activity as well as the environmental cues around you will help you to successfully overcome those sorts of challenges in the future.

- Become aware of your feelings of hunger and fullness. For many of us, eating is time-dependent, and we stop eating only when the food is gone (the "clean your plate" syndrome). Long years of "eating when it is time" instead of eating when it is necessary have cost us the ability to tell when we really are hungry and when we really are full. By training yourself to become more aware of the eating process, by learning to recognize hunger and the first signals that you have eaten enough, you will be able to manage your eating.
- Accept yourself. For many people, this is the most important aspect of successful weight management. It is important to keep your weight and body shape in perspective.
- Be physically active. Different people benefit from different types of physical activities. Just because your friends are into jogging or yoga does not mean that those types of physical activity are best for you. Select physical activities that you consider fun, not a daily form of punishment for overeating. Variety may be the key here. Planning physical activities that include friends and family may also improve your chances of success. It is important to remember that every little effort contributes toward long-term results.

CHECKLIST FOR CHANGE: MAKING COMMUNITY CHOICES

- Identify volunteer organizations that provide physically active opportunities for young adults.
- What opportunities for volunteering at nutrition- or weight-related programs does your campus provide?

CRITICAL THINKING

Until post-secondary school, your girlfriend Graziela had taken ballet very seriously, practising several hours a day. Now that the time pressures of school, a part-time job, and your relationship are starting to get to her, Graziela rarely has time to dance. You notice that she has consequently been more and more concerned about her weight. She rarely eats on your dates because she says she wants the two of you to save money for a trip during spring break. When you find a laxative hidden under her pillow, she says, "Doesn't everyone get constipated now and then?" Then a mutual female friend tells you that she's heard Graziela in the bathroom throwing up on several occasions after meals. Graziela denies it.

Using the DECIDE model in Chapter 1, decide how you can approach Graziela with your concern that she has an eating disorder. What help is available in your local area? Should you involve Graziela's family? If Graziela denies she has an eating disorder, what can you do?

From Atkins to the Glycemic Index: Getting the "Skinny" on Carbohydrates

Low-carbohydrate diets have attracted millions of North Americans with reports of massive, quick weight loss. Bookstores struggle to keep the latest editions of *The Atkins Diet, The South Beach Diet,* and other bestsellers on their shelves. Restaurants have added "low-carb" items to their menus, and a multimillion dollar industry of low-carb food products has emerged. The promise? Eliminate nearly all of the bread, pasta, sweets, and high-carbohydrate foods from your diet, eat red meat and other high-protein and high-fat foods until you are satisfied, and lose weight.

Many health professionals have spent the past 20 years criticizing low-carb diets as dangerous, ineffective, and unhealthy. The American Heart Association and the American Dietetic Association were just two of many professional health groups that issued warnings about the craze. Yet several well-designed clinical trials indicated that low-carbohydrate diets were as good as—and in many cases, better than—low-fat diets in helping very overweight people shed pounds.

In these studies, more people stayed with the low-carb diet than the low-fat one, and, although they ate more fat, they did not experience the harmful changes in blood cholesterol that many expected. In fact, their LDL ("bad") cholesterol and triglycerides were reduced and their HDL ("good") cholesterol increased.

However, these benefits were only short term, and reports of problems with low-carb diets eventually began to surface. A study by the Stanford University Medical Center in conjunction with researchers at Yale University found that although low-carbohydrate diets cause weight loss, it's the total caloric reduction and the duration of the reduction that causes the loss, not the reduction in carbohydrate intake per se. The take-home message was that any low-calorie diet that a person can stay on long enough will have similar results. Furthermore, people had difficulty with sticking to the rigid dietary requirements. When they lost weight, they gained it back nearly as quickly as they had lost it. People with diabetes had problems because whole grains, beans, and other fibre-rich foods were not allowed. And rather than remembering to cut back on saturated fats, people were gulping down bacon and eggs, eating huge steaks, and feeling good about the guilt-free diet.

A major problem with the Atkins and similar diets is that they assume that virtually any carbohydrate is bad for you. However, they do not account for the vast difference in nutrient value among carbohydrates and their *glycemic index,* a ranking of foods according to how quickly their sugars are released into the bloodstream. The body converts a food's sugars into glucose, which is released slowly or rapidly into the bloodstream. Insulin is secreted to counter glucose levels and return the body to healthy levels. The amount of insulin a food triggers is referred to as *glycemic load,* which considers both a food's glycemic index and how much carbohydrate the food delivers in one hit in a single serving.

Most fruits, vegetables, beans, and whole grains have low glycemic loads; their sugars enter the bloodstream gradually and trigger only a moderate rise in insulin. Sugar causes insulin levels to rise, triggering a chain of reactions that ultimately make you sluggish, bloated, and feeling hungry, driving you to eat more and continuing the cycle. Ultimately, these high insulin levels can lead to diabetes. Given this new understanding of carbohydrates, should you do what Atkins suggests and follow a diet that avoids most carbs? No. The bulk of scientific evidence suggests that you should choose foods with low glycemic loads and continue to reduce your total caloric intake and saturated fat intake.

A few examples of the glycemic load of common foods demonstrates the range you may find in your daily diet: a serving of high-quality orange juice has nearly three times the glycemic load (13) of an orange; a serving of cornflakes has five times the load (21) of a serving of All Bran (4). Listings for many foods can be found online, particularly in connection with diabetes resources.

However, instead of memorizing glycemic load values for all your favourite foods, try following these general guidelines:

- *Choose plants.* Pick the fruit rather than its sugar-laden juice counterpart. Eating the skin of apples adds fibre and slows the entry of glucose into the bloodstream. If you must eat potatoes, eat them with the skin on and cut back on other starches. Instead of potatoes and corn, try sweet potatoes and yams.

- *Forgo meat in favour of beans.* It isn't necessary to cut all meat-based protein from your diet. However, when you eat meat, opt for the lean cuts and choose poultry over pork or beef. Learn to cook and flavour beans. They are high in protein and other nutrients and have very little effect on blood sugar and insulin.

- *Go nuts several times a week.* Almonds, hazelnuts, peanuts, pecans, and others are healthy low-carbohydrate alternatives to snacking on chips and desserts made from white flour. They are not calorie free, though, so manage your intake based on exercise patterns and calorie needs.

- *Mix your carbs with other foods.* Eating carbohydrates with other foods such as monounsaturated oils (olive or canola) can slow the rate of carbohydrate absorption. Milk or yogurt with cereal is one example; bananas and cottage cheese in cereal is another.

- *Make whole-grain breads a staple.* Avoid white bread and look for brown breads with 100 percent whole wheat or other grains. Consider options such as brown rice and whole-wheat pizza dough and pasta. These are good choices for slowing your blood sugar.

- *Exercise regularly.* Most people would be shocked if they ate a normal meal, measured their blood sugar, then noted how dramatically their blood sugars go down after a 30-minute walk. It may seem simple, but one of the best ways to keep yourself healthy and still consume the carbs you want is through exercise. These recommendations hold true no matter what low-fat, low-carb, low-calorie diet or other plan you choose to follow.

Sources: W. Willet and P. Skerrett, "Going Beyond Atkins," *Newsweek,* January 19, 2004, 46; S. Conner et al., "Should a Low Fat, High-Carb Diet Be Recommended for Everyone?" *New England Journal of Medicine* 350 (2004): 1691–1692; F. F. Samaha et al., "A Low-Carbohydrate as Compared with a Low-Fat Diet in Severe Obesity," *New* England Journal of Medicine 348.21 (2003): 2074–2081; G. D. Foster et al., "A Randomized Trial of Low Carbohydrate Diet for Obesity," *New England Journal of Medicine* 348.21 (2003): 2082–2090; D. M. Bravata et al., "Efficacy and Safety of Low-Carbohydrate Diets," *Journal of the American Medical Association* 289.14 (2003): 1837–1850.

PEARSON
myhealthlab

Go to MyHealthLab at **www.pearsoned.ca/myhealthlab**. Here you will find self-assessments, case studies, links to health on the net, and much more.

DISCUSSION QUESTIONS

1. Differentiate the terms *overweight* and *obese*.

2. How is it possible that a person can be classified as obese (BMI ≥ 30) and yet not be overfat (that is, percentage of body fat within the healthy range)? Similarly, how can a person be overfat (that is, percentage of fat above the normal range) and not be classified as obese (that is, BMI < 30)? What is a better method of determining excessive fatness?

3. List the risk factors for developing obesity. Identify the factors that seem to be most important in determining whether you will be obese in middle age. Why these factors and not others?

4. Discuss the pressures, if any, you feel to change your body shape. Where do these pressures come from? How has the media influenced your thoughts about your body?

5. Create a plan for weight management. In what way would you have to modify this plan for your best friend? Your sister? Your brother?

6. Differentiate the eating disorders discussed in this chapter. Identify why females are more prone to eating disorders than males.

7. Why are popular diets not the best method for weight management? Which popular diets might have better long-term success? Why?

APPLICATION EXERCISE

Reread the "Consider This . . ." scenario at the beginning of the chapter and answer the following questions.

1. What motivates someone like Denzel to want to buff up and look good at certain times of the year? How could someone like Denzel change his behaviours so he can be healthier nutritionally and avoid the diet syndrome so many of us find ourselves in?

2. How can Eating Well with Canada's Food Guide and Canada's Physical Activity Guide help Denzel to manage his weight?

3. Why is dieting and excessive exercising to lose weight not a good idea in the long term?

MYSEARCHLAB EXERCISE

1. Log on to www.mysearchlab.com.

2. Retrieve article AN 28558637, "Review of the Use of the Health Belief Model for Weight Management," by Diane K. Daddario.

3. Read the article, then respond to the following:
   a. Briefly describe the Health Belief Model (HBM).
   b. According to the HBM, when are people more likely to change their behaviours?
   c. Which factors best predict dieting? Would you agree with this finding? Why or why not?
   d. In general, when are people most motivated to lose weight?
   e. Consider your personal beliefs regarding the HBM questions (that is, perceived susceptibility, perceived seriousness, perceived benefits of action, barriers to action, cues to action), how likely are you to take action to effectively manage your weight?

CHAPTER 7

HEALTHY RELATIONSHIPS AND SEXUALITY

Making Commitments

Jorge and Yasmin have been dating exclusively for more than two years and have talked about moving in together. Over time, Yasmin has noticed that Jorge has become possessive of her and jealous of any time she spends with others—regardless of whether they are male or female. As a result, they fight regularly about whom she does things with, potential threats to their relationship, and the like. Recently, Jorge took a weekend to go hunting with the guys while Yasmin stayed home to get caught up on her work. When Yasmin's friends called her to ask her to go to a party, she decided to go. When she talked to Jorge on the phone the next day, he asked her what she did the night before. Wanting to avoid a fight, she told him she stayed home and watched a movie. He responded angrily, "Liar! I tried to call you and you were not home!"

What should Yasmin say? What should she do? Why do you think she lied? Is dishonesty in a relationship justified? Why or why not? Is Jorge's jealousy a healthy, normal part of their relationship? Can a relationship based on mistrust, half-truths, and possessiveness survive? Why or why not?

CHAPTER OBJECTIVES

- Describe effective communication and the role it plays in intimate and nonintimate relationships.

- Clarify the characteristics of intimate relationships, the potential barriers to healthy relationships, and the factors important in maintaining intimate relationships.

- Describe the warning signs of a failing relationship, where you can get help, and factors that ultimately lead to the relationship failing.

- Differentiate sexual and gender identity. How are they developed? How does society help and/or hinder their development?

- Identify the various sexual dysfunctions as well as the treatment of each.

Humans are social beings—we have a basic need to belong and feel loved, appreciated, and wanted. We cannot live without relating to others in some way. In fact, research indicates that the ability to relate well with people, as well as give and receive love and support throughout your life, can have almost as much impact on your health as regular physical activity and consuming a diet that follows Eating Well with Canada's Food Guide.[1] All relationships involve a degree of risk and it is by taking these risks that we grow and truly experience all that life has to offer. By looking at our intimate and nonintimate relationships, components of sexual identity, gender roles, and sexual orientation, we will come to better understand who we are and increase our capacity to relate effectively with others and build better, stronger relationships.

COMMUNICATING: A KEY TO ESTABLISHING RELATIONSHIPS

From the moment of birth, we struggle to be understood. We flail our arms, cry, scream, smile, frown, and make sounds and gestures to attract attention, get a reaction from someone, or have someone understand what we want or need from them. By the time we enter adulthood, each of us has developed a unique way of communicating using gestures, words, expressions, and body positions. No two of us communicate in the exact same way or have the same need for connecting with others. Some are outgoing and quick to express emotions and thoughts. Others are quiet, reluctant to talk about feelings, and prefer to spend time alone.

Different cultures have not only distinct languages and dialects but also unique ways of expressing themselves and using body language to communicate.[2] Some cultures gesture wildly; others maintain a closed and rigid means of speaking. Some cultures are offended by apparent "fixed and dilated" staring, while others welcome a steady look in the eyes. Although people differ in the way they communicate, this doesn't mean that one sex, culture, or group is better or should be a model for the others. We have to be willing to accept differences and work to keep communication lines open and fluid. Appearing interested, actively engaged in the interaction, and open and willing to exchange ideas and thoughts is something that we typically learn with practice and hard work.

✳ Communicating How You Feel

Do you find it easy to express how much you care about friends and family members with hugs, kisses, and verbal expressions? If you are comfortable telling them you love them and that they mean a lot to you, chances are that you also will be able to tell them when you are feeling sad, disappointed, angry, or frustrated. However, it is important to realize that some people were not raised in affectionate families or a culture supportive of open expressions, do not readily discuss feelings or emotions, and sometimes struggle to find the right words for expressing what they feel.

When two people begin a relationship, they bring their communication styles with them.[3] How often have you heard someone say, "We just cannot communicate," or "You are sending mixed messages"? These exchanges occur regularly as people start relationships or work through communication problems in an existing relationship. Because communication is a process, our every action, word, facial expression, gesture, or body posture becomes part of our shared history and part of the evolving impression we make on others. If we are angry in our responses, others will be reluctant to interact with us. If we bring "baggage" from past bad interactions to new relationships, we may be cynical, distrustful, and guarded in our exchanges with others. If we are positive, happy, and share openly with others, they will be more likely to communicate openly with us. This ability to communicate assertively is an important skill in relationships (see Improving Communication Skills below). Assertive communicators are in touch with their feelings and values and able to directly and honestly communicate their needs or defend choices in a positive manner.

✔ Improving Communication Skills

Because people have such different ways of communicating, there is no recipe for how to communicate effectively in a given situation. At times, silence may be the best approach. However, there are things that each of us can do to become better communicators and to encourage and assist others in their attempts to interact with us.

Learning Appropriate Self-Disclosure

Sharing personal information with others is called **self-disclosure**. If you are willing to share personal information with others, they will likely share personal

Self-disclosure: Sharing personal information with others. ⌐

information with you. In other words, if you want to learn more about someone, you have to be willing to share parts of yourself with that person. Self-disclosure is not storytelling or sharing secrets; rather, it is revealing how you are reacting to the present situation and giving information about the past relevant to the other person's understanding of your current reactions.[4]

Self-disclosure can be a double-edged sword, for there is risk in divulging personal insights and feelings. If you sense that sharing feelings and personal thoughts will result in a closer relationship, you will likely take the risk. But if you believe that self-disclosure may result in rejection or alienation, you may not open up so easily. If the confidentiality of previously shared information has been violated, you are likely to hesitate to disclose yourself in the future.

Becoming a Better Listener

Listening is a vital part of interpersonal communication; it allows us to share feelings, express concerns, communicate wants and needs, and let our thoughts and opinions be known. We must do the necessary work to improve our speaking and listening skills, which will enhance our relationships, improve our grasp of information, and allow us to interpret more effectively what others say. We listen best when (1) we believe that the message is important and relevant to us, (2) the speaker holds our attention through humour, dramatic effect, use of media, or other techniques, and (3) we are in the mood to listen (free of

Listening is a key component of communication.

distractions and worries). When we listen effectively, we try to understand what people are thinking and feeling from their perspective. We not only hear the words, but we try to understand what is really being said. How many times have you been caught pretending to be listening when you were not? After several moments of nodding and saying "uh-huh," the person talking to you asks a question, and you do not have a clue about what he or she has been saying. Sometimes this tuned-out behaviour results because of a lack of sleep, stress, being preoccupied, having too much to drink, or being under the influence of drugs. Other times it is because the speaker is a person who talks for the sake of talking or you find the speaker and/or what he or she is talking about boring. Still, many of the most common listening difficulties are things that we can work to improve.

CHARACTERISTICS OF INTIMATE RELATIONSHIPS

There are many definitions of **intimate relationships**. One classic definition is "close relationships with another person in which you offer, and are offered, validation, understanding, and a sense of being valued intellectually, emotionally, and physically."[5] In this context, friends, family, lovers, partners, and even people you work with or interact with at the grocery store may be included in the sphere of intimate interactions. For the purposes of this chapter, we define intimate relationships in terms of three characteristics: behavioural interdependence, need fulfillment, and emotional attachment. Each of these characteristics may be related to interactions with family, close friends, and romantic relationships.[6]

Behavioural interdependence refers to the mutual impact that people have on each other as their lives and daily activities become intertwined. What one person does may influence what the other person may

Learning to Really Listen

Most of us lament that someone "never listens" and monopolizes the entire conversation. Although we are quick to recognize such flaws in others, we are often less likely to spot our own poor listening skills. On a daily basis, we have times when we simply "tune out." When a professor drones on about a subject we don't relate to or are not very interested in, we begin doodling and/or daydreaming. When a friend or colleague tells the same story again and again, we say "uh-huh"—and worry that we will be caught and asked a question. We grimace at the thought of certain people calling, but dash for the phone when the caller ID indicates that it is someone we love to talk with. What is the difference? Why do we tune out when some people speak and tune in for others? We gravitate toward those who seem to understand us and with whom we have fun and interesting interactions.

If truth be told, most of us are only mediocre listeners. What does it take to be a very good or excellent listener? Practise the following skills and consciously use them on a daily basis to improve your communication skills.

- Be present in the moment. Contrary to popular thought, good listeners do not just sit back with their mouths shut. They participate and acknowledge what the speaker is saying. (Nodding, smiling, saying "yes" or "uh-huh," and asking reflective questions at appropriate times are part of this. Take care, however, not to numbly say "uh-huh" too frequently since it can be distracting and convey insincerity.)

- Use positive body language and voice tone. Show that you are "with" the speaker by turning toward him or her and staying focused (wandering eyes are a sure sign that your mind is elsewhere). Avoid barrier gestures such as shaking your head "no," negative faces, or folding your arms; smile at appropriate times and maintain eye contact without staring. Voice tone, posture, and an attitude that conveys interest are important.

- Express empathy, not necessarily sympathy. Watch for verbal and nonverbal clues to the other person's feelings and try to relate to them. For example, saying, "That must have been really hard for you" can encourage the speaker to talk and feel more comfortable with you as an understanding and caring listener.

- Ask for clarification. If you are not sure what the speaker means, ask for clarification or paraphrase what you think you heard. This kind of feedback is invaluable in avoiding misinterpretation and lapses in overall communication. As a speaker, you may ask, "What did you think I was just saying?" so long as it is said in a nonthreatening manner.

- Control the desire to interrupt. Some people start nodding and gesturing before you even get a word out. If you are like that, squelch it, even if you have to put an inconspicuous—or conspicuous—hand over your mouth. Try taking a deep breath for two seconds, then hold your breath for another second and really listen to what is being said as you slowly exhale. Try not to be so enthusiastically empathetic that you finish speakers' sentences or put words in people's mouths.

- Avoid snap judgments based on what people look like or what they say. If you notice some strange mannerism, try to focus on what is being said, not on how it is being said. Avoid stereotyping or labelling, particularly with people who have a background different from yours.

- Resist the temptation to "set the other person straight." Control your urge to correct errors, be right, or react defensively. Listen without reacting or trying to rationalize what the speaker is trying to say.

- Try to focus on the speaker. Sometimes it is tough to listen to someone who is talking about a painful situation, especially if we are experiencing or have recently experienced something similar. Hold back the temptation to "tell all" about your own rendition. Each person experiences his or her situations in their own way. Give the speaker the moment and later, after he or she has finished talking, you may talk about your own experience as a way of validating the feelings expressed. Do not tell someone how to feel or react to a particular situation.

- Be tenacious. Stick with the speaker and try to stay on the topic. If he or she wanders, gently nudge him or her back by saying, "You were just saying . . ." Offer your thoughts and suggestions, and remember to advise only up to a certain point. Clarify with "this is my opinion" as a reminder that it is your thoughts, rather than fact.

want and can do. Such interdependence may become stronger over time to the point that each person would find a void in his or her life if the other person left.

Another characteristic of intimate relationships is that they fulfill psychological needs and, as such, are a means of need fulfillment. These needs, which may often be met only through relationships with others, are as follows:

- The need for approval and for a sense of purpose in life—requiring the sense that what we say and do matters.

Intimate relationships: Close relationships with other people in which you offer, and are offered, validation, understanding, and a sense of being valued intellectually, emotionally, and physically.

- The need for intimacy—requiring someone with whom we can share our feelings freely.
- The need for social integration—requiring someone with whom we can share our worries and concerns.
- The need for nurturing—requiring someone whom we can take care of.
- The need for being nurtured—requiring someone who can take care of us.
- The need for reassurance or affirmation of our own worth—requiring someone to tell us that we matter.

In other words, rewarding, intimate relationships, partners, or friends meet each other's needs. They disclose feelings, share confidences, and discuss practical concerns; they help each other and provide reassurance. They serve as major sources of social support and reinforce our feelings that we are important and serve a purpose in life.

In addition to behavioural interdependence and need fulfillment, intimate relationships involve strong bonds of emotional attachment, or feelings of love and attachment. The intimacy level experienced by any two people cannot easily be judged by those outside the relationship. Although sex can often be an important part of an intimate relationship, a relationship can also be very intimate without it. In fact, many satisfying and lasting intimate relationships go well beyond the need for sexual contact.

Emotional availability, the ability to give to and receive from others emotionally without fear of being hurt or rejected is another characteristic of intimate relationships. At times, all of us need to protect ourselves psychologically by making ourselves unavailable emotionally. For example, after the end of a relationship, a young person may close down emotionally and carefully avoid letting her- or himself feel too much. This allows time for regrouping and healing before reaching out to people again. It also reduces the risk of a rebound romance that is often doomed to failure as a result of unresolved personal hurts and issues.

Emotional bonding and other elements of intimate relationships are rooted in a caring, supportive family environment.

FORMING INTIMATE RELATIONSHIPS

Throughout our lives, we go through predictable patterns of relationships. In our early years, our most significant relationships are with our families. Gradually, our relationships widen to include friends, co-workers/classmates, and acquaintances. Ultimately, most of us develop one or more romantic or sexual relationships with another over our lifetime. Each of these relationships plays a significant role in our psychological, social, spiritual, and physical health.

Families: The Ties That Bind

Although many people consider the family the foundation of Canadian society and talk about a return to "family values" as a desirable objective, it is clear that the modern Canadian family looks quite different from families of previous generations. The *Leave It to Beaver* family model that was held up during the 1950s—Mom with her apron, staying at home, content in her role as mother and spouse; Dad with his briefcase, trying to move up the corporate ladder; and two or three happy, well-adjusted children—is no longer the norm. More than half of today's moms work outside the home, and many children are raised by single parents, grandparents, relatives, stepparents, nannies, day-care centre workers, and other "parents."

Regardless of the form or structure of each family, all families should care for, protect, love, and socialize with one another. Whether the family is related by birth or simply connected by a high level of love and regard, their living arrangement, or some other factor, the family network often provides the sense of security needed to develop into healthy adults. The definition of family changes dramatically from culture to culture and from place to place over time.

The Vanier Institute of the Family defines family as "any combination of two or more persons bound together over time by ties of mutual consent, birth or adoption/placement and who, together, assume responsibilities for variant combinations of the following: physical maintenance and care of family members; addition of new members; socialization of children; social control of members; production, consumption and distribution of goods and services; love and affective nurturance."[7]

Today's Family Unit

The United Nations defines seven basic types of families, including single-parent families, communal families (unrelated people living together for ideological, economic, or other reasons), extended families, and others. Most of us think of family in terms of the "family of origin" or the "nuclear family." The family of origin includes the people present in the household during a child's first years of life—usually parents and siblings. However, the family of origin may also include a stepparent, parents' lovers, or significant others such as grandparents, aunts, or uncles. The family of origin has a tremendous impact on the child's psychological, social, and spiritual development. The nuclear family consists of parents (usually, but not necessarily, married) and their offspring.

If parents are comfortable in sharing feelings, affection, and love with each other and their offspring, their children are likely to become emotionally connected adults. If the home environment provides stability and seems a safe place to be, it is likely that the children will learn to express feelings and develop intimacy skills. Sibling interactions provide a way to learn and practise interpersonal skills.[8] The family of origin and the nuclear family have the potential for encouraging significant positive interactions and growth. People can practise positive behaviours and learn the rights and wrongs of negative behaviours in a safe and nonjudgmental environment when the family itself is healthy. However, if the family is psychologically or physically unhealthy, it may pose significant barriers to later relationships.

Establishing Friendships

A Friend is one who knows you as you are
understands where you've been
accepts who you've become,
and still gently invites you to grow.

—*Author Unknown*

Although most of us have a fairly clear idea of the distinction between a friend and a lover, this difference is not always easy to verbalize. Some people believe that the major difference is that there is no intimate physical involvement between friends. Others have suggested that intimacy levels are much lower between friends than between lovers. But, as stated previously, people can be intimate with each other without being sexually involved. Confused? You are probably not alone. Surprisingly, there has not been a lot of research to clarify these terms. Beyond the fact that two people participate in a relationship as equals, friendships include the following (See also Figure 7.1):[9]

- Enjoyment. Friends enjoy each other's company, although there may be temporary states of anger, disappointment, or mutual annoyance.

- Acceptance. Friends accept each other as they are, without trying to change one another.

- Trust. Friends have mutual trust in that each assumes that the other will act in his or her friend's best interests.

- Respect. Friends respect each other in that each assumes that the other uses good judgment in making life choices.

- Mutual assistance. Friends are inclined to help and support one another. They can count on each other in times of need or duress as well as in positive times, worthy of celebration.

- Confiding. Friends share experiences and feelings with each other that they do not share with other people.

- Understanding. Friends know what is important to each other and usually understand each other's behaviour.

- Spontaneity. Friends feel free to be themselves in the relationship rather than play a role, wear a mask, or refrain from revealing their true self.

Significant Others, Partners, Couples

Although family and friends provide necessary intimate relationships, most people choose at some point whether or not to enter into an intimate sexual relationship with another person. Most couples fit into one of four categories of significant relationships: married heterosexual couples, cohabiting heterosexual couples, married lesbian or gay couples, and cohabiting

Emotional availability: The ability to give to and receive from other people emotionally without being inhibited by fears of being hurt.

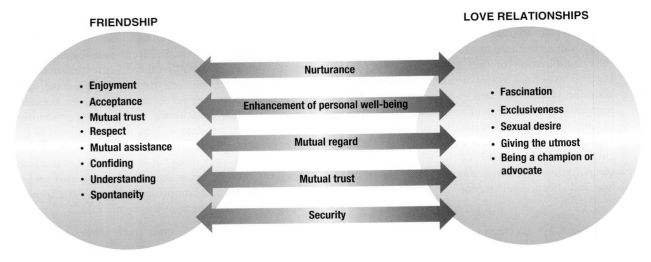

FIGURE 7.1

Common Bonds of Friends and Lovers

FRIENDSHIP

- Enjoyment
- Acceptance
- Mutual trust
- Respect
- Mutual assistance
- Confiding
- Understanding
- Spontaneity

Nurturance

Enhancement of personal well-being

Mutual regard

Mutual trust

Security

LOVE RELATIONSHIPS

- Fascination
- Exclusiveness
- Sexual desire
- Giving the utmost
- Being a champion or advocate

lesbian or gay couples. Love relationships in each of these four groups typically include the characteristics of friendship as well as the following related to passion and caring:[10]

- Fascination. Lovers tend to pay attention to the other person even when they should be involved in other activities. They are preoccupied with the other person and want to think about, look at, talk to, touch, or merely be with him or her.

- Exclusiveness. Lovers have a special relationship that usually precludes having the same relationship with a third party.

- Sexual desire. Lovers want physical intimacy with their partner, desiring to touch, hold, kiss, and engage in sexual activities. However, lovers may choose not to act on their sexual desire because of religious, moral, or other practical considerations.

- Giving the utmost. Lovers care enough to give the utmost when the other is in need, sometimes to the point of extreme self-sacrifice.

- Being a champion/advocate. The depth of lovers' caring may show up as an active, unselfish championing of each other's interests and a positive attempt to ensure that the other succeeds.

For obvious reasons, the best love relationships share friendships, and the best friendships include several love components. Both types of relationships share common bonds of nurturance, enhancement of personal well-being, and a genuine sense of mutual regard, trust, and security.

✳ This Thing Called Love

Love is a gift, not an obligation.

—*Author Unknown*

What is love? Defining love is more difficult than simply listing characteristics of a loving relationship. Love has been written about and engraved on walls; it has been the theme of countless novels, poems, movies, songs, and plays. There is no one definition of love, and the word means different things depending on cultural values, age, sex, education, experiences, and situation.

Many social scientists maintain that love may be of two kinds: companionate and passionate. Companionate love is a secure, trusting attachment, similar to what we often feel for family members or close friends. In companionate love, two people are attracted, have much in common, care about each other's well-being, and express reciprocal liking and respect. Passionate love involves a state of high arousal filled with the ecstasy of being loved or the agony of being rejected.[11] The person experiencing passionate love tends to be preoccupied with his or her partner and to perceive the loved person as perfect.[12] Passionate love will not occur unless three conditions are met.[13] First, the person must live in a culture in which the concept of "falling in love" is idealized. Second, a "suitable" person to love must be present. If the culture a person is immersed in—including influence from parents, movies, books, songs, peers, and the like—projects the need to seek a particular partner with a certain level of attractiveness or belonging to a certain ethnic or age group or with a certain socioeconomic status, and none is available, the "seeker" may find it difficult to allow him- or herself to find "love." Finally, for passionate love to happen there must be some type of physiologic arousal that occurs when a person is in the presence of the object of desire. Sexual excitement is often the way this arousal is expressed.

In the "triangular theory of love," love is clarified by isolating three key ingredients:

- Intimacy. The emotional component, which involves feelings of closeness.

- Passion. The motivational component, which reflects romantic, sexual attraction.

- Decision/commitment. The cognitive component, which includes the decisions you make about being in love and the degree of commitment to your partner.

According to this model, the greater the intimacy, passion, and commitment, the more likely a person is to be involved in a healthy, positive love relationship.

A second theory of love and attraction based on brain circuitry and chemistry is quite different from the Triangular Theory discussed above. In this theory, in regard to attraction and the process of falling in love, a fairly predictable pattern is followed based on (1) imprinting, in which our evolutionary patterns, genetic predispositions, and past experiences trigger romantic reaction; (2) attraction, in which neurochemicals produce feelings of euphoria and elation; (3) attachment, in which endorphins—natural opiates—cause lovers to feel peaceful, secure, and calm; and (4) production of a "cuddle chemical"—the brain secretes the chemical oxytocin, thereby stimulating sensations during lovemaking and eliciting feelings of satisfaction and attachment.[14]

Lovers who claim to be swept away by passion may not, therefore, be far from the truth:

> A meeting of the eyes, a touch of the hands or a whiff of scent may set off a flood that starts in the brain and races along the nerves and through the blood. The familiar results—flushed skin, sweaty palms, heavy breathing—are identical to those experienced when under stress. Why? Because the love-smitten person is secreting chemical substances such as dopamine, norepinephrine, and phenylethylamine (PEA) that are chemical cousins of amphetamines.[15]

Although attraction may in fact be a "natural high," with PEA levels soaring, this hit of passion loses effectiveness over time as the body builds tolerance to it, like it does for any other drug. Needing a continual fix, some people may become attraction junkies, seeking the intoxication of love in a way similar to a drug user who seeks a chemical high.[16] It has been speculated that PEA levels drop significantly over a three- to four-year period, thus eliciting the "four-year itch" that shows up in the peaking fourth-year divorce rates present in more than 60 cultures. Those romances that last beyond the four-year decline of PEA are influenced by another set of chemicals known as endorphins, soothing substances that give lovers a sense of security, peace, and calm.[17]

In another theory, researchers describe the first stage as the lust phase, in which our biological and genetic histories converge to pique our interest and intensity of response. In the lust phase, if someone comes into our range of awareness, a chemical surge triggers our enthusiastic response. Known as pheromones and said to be as unique as our fingerprints, these triggers are scent-infused chemicals found in perspiration under the arm. They trigger a unique sensory reaction in the nose and result in attraction if their producer is a match for you.[18] Following these pheromone triggers comes the attraction phase, often labelled the "falling in love" phase, and then the attachment phase. The two hormones most important in this last phase are oxytocin and vasopressin. Oxytocin increases the bond between lovers, is released by both sexes during orgasm, and is one of the chemicals responsible for contractions during childbirth and milk expression when breastfeeding. Scientists suspect vasopressin to be the chemical responsible for creating the desire to be monogamous with another person. One theory suggests that the more sex a couple has, the greater the bond between them.[19]

In addition to the possible chemical influences, our past experiences may significantly affect our attraction to others. Our parents' modelling of traits we believe to be desirable or undesirable may play a role in drawing us to people with similar traits. Many researchers investigated the possible link between heterosexual males seeking partners similar to their mothers and heterosexual females seeking partners similar to their fathers. For heterosexual males and females, it may be that we are attracted to what we are familiar with.

GENDER ISSUES

In any relationship, understanding and communication are important ingredients for success. Sometimes it may seem that the relating styles of men and women are so different that obtaining true understanding and open communication may be next to impossible. Men's and women's social conditioning is so different that it is almost as if they are raised in two different cultures.[20] Women are brought up to feel comfortable and share freely in their intimate relationships. As a result, they tend to be more nurturing and less afraid

Is It Love or Infatuation?

In the early stages, love and infatuation can be very similar. They both produce a characteristic rush of excitement as well as a strong desire to have more of the loved one's time, energy, and physical contact. The primary difference is that, with love, the feelings grow deeper as you get to know the person better and come to appreciate him or her more. With infatuation or a crush, you realize that Ms. or Mr. Right was not all you had thought. Taking the following test may help you determine whether it's the real thing or merely a case of infatuation. Respond honestly YES or NO to the following statements.

1. I knew I was in love with this person almost immediately.
2. Even though I have known this person for a while, I still really love his/her personality.
3. I wonder sometimes if the person has changed a lot since I have known him/her because he/she acts differently around me now.
4. The more I am with this person, the more I want to be around him/her.
5. I am less interested in the person sexually than I was in the beginning.
6. The more I know about this person, the more I want to know.
7. The more I know about this person, the less interested I am in him/her.
8. I feel really good associating with this person and being regarded as a couple.
9. I have begun to notice more things "wrong" with this person and spend a lot of time trying to get him/her to change.
10. Even though I have been with this person for a while, I am still as sexually interested as I was in the beginning.
11. I would just as soon do things with other people as with this person because I would probably have more fun.

12. I am able to share my feelings with this person and trust him/her completely.
13. I really love this person but do not feel good about sharing intimate feelings with him/her yet.
14. This person brings out the best in me and genuinely seems to care about me.
15. I love this person, but I do not respect him/her the way I respect others.

SCORING

There are no right or wrong responses to these statements. Answering YES to the even-numbered statements may indicate that your feelings are more likely to be love-directed. Answering YES to the odd-numbered statements may indicate a tendency toward infatuation. Count the number of YES responses to the even-numbered statements and the number of YES responses to the odd-numbered statements. Look carefully at each statement. Are these things that you feel are important enough to work on? Or are your responses telling you that another person may be a better choice?

to share their fears, anxieties, and emotions. It is okay if they cry, scream, or express wide emotional swings. Men are not supposed to cry—at least according to popular belief. Unlike their female counterparts, they are not to show emotions, and are brought up believing that being strong and independent is more important than close friendships. As a result, only 1 in 10 males has a close male friend to whom he divulges his innermost thoughts.[21]

Why the Differences?

Although there are various theories about why males and females relate the way they do, the basic difference lies in the development patterns of men and women.[22] According to this belief, men are less able to express emotions and achieve intimacy owing to the process of identity development in infancy, which is often more difficult for males than females. Males initially achieve

intimacy with a female caregiver, usually a mother, at a preverbal stage. By the time they develop verbal skills, boys have physically separated from their caregiver. Thus, for males, intimacy may consist of physical proximity rather than verbal sharing. Because females do not need to separate themselves from a female caregiver, they do not separate their feelings of intimacy from their verbal constructs. As a result, women are often able to express intimacy verbally, whereas men often are not. This male/female disparity in the ability to express emotions is the single greatest difference between the sexes and the greatest threat to intimacy in many relationships. This theory has received widespread acceptance among sociologists and psychologists. The disparity in the ability to express emotions may account for common female complaints about male attitudes toward sex; generally, emotion generates sexual feelings in women, whereas sexual feelings generate emotion in men. Sex, it seems, is one area in which men are allowed to contact deeper emotional states that may be hard for them to access in other circumstances. In fact, sexual activity carries the major burden of emotional expression for many males and may explain the urgency with which some men approach sex.

what do you THINK?

To whom do you feel most comfortable talking about personal issues? Do you talk equally with males and females about personal issues, or do you prefer one sex? Why? Similarly, who most frequently shares personal issues with you? Are males and females equally likely to open up to you, or just one sex? Why do you think this happens?

Picking Partners: Similarities and Differences between Genders

Just as males and females may find different ways to express themselves, the process of partner selection is also distinct. In males and females, more than chemical and psychological processes influence the choice of partners.[23] One factor is proximity, or being in the same place at the same time. The more you see a person in your hometown, at social gatherings, or at work, the more likely an interaction will occur. Thus, if you live in Winnipeg, you will probably choose another Winnipegger. If you live on Prince Edward Island, you will probably choose another Islander.

You also pick a partner on the basis of similarities (attitudes, values, intellect, experiences, interests); the adage that "opposites attract" usually is not true. Even though you may initially be attracted to someone extremely different from you, time tends to reveal that your lack of commonalities is too big a barrier to overcome. If your potential partner expresses interest or liking, you may react with mutual regard, known as reciprocity. The more you express interest, the safer it is for someone else to return the regard, and the cycle spirals onward.

Another factor that apparently plays a significant role in selecting a partner is physical attraction. Whether such attraction is caused by a chemical reaction or a socially learned behaviour, males and females appear to have different attraction criteria. Men tend to select their mates primarily on the basis of youth and physical attractiveness. Although physical attractiveness is an important criterion for women in mate selection, they tend to place greater emphasis on partners who are somewhat older, have good financial prospects, and are dependable and industrious. Good grooming is an almost universally desirable trait for

all. If you smell or appear less than squeaky clean, you may have problems in the partner arena regardless of your sex or sexual orientation.

BARRIERS TO INTIMACY

Obstacles to intimacy include lack of personal identity, emotional immaturity, and a poorly developed sense of responsibility. The fear of being hurt, low self-esteem, mishandled hostility, chronic "busyness" (and its attendant lack of emotional presence), a tendency to "parentify" loved ones, and a conflict of role expectations may be equally detrimental. In addition, individual insecurities and difficulties in recognizing and expressing emotional needs can lead to an intimacy barrier. These barriers to intimacy may have many causes, including the different emotional development of men and women and/or an upbringing in a dysfunctional family.

Dysfunctional Families

As noted earlier, the ability to sustain genuine intimacy is largely developed in the family of origin. Unfortunately, sharing, trust, and openness do not always occur in the family. In fact, the assumption that such intimacy exists in the family of origin may actually be unrealistic. As adults, we may discover that although we thought our family encouraged emotional intimacy, it was actually judgmental, full of expectations, controlling, and, in many ways, dysfunctional. A **dysfunctional family** is one in which the

The negative interactions in dysfunctional families that damage self-esteem and deter psychosocial growth do not exist in healthy families that encourage emotional intimacy.

Dysfunctional family: A family in which the interaction between family members inhibits rather than enhances psychological growth.

interaction between family members inhibits psychological growth rather than encouraging self-love, emotional expression, and individual growth. If you were to examine even the most pristine family under a microscope, you would likely find some type of dysfunction. No group of people who live together day in and day out can interact perfectly all the time. However, many people have begun to overuse the term *dysfunctional* to refer to even the smallest problems in the family unit. True dysfunctionality refers to settings where negative interactions are the norm rather than the exception. Children raised in these settings face tremendous obstacles to growing up to be healthy. Coming to terms with past hurts may take years. However, with careful planning and introspection support from loved ones, and counselling when needed, children from even the worst homes have proved to be remarkably resilient. Many are able to leave the past and focus on the future, developing into healthy, well-adjusted adults.[24] It is important to note that dysfunctional families are found in every social, ethnic, religious, and economic group.

For more than a decade, social scientists studied the impact of the alcoholic home environment on the sexual and intimate behaviours of adult children of alcoholics (ACOAs). A number of intimacy problems were identified as typical of ACOAs. Many ACOAs claim that they become involved in unhealthy relationships and have difficulty trusting others, problems in communicating with partners, and difficulty defining a healthy relationship.[25]

Another large group of people struggling with intimacy problems originating in the family of origin are survivors of childhood emotional, physical, or sexual abuse. Experiencing or witnessing physical, sexual, or emotional abuse as a child can have an impact on a person's intimate relationships as an adult. Domestic violence, whether directed at a child or another family member, can affect a child's ability to trust others and to maintain an intimate relationship later in life. Physical abuse may vary from spanking to violent beatings. Sexual abuse refers to any suggestive conversations, inappropriate kissing, touching, petting, oral, anal, or vaginal sex or any other kinds of sexual interaction between a child and an older child, adolescent, or adult. Emotional abuse includes name-calling and other tactics that damage a child's self-esteem.

Jealousy in Relationships

Jealousy is an aversive reaction evoked by a real or imagined relationship involving your partner and another person. Contrary to what many believe, jealousy is not a sign of intense devotion or of passionate love. Instead, jealousy is a sign of underlying problems that are a significant barrier to a healthy, intimate relationship. The roots of jealous feelings and behaviours may run deep and typically include

- Overdependence on the relationship. People who have few social ties and rely exclusively on their significant other tend to be excessively fearful of losing them.
- High value on sexual exclusivity. People who believe that sexual exclusiveness is a crucial indicator of a love relationship are more likely to become jealous.
- Severity of the threat. People may feel uneasy if a person with a fantastic body, stunning good looks, and a great personality appears interested in their partner.
- Low self-esteem. The underlying question that torments people with low self-esteem is, "Why would anyone want me?" People who feel good about themselves are less likely to feel unworthy and to fear that someone else is going to snatch their partner.
- Fear of losing control. Some people need to feel in control of the situation. Feeling that they may be losing the attachment of or control over a partner can cause jealousy.

For men and women, jealousy is related to the expectation that it would be difficult to find another relationship if the current one ends. For men, jealousy is related to self-evaluative dependence—that is, the degree to which the man's self-esteem is affected by his partner's judgments. A certain amount of jealousy is expected in any relationship. Communicating effectively about it will prevent the jealousy from causing any lasting damage.

---

what do you THINK?

"Jealousy is not a barometer by which the depth of love can be read. It merely records the depth of the lover's insecurity," observed anthropologist Margaret Mead. Do you agree with this statement? Why or why not? What other factors play a role in jealousy?

COMMITTED RELATIONSHIPS

Feelings of love or sexual attraction do not always equal commitment in a relationship. There can be love—or sex—without commitment. Commitment in a relationship refers to an intent to act over time in a way that perpetuates the well-being of the other person, you, and the relationship. A committed relationship involves tremendous diligence on the part of both partners. Over the years, partners learn about one another and adjust their relationship accordingly. What separates committed from uncommitted relationships is the willingness of the partners to dedicate themselves to acquiring and using the skills that will ensure a lasting relationship.

Marriage

Marriage is the traditional committed relationship in many societies around the world. For many people, marriage is the ultimate expression of an intimate relationship. When two people marry in Canada, they enter into a legal agreement that includes shared financial plans, property, and responsibility in raising children (should children become part of the relationship). For religious people, marriage is also a sacrament that stresses the spirituality, rights, and obligations of each person.

In 2007, of the total population in Canada 48.3 percent were legally married, living common law, or legally separated; 41.9 percent were single; 5.1 percent were divorced; and 4.8 percent were widowed.[26] There were 151 695 marriages in 2007, about 2000 more than in the previous year.[27] In 2003, the most recent year for which data are available, there were 70 828 divorces.[28]

Most people believe that marriage involves **monogamy**, or exclusive sexual involvement with one partner. The lifetime pattern for many Canadians appears to be **serial monogamy**, which means that a person has a monogamous sexual relationship with one partner for the duration of a relationship before moving on to another monogamous relationship. Some people prefer to have an **open relationship**, or open marriage, in which the partners agree that each person may be sexually involved outside their relationship.

Humans are not naturally monogamous; that is, most of us are capable of being sexually or emotionally involved with more than one person at a time. Yet Canadian society frowns on involvement with another person when in a committed relationship. Many people find themselves attracted to others while in a relationship and consciously try to stop subsequent interactions. Others find themselves involved unintentionally. Still others actively seek out extra-relationship affairs. Whether by choice or chance, sexual infidelity is a common factor in many divorces and break-ups. It seems that only those having exceptionally strong self-images and a dedication to the principles of open relationships are able to maintain nonmonogamy over a period of time.

As with all relationships, there are marriages that work well and bring satisfaction to the partners, and there are marriages that are unhealthy for the people involved. A good marriage can yield support and stability, not only for the couple but also for those involved in the couple's life. Considerable research also indicates that married people live longer, are happier, remain mentally alert longer, and suffer fewer bouts of physical and mental ailments. However, traditional marriage does not work for everyone and is not the only path to a happy and successful committed relationship.

Cohabitation

Cohabitation is defined as two unmarried people with an intimate connection who live together in the same household. The relationship can be stable, with a high level of commitment between the partners. In the latest Canadian census data available (2006), common-law couples comprised 10.5 percent of all legally married couples. In 2006, this category also included same-sex marriages.[29] The number of couples living common-law has risen steadily over the past 50 or 60 years such that there are now approximately 2.7 million couples. There is less marriage today as more young adults are choosing to live common-law.[30]

The increase in common-law marriages may be partly attributed to youth's inclination to question traditional values and the recognition that marriage may not be the only legitimate basis for sexual relations. The availability of cheaper, more effective birth control has probably been another factor, as has the notion that marriage is no longer a prerequisite for childbearing.[31] Many couples also believe that living together simply because they choose to may be more important than being bound by a legal document.

Although cohabitation is a viable alternative for some, many cohabitors eventually marry because of pressures from parents and friends, difficulties in obtaining insurance and tax benefits, legal issues over property, and a host of other reasons. The disadvantage of cohabitation lies in the lack of societal validation for the relationship and, in some cases, in the

Jealousy: An aversive reaction evoked by a real or imagined relationship involving a person's partner and another person.

Monogamy: Exclusive sexual involvement with one partner.

Serial monogamy: Monogamous sexual relationship with one partner before moving on to another.

Open relationship: A relationship in which partners agree that there can be sexual involvement outside the relationship.

Cohabitation: Living together without being married.

societal disapproval of living together without being married. Cohabiting partners do not usually experience the social incentives to stay together that they would if they were married. If they decide to separate, however, they do not experience the legal problems involved in obtaining a divorce. In most provinces, cohabitation that lasts more than six months is viewed as a **common-law marriage** in the eyes of the court on issues of child care and spousal support. It is not the same, however, as becoming legally married. Some laws treat common-law spouses the same as married spouses. For example, parents' responsibilities to their children are the same whether the parents are married to each other or not. On the other hand, some laws apply to married people and not to common-law couples, such as the one that divides matrimonial property. In still other situations, how the law treats a common-law couple depends on how long they have lived together. For example, Service Canada considers moving to be with a spouse a valid reason to quit a job, and, for this purpose, considers a couple who have been living together for at least one year to be spouses.[32]

Gay and Lesbian Partnerships

Most people seek intimate, committed relationships during their adult years. This is no different for homosexual couples. Lesbians and gay men are socialized like others in our culture and place a high value on relationships. They seek the same things in their primary relationships as heterosexual partners: friendship, communication, validation, companionship, and a sense of stability. Studies of lesbian couples indicate high levels of attachment and satisfaction and a tendency toward monogamous, long-term relationships. Gay men, too, tend to form committed, long-term relationships, especially as they age.[33]

Challenges to successful homosexual relationships often stem from the discrimination they face and from difficulties dealing with social, legal, and religious doctrines. On July 19, 2005, Canada redefined the legal and social boundaries of marriage to include same-sex couples. For details, see the Health in the Media box "It's a Quiet Thing: Equal Marriage Is Law."

✳ SUCCESS IN COMMITTED RELATIONSHIPS

Because the traditional marriage ceremony includes the vow "till death do us part," the definition of success in a relationship tends to be based on whether a couple stays together over the years. Marriage has become the model to which relationships must conform to be considered stable or healthy. One reason for the increase in cohabitation and other alternative relationships is the need for new forms in which people can express their love and commitment to one another and still have individual needs met adequately. Success in relating to another human being may have more to do with the quality of the interaction between two people than with the number of years they live together. Many social scientists agree that the ideal in relating to another person is to develop a committed bond, the boundaries and form of which can—and should—change to allow the maximum degree of growth over time.

Partnering Scripts

Most parents love their children and want them to be happy. They often believe that their children will achieve happiness by living much as they have.

HEALTH IN THE MEDIA

It's a Quiet Thing: Equal Marriage Is Law

Marriage for same-sex couples is the law in Canada. Bill C-38 was passed into law by the Canadian Senate on July 19, 2005. The following evening, Chief Justice Beverly McLaughlin gave the bill royal assent.

The law was debated for more than five years in courtrooms, cabinet rooms, and living rooms across the country. The language of the debate indicated that what was at stake was more than simply small wording changes to the marriage law, but how marriage would be defined. Specifically, many debates were over whether individuals in same-sex unions formed families. Undoubtedly, the law indicated that such unions can and do form families.

The lack of "noise" made over this historic law in Canada (158 voted in favour and 133 against) indicates that the world simply continues, as it should.

Source: Adapted from K. Bourassa and J. Varnell, "It's a Quiet Thing: Equal Marriage Is Law: Marriage Receives Senate Approval & Royal Assent." Retrieved on May 9, 2006, from www.samesexmarriage.ca/legal/qui210705.htm.

Accordingly, children are raised with a very strong script for what is expected of them as adults. Each group in society has its own partnering script that prescribes standards regarding sex, age, social class, ethnicity, religion, physical attributes, and personality types. By adolescence, boys and girls generally know exactly what type of person they are expected to befriend or to date.

Society provides constant reinforcement for traditional couples. People who choose an "appropriate" partner usually have plenty of validation for the relationship. The love and support they feel from friends and family is genuine. It also comes with expectations of what will occur within the relationship. Decisions that the couple feels should be exclusively theirs may provoke unsolicited advice from friends and family.

As Canadian society becomes increasingly multicultural, in-group partnering is giving way to more frequent mixing of cultures, backgrounds, and ethnicities. Nonetheless, a relationship between people of different cultural and ethnic backgrounds often brings increased tension partly because of the lack of societal reinforcement. In addition to a lack of recognition given to non-traditional couples, friends and family often blame the non-traditional nature of the pairing if the relationship fails.

---

what do you THINK?

By which partnering script were you raised? Would your parents be happy if you brought a same-sex partner into your home? Or a partner of a different religion, cultural background, or ethnicity?

The Importance of Self-Nurturance

It is often stated that you must love yourself before you can love someone else. What does this mean? Learning how you function emotionally and how to nurture yourself through all life's situations is a lifelong task. There seems to be a certain level of individual maturity that needs to be reached before a successful intimate relationship becomes possible. One can look to age of marriage and divorce rates for support. Someone marrying in their teens faces a risk of marital breakdown twice as high as someone who marries between the ages of 25 and 29 years.[34] People who wait until their mid 30s to marry have a 43 percent reduced risk of marital break up.

Two concepts especially important to knowing yourself and maintaining a good relationship are accountability and self-nurturance. **Accountability** means that both partners see themselves as responsible for their decisions and actions. The other person is not held responsible for the positive or negative experiences in life. Each and every choice is one's own responsibility. When two people are accountable for their own emotional states, partners can be angry, sad, or frustrated without the other person taking it personally. Accountable people may even say something like, "This has nothing to do with you; I just happen to be angry right now."

Self-nurturance goes hand-in-hand with accountability. In order to make good choices in life, a person needs to maintain a balance of sleeping, healthy eating, being physically active, working, relaxing, and socializing. When the balance is disrupted, as it will inevitably be, self-nurturing people are patient with themselves and sort these things out to get back on track. When they make bad choices, as all people do, self-nurturing people learn from the experience. Learning to live in a balanced and healthy way is a lifelong process. Two people on a path of accountability and self-nurturance together have a much better chance of maintaining a satisfying relationship.

Elements of Good Relationships

Satisfying and stable relationships share certain elements. Some of these are achieved through conscious efforts and communication; others evolve over time. People in healthy, committed relationships trust one another. Without trust, intimacy will not develop and the relationship will experience trouble and possible failure. **Trust** can be defined as the degree of confidence felt in a relationship. Trust includes three fundamental elements: predictability, dependability, and faith.

- Predictability means that you can predict your partner's behaviours. This sense of predictability is based on the knowledge that your partner acts in consistently positive ways.

- Dependability means that you can rely on your partner to give support in all situations, particularly in those in which you feel threatened with hurt or rejection.

- Faith means that you feel absolutely certain about your partner's intentions and behaviours.

Trust and intimacy are the foundation of healthy, committed relationships. Spouses who like and enjoy

---

Common-law marriage: Cohabitation lasting at least six months.

Accountability: Accepting responsibility for personal decisions, choices, and actions.

Self-nurturance: Taking care of oneself as needed.

Trust: The degree of confidence felt in a relationship.

one another as people and find each other interesting frequently are happier than those who do not. Many spouses describe their partners as their best friends. Although most marriages have their share of ups and downs, successful couples are able to communicate and touch one another in an atmosphere of caring. They value a good sense of humour and exhibit communication, cooperation, and the ability to resolve conflicts constructively.

Sexual intimacy is also a major part of healthy relationships, but sex is not the major reason the relationship exists. Some couples admit to sexual dissatisfaction but feel the relationship is more important. Rather than seek an outlet in an extramarital affair, those who are dissatisfied with their sex lives adjust and spend little energy worrying about it because the relationship is satisfying in other, important ways. Many couples report that as communication and trust increase in a long-term, committed relationship, their sexual relationship also improves.

STAYING SINGLE

While many people choose to marry and have children, increasing numbers of young and older adults remain single. As previously noted, 41.9 percent of the population is single; 53.6 percent of which is male.[35] While many of these people seek or have sought committed relationships, they find being single preferable. Singles clubs, social outings arranged by communities and churches, extended-family environments, and a large number of social services support the single lifestyle. Although some research indicates that single people live shorter lives, are less happy, more likely to be financially distressed, and more prone to illnesses than their married counterparts, other studies contradict these findings. At least one Canadian study noted it was social isolation (as measured by the social network index), not marital status, that had an impact on self-reported health.[36]

✳ HAVING CHILDREN

When a couple decides to have children, their relationship changes. Resources of time, energy, and money are split many ways, and the partners no longer have each other's undivided attention. Babies and young children do not time their requests for food, sleep, and care to the convenience of adults. Therefore, individuals or couples whose basic needs for security, love, and purpose are met make better parents. Any stresses that

already exist in a relationship are further accentuated when parenting is added to the list of responsibilities. Having a child does not "fix" a bad relationship and, in fact, may compound problems that already exist. A child cannot and should not be expected to provide the parents with self-esteem and security.

Changing patterns in family life affect the way children are raised. In modern society, it is not always clear which partner will adjust his or her work schedule to provide the primary care. Remarriage creates a new family of stepparents and stepsiblings. An increasing number of individuals are choosing to have children in a family structure other than a male/female couple. Single women or lesbian couples can choose adoption or alternative (formerly "artificial") insemination as a way to create a family. Single men or gay couples can choose to adopt or obtain the services of a surrogate mother. Regardless of the structure of the family, certain factors remain important to the well-being of the unit: consistency, communication, affection, and mutual respect.

Some people become parents without a lot of forethought and some children are born into a relationship that does not last. This does not mean it is too late to do a good job of parenting. Attention, consistency, and caring can be provided by other adults if a parent cannot be physically or emotionally present for a period of time. Children are resilient and forgiving if parents show respect to them and communicate about household activities that affect their lives. Even children who grow up in a household of conflict can feel loved and respected if the parents treat them fairly. This means that parents take responsibility for any of their own conflicts and make it clear to the children that they are not the reason for the conflict. Further, these parents do not bring their children into the conflict, nor do they use them as pawns against one another.

Changes in the traditional family structure have forced society to examine alternative means of raising children. Day-care centres, extended families, and live-in babysitters or nannies are becoming important alternatives to the traditional "nuclear family" unit.

what do you THINK?

What are the essential characteristics of a healthy "family" environment? How is such an environment important to the future development of our children? Do you think that day-care centres, extended family units, and full-time babysitters or nannies are equally capable of providing a positive environment for a child's personal growth? Why or why not?

ENDING A RELATIONSHIP

The Warning Signs

The symptoms of a troubled relationship are relatively easy to recognize. Many couples choose to ignore them, however, until the situation erupts into some type of emotional confrontation. By then, the relationship may be beyond salvaging. Breakdowns in relationships usually begin with a change in communication, however subtle. Either partner may stop listening, ceasing to be emotionally present for the other. In turn, the other feels ignored, unappreciated, or unwanted. Unresolved conflicts may increase, and unresolved anger can cause problems in sexual relations.

When a couple who previously enjoyed spending time alone together find themselves continually in the company of others, spending time apart, or preferring to stay home alone, it may be a sign that the relationship is in trouble. Of course, the need for individual privacy is not a cause for worry—it's essential to health. If, however, a partner decides to make a change in the amount and quality of time spent together without the input or understanding of the other, it may be a sign of hidden problems.

Post-secondary students, particularly those who are socially isolated because they are far from family and hometown friends, may be particularly vulnerable to remaining in unhealthy relationships. They may become emotionally dependent on a partner for everything from eating meals to recreational and study time: mutual obligations such as shared rental arrangements, transportation, and child care can make it difficult to leave. It is also easy to mistake unwanted sexual advances for physical attraction or love. Without a network of friends and supporters with whom a student can talk, obtain validation for feelings, or share concerns, he or she may feel stuck in a relationship headed nowhere.

Honesty and verbal affection are usually positive aspects of a relationship. In a troubled relationship, however, they can be used to cover up irresponsible or hurtful behaviours. "At least I was honest" is not an acceptable substitute for acting in a trustworthy way. The words "But I really do love you" should not be used as a licence to be inconsiderate, rude, or hurtful to a partner.

Seeking Help: Where to Look

The first place some people look for help when there are problems in a relationship is a trusted friend. Although friends can offer needed support during these difficult times, few have the training and detachment necessary to help you to resolve your problems. Others find that they do not have the type of friendships that lend themselves to divulging these kinds of problems.

As previously mentioned, most communities have private practitioners trained to counsel married or committed couples. Community mental health centres usually have trained counsellors as well. These practitioners may be psychiatrists, licensed psychologists, social workers, or counsellors with advanced degrees. These counsellors are often specially equipped to deal with the unique needs of young adults with relationship, sexual, emotional, financial, or other concerns. Most student health centres or counselling centres on campus have reduced student fees or no fees for students who need help. If you are unaware of such services, talk with your instructor and ask for his or her advice about where someone with your type of problem may get help.

Trial Separations

Sometimes a relationship becomes so dysfunctional that even counselling cannot bring about significant change. Moving apart for a period of time may allow some preliminary healing and give both parties an opportunity to reassess themselves and their commitment to the relationship. Trial separations do not guarantee that the situation will improve, nor do they mean the relationship is ending. If both people are involved in counselling or have other support systems and mutually agree on the need for a trial separation, it may be a way to regroup and save a failing relationship.

Unresolved conflicts and frequent emotional confrontations are signs of a troubled relationship. If each partner is committed to staying together, counselling may bring about positive change.

Building Healthy Relationships

Couple and family therapy often helps those who experience difficulty in their relationships. All communities have a variety of services that couples, individually or together, can use to better understand and strengthen their relationship. Below are some frequently asked questions:

What can I do if my relationship is in trouble?

Do not put it off—get professional help now. Often couples are afraid to admit that there is a problem, and wait too long. The distancing increases and things are said and done that are hard to take back. The right time to start improving the relationship is now, not later.

What kind of help is available?

Many different professionals can help: clergy, medical doctors, psychologists, psychiatrists, and social workers who have taken specialized training in couple and family therapy. Most communities have a Community Information Service that lists social service agencies and therapists whose specialty is couple and family therapy. Marriage and family therapists are also listed in the yellow pages.

What do couple and family therapists do?

Talking about your situation with a therapist can help you to gain a new perspective on the issues you are dealing with. You can also improve your level of communication so that the thoughts and feelings that have previously been unspoken are brought out into the open. The tension level is lowered so that old issues can be resolved.

How do I choose a couple and family therapist?

Since you will be sharing intimate details of your relationship with your therapist, you want to make sure that there is a good match, and that you feel safe. Feel free to call several offices and get a feel for the therapist. Most therapists should be willing to have a five-minute discussion on the phone with you while you are searching for the right match.

What kind of questions should I ask?

You are looking for two things: professional competence and personal style. For competence issues you will want to know what professional training therapists have, what professional associations they belong to, and if they are registered in their profession. Couple and family therapists must have at least a master's degree in relationship counselling and have been supervised for a minimum of 1000 client hours before they

can be registered. All provinces have an Association of Marriage and Family Therapists and an Association of Social Workers. They can provide you with a list of therapists in your area. You can also contact the Canadian Guidance Counsellors Association.

How long does therapy take?

Each situation is unique. Usually the therapist will set one appointment each week for the first few weeks. Each session is generally about 50 minutes, with an average of 8 to 10 sessions. Often by that time significant changes have been made in the relationship and you are ready to make a go of it on your own.

How much does therapy cost?

Costs can vary from $50 to $125 per session. Registered psychologists usually charge more than $100 per session. Public health insurance does not cover the cost of therapy unless the therapy is provided by a psychiatrist. Many employee benefit plans will cover all or portions of the cost of couple and family therapy. Check with your service provider to see what assistance you can receive.

You can expect to pay around $500 for couple therapy. Given that the cost of an uncontested divorce is about $1300 and one that is contested can cost much more, working on the relationship may provide savings in more than one way!

How long do I have to wait to get an appointment?

Usually you will be seen within a week or two. It depends, however, on how flexible you can be. Most therapists will have some evening hours, but these usually fill up quickly. If you require an evening appointment, you might have to wait a little longer.

Who should come to the appointment?

Whoever is involved! If it is a marital issue it is best if both partners attend. If it is a family issue, the therapist may ask the whole family to attend. This helps the therapist to see the situation in its full context and for each person involved to present how they experience the issue.

What if my partner won't come?

The therapist may suggest some helpful strategies to lower your partner's anxiety and make it easier for him or her to attend. If, however, your partner chooses not to participate, it is still possible to proceed on your own.

Why Relationships End

Although there was a gradual decrease in the number of Canadian couples experiencing divorce from the 1990s to the 2000s, the number of divorces now remains steady. As noted previously, there were 70 828 divorces in 2003 (the most recent data available).[37] The reasons for divorce and relationship breakdown are numerous. One contributing factor may be the lack of communication and cooperation between partners under the additional stress of tragedies such as the death of a child, serious illness of one partner, severe financial difficulties, and career failures. What about breakups between people who have not experienced these tragedies? These breakups also arise from poor communication and cooperation between partners along with unmet expectations regarding marriage or relationships in general or personal roles within the relationship. Many people enter marriage with unrealistic expectations about what marriage will be like and how they and their partner will behave. Many people enter relationships looking for someone to fill the empty spots in their lives. Failure to communicate such expectations to your partner can lead to resentment and disappointment. Because many premarital expectations may be unreasonable, early exploration of these expectations is important. This exploration may take place together or within a support program.

Differences in sexual needs may also contribute to the demise of a relationship. Many partners find that their spouses desire sex at different times or in different styles and frequencies than they do. Unless sexual differences are resolved, one or both partners may begin to feel used and resent sexual activity.

The bottom line is that if couples do not grow together, they often grow apart. Reality dictates a need to change or adapt to life's experiences as we grow older, our careers change, we develop new friendships, or our family life changes, first with the addition of children and then later when they move away from home. Without a commitment to working on their differences and continuing to build a life together, many people choose to move on, and this decision—as difficult as it may be—could be the best for all concerned.

Deciding to Break Up

At some point, troubled couples may feel that their relationship is not worth saving. The decision to end the relationship is usually difficult, even for couples whose relationship was over long before the decision was made. Choosing to leave is not an easy decision, nor is formally separating and/or divorcing.

For married couples, wading through divorce or dissolution proceedings may be painful as they decide child-custody issues, alimony questions, and division of property. Finding legal assistance may be difficult, because painful emotions usually affect judgment. Cohabiting couples also experience difficulty in separating. Legal problems involving property, children, and alimony are often more ambiguous than in a marriage. Some couples expend much time, money, and energy working out settlements with lawyers who specialize in problems following the breakup of a common-law relationship.

Aside from legal worries, many newly separated or divorced people experience painful emotions of anger, guilt, rejection, and unworthiness. No matter how miserable the relationship, feelings of failure are not uncommon or abnormal following a divorce or breakup, and the emotional wounds take varying amounts of time to heal. Counsellors familiar with loss and grieving estimate that it takes at least a year and often longer to recover from the loss of a major relationship, whether by death or separation. With time, support from others, and community or professional help, most people do recover and establish new relationships.

Coping with Loneliness

Some people find establishing and maintaining relationships difficult. Others find that through death, illness, or distance, their relationships disappear or grow dim with time. Loneliness, or the unfulfilled desire to engage in a close personal relationship, is a difficult emotion to experience, even for the most determined person.

The loss of a committed relationship is usually too painful for a person to want to repeat. Reflecting on the beginning, the middle, and the ending of the relationship and identifying where there were problems can help you avoid similar mistakes in the future. Concentrating on the negative aspects of past behaviours of an ex-partner is a natural tendency, and may be helpful in getting in touch with emotions or in learning from the situation. It is equally important to spend time remembering what was loved in the other person and what is lovable about yourself. Intimacy, love, and commitment between people always change the lives of those involved. It is through relationships that we give and receive our greatest support and validation as worthwhile human beings. When we accept the risk and challenge of close relationships, we accept one of the greatest gifts life has to offer.

YOUR SEXUAL IDENTITY

Although you are a sexual being from birth, you are not born with complete knowledge about your sexuality. Learning about and becoming comfortable with your sexual self is a lifelong process. Taboos, mores, laws, and sexual myths abound and often hinder the process of learning about your sexual self. Family, friends, and the media—including print and electronic forms, music, religion, and educational institutions—provide you with information about your sexuality and how you should or should not express it.

In the end, it is up to you to blend all of this information with your personal experience and values to create your own sexual identity.

Your **sexual identity** is determined by a complex interaction of genetic, physiological, and environmental factors. The beginning of your sexual identity occurs at conception, with the combining of chromosomes that determine your sex. Actually, it is your biological father who determines whether you will be a boy or a girl. Here's how it works. All eggs (ova) carry an X sex chromosome; sperm carry either an X or a Y chromosome. If a sperm carrying an X chromosome fertilizes an egg, the resulting combination of sex chromosomes (XX) creates the blueprint to produce a female. If a sperm carrying a Y chromosome fertilizes an egg, the XY combination produces a male (see Figure 7.2). The genetic instructions included in the sex chromosomes lead to the differential development of male and female **gonads** at about the eighth day in utero. Once the male gonads (testes) and the female gonads (ovaries) are developed, they play a key role in all future sexual development because they are responsible for the production of sex hormones. The primary sex hormones produced by females are estrogen and progesterone. In males, the hormone of primary importance is testosterone. The release of testosterone in a maturing fetus signals the development of a penis and other male genitals. If no testosterone is produced, female genitals form.

During **puberty**, sex hormones play major roles in further development. Hormones released by the **pituitary gland**, called gonadotropins, stimulate the testes and ovaries to make appropriate sex hormones. The increased production of estrogen in females and testosterone in males leads to the development of **secondary sex characteristics**. Secondary sex characteristics in males include deepening of the voice, development of facial and body hair, and genital (penis and testes) development. In females, secondary sex characteristics include growth of the breasts, menarche, widening of the hips, and the development of pubic and underarm hair.

✳ Gender Identity and Roles

Thus far, we have described sexual identity only in terms of a person's sex. Sex simply refers to the biological condition of being male or female based on physiological and hormonal differences. **Gender**, on the other hand, refers to your sense of masculinity or femininity as defined by the society in which you live. Each of us expresses our maleness or femaleness to others on a daily basis through the **gender roles** we play. **Gender identity** refers to your personal sense or awareness of being masculine or feminine, a male or a female. It may sometimes be difficult for you to express your true sexual identity because you feel bound by existing gender-role stereotypes. **Gender-role stereotypes** refer to generalizations about how males and females should express themselves and the characteristics each possesses. Traditional sex roles are examples of gender-role stereotyping. Men are thought to be independent, aggressive, better in math and science, logical, and in control of their emotions. Women, on the other hand, are expected to be passive, nurturing, intuitive, sensitive, and emotional. **Androgyny** is the combination of traditional masculine and feminine traits in a single person. Androgynous people do not always follow traditional sex roles but, rather, act according to the given situation. The process by which a society transmits behavioural expectations to its individual members is called **socialization**. Gender roles are shaped or socialized by our parents, peers, education, and many forms of media including television, advertisements, the internet, music, video games, and movies. Think about the current television shows or movies you watch. Do the characters play traditional gender roles?

By now you can see that defining your sexual identity is not a simple matter. Your sexual identity is made up of the unique combination of your sex, gender identity, chosen gender roles, sexual preference, and personal experiences. No other person is exactly like you, and it is up to you to take every opportunity to get to know and like yourself so that you may enjoy your life to the fullest. Sex is what you are born with, while sexuality reflects who you are.

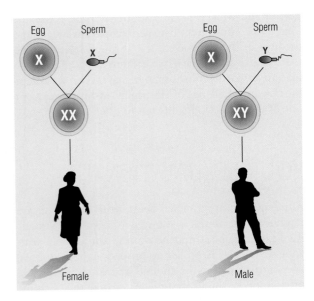

FIGURE 7.2
How Sex Is Determined

what do you THINK?

In what ways do you feel masculine or feminine? In what ways are you limited or bound by existing gender-role stereotypes? Do you challenge these stereotypes? In what way? What else can you do?

REPRODUCTIVE ANATOMY AND PHYSIOLOGY

An understanding of the functions of the male and female reproductive systems will help you derive pleasure and satisfaction from your sexual relationships, be sensitive to your partner's wants and needs, and be more responsible in your choices regarding your sexual health.

Female Reproductive Anatomy and Physiology

The female reproductive system includes two major groups of structures: the external and internal genitals (see Figures 7.3 and 7.4). The **external female genitals** include the outwardly visible structures often referred to as the vulva. The **vulva**, includes the mons pubis, the labia minora and majora, the clitoris, the urethral and vaginal openings, and the vestibule of the vagina. The **mons pubis** is a pad of fatty tissue covering the pubic bone. The mons protects the pubic bone, and during puberty becomes covered with coarse hair. The **labia minora** are folds of mucous membrane and the **labia majora** are folds of skin and erectile tissue that enclose the urethral and vaginal openings. The labia minora are found just inside the labia majora.

The **clitoris** is the female sexual organ whose only known function is sexual pleasure. It is located at the upper end of the labia minora and beneath the mons pubis. Directly below the clitoris is the **urethral opening** through which urine leaves the body. Below the urethral opening is the opening of the **vagina**. In some women, the vaginal opening is covered by a thin membrane called the **hymen**. It is a myth that an intact hymen is proof of virginity. The **perineum** is the area between the vulva and the anus. Although not technically part of the external genitalia, the tissue in this area has many nerve endings and is sensitive to touch; it can play a part in sexual excitement.

The **internal female genitals** of the reproductive system include the vagina, uterus, fallopian tubes, and ovaries. The vagina is a tubular passageway from the uterus to the outside of a female's body. This passageway allows menstrual flow to exit from the uterus during a woman's monthly cycle and serves as the birth canal. The vagina also receives the penis during intercourse. The **uterus**, also known as the womb, is a hollow, muscular, pear-shaped organ. Hormones acting on the

Sexual identity: Our recognition of ourselves as sexual beings; a composite of sex, gender, gender roles, sexual preference, body image, and sexual scripts.

Gonads: The reproductive organs in a male (testes) and female (ovaries).

Puberty: The period of sexual maturation.

Pituitary gland: The endocrine gland controlling the release of hormones from the gonads (ovaries and testes).

Secondary sex characteristics: Characteristics associated with sex developed during puberty such as vocal pitch, degree of body hair, and genital development.

Gender: Your sense of masculinity or femininity as defined by the society in which you live.

Gender roles: Daily expression of maleness or femaleness.

Gender identity: Your personal sense or awareness of being masculine or feminine, a male or a female.

Gender-role stereotypes: Socialized generalizations concerning how males and females should be and how they express themselves.

Androgyny: Combination of traditional masculine and feminine traits in a single person.

Socialization: Process by which a society identifies attitudinal and behavioural expectations to its individual members.

External female genitals: The outwardly visible structure or vulva.

Vulva: Includes the mons pubis, labia majora and minora, clitoris, urethral and vaginal openings, and vestibule of the vagina and its glands.

Mons pubis: Fatty tissue covering the pubic bone in females; in physically mature women, the mons is covered with coarse hair.

Labia minora: "Inner lips" or folds of tissue just inside the labia majora.

Labia majora: "Outer lips" or folds of tissue covering the female sexual organs.

Clitoris: A pea-sized nodule of tissue located at the top of the labia minora.

Urethral opening: The opening through which urine is released.

Vagina: The passage leading from the vulva to the uterus.

Hymen: Thin tissue covering the vaginal opening.

Perineum: Tissue extending from the vulva to the anus.

Internal female genitals: The vagina, uterus, fallopian tubes, and ovaries.

Uterus (womb): Hollow, pear-shaped muscular organ whose function is to house the developing fetus.

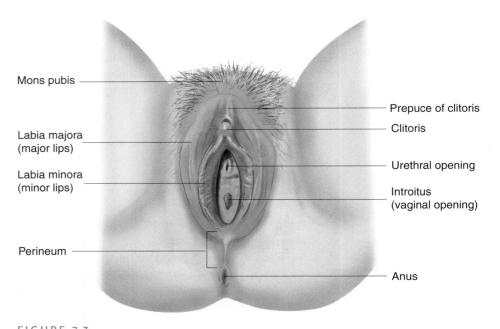

FIGURE 7.3

External Female Genital Structures

Source: R. D. McAnulty and M. M. Burnette, *Exploring Human Sexuality: Making Healthy Decisions* (Boston: Allyn & Bacon, 2001). Copyright © 2001 by Pearson Education.

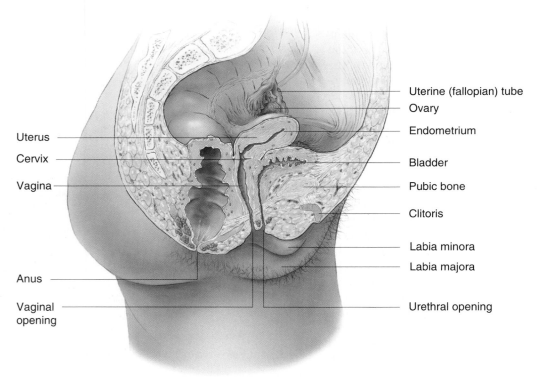

FIGURE 7.4

Side View of the Female Reproductive Organs

inner lining of the uterus, called the **endometrium**, either prepare the uterus for implantation and development of a fertilized egg or signal that no fertilization has taken place, in which case the endometrium deteriorates and becomes menstrual flow.

The lower end of the uterus is called the **cervix** and extends down into the vagina. The **ovaries** are almond-sized structures suspended on either side of the uterus. The ovaries produce the hormones estrogen and progesterone and are the reservoir for immature eggs. All the eggs a female will ever have are present in her ovaries at birth. Eggs mature and are released from the ovaries in response to hormones. Extending from the upper end of the uterus are two thin, flexible tubes called the **fallopian tubes**. The fallopian tubes are where the sperm and egg meet and fertilization takes place. Following fertilization, the fallopian tubes serve as the passageway to the uterus, where the fertilized egg implants and development continues.

The Onset of Puberty and the Menstrual Cycle

During puberty, the female reproductive system matures and secondary sex characteristics transform girls into women. Under the direction of the endocrine system, the pituitary gland, the hypothalamus, and the ovaries secrete hormones that act as the chemical messengers among them. Working in a feedback system, hormonal levels in the bloodstream act as the trigger mechanism for release of more or different hormones (see Figure 7.5).

At the beginning of puberty in females, the **hypothalamus** receives the message to begin secreting **gonadotropin-releasing hormone (GnRH)**. The release of GnRH in turn signals the **pituitary gland** to release hormones called gonadotropins. **Follicle-stimulating hormone (FSH)** and **luteinizing hormone (LH)** are two gonadotropins, and their role is to signal the gonads, in this case the ovaries, to start producing **estrogen** and **progesterone**. Increased estrogen directs the development of female secondary sex characteristics. In addition, estrogen is responsible for regulating the reproductive cycle. The usual age range for the onset of the first menstrual period, termed **menarche**, is 10 to 16 years, with the average age in Canada around 12 or 13 years.

The average menstrual cycle is 28 days and is divided into three phases: the proliferatory phase, the secretory phase, and the menstrual phase. During the proliferatory phase, the pituitary gland releases FSH and LH. The FSH acts on the ovaries to stimulate the maturation process of several **ovarian follicles (egg sacs)**. These follicles secrete estrogen and, in response, the lining of the uterus, the endometrium, begins to

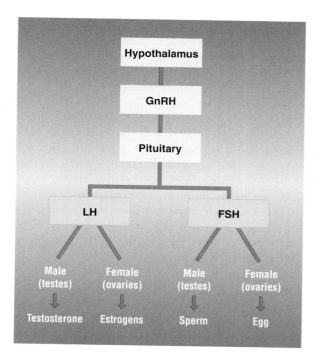

FIGURE 7.5

Hormonal Direction of the Human Reproductive System

Endometrium: Soft, spongy matter that makes up the uterine lining.

Cervix: Lower end of the uterus that opens into the vagina.

Ovaries: Almond-sized organs that house developing eggs and produce hormones.

Fallopian tubes: Tubes that extend from the ovaries to the uterus.

Hypothalamus: An area of the brain located near the pituitary gland. The hypothalamus works with the pituitary gland to control reproductive functions.

Gonadotropin-releasing hormone (GnRH): Hormone that signals the pituitary gland to release gonadotropins.

Pituitary gland: A gland located deep within the brain; controls reproductive functions.

Follicle-stimulating hormone (FSH): Hormone that signals the ovaries to prepare to release an egg and to begin producing estrogen.

Luteinizing hormone (LH): Hormone that signals the ovaries to release an egg and to begin producing progesterone.

Estrogen: Hormones that control the menstrual cycle.

Progesterone: Hormone secreted by the ovaries; helps keep the endometrium developing in order to nourish a fertilized egg; also helps maintain pregnancy.

Menarche: The first menstrual period.

Ovarian follicles (egg sacs): Areas within the ovary in which individual eggs develop.

grow and develop. The inner walls of the uterus become coated with a thick, spongy lining composed of blood and mucus. In the event of fertilization, the endometrial tissue will become a nesting place for the developing embryo. The increased estrogen level also signals the pituitary to slow down FSH production and to increase LH secretion. Of the several follicles developing in the ovaries, only one each month normally reaches complete maturity. Under the influence of LH, this one ovarian follicle rapidly matures, and on or about the fourteenth day of the proliferatory phase it releases an ovum into the fallopian tube—a process referred to as **ovulation**. Just prior to ovulation, the mature egg's follicle begins to increase secretion of progesterone, the first function of which is to spur the addition of further nutrients to the developing endometrium.

After ovulation, the ovarian follicle is converted into the corpus luteum, or yellow body, which continues to secrete estrogen and progesterone but in decreasing amounts. In addition, FSH falls back to its preproliferatory levels. Essentially, the woman's body is "waiting" to see whether fertilization occurs. During the time after ovulation, LH declines, and progesterone levels begin to rise, causing additional tissue growth in the endometrium. This phase of the cycle is called the secretory phase.

If fertilization takes place, cells surrounding the developing embryo release a hormone called **human chorionic gonadotropin (HCG)**. This hormone leads to increased levels of estrogen and progesterone secretion, which maintains the endometrium while signalling the pituitary gland not to start a new menstrual cycle. If fertilization does not occur, the egg gradually disintegrates in about 72 hours. The corpus luteum gradually becomes nonfunctional, causing levels of progesterone and estrogen to decline. As hormonal levels decline, the endometrial lining of the uterus loses its nourishment, dies, and is sloughed off as menstrual flow. Menstruation is the third phase of the menstrual cycle.

Menopause

Just as menarche signals the beginning of a woman's potential reproductive years, **menopause**—the permanent cessation of menstruation—signals the end. Generally menopause occurs between the ages of 40 and 60 years and results in decreased estrogen levels. Reduced estrogen typically results in a decrease in vaginal lubrication, hot flashes, headaches, dizziness, and joint pain. As a woman's body adjusts to the decreased level of estrogen, these symptoms abate.

Hormones such as estrogen and progesterone have been prescribed as hormone replacement therapy (HRT) to relieve menopausal symptoms and reduce the risk of heart disease and osteoporosis. However, the results from some studies indicate that hormone therapy may actually do more harm than good. In particular, HRT may increase risk of breast cancer, heart attack, stroke, blood clots, and other health problems.[38] A woman needs to discuss the risks and benefits of HRT with her health-care provider and come to an informed decision. Certainly lifestyle changes such as regular physical activity and a dietary intake low in fat and adequate in calcium can also help protect postmenopausal women from heart disease and osteoporosis. Engaging in regular physical activity may also alleviate the symptoms experienced from reduced estrogen.

> ## what do you THINK?
>
> Why is it important to understand the design and function of our sexual anatomy? Should men learn about the menstrual cycle too? Why or why not?

Male Reproductive Anatomy and Physiology

The structures of the male reproductive system may be divided into external and internal genitals (see Figure 7.6). The penis and the scrotum make up the **external male genitals**. The **internal male genitals** include the testes, epididymides, vasa deferentia, urethra, and three other structures—the seminal vesicles, the prostate gland, and the Cowper's glands—that secrete components that, with sperm, make up semen. These three structures are sometimes referred to as the **accessory glands**.

The **penis** is the organ that releases sperm during ejaculation. The urethra, which passes through the centre of the penis, acts as the passageway for semen and urine to exit the body. During sexual arousal, the spongy tissue in the penis becomes filled with blood, making it erect. Further sexual excitement leads to **ejaculation**, a series of rapid spasmodic contractions that propel semen out of the penis.

Situated behind the penis outside the body is a sac called the **scrotum**. The scrotum protects the testes and helps control the temperature within the testes, which is vital to sperm production. The **testes** (singular: testis) are egg-shaped structures in which sperm are manufactured. The testes also contain cells that manufacture **testosterone**, the hormone responsible for male secondary sex characteristic development.

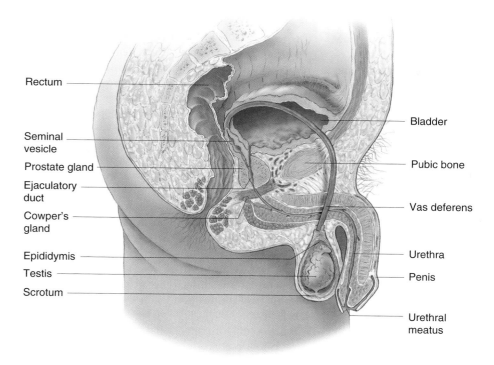

Rectum

Seminal vesicle

Prostate gland

Ejaculatory duct

Cowper's gland

Epididymis

Testis

Scrotum

Bladder

Pubic bone

Vas deferens

Urethra

Penis

Urethral meatus

FIGURE 7.6

Side View of the Male Reproductive Organs

Spermatogenesis describes the development of sperm. Like the maturation of eggs in the female, this process is governed by the pituitary gland. Follicle-stimulating hormone (FSH) is secreted into the blood-stream to stimulate the testes to manufacture sperm. Immature sperm are released into a comma-shaped structure on the back of each testis called the **epididymis** (plural: epididymides), where they reach full maturity.

The epididymis contains coiled tubules that gradually "unwind" and straighten to become the **vas deferens**. The two vasa deferentia, as they are called in the plural, make up the tubular transportation system with the sole function to store and move sperm. Along the way, the **seminal vesicles** provide sperm with nutrients and other fluids that compose **semen**.

The vasa deferentia eventually connect each epididymis to the ejaculatory ducts, which pass through the **prostate gland** and empty into the urethra. The prostate gland contributes more fluids to the semen, including chemicals to aid the sperm in fertilization of an ovum, and, more importantly, a chemical that neutralizes the acid in the vagina to make its environment more conducive to sperm motility (ability to move) and potency (potential for fertilizing an ovum).

Ovulation: The point of the menstrual cycle at which a mature egg ruptures through the ovarian wall.

Human chorionic gonadotropin (HCG): Hormone that calls for increased levels of estrogen and progesterone secretion if fertilization has taken place.

Menopause: The permanent cessation of menstruation.

External male genitals: The penis and scrotum.

Internal male genitals: The testes, epididymides, vasa deferentia, ejaculatory ducts, urethra, and accessory glands.

Accessory glands: The seminal vesicles, prostate gland, and Cowper's glands.

Penis: Male sexual organ.

Ejaculation: The propulsion of semen from the penis.

Scrotum: Sac of tissue that encloses the testes.

Testes: Two organs, located in the scrotum, that manufacture sperm and produce testosterone.

Testosterone: The male sex hormone manufactured in the testes.

Spermatogenesis: The development of sperm.

Epididymis: A comma-shaped structure atop the testis where sperm mature.

Vas deferens: A tube that transports sperm toward the penis.

Seminal vesicles: Storage areas for sperm where nutrient fluids are added.

Semen: Fluid containing sperm and nutrients that increase sperm viability and neutralize vaginal acid.

Prostate gland: Gland that secretes nutrients and neutralizing fluids in the semen.

Just below the prostate gland are two pea-shaped nodules called the Cowper's glands. Their primary function is to secrete a fluid that lubricates the urethra and neutralizes any acid that may remain in the urethra after urination. Urine and semen do not come into contact with each other. During ejaculation of semen, the tube to the urinary bladder is closed off by a small valve.

Circumcision: Risk versus Benefit

Parents decide whether their male infant will be circumcised. Circumcision involves the surgical removal of the **foreskin**, a flap of skin covering the tip of the penis. Most circumcisions are performed for religious or cultural reasons or because of concerns about hygiene. In the uncircumcised male, oily secretions and sloughed-off dead cells (smegma) can collect under the foreskin and create an irritation or a breeding ground for infection. Removing the foreskin makes cleansing the penis easier. Today, infants can be given a local anesthetic, and circumcisions can be performed with little or no pain. This does not mean, however, that the procedure itself is without risk. All surgery involves some risk. If circumcision is performed later in life under a general anesthetic, the risk of complications is greater. Like all other elective surgical procedures, careful consideration of the risks and benefits of circumcision should be made prior to making a decision.

EXPRESSING YOUR SEXUALITY

Finding healthy ways to express your sexuality is an important part of developing sexual maturity. Many avenues of sexual expression are available.

Human Sexual Response

Sexual response is a physiological process that involves different stages. The biological goal of the response process is the reproduction of the species. Human psychological traits greatly influence sexual desire and response. Thus, we may find relationships with one partner vastly different from those we experience with another partner.

Sexual response generally follows a pattern, though individual differences are common. Men and women each exhibit four common stages: excitement/arousal, plateau, orgasm, and resolution. In addition, some men may experience a fifth stage, the refractory period. Regardless of the type of sexual activity (stimulation by a partner or self), the response stages are the same.

During the first stage, excitement/arousal, genital responses are caused by **vasocongestion**, or increased blood flow in the genital region. Increased blood flow to these organs causes them to swell. The vagina begins to lubricate in preparation for penile penetration and the penis becomes partially erect. Both sexes may exhibit a "sex flush," or light blush all over their bodies. Excitement/arousal can be generated by touching, kissing, talking, through fantasy, viewing films or videos, or reading erotic literature.

The plateau phase is characterized by an intensification of the initial responses. Voluntary and involuntary muscle tensions increase. The woman's nipples and the man's penis become erect. A few drops of semen, which may contain sperm, are secreted from the penis at this time. The women's genitalia also become "wet" at this point as her vagina continues to lubricate.

During the orgasmic phase, vasocongestion and muscle tensions reach their peak, and rhythmic contractions occur through the genital regions. In women, these contractions are centred in the uterus, the outer vagina, and the anal sphincter. In men, the contractions occur in two stages. First, contractions within the prostate gland begin propelling semen through the urethra. In the second stage, the muscles of the pelvic floor, the urethra, and the anal sphincter contract. Usually, but not always, semen is ejaculated from the penis. In both sexes, spasms in other major muscle groups also occur, particularly in the buttocks and abdomen. Feet and hands may also contract, and facial features often contort.

Muscle tension and congested blood subside in the resolution phase, as the genital organs return to their pre-arousal states. Both sexes usually experience deep feelings of well-being, satisfaction, and profound relaxation.

As previously noted, some men experience a fifth phase—the refractory phase. In this phase, men experience a period of time in which their systems are incapable of subsequent arousal. This refractory period may last from a few minutes to several hours. The length of the refractory period increases with age. Following orgasm and resolution, many women are capable of being aroused and brought to orgasm again, though subsequent orgasms are typically less intense. Men and women experience the same stages in the sexual response cycle; however, the length of time spent in any one stage is variable. Thus, one partner may be in the plateau phase while the other is in the excitement or orgasmic phase. Such variations in response rates are entirely normal. Some couples believe that simultaneous orgasm is desirable for sexual satisfaction. Although simultaneous orgasm is pleasant, so are orgasms achieved at different times.

Sexual pleasure and satisfaction are also possible without orgasm or intercourse. Achieving sexual maturity includes learning that sex is not a contest with a real or imaginary opponent. The sexually mature person enjoys sexual activity whether or not orgasm occurs. Expressing love and sexual feelings for another person involves many pleasurable activities, of which intercourse and orgasm may be only a part.

what do you THINK?

Do men and women perceive the "orgasmic" phase of sex in the same way? Why or why not? Should there be a "psychological phase" added to descriptions of the sexual response cycle? Why or why not?

Sexual Orientation

An essential part of your sexual identity is your sexual orientation. **Sexual orientation** refers to a person's potential to respond with sexual excitement to another person.[39] You may be primarily attracted to members of the opposite sex (**heterosexual**), the same sex (**homosexual**), or both sexes (**bisexual**).

Homosexuality refers to emotional and sexual attachment to persons of your same sex. Many homosexuals prefer the terms *gay* and *lesbian* to describe their sexual orientation, as these terms go beyond the exclusively sexual connotation of the term *homosexual*. Although the term *gay* can be applied to men and women, the term *lesbian* is applied only to women.

Most researchers today agree that sexual orientation is best understood using a multifactorial model, which incorporates biological, psychological, and socioenvironmental factors. Biological explanations focus on research into genetics, hormones (perinatal and postpubertal), and differences in brain anatomy, while psychological and socioenvironmental studies examine parent–child interactions, sex roles, and early sexual and interpersonal interactions. Collectively, this growing body of research suggests that the origins of homosexuality, like heterosexuality, are complex. To diminish the complexity of sexual orientation to "a choice" is a clear misrepresentation of current research. Homosexuals do not "choose" their sexual orientation any more than heterosexuals do.

Irrational fear or hatred of homosexuality creates antigay prejudice, termed **homophobia**. Homophobia

is expressed in many subtle and not so subtle ways. Homophobic behaviours range from avoiding hugging same-sex friends to "gay bashing" (physical and verbal attacks on gays). The emergence of AIDS (acquired immune deficiency syndrome) magnified homophobic feelings in some, due to the erroneous assumption that homosexuality, rather than high-risk behaviours, was responsible for it.

Bisexuality refers to emotional attachment and sexual attraction to members of both sexes. Bisexuals may face great social stigma, as they are often ostracized by homosexuals as well as by heterosexuals. Little research has been done on this segment of the population, and many bisexuals remain hidden or closeted.

what do you THINK?

What is at the root of homophobia? Has homophobia increased or decreased in recent years? Why? What can you do to prevent homophobia?

Developing Sexual Relationships

Perhaps the most important part of developing mature sexuality is learning to develop rewarding sexual relationships. Like all skills, developing relationships takes time, patience, and practice. Your sexual education begins with yourself, your family, and your close friends. You watch the significant adults in your life and pattern your attitudes and behaviours after theirs. At puberty, when extrafamilial elements, peers, and the media become more important, you adapt some of

Foreskin: Flap of skin covering the end of the penis.

Vasocongestion: The engorgement of the genital organs with blood.

Sexual orientation: Attraction to and interest in members of the opposite sex, the same sex, or both sexes in emotional, social, and sexual situations.

Heterosexual: Refers to attraction to and preference for sexual activity with people of the opposite sex.

Homosexual: Refers to attraction to and preference for sexual activity with people of the same sex.

Bisexual: Refers to attraction to and preference for sexual activity with people of both sexes.

Homophobia: Irrational hatred or fear of homosexuals or homosexuality.

TABLE 7.1

Analyzing Sexual Preferences

To complete this worksheet, use the scales provided below and choose a number for each of the three aspects of your life: your past, your present, and your ideal. Remember that there are no right or wrong answers. Comparing your scores in each column may indicate your maturation in understanding yourself and your sexuality. You should work toward your "Present" and "Ideal" scores being the same.

Variable	Past (your entire life up until one year ago)	Present (the last 12 months)	Ideal (if you could order your life any way you wanted)
A. SEXUAL ATTRACTION: To whom are you sexually attracted?	_____	_____	_____
B. SEXUAL BEHAVIOUR: With whom do you have sex?	_____	_____	_____
C. SEXUAL FANTASIES: Whom do you fantasize about?	_____	_____	_____
D. EMOTIONAL PREFERENCE: Whom do you feel drawn to or close to emotionally?	_____	_____	_____
E. SOCIAL PREFERENCE: With whom do you spend most of your social life?	_____	_____	_____
F. LIFESTYLE PREFERENCE: In which community (gay, straight, mixed) do you prefer to spend your time or feel most comfortable?	_____	_____	_____
G. SELF-IDENTIFICATION: How do you label or identify yourself?	_____	_____	_____

SCALE FOR A–E

0 = other sex only
1 = other sex mostly
2 = other sex somewhat more
3 = both sexes equally
4 = same sex somewhat more
5 = same sex mostly
6 = same sex only

SCALE FOR F AND G

0 = heterosexual only
1 = heterosexual mostly
2 = heterosexual somewhat more
3 = equally heterosexual and homosexual
4 = homosexual somewhat more
5 = homosexual mostly
6 = homosexual only

Source: From F. Klein, *The Bisexual Option*. Copyright © 1978 The Haworth Press, Inc. Used with permission.

---

try it NOW!

Sexual orientation is often viewed as a simple concept based entirely on whom one has sex with. This is not only inaccurate, it oversimplifies reality. A questionnaire was developed (see Table 7.1) that examines whom you are attracted to, fantasize about, and actually have sex with. It also considers factors such as whom you feel more close to emotionally, like to socialize with, and in which "community" you feel most comfortable. Respond to the questions. This should help you to see a range of complex, interacting, and fluid factors that influence your sexuality over time.

their standards to your behaviours. Your shyness, aggressiveness or assertiveness, passiveness, and levels of comfort with your sexuality come from your personality and from what you have learned from others.

You bring not only your history to your sexual relationships, but also your peculiar chemistry. The human potential for passionate sexual love has been defined as **limerence**. The word *limerence* is derived from the name of the portion of the brain that controls sexual response, the limbic cortex. Limerence is what makes us feel sexually "turned on" by another person. This powerful feeling can overshadow common sense. Sexual relationships based on limerence may or may not develop into long-lasting or committed relationships. Limerence is thought to last two years at most. Relationships based upon a love that has taken time to mature are much more likely to last. The following are some "symptoms" of limerence:[40]

- Intrusive thoughts about the object of desire.
- Dependence of mood on love object's actions.
- Fear of rejection, along with an almost incapacitating shyness.
- Sharp sensitivity to interpret the desired person's actions favourably and ability to interpret any signs from the other as hidden passion.

- Buoyant, walking-on-air feeling when reciprocation is evident.
- Intensity of feelings that leaves other concerns in the background.
- Ability to emphasize what is admirable in the love object and to avoid dwelling on the negative—or even ability to reconceptualize the negative into a positive attribute.

Sexual Expression: What Are Your Options?

The range of human sexual expression is virtually infinite. What you find personally satisfying and enjoyable may not work for someone else. Further, the ways you choose to meet your sexual needs today may be very different two weeks or two years from now. Knowing and accepting yourself as a sexual person with individual desires and preferences is the first step in achieving sexual satisfaction. Further, understanding that learning about your sexuality, including your sexual expression, is a lifelong process is another step in achieving short and long term sexual satisfaction.

In a society where anti-homosexual attitudes prevail, a gay person's decision to make his or her sexual preference known to the public, as Olympic diver Greg Louganis did, involves courage and a strong belief in oneself.

what do you THINK?

Do you know anyone who has used an online dating service? What impact has technology made on dating in Canada? How will these changes have an impact on the psychosocial health of the Canadian public? What safety precautions should be taken by those who use online dating services?

Celibacy

Celibacy is avoidance of or abstention from sexual activities with others. A completely celibate person also does not engage in masturbation (self-stimulation), whereas a partially celibate person avoids sexual activities with others but engages in autoerotic behaviours such as masturbation. Some individuals choose to be celibate for religious or moral reasons. Others may be celibate for a period of time due to illness, the break-up of a long-term relationship, or lack of an acceptable partner. For some, celibacy is a lonely, agonizing state, but others find that it can be a time for introspection, value assessment, and personal growth.

Autoerotic Behaviours

The goal of **autoerotic behaviours** is sexual self-stimulation. Sexual fantasy and masturbation are the two most common autoerotic behaviours. **Sexual fantasies** are sexually arousing thoughts and dreams. Fantasies may reflect real-life experiences or forbidden desires or may provide the opportunity for practice of new or anticipated sexual experiences. The fact that you may fantasize about a particular sexual experience does not mean that you want to, or have to, act out that experience. Sexual fantasies are just that—fantasy. **Masturbation** is self-stimulation of the genitals. Although many people feel uncomfortable discussing masturbation, it is a common sexual practice across the life span. Masturbation is a natural, pleasure-seeking behaviour in infants and children. It is a valuable and important means for adolescent males and females, as well as adults, to explore their sexual feelings and responsiveness. In addition, masturbation is an important means of sexual expression for older

Limerence: The quality of sexual attraction based on chemistry and gratification of sexual desire.

Celibacy: Not engaging in sexual activity.

Autoerotic behaviours: Sexual self-stimulation.

Sexual fantasies: Sexually arousing thoughts and dreams.

Masturbation: Self-stimulation of genitals.

Online Dating Becoming Common: Love and Lies Are Alive on the Internet, Canadian Study Reveals

By Marlene Habib—The Canadian Press

Online dating has become so common it is being studied by experts in human behaviour and the financial stakes are rising. Sociologists Robert Brym and Rhonda Lenton call internet use "the birth of a new society."

The study says internet dating began about five years ago. In North America, the dating-services industry was estimated to be worth $1 billion US in 1998 and is projected to reach $1.5 billion US by 2003, says the Computer Industry Almanac. "The main important finding that has emerged from this study for us is how mainstream online dating has become," says Lenton, a professor at McMaster University in Hamilton.

Among the results: 68 percent of respondents were men, 63 percent said they had sex with someone they met online, 60 percent formed at least one long-term relationship, 27 percent met at least one partner, and 3 percent eventually married.

There is a downside and some cautionary advice for those looking for real love: 18 percent of online dating users were already married or living common-law, and of that group, most were men.

As well, Lenton noted, many online daters misrepresent themselves. For instance, more than 25 percent of respondents said they had given inaccurate information in their online personal ads, with many lying about their age, marital status, and appearance.

And 26 percent of respondents said they had been pestered after a date, while 10 percent said they had felt frightened at least once. "We would recommend that people using online dating follow the same common-sense precautions as [with] someone they had met at a bar," Lenton warned in an interview.

While acknowledging the pitfalls, Lenton and Brym, a professor at the University of Toronto, say online dating is booming because most experiences are positive and it is as viable a way to meet people as any other.

The convenience of connecting online appeals to a growing proportion of the population that is single, career-driven, and short on time. The report offers safety tips such as using an anonymous email address, arranging a first meeting during the day in a public place, and not giving out phone numbers or addresses until trust has been established.

Judy Farrant and Mark Nesbitt are mid-40s newlyweds who met on Webpersonals and who agreed to tell their story. They said their busy lives made dating difficult. So they turned to the internet because it was convenient and they could remain anonymous.

Farrant, a flight attendant, said she began her cybersearch in 1997. She did not tell her two children at first "because I did not want them to know." She met 14 men before responding to Nesbitt's ad, "which was distinctive and different from anything else I had ever seen."

"I had become fussier, so I cut to the chase," Nesbitt said. In his online profile, he stated exactly who he was and what kind of woman he was looking for.

There is, of course, a cost for using online dating services: some companies have membership subscriptions. Webpersonals sells blocks of credits. Paul Gallucci, a Webpersonals spokesman, would not say how much revenue the service generates, but added that "it is a multimillion-dollar business."

Source: The Canadian Press.

adults whose lifelong companion has died or has a prolonged illness.

Kissing and Erotic Touching

Kissing and erotic touching are two very common forms of nonverbal sexual communication or expression. Men and women have **erogenous zones**, or areas of the body that when touched lead to sexual arousal. Erogenous zones may include genital as well as nongenital areas, such as the earlobes, mouth, breasts, and inner thighs. Almost any area of the body can be conditioned to respond erotically to touch. Spending time with your partner exploring and learning about his or her erogenous areas is another pleasurable, safe, and satisfying means of sexual expression.

Oral–Genital Stimulation

Cunnilingus is the term used for oral stimulation of a woman's genitals, and **fellatio** refers to oral stimulation of a man's genitals. Many partners find oral–genital stimulation an intensely pleasurable means of sexual expression. For others, oral sex is not an option because of moral or religious beliefs. It is important to remember that HIV and other sexually

Kissing can be a nonverbal form of sexual communication.

transmitted infections (STIs) can be transmitted via unprotected oral–genital sex. Use of an appropriate barrier device is strongly recommended if either partner's disease status is in question or unknown or if either partner is not monogamous.

Anal Intercourse

The anal area is highly sensitive to touch, and some find pleasure in its stimulation. **Anal intercourse** refers to the insertion of the penis into the anus. Stimulation of the anus by mouth or with the fingers is also practised. If you do enjoy this form of sexual expression, remember to use condoms to prevent STIs. Also, anything inserted into the anus should not be directly inserted into the vagina, as bacteria commonly found there can cause infections when introduced into the vagina.

Vaginal Intercourse

The term *intercourse* generally refers to **vaginal intercourse**, or insertion of the penis into the vagina. *Coitus* is another term for vaginal intercourse, the most often practised form of sexual expression. A great variety of positions can be used during coitus. Examples include the "missionary position" (man on

top facing the woman), woman on top, side by side, or man behind (rear entry). Many partners enjoy changing and experimenting with different positions. Sexual intercourse can take on different meanings under different circumstances. It can be a hurried, unplanned event involving little communication in the back seat of a car or an erotic, sensual experience including the exchange of love and mutual emotions in a private setting. Knowledge of yourself and your body, along with your ability to communicate effectively with others, will play a large part in determining the enjoyment or meaning of intercourse for you and your partner. Whatever your circumstance, you should practise safe sex to avoid STIs or unwanted pregnancy.

What Is Right for Me?

Invariably, whenever people talk about the spectrum of sexual behaviours, someone in the group will bring up the issue of normality. In *The Joy of Sex*, Alex Comfort summarizes "normality" succinctly:

> Accordingly, if you must talk about "normality," any sex behavior is normal which (1) you both enjoy, (2) hurts nobody, (3) isn't associated with anxiety, (4) doesn't cut down your scope. . . . "Normal" implies there is something which sex ought to be. That is, it ought to be a wholly satisfying link between two affectionate people, from which both emerge unanxious, rewarded, and ready for more.[41]

Many couples worry that they do not have sex often enough. Popular magazines frequently give the "average" number of times couples engage in sex every week. Such numbers are meaningless. Rather than compare yourself to these statistics, you would be wise simply to follow your own feelings. The bottom line is that you must decide what is right for you and your partner.

Variant Sexual Behaviour

Variant sexual behaviour is the term used to describe sexual behaviours not engaged in by most people. The

---

Erogenous zones: Areas in the body that, when touched, lead to sexual arousal.

Cunnilingus: Oral stimulation of a woman's genitals.

Fellatio: Oral stimulation of a man's genitals.

Anal intercourse: The insertion of the penis into the anus.

Vaginal intercourse: The insertion of the penis into the vagina.

Variant sexual behaviour: A sexual behaviour not engaged in by most people.

following list of variant sexual behaviours includes behaviours illegal in some provinces and territories and actions that could be harmful to others:

- Group sex. Sexual activity involving more than two people. Participants in group sex run a high risk of STIs, including HIV.

- Transvestitism. The wearing of clothing of the opposite sex. Most transvestites are men, heterosexual, and married.

- Transsexualism. Strong identification with the opposite sex in which men or women feel "trapped in the wrong body." In some cases, transsexuals undergo sex-change operations.

- Fetishism. Sexual arousal achieved by looking at or touching inanimate objects, such as underclothing or shoes.

- Exhibitionism. The exposure of one's genitals to strangers in public places. Most exhibitionists are seeking a reaction of shock or fear from their victims.

- Voyeurism. Observing other people for sexual gratification. Most voyeurs are men who attempt to watch women undressing or bathing. Voyeurism is illegal and an invasion of privacy.

- Sadomasochism. Sexual activities in which gratification is received by inflicting pain (verbal or physical abuse) on a partner or by being the object of such infliction. A sadist is a person who receives gratification from inflicting pain, and a masochist is a person who receives gratification from experiencing pain.

- Pedophilia. Sexual activity or attraction between an adult and a child. Any sexual activity involving a minor, including creating, possessing, or selling child pornography, is illegal in Canada.

- Autoerotic asphyxiation. The practice of reducing or eliminating oxygen to the brain, usually by tying a cord around one's neck, while masturbating. Tragically, some individuals accidentally hang themselves in the process.

---

what do you THINK?

How does our society decide what sexual behaviours are normal and which are variant? Are some sexual behaviours that we consider normal looked upon as abnormal or perverse by others of a different religion, ethnicity, or culture? Why are some individuals willing to try various sexual behaviours while others are not? Where do you "draw the line" for your sexual experiences?

✳ DIFFICULTIES THAT CAN HINDER SEXUAL FUNCTIONING

Research indicates that problems that hinder sexual functioning are quite common in Canada. The label given to the various problems that interfere with sexual pleasure is **sexual dysfunction**. You should not be embarrassed if you experience a sexual dysfunction at some point in your life. The sexual part of yourself does not come with a lifetime warranty. You can have breakdowns involving your sexual function just as you can have breakdowns in any of your other body systems. Sexual dysfunctions can be divided into four major classes: sexual desire disorders, sexual arousal disorders, orgasm disorders, and sexual pain disorders. In most cases, sexual dysfunctions can be treated successfully if both partners are willing to work together to solve the problem.

Sexual Desire Disorders

The most frequent reason people seek a sex therapist is **ISD**, or **inhibited sexual desire**.[42] ISD is the lack of a sexual appetite or simply a lack of interest and pleasure in sexual activity. In some instances, it can result from stress or boredom with sex. **Sexual aversion disorder** is another type of desire dysfunction, characterized by sexual phobias (unreasonable fears) and anxiety about sexual contact. The psychological stress of a punitive upbringing, rigid religious background, or a history of physical or sexual abuse may be a source of these desire disorders.

Sexual Arousal Disorders

The most common disorder in this category is **erectile dysfunction**. Erectile dysfunction, or impotence, refers to difficulty in achieving or maintaining a penile erection sufficient for intercourse. At some time in his life, every man experiences impotence. Causes are varied and include underlying diseases, such as diabetes or prostate problems, reactions to some medications (for example, medication for high blood pressure), depression, fatigue, stress, alcohol, performance anxiety, and guilt over real or imaginary problems (such as when a man compares himself to his partner's past lovers). Impotence generally becomes more of a problem as men age, affecting one in four men over the age of 65.[43]

Chronic impotence (impotence lasting more than three months) should be treated by a physician. A complete medical examination and history are necessary to rule out physical causes. Viagra (sildenafil citrate), Levitra, and Cialis are used as treatments for

Building Better Relationships

After reading this chapter, it should be apparent that relationships involve complex interactions between individuals. To build strong and effective relationships, you must carefully assess the values you put on friendships, significant others, and other forms of interpersonal interactions. Healthy relationships involve developing intimacy in several dimensions. It may be helpful for you to take a personal inventory of your relationships to determine how healthy they are.

MAKING DECISIONS FOR YOU

Think about the most important relationship in your life. Why is this relationship important to your overall health and well-being? Are there any attitudes and/or behaviours that you should change to strengthen this relationship? To make such a change, begin by listing the reasons why the change is important. Who will benefit from this change? What steps will you take to make this change occur? What will you do to make sure that you keep up with or maintain this behaviour change?

CHECKLIST FOR CHANGE: MAKING PERSONAL CHOICES

- What relationships are most important to you right now?
- How have these relationships affected your relationships with others? Are you giving enough time to your other relationships?
- Have you thought about how good your relationships are from an emotional perspective? A psychological perspective? A physical perspective? A spiritual perspective? Which of these factors is the most important to you? Why?
- What would an ideal set of relationships look like for you? How many close interactions would you want to make time for? What would be the nature and extent of these relationships?
- Are you comfortable with yourself sexually? Are you satisfied with your current choice(s) of sexual expression?
- What do you expect in a committed relationship? What would you be willing to accept in terms of attitudes and/or behaviours from your committed partner? What do you expect of yourself?
- What do you think are the three most important attributes of a friend? Do you display these attributes with your friends?
- How are you limited or bound by gender-role stereotypes?
- Have you considered your values or beliefs about what is most important to you in a prospective lifelong partner? Are you asking for the same attributes that you would be able to give to a partner?

CHECKLIST FOR CHANGE: MAKING COMMUNITY CHOICES

- Do you make a habit of putting yourself in the other person's shoes when discussing how your actions may have made that person feel or how that person may be feeling in general?
- Do you take time to listen to your friends? Your parents? Your acquaintances? Your professors? Do you find yourself thinking about your own problems, thoughts, or issues when someone is trying to tell you about his or her problems?
- Do you reach out to friends having problems in their relationships?
- Are you supportive of couples having problems in their relationship without being judgmental or taking sides?
- Do you try to work through your problems with others, or do you run from, avoid, or get angry rather than try to talk through your difficulties?
- Are you supportive of counselling services and other campus and community services that offer help for people who have troubled relationships?
- Do you listen carefully to what your legislators propose in the way of family and individual policies and programs that may unfairly harm others?

CRITICAL THINKING

After leading what you consider a normal sex life, which has included several intimate sexual relationships, you meet that special person. When you first started dating you learned that this person was a practising member of an Eastern religion, but you never really gave much thought to what that meant to your relationship. Now, several months later, as you want to become intimate, you realize that this religion does not accept any sexual activity before marriage.

You feel sexually frustrated. But at the same time, you believe you are in love and that this relationship could lead to marriage. Using the DECIDE model in Chapter 1, think about what the two of you could do to satisfy physical, sexual, and emotional feelings.

---

erectile dysfunction. Taken orally one hour before sexual activity, Viagra is reported to manage erectile dysfunction successfully in 60 to 80 percent of cases.[44] The most commonly reported side effects of Viagra include headache, flushing, stomach ache, urinary tract infection, diarrhea, dizziness, rash, and mild and temporary visual changes.[45] There also have been several deaths among Viagra users, prompting more

Sexual dysfunction: Problems associated with achieving sexual satisfaction.

Inhibited sexual desire (ISD): Lack of sexual appetite or simply a lack of interest and pleasure in sexual activity.

Sexual aversion disorder: Type of desire dysfunction characterized by sexual phobias and anxiety about sexual contact.

Erectile dysfunction: Also called impotence; difficulty in achieving or maintaining a penile erection sufficient for intercourse.

caution in prescribing it to patients with known cardiovascular disease and those taking commonly prescribed short- and long-acting nitrates, such as nitroglycerin. Impotence due to psychological factors can be treated with psychotherapy. Such treatment is effective in 90 percent of cases.

Orgasm Disorders

Up to 50 percent of the male population is affected by premature ejaculation at some time in their lives. **Premature ejaculation** is ejaculation that occurs prior to or very soon after the insertion of the penis into the vagina. Another orgasm disorder in males is **retarded ejaculation,** or the inability to ejaculate once the penis is erect. Treatment for premature ejaculation involves a physical examination to rule out organic causes. If the cause of the problem is not physiologic, therapy is available to help a man learn how to control the timing of his ejaculation. Fatigue, stress, performance pressure, and alcohol can be contributing factors to these orgasmic disorders in men.

When a woman is unable to achieve orgasm with her partner, she often blames herself and fakes orgasm to preserve her partner's ego. Researchers reported that up to 66 percent of women have faked an orgasm at one time or another.[46] Until recently, societal norms were that women were not supposed to enjoy sex but rather "do it" to fulfill their "marital duty." The Kinsey reports in the 1950s and Masters and Johnson's findings in the 1960s and 1970s raised questions about these sexual myths. We recognize today that women enjoy sexual activity as much as men. In the past, women who did not experience orgasm were called "frigid." This term is no longer used because it implies that a woman is at fault. Instead, the term **preorgasmic** is used, since many women can learn to become orgasmic.

For women whose sexual pleasure is hampered, therapy is available. A physical examination to rule out organic causes is generally the first step. Masturbation is usually a primary focus in helping a woman to become orgasmic. Through masturbation, a woman can learn how her body responds sexually to various types of touch. Once a woman has become orgasmic through masturbation, she must learn to communicate her needs to her partner. The investment of time and caring by both partners is usually worth the effort, for 70 percent of preorgasmic women can be helped.

Sexual Pain Disorders

Two common disorders in the category of sexual pain disorders are dyspareunia and vaginismus. **Dyspareunia** is pain experienced by a female during intercourse. This pain may be caused by endometriosis, uterine tumours, chlamydia, gonorrhea, or urinary tract infections. Damage to tissues during childbirth and insufficient lubrication during intercourse may also cause pain or discomfort. Dyspareunia can also be psychological in origin. As with other problems, dyspareunia can be treated with good results. The first step in treatment is a thorough pelvic examination to rule out physical disease. Diseases or disorders can usually be cured with medication or surgery. Vaginal lubricants can be purchased to help with inadequate lubrication. Psychologically caused dyspareunia is much more difficult to treat.

Vaginismus is the involuntary contraction of vaginal muscles, making penile insertion painful or impossible. Most cases of vaginismus are related to fear of intercourse or to unresolved sexual conflicts. Treatment of vaginismus involves teaching a woman to achieve orgasm through nonvaginal stimulation. Becoming orgasmic is important because research has indicated that treatment for vaginismus is more successful in orgasmic women. The woman and her partner are then taught methods for dilating the vagina, either with fingers or a vibrator. As dilation is achieved, the woman is taught to relax in order to allow penetration. Cure rates are close to 100 percent.

> ## what do you THINK?
> Why do we find it so difficult to discuss sexual dysfunction in our society? Do you think it is more difficult for men? Why or why not? If you were experiencing sexual dysfunction, what would you tell your partner?

Drugs and Sex

Because psychoactive drugs affect our entire physiology, they affect our sexual behaviours. Promises of increased pleasure make drugs very tempting to those seeking greater sexual satisfaction. Too often, however, drugs become central to sexual activities and damage the relationship. Alcohol is notorious for reducing inhibitions and giving increased feelings of well-being and desirability. At the same time, alcohol inhibits sexual response; thus, the mind may be willing, but not the body. Perhaps the greatest danger associated with use of drugs during sex is the tendency to blame the drug for negative or irresponsible behaviours: "I can't help what I did last night because I was stoned" is a response that demonstrates sexual immaturity. A sexually mature person carefully examines risks and benefits and makes decisions accordingly. If drugs are necessary to increase erotic feelings, it is likely that the partners are being dishonest about their feelings for each other. Good sex is not dependent on chemical substances.

Premature ejaculation: Ejaculation that occurs prior to or almost immediately following penile penetration.

Retarded ejaculation: The inability to ejaculate once the penis is erect.

Preorgasmic: In women, the state of never having experienced an orgasm.

Dyspareunia: Pain experienced by women during intercourse.

Vaginismus: A state in which the vaginal muscles contract so forcefully that penetration cannot be accomplished.

Go to MyHealthLab at **www.pearsoned.ca/myhealthlab.** Here you will find self-assessments, case studies, links to health on the net, and much more.

DISCUSSION QUESTIONS

1. What is the role of communication in nonintimate and intimate relationships? How can you become a better listener? Speaker?
2. What are behavioural interdependence, need fulfillment, and emotional attachment, and why is each of these important in subsequent relationship development?
3. What are the common types of intimate relationships? Which of these do you think is most important to you right now? Why?
4. Why are your relationships with your family important? Explain how your family unit is similar to or different from the family unit of the early 1900s. Who made up your family of origin? Your nuclear family?
5. How can you tell the difference between a love relationship and one that is based primarily on attraction? What common characteristics do love relationships share?
6. What prevents intimacy? What can you do to reduce or remove these barriers?
7. What are the common elements of good relationships?
8. What actions can you take to improve your interpersonal relationships?
9. What are the functions of the various hormones during puberty? What physical changes are brought about by menopause?
10. What are "normal" sexual behaviours? Do men and women differ in sexual response? In their preference for sexual behaviours?
11. Do drugs and alcohol enhance sexual performance? What risks are involved in such experimentation?

APPLICATION EXERCISE

Reread the "Consider This . . ." scenario at the beginning of the chapter and answer the following questions.

1. From what you have read in this chapter, what problems do Jorge and Yasmin have in their relationship?
2. Why do you think people feel forced to tell lies or half-truths in their relationships with others?
3. Are there times with your partner when it is okay to be dishonest or to not tell the truth, or should you always be totally honest and truthful about your actions?
4. Do you believe that you should tell your partner about all of your previous sexual experiences? Why or why not?

MYSEARCHLAB EXERCISE

1. Log on to www.MySearchLab.com.

2. Retrieve article AN 34125059, "Why Do We Flirt?" by David Dryden Henningsen, Mary Braz, and Elaine Davies.

3. Read the article and prepare responses to the following questions:

   a. Why do men flirt?
   b. Why do women flirt?
   c. How do our reasons for flirting differ depending on our stage of life (student versus gainfully employed, single versus married, etc.)
   d. What are your typical flirting behaviours?
   e. Are you aware when/where you flirt? Is it always intentional?

4. Form a small group (that is, three to five people) of men and women and share your responses. Compare the responses of the men and women. Is there any difference based on gender?

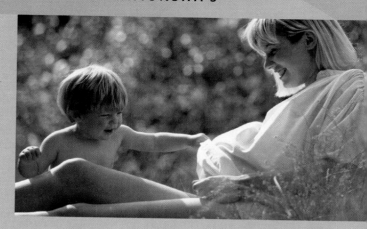

CHAPTER 8

BIRTH CONTROL, PREGNANCY, AND CHILDBIRTH

Managing Your Fertility

CONSIDER THIS . . .

Jamila and Karim have been dating for several months. After a wonderful evening together, they go back to Karim's place with the intention of having sex. When they arrive at Karim's, they discover that neither of them has a condom. Karim thought that Jamila was taking the birth control pill. Jamila thought Karim would have condoms. Rather than spoil the evening, Jamila and Karim have unprotected sex. The next day, they argue over who is responsible for the birth control.

What mistakes were made in this relationship? When should a couple talk about this responsibility as well as the issue of preventing sexually transmitted infections? Who is responsible for providing birth control? Who is responsible for protection from sexually transmitted infections? What were the risks involved in engaging in unprotected sex? What were the alternatives?

CHAPTER OBJECTIVES

- Describe the various contraceptive methods available, including their effectiveness in preventing pregnancy and sexually transmitted infections.

- Identify the emotional health, maternal health, financial evaluation/planning, and contingency planning to be considered when planning to become a parent.

- Explain the importance of prenatal care in the process of pregnancy.

- Summarize the basic stages of childbirth as well as complications that can arise during labour and delivery.

- Review the primary causes of and possible solutions to infertility.

Fertility is a mixed blessing for women. The ability to participate in the miracle of birth is an incredible experience for many. Yet the responsibility for controlling one's fertility can also be overwhelming. Today, we not only understand the intimate details of reproduction but also possess technologies designed to control or enhance our fertility. Along with information and technological advance comes choice, and choice goes hand-in-hand with responsibility. Choosing if and when to have children is one of the most important decisions we have to make. A woman and her partner have much to consider before planning or risking a pregnancy. Children, whether planned or unplanned, change people's lives. They require a lifelong personal commitment of love and nurturing.

Before you plan or risk a pregnancy, you have the responsibility to make certain you are physically, emotionally, and financially prepared to care for another human being. One measure of maturity is the ability to discuss reproduction, birth control, and sexually transmitted infection (STI) protection with your sexual partner before giving in to sexual urges. If you cannot discuss birth control or STI protection then you may not be mature enough to engage in sex. Men often assume that their partner is taking care of birth control. Women often feel that if they bring up the subject, it implies that they are "easy" or "loose." You will find embarrassment-free discussion a lot easier if you understand human reproduction and contraception and thoroughly consider your attitudes toward these matters before you get into compromising situations.

MANAGING YOUR FERTILITY

Conception refers to the fertilization of an ovum by a sperm. The sperm enters the ovum. Its tail breaks off, and a protective chemical barrier secreted by the ovum surrounds the sperm and prevents other sperm from entering. A viable egg, a viable sperm, and possible access to the egg by the sperm are necessary conditions for conception.

Contraception refers to methods of preventing conception. Society has and continues to search for a simple, infallible, and risk-free method of preventing pregnancy. Our present methods of contraception fall into two categories: reversible methods, such as the pill, condoms, and abstinence; and permanent methods, such as vasectomy (for men) and tubal ligation (for women).

Reversible Contraception

Abstinence and "Outercourse"

Strictly defined, abstinence means not engaging in intercourse. Traditionally, individuals could still

For couples who want to avoid pregnancy, a wide variety of contraceptives are available, including male and female condoms, IUDs, cervical caps, diaphragms, and different types of pills.

engage in such forms of sexual intimacy as massage, kissing, and solitary masturbation and consider themselves abstainers. However, many people today have broadened the definition of abstinence to include all forms of sexual contact, even those that do not culminate in sexual intercourse.

Couples who go a step farther than massage and kissing and engage in such activities as oral–genital sex and mutual masturbation are sometimes said to be engaging in "outercourse." Like abstinence, outercourse can be 100-percent effective for birth control as long as the male does not ejaculate near the vaginal opening. Unlike abstinence, however, there is still a risk of STIs. Oral–genital contact can result in transmission of an STI, although the risk can be reduced by using a condom on the penis or a dental dam on the vaginal opening.

Condoms

The **condom** is a strong sheath of latex rubber or other material designed to fit over an erect penis (Figure 8.1). The condom catches the ejaculate, thereby preventing sperm migration toward the egg. The condom is the only temporary means of birth control available for men and the only barrier that effectively prevents the spread of STIs, including HIV. Regardless of your preferred method of birth control, you should always use a condom. Condoms come in a wide variety of styles: coloured, ribbed for "extra sensation," lubricated, nonlubricated, and with or without reservoirs at the tip. They also can be purchased with or without spermicide in pharmacies, in some schools, and in some public washrooms. Some health clinics, including those on many college and university campuses, provide condoms free of

FIGURE 8.1

How to Use a Condom

The condom should be rolled over the erect penis as soon as it is erect (even during outercourse). A small space (about 1 cm) should be left at the end of the condom to collect the semen after ejaculation. Hold the tip of the condom, and unroll it all the way to the base of the penis. Hold the base of the condom before withdrawal to avoid spilling any semen.

charge. A new condom must be used for each act of intercourse or oral sex.

Condoms help prevent the spread of some STIs, including genital herpes and HIV. They may also slow or reduce the development of cervical abnormalities in women that can lead to cancer. The theoretical **perfect-use effectiveness rate** for condoms is 98 percent, meaning that when they are used correctly and consistently, 2 out of 100 women who use them will become pregnant in one year. In reality, however, their effectiveness, or **typical-use rate**, is only 85 percent (15 out of every 100 women who use condoms will become pregnant in one year) because they are so often used incorrectly or inconsistently. The unintended pregnancies or failure rates of contraceptives are shown in Table 8.1 according to typical and perfect-use rates. Condoms should always be used for vaginal, anal, and oral sex. They must be rolled on the erect penis before the penis touches the vagina, leaving about a 1-centimetre space at the tip to collect ejaculated semen (see Figure 8.1). After ejaculation, the condom should be held at the base of the penis before withdrawal, to avoid spillage. For greatest efficacy, condoms should be used with a spermicide containing nonoxynol-9.

Another reason why condoms are not as effective in real life as in theory is that they can break during intercourse, especially if they are old or poorly stored. They must be stored in a cool place (not in a wallet, hip pocket, or in the glove box of your car!) and should be inspected before use for small tears.

Some people claim that a condom ruins the spontaneity of sex; stopping to put it on breaks the mood for them. Others report that the condom decreases sensation. These perceived inconveniences contribute to improper use. As mentioned, the condom should be put on the penis as soon as it is erect, so that should not interrupt the mood. Couples can also put the condom on together as part of foreplay, thus enhancing the mood and generally leading to more successful birth control and STI protection.[1]

Oral Contraceptives

Oral contraceptive pills were first marketed in Canada in 1961 and quickly became the most widely used reversible method of fertility control. Most oral contraceptives work through the combined effects of synthetic estrogen and progesterone. Because the levels of estrogen in the pill are higher than those produced by the body, the pituitary gland is not signalled to produce follicle-stimulating hormone (FSH), without which ova will not develop in the ovaries. Further, progesterone in the pill prevents growth of the uterine lining and thickens the cervical mucus, forming a barrier against sperm.

Pills are meant to be taken in a cycle. At the end of each three-week cycle, the user discontinues the drug or takes a placebo pill for one week. The resultant drop in hormones causes the uterine lining to disintegrate, and the user will have menstrual flow, usually within one to three days. The same cycle is repeated every 28 days. Menstrual flow is generally lighter than in a non–pill user because the hormones in the pill prevent thick endometrial build-up.

Fertility: The ability to reproduce.

Conception: The fertilization of an ovum by a sperm.

Contraception: Methods of preventing conception.

Condom: A sheath of thin latex or other material designed to fit over an erect penis to collect semen upon ejaculation.

Perfect-use effectiveness rate: The percentage rate of women who will become pregnant in one year when a contraceptive method is used correctly and consistently.

Typical-use effectiveness rate: The percentage of women who will become pregnant in one year considered that a contraceptive method is often used incorrectly or inconsistently.

Oral contraceptive pills: Pills taken daily for three weeks of the menstrual cycle that prevent ovulation by regulating hormones.

TABLE 8.1

Contraceptive Effectiveness

	Number of Unintended Pregnancies per 100 Women during the First Year of Use	
	Typical Use	**Perfect Use**
Continuous abstinence*	0	0
Female sterilization	0.5	0.5
Male sterilization	0.15	0.1
Implanon	0.05	0.05
IUD (intrauterine device)		
ParaGard (copper T)	0.8	0.6
Mirena (LNG-IUS)	0.2	0.2
Depo-Provera	3	0.3
Oral contraceptives (combined pill and progestin-only pill)	8	0.3
Ortho Evra patch	8	0.3
NuvaRing	8	0.3
Male condom[†] (without spermicides)	15	2
Diaphragm[†] (with spermicidal cream or jelly)	16	6
Sponge		
Women who have never given birth	16	9
Women who have given birth	32	20
Female condom[†] (without spermicides)	21	5
Fertility awareness methods	25	12
Withdrawal	27	4
Spermicides[†] (foams, creams, gels, vaginal suppositories, and vaginal film)	29	18
No method	85	85
Emergency contraceptive pill	Treatment initiated within 72 hours after unprotected intercourse reduces the risk of pregnancy by 75–89 percent (with no protection against STIs).	

*Indicates complete protection from STIs.
[†]Indicates limited protection from STIs.
Note: "Typical Use" refers to failure rates for men and women whose use is not consistent or always correct. "Perfect Use" refers to failure rates for those whose use is consistent and always correct.

Source: R. Hatcher et al., *Contraceptive Technology*, 19th rev. ed. Copyright © 2007 Contraceptive Technology Communications, Inc. Used with permission.

Talking with Your Partner about Using Condoms

Knowing what is best for our health and doing something about it can be two different things. Talking about condoms can be hard—especially the first time. It is a sign of maturity and readiness for sexual activity if you can bring the subject up and talk effectively about it. Here are some suggestions:

1. Think about what you want to say ahead of time. Sort out your feelings about using condoms before you talk with your partner.

2. Choose a time to talk before your first intimate moment. Getting things straight before you engage in sexual activity means you will both be prepared and relaxed.

3. Decide how you want to start the conversation. You might say, "I need to talk with you about something that is important to both of us," or, "I have been hearing a lot lately about safer sex. Have you ever used condoms?" or, "I feel kind of embarrassed, but I care too much about you and myself not to talk about this."

4. Remember, starting to talk is the hardest part. Do not be surprised if your partner responds with, "I am glad you brought it up. I was worried too," or, "I like sharing the responsibility of sex. I appreciate a woman who is willing to let me."

5. Once you have agreed to use condoms, do something positive and fun. Go to the store together. Buy lots of different brands and colours. Plan a special day when you can experiment. Just talking about how you will use all those condoms can be a turn-on.

Today's pill is different from the one introduced more than three decades ago. The original pill contained large amounts of estrogen, which increased health risk whereas the current pill contains the minimal amount of estrogen necessary to prevent pregnancy.

Because the chemicals in oral contraceptives change the way the body metabolizes certain nutrients, all women using the pill should check with their prescribing practitioners regarding dietary supplements. The nutrients of concern include vitamin C and the B-complex vitamins—B2, B6, and B12. A nutritious diet that includes whole grains, fresh fruits and vegetables, lean meats, fish and poultry, and nonfat dairy products is advised (See also Chapter 5). Oral contraceptives can interact negatively with other drugs. Some antibiotics diminish the pill's effectiveness, as can the 24-hour flu or diarrhea. A backup contraceptive should be used for the rest of the pill pack if these circumstances occur. Women in doubt should check with their prescribing practitioners, their pharmacists, or other knowledgeable health professionals. You can learn more about health methods and contraceptive choice in the Skills for Behaviour Change box.

Although return of fertility may be delayed after discontinuing the pill, it is not known to cause infertility. Women who had irregular menstrual cycles before going on the pill are more likely to have problems conceiving, regardless of pill use.

The perfect-use effectiveness rate of oral contraceptives is 99.7 percent, making them one of the most effective reversible methods of fertility control. Using the pill is convenient and does not interfere with sexual activity. It may lessen menstrual difficulties, such as cramps and premenstrual syndrome (PMS). Women using oral contraceptives have lower risks for developing endometrial and ovarian cancers. They are also less likely than nonusers to develop fibrocystic breast disease. In addition, pill users have lower incidences of ectopic pregnancies, ovarian cysts, pelvic inflammatory disease, and iron deficiency anemia.[2] Possible serious health problems associated with the pill include the tendency for pill users' blood to form clots and an increased risk for high blood pressure in a few women. Clotting can lead to strokes or heart attacks. The risk is low for most healthy, non-smoking women under 35; it increases with age and, especially, with cigarette smoking.

Although the perfect-use rate of oral contraceptives is 99.7 percent, the typical-use effectiveness is only 92 percent. The typical-use rate may relate to the fact that the pill must be taken every day. If a woman misses taking one pill, she is advised to use an alternative form of contraception for the remainder of that cycle. The cost of the pill may also be a problem for some women. Finally, some younger teenagers report that the requirement to have a complete gynecological examination in order to get a prescription for the pill

Choosing a Contraceptive

Part of sexual maturity is taking responsibility for your personal health regarding contraceptives and STI protection. Aside from simply worrying about contraceptive effectiveness and convenience, you need to consider the effects that your birth control method may have on your health now and in the future. Here are some things to keep in mind when you decide on your contraceptive method:

1. Talk to your medical professional about your and your family's medical history. Is there anything that would encourage the use of one method over another? Some contraceptive methods may have serious side effects according to your medical history (for example, if there is a history of high blood pressure in your family, you may choose not to use oral contraceptives).

2. Learn about the potential side effects. If you find yourself experiencing the side effects of a contraceptive, you should talk to your doctor immediately. Your doctor may suggest switching to a different contraceptive or may simply assure you that the "side effects" do not appear related to contraceptive use.

3. Devise a method to ensure that you can not miss using it. If you take the pill, take it at the same time every day. Associating it with a certain time or event (for instance, taking a morning shower) will reinforce your memory. If you use condoms, you might keep some in your coat pocket so they will be there when you need them. Or you might keep your diaphragm packed in your overnight bag.

4. Learn how to talk to your partner about your choice of contraception and STI protection. Decisions about contraceptives should be made as a couple, taking each person's health and desires into account.

5. Learn about drug interactions with your birth control method. While we will discuss this in more detail in Chapter 9, it is important to know what medications may interact with your method of birth control. For example, interactions may occur between alcohol and contraceptive pills or between antibiotics and contraceptive pills. Specifically, alcohol and antibiotics may diminish the effectiveness of birth control pills in some women. Ask your doctor or pharmacist about drug interactions if you receive a prescription drug. If there is a potential for diminished effectiveness of your contraceptive, ask when you can resume normal sexual relations without taking added precautions.

---

is an obstacle. In fact, 69 percent of female teenagers think that this requirement frightens their peers away from use of the pill.[3] Educating young women about what goes on in a gynecological exam may ease their anxiety, along with confirmation that their examination and prescription remains confidential.

Progestin-Only Pills

Progestin-only pills (or minipills) contain small doses of progesterone. Women who feel uncertain about using estrogen pills, who suffer from side effects related to estrogen, or who are nursing may want to take these pills rather than combination pills. There is still some question about the specific ways progestin-only pills work. Current thought is that they change the composition of the cervical mucus, thus impeding sperm travel. They may also inhibit ovulation in some women. The perfect use effectiveness rate of progestin-only pills is 96 percent, which is lower than that of estrogen-containing pills. Also, their use usually leads to irregular menstrual bleeding.

Birth Control Patch (Ortho-Evra)

In Canada, since January 2003, Canadian women have been able to obtain a dermal patch that may be applied to the skin by prescription and use it in place of birth control pills or injections. The patch contains the hormones progestin and estrogen, two ingredients also found in birth control pills. It works like a smoking

Ortho Evra, the contraceptive patch.

cessation patch, releasing medication through the skin into the bloodstream. The patch can be worn on the buttocks, upper outer arm, abdomen, back, or stomach. A new patch is applied every week for three weeks each month. During the fourth week, no patch is worn to allow for menstruation. If a patch falls off at any time you must replace it within a 24-hour period to maintain your normal birth control cycle.

While the patch will not protect you from STIs, it may be an alternative worth considering for those who frequently forget to take birth control pills and who do not like injections. The patch has similar effectiveness rates as the pill: perfect use is 99.7 percent and typical use is 92 percent. A small percentage of women may find that they are not able to use the patch because it irritates the skin.

Depo-Provera

Depo-Provera is a long-acting synthetic drug injected intramuscularly every three months. Although used in other countries for years, the Health Protection Branch did not approve it for use in Canada until 1997. Researchers believe that the drug prevents ovulation. Its perfect use effectiveness in preventing pregnancy is greater than 99 percent while its typical use is 97 percent. Its use may prevent menstrual blood loss, iron deficiency anemia, premenstrual tension, and endometriosis. The main disadvantage is irregular bleeding, which can be troublesome at first, but within a year most women are amenorrheic (have no menstrual cycles). Weight gain (an average of 2.5 kg in the first year) is also common and may be of concern for women who already have issues with weight control (see Chapter 6). Other potential disadvantages include fatigue, mood disturbances, loss of libido, and increased risk of osteoporosis and diabetes. Dizziness, nervousness, and headache are other possible side effects. Unlike other methods of contraception, this method cannot be stopped immediately if problems arise. In addition, fertility may not return immediately after Depo-Provera use is discontinued.

NuvaRing

Introduced in 2002, this effective contraceptive offers protection for four weeks at a time when used as prescribed. Perfect use results in a 99.7 percent effectiveness rate. Typical use results in 92 percent effectiveness at preventing pregnancy. **NuvaRing** is a soft flexible ring about 5 centimetres in diameter that the user inserts into the vagina and leaves in place for three weeks. The user removes it for one week during her menstrual cycle. Once the ring is inserted, it continuously releases estrogen and progestin. See the photo included to the right.

Advantages to NuvaRing include protection against pregnancy for one month; no pill to take daily; no requirement to be fitted by a clinician; no requirement to use spermicide; and the quick return of the ability to become pregnant when no longer in use. Possible side effects include increased vaginal discharge and vaginal irritation or infection. Oil-based vaginal medicine to treat yeast infections cannot be used when the ring is in place, and a diaphragm or cervical cap cannot be used as a backup method.

Emergency Contraceptive Pills

Emergency contraceptive pills can be used when a condom breaks, after a sexual assault, or any time unprotected sexual intercourse occurs. Although often referred to as "the morning-after pill," they can be taken up to three days after unprotected intercourse to reduce the risk of pregnancy by 75 percent. It is not clear how emergency contraceptive pills prevent pregnancy, but it may be that they prevent ovulation rather than implantation of a fertilized egg. The most common emergency contraceptive pill prescribed is a combination of estrogen and progesterone. Nausea, vomiting, menstrual irregularities, breast tenderness,

NuvaRing (actual size).

Depo-Provera: An injectable method of birth control that lasts for three months.

NuvaRing: A soft, flexible ring inserted into the vagina for three weeks at a time to prevent pregnancy in the same way that the pill does.

Emergency contraceptive pills: Drugs taken up to three days after intercourse to reduce the risk of pregnancy.

headaches, abdominal pain and cramps, and dizziness are the most likely side effects.

Preven was approved by Health Canada in November 1999. It contains two hormones that stop or delay ovulation and may prevent a fertilized egg from implanting in the uterus. Two pills are to be taken within 24 hours of intercourse and another two 12 or more hours after that. This drug is intended for a woman who uses a method that fails or a woman who has experienced non-consensual sex. It is not "the abortion pill." Nor should it be considered a preferred method of contraception over the long term; it is meant to be used only in cases of emergency. Side effects are as listed above.

Foams, Suppositories, Jellies, and Creams

Like condoms, these contraceptive preparations are available without a prescription. Chemically, they are referred to as **spermicides**—substances designed to kill sperm.

Jellies and creams are packaged in tubes, and foams are available in aerosol cans. They must be inserted far enough into the vagina to cover the cervix, providing both a chemical barrier that kills sperm and a physical barrier that stops sperm from continuing toward an egg (Figure 8.2).

Suppositories are waxy capsules placed deep in the vagina that melt once they are inside. They must be inserted 10 to 20 minutes before intercourse to have time to melt, but no longer than one hour prior to intercourse or they lose their effectiveness. Similar to condoms, additional contraceptive chemicals must be applied for each subsequent act of intercourse. They help prevent the spread of certain sexually transmitted infections. Jellies and creams are designed to be used with a diaphragm or condom. When used with another method of contraception, their effectiveness improves. Used alone, the perfect-use effectiveness of foams, creams, gels, vaginal suppositories, and vaginal film is 82 percent. Typical use effectiveness is only 71 percent.

Female Condoms

The **female condom** is a single-use, soft, loose-fitting polyurethane sheath. It is designed as one unit, with two diaphragm-like rings. One ring, which lies inside the sheath, serves as an insertion mechanism and internal anchor. The other ring, which remains outside the vagina once the device is inserted, protects the labia and the base of the penis from infection. Perfect use effectiveness of the female condom is less than for the male condom, at 95 percent. Typical use is also lower, at 79 percent. Still, many women like the female condom because it gives them more control over their reproduction.

Diaphragm with Spermicidal Jelly or Cream

Invented in the mid-nineteenth century, the **diaphragm** was the first widely used birth control method for women. Before that, most women relied on their partner to use a condom or to withdraw before ejaculation. The diaphragm is a soft, shallow

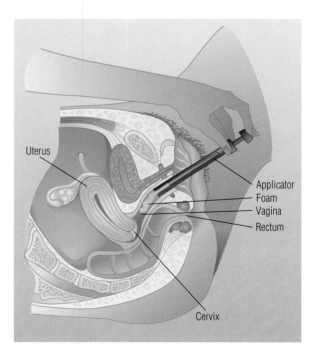

FIGURE 8.2

The Proper Method of Applying Spermicide within the Vagina

The female condom.

Place spermicide inside and around the rim of the diaphragm

Insertion: squeeze rim together; insert with spermicide-side up

Check placement, making certain cervix is covered

FIGURE 8.3

The Proper Use and Placement of a Diaphragm

cup made of thin latex rubber. Its flexible, rubber-coated ring is designed to fit snugly behind the pubic bone in front of the cervix and over the back of the cervix on the other side. Diaphragms are manufactured in different sizes and must be fitted to the woman by a trained practitioner. The practitioner should also be certain that the user knows how to insert her diaphragm correctly before she leaves his or her office.

Diaphragms must be used with spermicidal cream or jelly. The spermicide is applied to the inside of the diaphragm before insertion. The jelly or cream is held in place by the diaphragm, creating a physical and chemical barrier against sperm. Additional spermicide must be applied before each subsequent act of intercourse, and the diaphragm must be left in place for six to eight hours after intercourse to allow the chemical to kill any sperm remaining in the vagina (see Figure 8.3).

The typical-use effectiveness rate of the diaphragm with spermicidal cream or jelly is 84 percent; perfect-use effectiveness is 94 percent. Further, using the diaphragm during menstruation or leaving the diaphragm in place beyond the recommended time increases the risk of developing **toxic shock syndrome (TSS)**. TSS results from the multiplication of a type of bacteria that spreads to the bloodstream and causes sudden high fever, rash, nausea, vomiting, diarrhea, and a sudden drop in blood pressure. If not treated, TSS can be fatal. The diaphragm (as well as tampons left in place too long) creates conditions conducive to the growth of these bacteria. To reduce the risk of TSS, women should wash their hands carefully with soap and water before inserting or removing the diaphragm.

Another problem with the diaphragm is that it can put undue pressure on the urethra, blocking urinary flow and predisposing the user to bladder infections. A further disadvantage is that inserting the device can be awkward, especially if the woman is rushed. When inserted incorrectly, the effectiveness rate of the diaphragm decreases.

Contraceptive Sponge

First manufactured in 1983, the contraceptive sponge increased in popularity among young women during the 1980s and early 1990s. Plagued by problems with reliability, allergic reactions, and other serious concerns, the original sponge was discontinued. In Canada, a new sponge is available called Protectaid. The sponge—as depicted in the photograph on the next page—is made of a polyurethane foam and contains nonoxynol 9. It fits over the cervix and provides a physical barrier against sperm. A main advantage is convenience as the sponge does not have to be fitted by a medical practitioner. Protection begins upon insertion and lasts for up to 24 hours. Unlike other methods, there is no need to reapply spermicide or insert a new sponge for subsequent acts of intercourse within the same 24-hour time frame; it must be left in place

Spermicides: Substances designed to kill sperm.

Female condom: A single-use polyurethane sheath for internal use by women.

Diaphragm: A latex, saucer-shaped device designed to cover the cervix and block access to the uterus; should be used with spermicide.

Toxic shock syndrome (TSS): A potentially life-threatening disease that occurs when specific bacterial toxins are allowed to multiply unchecked in wounds or through improper use of tampons or diaphragms.

The contraceptive sponge.

for at least six hours after the last intercourse. Disadvantages include the limited protection from STIs and limited typical-use effectiveness with 84 percent for women who have never had a child and only 68 percent for women who have given birth; perfect-use effectiveness is 91 percent for women who have not given birth and 80 percent for women who have. Allergic reactions and vaginal irritations are common side effects with the sponge. Further when the vaginal lining becomes irritated, the risk of yeast infections and STIs increases as well. Similarly, there is an increased risk of TSS.

Cervical Cap

Cervical caps are one of the oldest methods used to prevent pregnancy. Early caps were made from beeswax, silver, or copper. The modern cervical cap was approved for use in Canada by the Health Protection Branch in 1982. The cervical cap is a small cup made of latex designed to fit snugly over the entire cervix. It must be fitted by a practitioner and is designed for use with contraceptive jelly or cream. It is somewhat more difficult to insert than a diaphragm because of its smaller size.

The cap keeps sperm out of the uterus. It is held in place by suction created during application. Insertion may take place any time up to two days prior to intercourse, and the device must be left in place for six to eight hours after intercourse. The maximum length of time the cap can be left on the cervix is 48 hours. If removed and cleaned, it can be reinserted immediately. Some women report unpleasant vaginal odours

after use. Because the device can become dislodged during intercourse, placement must be checked frequently. It cannot be used during the menstrual period and there is increased risk of TSS.

Intrauterine Device

Widespread use of **intrauterine devices (IUDs)** for contraception began in the mid-1960s, when they were advertised as less risky and more convenient than the pill. The devices fell out of favour in the mid-1970s, following negative publicity about the Dalkon Shield, a device associated with pelvic inflammatory disease and sterility. The manufacturer stopped making Dalkon Shields in 1975. We are not certain how IUDs work, despite the fact that women have been using them since 1909. Although it was once thought that IUDs act by preventing implantation of a fertilized egg, most experts now believe that they interfere with the sperm's fertilization of the egg.

A physician must fit and insert the IUD. For insertion, the device is folded and placed into a long, thin plastic applicator. The practitioner measures the depth of the uterus with a special instrument and then uses these measurements to place the IUD accurately. When in place, the arms of the T open out across the top of the uterus. One or two strings extend from the IUD into the vagina so the user can check to make sure that her IUD is in place. The device is removed by a practitioner when desired.

Although IUDs have a perfect- and typical-use rate greater than 99 percent, the discomfort and cost of insertion may be a disadvantage. When in place, the device can cause heavy menstrual flow and severe cramps. There is also risk of uterine perforation. Women using IUDs have a higher risk of ectopic pregnancy, pelvic inflammatory disease, infertility, and tubal infections. If a pregnancy occurs while the IUD is in place, the chance of miscarriage ranges from 25 to 50 percent. Removal of the device as soon as the pregnancy is known is advised. Doctors often offer therapeutic abortion to women who become pregnant while using an IUD because of the serious risks (including premature delivery, infection, and congenital abnormalities) associated with continuing the pregnancy.

Withdrawal

The **withdrawal** method is a not very effective method of birth control that involves withdrawing the penis from the vagina just prior to ejaculation. Because there can be up to half a million sperm in the drop of fluid at the tip of the penis before ejaculation, this method is unreliable and ineffective at preventing pregnancy and the spread of STIs. Timing withdrawal is also difficult; males concentrating on accurate timing may not be able to relax and enjoy intercourse. The typical-use effectiveness rate for the withdrawal method is 73 percent; perfect-use effectiveness is 96 percent.

Oral Contraceptives for Men?

The development of an oral contraceptive for men has been slow. Evidently, the mechanisms involved in the manufacture and release of sperm are not as easy to manipulate as the female ovulatory and uterine cycles. Some oral contraceptives for men have been tested, but they produced unpleasant side effects such as diminished sex drive and impotence. At the present time, research into the development of new male contraceptives is being carried on in various countries. One compound undergoing research is gossypol, a substance derived from the cotton plant. Chinese and Canadian researchers have found that gossypol inhibits sperm production, causing infertility. Difficulties in reversing the effects of the drug are presenting problems, as are concerns over long-term health consequences and possible genetic effects.

Other researchers are investigating the possibility of using ultrasound as a male contraceptive. In this method, a high-frequency sound machine is placed in contact with the scrotum. The device emits sound waves that slow sperm production, thereby lowering sperm counts. In some cases, sperm counts have remained lowered for up to two years after the procedure. Reduced sperm count, as opposed to total destruction of sperm, may suffice as a contraceptive measure because a minimum number of sperm are needed for fertilization. Before this method can be made available, the risks for testicular cancer and genetic damage must be thoroughly explored.

Fertility Awareness Methods (FAM)

Methods of fertility control that rely upon the alteration of sexual behaviours are called **fertility awareness methods (FAM)**. These methods include observing female "fertile periods" by examining cervical mucus or keeping track of internal temperature and then abstaining from vaginal intercourse during these fertile times.

Although the "rhythm method" is often the object of ridicule because of its low effectiveness rates, it is the only method of birth control available to women belonging to religious denominations that forbid the use of oral contraceptives, barrier methods, and sterilization. Our present reproductive knowledge enables women and their partners to use natural methods of birth con-

trol better with fewer risks of pregnancy, although these methods remain less effective than others.

Fertility awareness methods of birth control rely upon basic physiology. A released ovum can survive for up to 48 hours after ovulation. Sperm can live for as long as five days in the vagina. Natural methods of birth control help women to learn more about their bodies in addition to learning how to recognize their fertile times. Changes in cervical mucus prior to and during ovulation and a rise in basal body temperature are two indicators frequently used in natural contraceptive techniques. Another method involves charting a woman's menstrual cycle and ovulation times on a calendar. Any combination of these methods may be used to determine fertile times more accurately. The effectiveness of any of the methods listed below is highly dependent upon the woman's knowledge and understanding of her body as well as diligence in following the recommended guidelines. There are numerous agencies, including churches—of which you do not necessarily need to be a member—willing to assist women in learning about these methods of fertility control.

Cervical Mucus Method

The **cervical mucus method** requires women to examine the consistency and colour of their normal vaginal secretions. Before ovulation, vaginal mucus becomes gelatinous and stringy, and normal vaginal secretions may increase. Sexual activity involving penis–vagina contact must be avoided while this "fertile mucus" is present and for several days after.

Body Temperature Method

The **body temperature method** relies on the fact that the female's basal body temperature rises between 0.4 and 0.8 degrees after ovulation. For this method to be

Cervical cap: A small cup made of latex designed to fit snugly over the entire cervix.

Intrauterine device (IUD): A T-shaped device implanted in the uterus to prevent pregnancy.

Withdrawal: A method of contraception that involves withdrawing the penis from the vagina before ejaculation.

Fertility awareness methods (FAM): Several types of birth control that require alteration and/or abstinence of sexual behaviours based upon awareness of a woman's fertile time.

Cervical mucus method: A FAM that relies upon changes in cervical mucus to determine when the woman is fertile so the couple can abstain from intercourse during those times.

Body temperature method: A FAM that requires a woman to monitor her body temperature for the rise that signals ovulation and to abstain from intercourse around this time.

effective, the woman must chart her temperature for several months to recognize her body's temperature fluctuations. Abstinence from intercourse and any other penis–vagina contact must be observed preceding the temperature rise and until several days after the temperature rise was first noted.

Calendar Method

The **calendar method** requires women to record the exact number of days in their menstrual cycle. Since few women menstruate with complete regularity, a record of the menstrual cycle must be kept for 12 months, during which some other method of birth control must be used. The first day of a woman's period is counted as day one. To determine the first fertile unsafe day of the cycle, she subtracts 18 from the number of days in the shortest cycle. To determine the last unsafe day of the cycle, she subtracts 11 from the number of days in the longest cycle. This method assumes that ovulation occurs during the midpoint of the cycle (see Figure 8.4). The couple must abstain from penis–vagina contact during the fertile time. Given the

assumptions of the calendar method (that is, that ovulation always occurs at midpoint of the cycle, the cycle is regular and predictable, etc.), the calendar method is the least effective of the FAM methods.

Women interested in FAM of birth control are advised to take supervised classes. The risks of an unwanted pregnancy are great for the untrained woman. Reading a book or watching a film on the subject or talking to the proprietor of the local health food store will not likely provide the necessary training to ensure maximum effectiveness. Incidentally, information on these methods can also be helpful to couples who are trying to conceive.

Permanent Contraception

Sterilization, permanent fertility control achieved through surgical procedures, has become a popular method of contraception for women and men. Although some of the newer surgical techniques make reversal of sterilization theoretically possible, anyone considering sterilization should assume that the operation is not reversible. Before becoming sterilized,

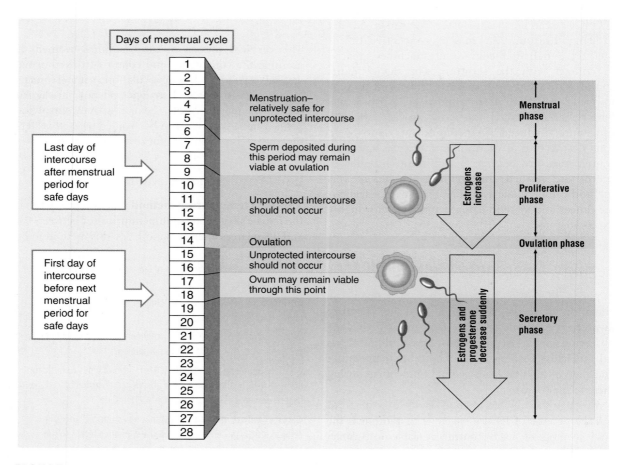

FIGURE 8.4
The Fertility Cycle

people should think through such possibilities as divorce and remarriage or a future improvement in their financial status that may make them want a larger family.

Female Sterilization

One method of sterilization in females is called **tubal ligation**. It is achieved through a surgical procedure that involves tying the fallopian tubes closed or cutting them and cauterizing (burning) the edges to seal the tubes so that an egg can no longer be fertilized. The operation is usually done in a hospital on an outpatient basis. First, the abdomen is inflated with carbon dioxide gas through a small incision in the navel. The surgeon then inserts a laparoscope into another incision just above the pubic bone. This specially designed instrument has a fibre-optic light source that enables the physician to see the fallopian tubes clearly. Once located, the tubes are cut and tied or cauterized.

> ## try it NOW!
>
> Be prepared. Any method of contraception can fail. Take steps to protect yourself from unintended pregnancy and STIs at all times. Whether you are on the pill or rely on condoms or other barriers, always have a backup plan in mind and supplies available in case the condom tears or you forget to take the pill. An extra pack of condoms and spermicidal jelly, foam, or film are good items to have on hand.

Ovarian and uterine functions are not affected by a tubal ligation. The woman's menstrual cycle continues, and released eggs simply disintegrate and are absorbed by the lymphatic system. As soon as her incision is healed, the woman may resume sexual intercourse with no fear of pregnancy.

As with any kind of surgery, there are risks. Some patients are given general anesthesia, which presents a small risk; others receive local anesthesia. The procedure itself usually takes less than an hour, and the patient is generally allowed to return home within a short time after waking up. Women considering a tubal ligation should thoroughly discuss all the risks with their physician before the operation.

A **hysterectomy**, or removal of the uterus, is a method of sterilization requiring major surgery. It is usually done only when the patient's uterus is diseased or damaged.

Male Sterilization

Sterilization in men is less complicated than in women. The procedure, called a **vasectomy**, is usually done on an outpatient basis using a local anesthetic. The surgeon makes an incision on each side of the scrotum. The vas deferens on each side is then located, and a piece is removed from each. The ends are often cauterized, then tied or sewn shut.

After a vasectomy, there is usually some discomfort, local pain, swelling, and discolouration for about a week. In a small percentage of cases, more serious complications occur: formation of a blood clot in the scrotum (which usually disappears without medical treatment), infection, and inflammatory reactions. Because sperm are stored in other areas of the reproductive system besides the vas deferens, couples must use alternative methods of birth control for at least one month after the vasectomy. The man must check with his physician (who will do a semen analysis) to determine when unprotected intercourse can take place. The pregnancy rate in women whose partners had vasectomies is about 15 in 10 000.

Many men are reluctant to consider sterilization because they fear the operation will affect their sexual performance and/or drive. Such fears are unfounded and can be alleviated by talking to men who have already had a vasectomy. A vasectomy in no way affects sexual response. Because sperm constitute only a small percentage of the semen, the amount of ejaculate is not changed significantly. The testes continue to produce sperm, but the sperm are prevented from entering the ejaculatory duct because of the surgery. After a time, sperm production may diminish. Any sperm manufactured disintegrate and are absorbed into the lymphatic system.

Although a vasectomy should be considered a permanent procedure, surgical reversal is sometimes successful in restoring fertility. Improvements in microsurgery techniques have resulted in annual pregnancy rates of between 40 and 60 percent for women whose partners have had reversals. The two major factors influencing the success rate of reversal are the doctor's expertise and the time elapsed since the vasectomy.

Calendar method: A FAM that requires mapping the woman's menstrual cycle on a calendar to determine presumed fertile times and abstaining from intercourse and any other penis–vagina contact during those times.

Sterilization: Permanent fertility control achieved through surgical procedures.

Tubal ligation: Sterilization of the female that involves cutting and tying off of the fallopian tubes.

Hysterectomy: The removal of the uterus.

Vasectomy: Sterilization of the male that involves the cutting, cauterizing, and tying off of the vasa deferentia.

Contraceptive Comfort and Confidence Scale

These questions will help you assess whether the method of contraception you are using now or may consider using in the future will be effective for you. Answering yes to any of these questions predicts potential problems. Most individuals will have a few yes answers. If you have more than a few yes responses, however, you may want to talk to a health-care provider, counsellor, partner, or friend to decide whether to use this method or how to use it so that it will really be effective. In general, the more yes answers you have, the less likely you are to use this method consistently and correctly with every act of intercourse.

Method of contraception you use now or are considering:

_____

Length of time you have used this method:

_____

Answer yes or no to the following questions:	Yes	No
1. Have I ever had problems using this method?	❑	❑
2. Have I ever become pregnant while using this method?	❑	❑
3. Am I afraid of using this method?	❑	❑
4. Would I really rather not use this method?	❑	❑
5. Will I have trouble remembering to use this method?	❑	❑
6. Will I have trouble using this method correctly and consistently?	❑	❑
7. Do I still have unanswered questions about this method?	❑	❑
8. Does this method make menstrual cycles longer, heavier, or more painful?	❑	❑
9. Does this method cost more than I can afford?	❑	❑
10. Could this method cause serious complications?	❑	❑
11. Am I opposed to this method because of any religious or moral beliefs?	❑	❑
12. Is my partner opposed to this method?	❑	❑
13. Am I using this method without my partner's knowledge?	❑	❑
14. Will using this method embarrass my partner?	❑	❑
15. Will using this method embarrass me?	❑	❑
16. Will I enjoy intercourse less because of this method?	❑	❑
17. If this method interrupts lovemaking, will I avoid using it?	❑	❑
18. Has a nurse or doctor ever told me not to use this method?	❑	❑
19. Is there anything about my personality that could lead me to use this method incorrectly?	❑	❑
20. Am I at risk of being exposed to HIV (the human immunodeficiency virus) or other sexually transmitted infections (STIs) if I use this method?	❑	❑

Total number of yes answers: _____

MAKE IT HAPPEN!

Making a Change: In order to change your behaviours, you need to develop a plan. Follow these steps and complete your Behaviour Change Contract to take action.

1. Evaluate your behaviours, and identify patterns. What can you change now? What can you change in the near future?

2. Select one pattern of behaviour that you want to change.

3. Fill out a behaviour change contract. It should include your long-term goal for change, your short-term goals, the rewards you will give yourself for reaching these goals, potential obstacles along the way, and strategies for overcoming these obstacles. For each goal, list the small steps and specific actions that you will take.

4. Chart your progress in a journal. At the end of a week, consider how successful you were in following your plan. What helped you to be successful? What made change more difficult? What will you do differently next week?

5. Revise your plan as needed: Are the short-term goals attainable? Are the rewards satisfying?

Example: Afua had been using a diaphragm as her form of birth control. When she completed the self-assessment, she discovered that there were several aspects of it that made her uncomfortable. The questions to which she answered "yes" showed that she sometimes forgot to bring her diaphragm when she planned to see her boyfriend, Ben, and she disliked using it because it interrupted her sexual activity. She also was embarrassed to use it because she did not like inserting it in front of Ben. She decided she should investigate other birth control options and discuss them with Ben. Her first step was to visit her student health centre and, based on her likes and dislikes, to choose one or two alternatives. Among the options suggested to her were the contraceptive patch (Ortho Evra) and the vaginal ring (NuvaRing), both of which she would not have to remember to use and would not interrupt sexual activity. Afua's next step was to talk to Ben about his likes and dislikes and then to make a final decision based on her confidence in the method, its convenience, and its cost.

Source: From R. A. Hatcher et al., *Contraceptive Technology*, 17th ed. (New York: Ardent Media, 1998), 238. Reprinted by permission of Ardent Media.

Decision Making about Unplanned Pregnancy

Making decisions about an unplanned pregnancy is difficult. For many women, an unplanned pregnancy can be one of the first times that they have to deal with a decision about their health and the course of their life.

If you experience an unplanned pregnancy you have three options:

* continue the pregnancy and raise the child
* continue the pregnancy and place the child for adoption
* end the pregnancy with an abortion

Consider the various aspects of your life when considering these options. Unplanned pregnancy can happen at different stages of a woman's life. Often the decision is about what is best at this time; at another point in your life the decision might be different.

You may:

* think about your personal beliefs, values, and practices and those of others in your life
* assess your existing relationships (partners, family, friends) and the support that these relationships need and can provide
* evaluate financial and social realities
* consider your living conditions and life circumstances
* examine your feelings about becoming a mother and parenting
* explore spiritual, religious, and cultural beliefs

As with any decision, you need to come to grips with making a decision and living with that decision. It is very common for women to have a variety of emotional reactions to an unplanned pregnancy. Dealing with your feelings is an important part of making a decision you can live with. Each woman is unique and the time and effort needed to make a decision will be different for each one.

WHOM TO TALK TO

Weighing the pros and cons of such a personal decision can feel reassuring, stressful, and challenging. You may wish to seek advice before making this decision. Whom a woman chooses to talk to varies; each of us has individual needs for privacy and for emotional, physical, economic, and spiritual support. You may look for people to help you in the decision-making process who are:

* knowledgeable (able to provide information or referrals)
* non-judgmental
* able to provide support whatever the decision
* someone you feel comfortable talking to

Some women only want to talk to health-care providers; others want to include a partner or family member, a friend, or a member of the clergy. Whomever you talk to, you should never feel coerced or forced to make a decision that is not your own.

Source: "Decision-Making about Unplanned Pregnancy," Sexual Health Centre, at www.womenshealthmatters.ca. Brought to you by Sunnybrook and Women's Health Sciences Centre.

� ABORTION

The law on **abortion** has seen a number of changes in Canada and much activity federally and provincially. In 1869, two years after Confederation, a law was enacted that prohibited abortion and the penalty was life imprisonment. Those who oppose abortion believe that the embryo or fetus is a human being with rights that must be protected. Others have worked to get easier access to abortion for women. In 1967, the Federal Standing Committee on Health and Welfare began considering proposed amendments to the Criminal Code relating to abortion. Dr. Henry Morgentaler, an abortion activist and physician, appeared "on behalf of the Humanist Fellowship of Montreal, urging the repeal of the abortion law and freedom of choice on abortion."[4] In 1969, Dr. Morgentaler closed his general practice and opened a clinic in Montreal to specialize in abortion, using the vacuum aspiration method. In 1970, 1971, and 1973, 13 charges of illegal abortion were brought against Dr. Morgentaler. On November 13, 1973, a jury acquitted him. The next year, however, he was convicted by the Quebec Court of Appeal. Dr. Morgentaler appealed to the Supreme Court of Canada but in 1975 the appeal was dismissed and he served 10 months in jail. In 1983, Dr. Morgentaler opened clinics in Toronto and Winnipeg and was again charged, along with other clinic doctors and the head nurse. Appeal procedures and renewed charges continued through 1986.

what do you THINK?

Do you feel comfortable discussing birth control with your partner? Why or why not? Have you discussed with your partner what you would do if you became pregnant? Why or why not?

Abortion: The medical means of terminating a pregnancy.

In 1988 the Supreme Court of Canada ruled that Canada's abortion law was unconstitutional because it violated Canada's Charter of Rights and Freedoms and a woman's right to "life, liberty and security of the person."[5] In an attempt to recriminalize abortion, Bill C-43 was introduced in Parliament. This bill, which sought to prohibit abortion unless a physician deemed it necessary for the mother's physical, mental, or psychological health, was defeated by the Senate in 1991. Harassment and threats of violence by anti-abortion protesters have caused some physicians to stop performing abortions. On May 8, 1992, a firebomb destroyed the Morgentaler clinic in Toronto. On November 8, 1992, in Vancouver, abortion provider Dr. Garson Romalis was shot and seriously wounded at his home.

Another focus of debate is who will pay for abortions. Abortions conducted in hospitals are covered by public health insurance. Clinics, though, may be fully covered, partly covered, or not covered at all.[6] In 1995, the federal government ruled that if the provinces accept that abortion is medically necessary, they must pay the full cost of abortions or lose money from federal transfer payments under the Canada Health Act.[7]

In 2005 (the latest data available), there were 97 254 (or 13.7 per 1000 women) abortions performed in a hospital or clinic in Canada.[8] There was a 3.2 percent decrease in abortions compared to the previous year, with the greatest decline found in women under the age of 20.[9] The highest rate of abortions occurs in the Yukon, with 43.8 per 100 live births, followed by Quebec (38.3), British Columbia (35.4), and Alberta (25.8).[10] The lowest rate of abortions occurs on Prince Edward Island (9.4), in New Brunswick (13.7), Saskatchewan (15.2) and Manitoba (15.8). Women between the ages of 20 and 24 have the highest rate of abortions, with 27.7 per 1000 women. The next highest rate is found in women between the ages of 25 and 29 years, at 19.7 per 1000 women.[11]

Even the best birth control methods can fail. Pregnancies do occur despite due diligence. Women may be raped. When an unwanted pregnancy occurs, the decision whether to terminate, to carry to term and keep the baby, or to carry to term and give the baby up for adoption must be made. This is a personal decision each woman must make according to her personal beliefs, values, and resources after carefully considering the alternatives. There are resources available to help women with this decision.

Methods of Abortion

The type of abortion procedure used is determined by how many weeks pregnant the woman is. Pregnancy length is calculated from the first day of a woman's last menstrual period. If performed during the first trimester of pregnancy, abortion presents a relatively low risk to the mother. The most commonly used method of first-trimester abortion is **vacuum aspiration**. The procedure is usually performed with a local anesthetic. The cervix is dilated with instruments or by placing laminaria, a sterile seaweed product, in the cervical canal. The laminaria is left in place for a few hours or overnight and slowly dilates the cervix. After it is removed, a long tube is inserted into the uterus through the cervix. Gentle suction is then used to remove the fetal tissue from the uterine walls.

Pregnancies that progress into the second trimester can be terminated through **dilation and evacuation (D&E)**, a procedure that combines vacuum aspiration with a technique called **dilation and curettage (D&C)**. For this procedure, the cervix is dilated with laminaria for one to two days and a combination of instruments and vacuum aspiration is used to empty the uterus (see Figure 8.5). Second-trimester abortions are frequently done under general anesthetic. Both procedures can be performed on an outpatient basis (usually in the physician's office) with or without pain medication. Generally, the woman is given a mild tranquillizer to help her relax. Both procedures may cause moderate to severe uterine cramping and blood loss.

The **hysterotomy**, or surgical removal of the fetus from the uterus, may be used during emergencies or when the mother's life may be in danger and when other types of abortions are deemed too dangerous.

The risks associated with abortions include infection, incomplete abortion (when parts of the placenta

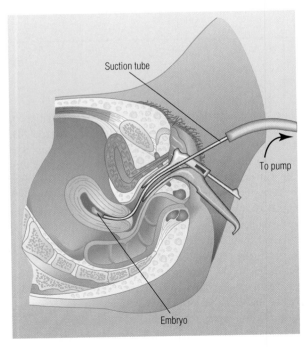

Suction tube

To pump

Embryo

FIGURE 8.5

Vacuum Aspiration Abortion

what do you THINK?

If you or your partner unexpectedly became pregnant, would you choose to terminate the pregnancy? What factors would you consider in making your decision? How might an abortion affect your relationship? How would your decision be different if you were married?

what do you THINK?

Do you know someone who has put off starting a family? Why have they decided to wait? What impact will this shift have upon the Canadian population? How will these changes affect our society?

remain in the uterus), missed abortion (when the fetus is not actually removed), excessive bleeding, and cervical and uterine trauma. Follow-up and attention to dangerous signs decrease the chances of any long term problems. The mortality rate for first-trimester abortions is 0.8 per 100 000 women. The rate for second-trimester abortions is higher, at 4.3 per 100 000 women. This higher rate is due to the increased risk of uterine perforation, bleeding, infection, and incomplete abortion due to the fact that the uterine wall becomes thinner as the pregnancy progresses.

Two other methods used in second-trimester abortions, though less commonly than the D&E method, are prostaglandin or saline **induction abortions**. In these methods, prostaglandin hormones or a saline solution is injected into the uterus. The injected solution kills the fetus and causes labour contractions to begin. After 24 to 48 hours the fetus and placenta are expelled from the uterus.

❋ PLANNING A PREGNANCY

The technological ability to control your fertility gives you choices not available when your parents were born. The loosening of social restrictions in the areas of marriage and parenting also affords single men and women, and gay and lesbian couples the opportunity to become parents. Regardless of your marital status, the preparation to become a parent involves similar considerations and decisions. If you are in the process of deciding whether to have children, you need to take the time to evaluate your emotions, finances, and health.

Emotional Health

First and foremost, consider why you want to have a child: To fulfill an inner need to carry on the family? Out of loneliness? Any other reasons? Can you care for this new human being in a loving and nurturing manner? Are you ready to make the sacrifices necessary to bear and raise a child? You can prepare yourself for this change in your life in several ways. Reading about

pregnancy and parenthood, taking classes, talking to parents of children of all ages, and joining a support group are helpful forms of preparation. If you choose to adopt, you will find many support groups available to you as well.

Maternal Health

Before becoming pregnant, a woman should have a thorough medical examination. **Preconception care** should include assessment of possible pregnancy complications. Medical problems such as diabetes and high blood pressure should be discussed, as should any genetic disorders that run in either family. Additional suggestions for a healthy pregnancy include:

- engage in regular physical activity (see also Chapter 4)
- eat a healthy diet, according to Eating Well with Canada's Food Guide (see also Chapter 5)
- maintain a normal weight (see also Chapter 6)
- do not smoke, drink alcohol, or use other illicit drugs
- reduce or eliminate caffeine intake
- avoid exposure to X-rays and environmental chemicals such as lawn and garden chemicals
- prior to becoming pregnant, have your annual dental X-rays and your regular checkup

Vacuum aspiration: The use of gentle suction to remove fetal tissue from the uterus.

Dilation and evacuation (D&E): An abortion technique that combines vacuum aspiration with dilation and curettage; fetal tissue is sucked and scraped out of the uterus.

Dilation and curettage (D&C): An abortion technique in which the cervix is dilated with laminaria for one to two days and the uterine walls are scraped clean.

Hysterotomy: The surgical removal of the fetus from the uterus.

Induction abortion: A type of abortion in which chemicals are injected into the uterus through the uterine wall; labour begins and the woman delivers a dead fetus.

Preconception care: Medical care received prior to becoming pregnant that helps a woman assess and address potential maternal health.

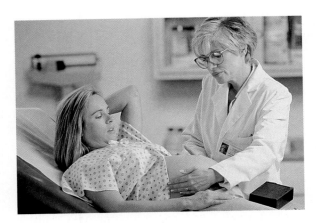
Good prenatal care involves regular medical checkups by a practitioner with whom the mother feels she can communicate freely.

Paternal Health

It is common wisdom that mothers-to-be should steer clear of toxic chemicals that can cause birth defects. Even women trying to conceive are cautioned to avoid toxic environments and to eat a nourishing diet, to stop smoking and drinking alcohol, and to avoid most medications. Now similar precautions are recommended for fathers-to-be. New research suggests that a man's exposure to chemicals influences not only his ability to father a child but also the future health of his child.

Fathers-to-be have been overlooked in the past for several reasons. Researchers assumed that the genetic damage leading to birth defects and other health problems always occurred while a child was in the mother's womb or was caused by random errors of nature. Scientists have recently discovered that how sperm look has little to do with how they act. Misshapen sperm can penetrate an egg, and they do not necessarily carry defective genetic goods. Moreover, sperm that look healthy and swim well can be the true genetic culprits. DNA fluorescent markers have identified normal-looking yet genetically flawed sperm that carry too many or too few chromosomes. Fathers contribute the extra chromosome 21 in about 6 percent of children with Down syndrome, which causes learning disabilities; the extra X chromosome in 50 percent of boys with Klinefelter's syndrome, which causes abnormal sexual development; and the shortened chromosome 15 in about 85 percent of children with Prader-Willi syndrome, a disorder characterized by physical and learning disabilities and obesity.

Although some birth defects are caused by the random errors of nature, it now appears that some disorders can be traced to sperm damaged by chemicals. Sperm are naturally vulnerable to toxic assault and genetic damage. Many drugs and ingested chemicals can readily invade the testes from the bloodstream;

others ambush sperm after they leave the testes and pass through the epididymides, where they mature and are stored. By one route or another, half of 100 chemicals studied so far (including by-products of cigarette smoke) apparently harm sperm. Some researchers believe that vitamin C is nature's way of protecting sex cells from damage. Poor dietary intake, exposure to toxic chemicals, cigarette smoking, and not enough foods rich in vitamin C are probably the biggest culprits in sperm damage.[12]

Financial Evaluation

You also need to evaluate your finances. Both partners should find out about their employers' policies concerning parental leave, including length of leave available and conditions for returning to work.

Raising a child exacts a tremendous strain on most families' finances. Expenses during the first year of life average to at least $10 000. The expense of raising a child from birth to 18 years of age (in 2004 dollars) was estimated to be more than $166 000—not including the cost of post-secondary education!

Parents should decide if either of them is willing to put their career on hold and spend the formative years raising their child(ren). The financial implications of this decision should be considered as well. Alternatively, the cost and availability of quality child care should be considered. Prospective parents should realistically assess how much family assistance they can expect with a new baby, as well as the availability and cost of nonfamily child care should staying at home to raise their child(ren) not be considered a viable option.

Contingency Planning

A final consideration is how to provide financially and practically for your child should something happen to you and/or your partner. If both of you were to die while the child is young, do you have relatives or close friends who would raise the child?

If you have more than one child, would they have to be split up or could they be kept together? What sort of financial situation would your child(ren) be in? Unpleasant though it may be to think about, this sort of contingency planning is extremely important.

what do you THINK?

Do most parents plan when they have their children? At what point in your life do you think you will be ready to take on the responsibilities of becoming a parent? What influences your decision? Why? What are your biggest concerns about parenthood?

The Impact of a Reduced Fertility Rate on Women's Health

Total fertility rates (number of children each woman has, on average) have decreased worldwide and in particular in Canada over the past 40 years. In fact, the Canadian fertility rate dropped from 3.90 children per woman in 1960 to 1.49 in 2000. Although there have been improvements in maternal and reproductive health over this time period, such as decreases in mortality and other pregnancy complications, little is known about the impact of reduced fertility, delayed fertility, and births to unmarried women.

Data from the General Social Survey Cycle 10–The Family (1995) were used to examine:

- the relationship between family size and specific determinants of health,
- the distribution of family and work attitudes by age and education, and
- the relationship between attitude and intention to have one or more children in the future.

The results indicated that total fertility rates decreased over the last 40 years, with considerable variation according to geographic location and socio-demographic subgroup. Further results indicated that the relationships between family size and selected determinants of health (marital status, education, employment, home ownership, and self-perceived health) were different for men and women. Specifically, a woman with one child was four times more likely to be "coupled" than a childless woman. Women with two children were as likely to be "coupled" as a woman with one child. Men were five times more likely to be married than their childless counterparts regardless of the number of children. In regard to education, women with two or more children were more likely to have not completed high school compared to their childless counterparts. A similar, but less strong relationship was noted in men. For employment, there was a negative relationship between number of children and employment status (that is, the more children they had, the less likely women were to be employed outside the home). In men, this relationship existed only with five or more children (that is, a man was less likely to be employed outside the home if he had five or more children). In regard to home ownership, there was a direct, positive relationship regardless of the number of children in men and only with two children in women. No clear relationships existed with self-perceived health and number of children in either women or men. In the analysis of the associations between attitude and intention to have one or more children in the future, similarities were found among men and women, though differences existed by age group and level of education. Specifically, women who intended to have one or more children in the future were older, had a higher level of education, were employed, and believed that having a child and home were an important part of their happiness. In men, the intention to have one or more children in the future was related to their age, a better than high school education, not being employed full time, the belief that a child is important to happiness, and the belief that what a women really wants is a home and children.

Source: Adapted from J. Payne, Public Health Agency of Canada (PHAC), "The Impact of a Reduced Fertility Rate on Women's Health." Retrieved May 16, 2006, from www.phac-aspc.gc.ca/publicat/whsr-rssf/chap_10_e.html.

PREGNANCY

✳ Prenatal Care

A successful pregnancy requires the mother's ability to take care of herself and her unborn child. It is essential to have regular checkups with a doctor or midwife, beginning as soon as possible (certainly within the first three months). Early detection of fetal abnormalities and identification of high-risk mothers and infants are the major purposes of prenatal care. On the first visit, the practitioner should obtain a complete medical history of the mother and her family and note any hereditary conditions that could put a woman or her fetus at risk.

Regular appointments to measure weight gain and blood pressure and monitor the size and position of the fetus should continue throughout the pregnancy. This early care reduces infant mortality and low birth-weight. Experts recommend obstetrical visits once a month to 28 weeks, biweekly to 36 weeks, and weekly to 40 weeks.

Additional concerns include the mother's physical condition, her level of nutrition, her confidence in her ability to give birth, her use of drugs and medications, and the availability of a skilled practitioner (midwife or doctor) who can oversee the pregnancy and delivery. A woman planning a pregnancy also needs a support system (spouse or partner, family, friends, community groups) willing to give her and her child the love and emotional support needed during and after her pregnancy. In most areas prenatal classes are available, including some for pregnant teens.

Choosing a Practitioner

A woman should carefully choose a practitioner who will attend her pregnancy and delivery, although in some localities physicians, midwives, and specialists may be in short supply. If possible, this choice should be made before she becomes pregnant. Recommendations from friends satisfied with the care they received during pregnancy may be a good starting point. The woman's family physician may also be able to recommend a midwife or specialist. The pregnant woman needs to find a practitioner she can trust with her own life and that of the baby and with whom she can communicate freely.

When choosing a practitioner, parents should ask a number of questions concerning credentials and professional qualifications. Besides this information, a pregnant woman must ask questions specific to her condition. Prospective parents should also inquire about the practitioner's experience in handling various complications, commitment to being at the mother's side during delivery, and beliefs and practices concerning the use of anesthesia, fetal monitoring, induced labour, and forceps delivery. What are the practitioner's attitudes toward circumcision and alternative birthing procedures? Finally, the parents must learn under what circumstances the practitioner would perform a Caesarean section.

Two types of physicians can attend pregnancies and deliveries. The obstetrician-gynecologist (ob-gyn) is an MD who specializes in obstetrics (pregnancy and birth) and gynecology (care of women's reproductive organs). These practitioners are trained to handle all types of pregnancy- and delivery-related emergencies. A family practitioner is a licensed MD who provides comprehensive care for people of all ages. The majority of family practitioners have obstetrical experience but will refer a patient to a specialist if necessary. Unlike the ob-gyn, the family practitioner can serve as the baby's physician after attending the birth.

A third option many women are choosing is to have their prenatal, delivery, and postnatal care given by a midwife, who is also an experienced practitioner trained to attend pregnancies and deliveries. Some of the reasons for choosing midwifery care are

- knowing that the person who has cared for you throughout your pregnancy will be with you during the labour and delivery
- having more time to ask questions and express your concerns during appointments (midwives typically schedule a longer time for appointments and are willing to discuss any concerns, personal or medical, that arise during pregnancy)
- the ability to reach your midwife with questions or problems between visits

- a postpartum home visit and other home visits if necessary
- breastfeeding support

Midwives are trained to recognize situations that call for the opinion—or the intervention—of a physician and will refer their clients to specialists—or even ask a physician to take over care (for instance, if an emergency C-section is required) when necessary. So a woman may go for one or more consultations with a doctor (about her blood sugar, her weight, or age-related concerns, for instance) while still having the care of a midwife throughout her pregnancy. Further, many midwives have "admitting privileges" at a hospital, which means they can supervise hospital births as well as home births.

Alcohol and Drugs

A woman should avoid all drugs during pregnancy unless prescribed by a doctor—and then she should ask whether the medication is really necessary and whether there is a safer alternative. Always tell a physician, dentist, or other practitioner if you are pregnant or think you might be pregnant. Even common over-the-counter medications such as Aspirin and beverages such as coffee and tea can damage a developing fetus. The fetus is particularly susceptible to the **teratogenic** (birth-defect-causing) effects of some chemical substances during the first three months of pregnancy. The fetus can also develop an addiction to or tolerance for drugs that the mother is using.

Of particular concern to medical professionals is the use of tobacco and alcohol during pregnancy. Women who drink heavily may have normal first babies and then subsequently deliver children with a fetal alcohol spectrum disorder. **Fetal alcohol spectrum disorder (FSAD)** describes a number of disorders related to alcohol consumption during pregnancy, including fetal alcohol syndrome, fetal alcohol effects, partial fetal alcohol effects, alcohol-related neurodevelopmental disorders, and neurobehavioural disorder–alcohol exposed. FSAD manifests in lifelong developmental and cognitive disabilities in children. The exact amount of alcohol necessary to cause FASD is not known, but researchers doubt that any level of alcohol consumption is safe. Therefore, total abstinence from alcohol during pregnancy—and when trying to get pregnant—is recommended. Table 8.2 provides a list of teratogenic effects of alcohol and other drugs ingested by the mother.

Cigarette smoking during pregnancy has more predictable effects than alcohol. Studies indicate a 25 to 50 percent higher rate of fetal and infant deaths among women who smoke during pregnancy than among those who do not.[13] Women who smoke more

TABLE 8.2

Teratogenic Effects of Drugs

Drug	Effect
Alcohol	Cognitive disabilities; growth retardation; increased spontaneous abortion
Amphetamines	Suspected nervous system damage
Aspirin	Newborn bleeding
Cocaine	Uncontrolled jerking motions; paralysis; depressed interactive behaviour; poor organizational response to environmental stimuli
Opioids	Immediate withdrawal in newborns; permanent learning disabilities
Tetracycline	Tooth discolouration
Sulfa drugs	Facial and skeletal abnormalities
Barbiturates	Congenital malformations
Streptomycin	Deafness
Accutane	Small or absent ears; small jaw; heart defects
Valium	Possible congenital anomalies

Source: Mike Samuels, M.D. and Nancy Samuels, The Well Pregnancy Book (New York: Summit Books, 1986) 131.

than 10 to 15 cigarettes a day during pregnancy have higher rates of miscarriage, stillbirth, premature births, and low-birthweight babies than nonsmokers. Fetal research on the effects of "secondhand" or sidestream smoke (inhaling smoke produced by others) is inconclusive, but babies whose parents smoke can be twice as susceptible to pneumonia, bronchitis, and related illnesses as other babies.

X-Rays

X-rays present a clear danger to the fetus. Although most diagnostic x-rays produce minimal amounts of radiation, even low levels may cause birth defects or other problems, particularly if several low-dose X-rays occur over a short time period. Pregnant women are advised to avoid X-rays unless absolutely necessary.

Nutrition and Physical Activity

Pregnant women have additional needs for water, protein, calories, and certain vitamins and minerals, so their dietary intake should be carefully monitored by a qualified practitioner. Special attention should be paid to getting enough folic acid (found in dark leafy greens and in fortified grains), iron (dried fruits, meats, legumes, liver, egg yolks), calcium (nonfat or low-fat dairy products, some canned fish), and fluids. Vitamin supplements can alleviate some deficiencies, but there is no substitute for a well-balanced dietary intake. Babies born to mothers whose nutrition has been poor run high risks of substandard mental and physical development (see Table 8.3).

Weight gain during pregnancy helps nourish a growing baby. For a woman of normal weight before pregnancy, the recommended weight gain during pregnancy ranges from 11 to 16 kilograms (25–35 pounds); a woman carrying twins should gain about 16 to 20 kilograms (35–45 pounds). Usually the mother can expect to gain about five kilograms (~12 pounds) during the first 20 weeks and about 0.5 kilograms (approximately 1 pound) per week during the rest of the pregnancy.

Of the total number of kilograms gained during pregnancy, about three to four are the baby's weight.

Teratogenic: Causing birth defects; may refer to drugs, environmental chemicals, X-rays, or diseases.

Fetal alcohol spectrum disorders (FASD): A number of disorders related to alcohol consumption during pregnancy–including fetal alcohol syndrome, fetal alcohol effects, partial fetal alcohol effects, alcohol-related neurodevelopmental disorders, and neurobehavioural disorder–alcohol exposed–that result in lifelong developmental and cognitive disabilities in children.

Doctor-approved physical activity during pregnancy helps the mother control her weight and contributes to easier deliveries and healthier babies.

The baby's birthweight is important, since a low weight can lead to health problems during labour and the baby's first few months. Eating right and gaining enough weight help reduce the chances of having a low-birthweight baby. If a woman gains an appropriate amount of weight while pregnant, chances are that her baby will gain weight properly, too. Pregnancy is not a time to think about losing weight—losing weight at this time may endanger the baby.[14]

As in all other stages of life, physical activity is an important factor in overall maternal health as well as in weight control during pregnancy. Regular, moderate-intensity physical activity of 45 minutes, three days per week has been associated in one study with heavier-birthweight babies, fewer surgical births, and shorter hospital stays after birth.[15] Other recommendations are for women to continue with their exercise regime during their pregnancy while paying extra attention to their changing body weight and shape and adapting their regime as needed. It is generally not recommended for women to engage in a new routine to build physical fitness at this time. Pregnant women should consult with their physicians or midwives before starting any new physical activities. See also the Health in the Media textbox.

TABLE 8.3

Nutrient Deficiency Effects

Nutrient	Deficiency Effect
Overall caloric intake	Low infant birthweight
Protein	Reduced infant head circumference, low infant birthweight
Folic acid	Miscarriage and neural tube defects
Vitamin D	Decreased infant bone density
Calcium	Decreased infant bone density
Iron	Low infant birthweight and premature birth
Iodine	Varying degrees of mental and physical disabilities
Zinc	Congenital malformations

Source: From ROLFES/DEBRUYNE/WHITNEY. Life Span Nutrition, 2E. © 1998 Brooks/Cole, a part of Cengage Learning, Inc. Reproduced by permission. www.cengage.com/permissions.

Researchers Develop Exercise Guidelines for Pregnancy

by Marlene Habib—The Canadian Press

Super-fit Beth Sweeney began worrying about how much exercise she should be doing when she learned she was pregnant.

Sweeney, a 30-year-old fitness instructor in the resort town of Grand Bend, Ontario, did not want to take chances with her first pregnancy. So she enrolled in a study at the University of Western Ontario in London assessing how much exercise extremely fit pregnant women should be doing.

The study, by Michelle Mottola of the University of Western Ontario and Larry Wolfe of Queen's University in Kingston, Ontario, aimed to develop exercise guidelines for pregnant women like aerobics instructors, military personnel, police officers and firefighters who are intense exercisers or engage in heavy work.

Early findings from the study indicated that super-active pregnant women can continue their regimens with proper monitoring.

Sweeney's body fat, blood pressure, weight and blood-sugar levels were recorded 16 weeks into her pregnancy. She was also given a 45-minute treadmill test to determine her maximum heart rate and fitness level.

Sweeney then continued exercising with the same intensity throughout much of her pregnancy, measuring her heart rate while instructing or doing other exercise to ensure it was not beyond the safe level determined by Mottola.

Sweeney felt so good that she was scheduled to teach an aerobics class the day she gave birth—nine days earlier than expected. She returned to lead aerobics classes in Grand Bend just five weeks postpartum.

The study by Mottola and Wolfe breaks new ground for exercising mums-to-be. Currently, there are only national guidelines for mild to moderate physical activity.

Avid exercisers like Sweeney are not covered under these guidelines. She is among the five fit women who have been followed through their pregnancies so far by Mottola. The researcher plans to recruit a few dozen more to monitor their energy changes and other fitness aspects before the first phase ends. "We are finding a lot of really active women cut back on their activity when they do not have to," Mottola said in a telephone interview. The Canadian Forces Personnel Support Agency is funding the study. It hopes the findings will help women taken off active duty when they become pregnant keep in shape so they can return to work after maternity leave.

General safety considerations for physically active pregnant women.

- Avoid prolonged or strenuous exertion during the first trimester.
- Avoid isometric exercise or straining while holding your breath.
- Maintain adequate nutrition and hydration—drink liquids before, during, and after exercise.
- Limit exercise in warm or humid environments.
- Avoid exercise while lying on your back past the fourth month of pregnancy.
- Avoid exercises which involve physical contact or danger of falling.
- Periodic rest periods may help to minimize possible low oxygen or temperature stress to the fetus.
- Know the reasons to stop exercise and consult a qualified physician immediately if they occur.

Source: The Canadian Press.

Other Factors

A pregnant woman should avoid exposure to toxic chemicals, heavy metals, pesticides, gases, and other hazardous compounds. She should not clean cat-litter boxes because cat feces can contain organisms that cause a disease called toxoplasmosis. If a pregnant woman contracts this disease, her baby may be stillborn or have cognitive disabilities or other birth defects.

Before becoming pregnant, a woman should be tested to determine if she has had rubella (German measles). If she has not had it, she should be immu- nized for it and wait the recommended length of time before becoming pregnant. A rubella infection can kill the fetus or cause blindness or hearing disorders in the infant. If a woman has ever had genital herpes, she should inform her midwife or physician. Contact with an active herpes infection during birth can be fatal to the infant. If a pregnant woman knows she has herpes, she may be prescribed anti-virals before delivery to reduce the likelihood of her having an outbreak; if she has active lesions at the time of delivery, the practitioner will recommend delivering the baby by Caesarian section.

A Woman's Reproductive Years

More than half of the average Canadian woman's expected life span is spent between menarche (first menses) and menopause (last menses), a period of approximately 40 years. During this 40-year period, she must make many decisions about her reproductive health. Deciding if and when to have children, as well as how to prevent pregnancy when necessary, are long-term concerns.[16]

Today, a pregnant woman over 35 has plenty of company. While births to women in their 20s are declining, the rate of first births to women between the ages of 30 and 39 has doubled in the past decade, and births to women over 39 have increased by more than 50 percent. Many women who wait until their 30s to consider having a child find themselves wondering, "Am I too old to have a baby?" Researchers believe that there is a decline in the quality and viability of eggs produced after age 35, which has resulted in an increase in the number of women struggling with fertility issues and a concomitant increase in the use of fertility clinics. Statistically, the chances of having a miscarriage or a baby with birth defects do rise after the age of 35. **Down syndrome**, a genetic anomaly characterized by mild to severe cognitive disabilities and a variety of physical abnormalities, is the most common birth defect found in babies born to older mothers. The incidence of Down syndrome in babies born to mothers aged 20 is 1 in 10 000 births; it rises to 1 in 365 births when the mother is 35, to 1 in 109 when she is 40, and to 1 in 32 when she is 45. Women who choose to delay motherhood until their late 30s also worry about their physical ability to carry and deliver their babies. For these women regular moderate intensity physical activity will help to maintain good posture and promote a successful delivery.

Pregnancy Testing

A woman may suspect she is pregnant before she has a pregnancy test. A typical sign is a missed menstrual period, yet this is not always an accurate indicator. A woman can miss her period for a variety of reasons: stress, excessive physical activity without an adequate dietary intake, or emotional upset. Another common sign is sore breasts. This too, can be caused by other health issues. Confirmation of a pregnancy should be obtained from a pregnancy test scheduled in a medical office or birth control clinic.

Women who wish to know immediately whether or not they are pregnant can purchase home pregnancy test kits. These kits, sold over the counter in drugstores, are about 85 to 95 percent reliable. A positive test is based on the secretion of **human chorionic gonadotropin**

(HCG) found in the woman's urine. Home test kits come equipped with a small sample of red blood cells coated with HCG antibodies, to which the user adds a small amount of urine. If the concentration of HCG is great enough, it will clump together with the HCG antibodies, indicating that the user is pregnant.

If taken too early in the pregnancy, the test may show a false negative. Other causes of false negatives are unclean test tubes, ingestion of certain drugs, and vaginal or urinary infections. Accuracy also depends on the quality of the test itself and the user's ability to perform it and interpret the results. Blood tests administered and analyzed by a medical laboratory give more accurate results.

The Process of Pregnancy

Pregnancy begins the moment a sperm fertilizes an ovum in the fallopian tubes (see Figure 8.6). From there, the single cell multiplies, becoming a sphere-shaped cluster of cells as it travels toward the uterus, a journey that may last three to four days. Upon arrival, the embryo burrows into the thick, spongy endometrium and is nourished from this carefully prepared lining.

Early Signs of Pregnancy

The first sign of pregnancy is usually a missed menstrual period (although some women "spot" in early pregnancy, and such spotting may be mistaken for a period). Other signs of pregnancy include

- breast tenderness
- extreme fatigue
- sleeplessness
- emotional upset
- nausea
- vomiting (especially in the morning)

A pregnancy typically lasts 40 weeks. The due date is calculated from the expectant mother's last menstrual period. Pregnancy is typically divided into three phases, or **trimesters**, of approximately three months each.

The First Trimester

During the first trimester, there are few noticeable changes in the maternal body. The expectant mother may urinate more frequently and experience morning sickness, swollen breasts, or undue fatigue. These symptoms may not be frequent or severe, so she may not realize she is pregnant at this time unless she has a pregnancy test.

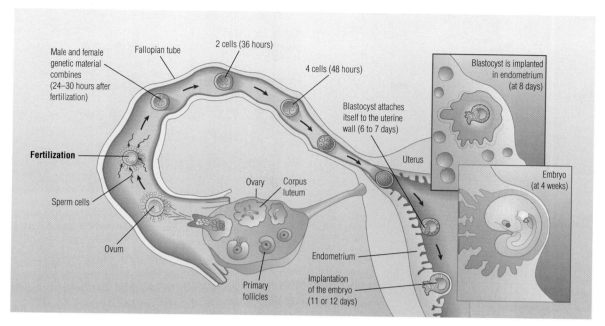

FIGURE 8.6

Fertilization

During the first two months after conception, the **embryo** differentiates and develops its various organ systems, beginning with the nervous and circulatory systems. At the start of the third month, the embryo is called a **fetus**, indicating that all organ systems are in place. For the rest of the pregnancy, growth and refinement occur in each major body system so that they can function independently, yet in coordination, at birth.

The Second Trimester

At the beginning of the second trimester, physical changes in the mother become more visible. Her breasts swell and her waistline thickens. During this time, the fetus makes greater demands upon the mother's body. In particular, the **placenta**, the network of blood vessels that carry nutrients and oxygen to the fetus and fetal waste products to the mother, becomes well established.

The Third Trimester

This is the period of greatest fetal growth. The fetus gains most of its weight during these last three months. During the third trimester, the fetus must get large amounts of calcium, iron, and nitrogen from the food the mother eats. Approximately 85 percent of the calcium and iron the mother digests goes into the fetal bloodstream. Although the fetus may live if it is born during the seventh month, it needs the layer of fat usually acquired during the eighth month and time for the organs (especially the respiratory and digestive organs) to develop to their full potential. Babies born prematurely usually require intensive medical care.

Prenatal Testing and Screening

Modern technology enables medical practitioners to detect health defects in a fetus as early as the 14th to 18th weeks of pregnancy. One common testing procedure, **amniocentesis**, which is strongly recommended for women over the age of 35, involves

Down syndrome: A genetic anomaly characterized by cognitive disabilities and a variety of physical abnormalities.

Human chorionic gonadotropin (HCG): Hormone detectable in blood or urine samples within the first few weeks of pregnancy.

Trimester: A three-month segment of pregnancy, useful in describing different developmental stages.

Embryo: The fertilized egg from conception until the end of two months' development.

Fetus: The name given the developing baby from the third month of pregnancy until birth.

Placenta: The network of blood vessels that carries nutrients to the developing infant and carries wastes away; it connects to the umbilical cord.

Amniocentesis: A medical test in which a small amount of fluid is drawn from the amniotic sac; usually used to detect genetic diseases.

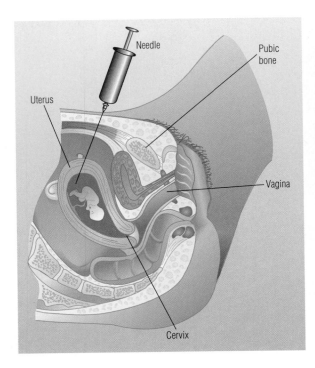

FIGURE 8.7
Amniocentesis

The process of amniocentesis can detect certain congenital problems as well as the sex of the fetus.

Ultrasound testing can reveal defects in the developing fetus, and, as the time of delivery nears, it can provide useful information about the size and position of the unborn child.

inserting a long needle through the mother's abdominal and uterine walls into the **amniotic sac**, the protective pouch surrounding the baby (see Figure 8.7). The needle draws out 15 to 20 mL of fluid, which is analyzed for genetic information about the baby. This test can reveal the presence of 40 genetic abnormalities, including Down syndrome, Tay-Sachs disease (a fatal disorder of the nervous system common among Jewish people of Eastern European descent), and sickle-cell anemia (a debilitating blood disorder found primarily among individuals of African descent). Amniocentesis can also reveal the sex of the child. Although widely used, amniocentesis is not without risk. Chances of fetal damage and miscarriage as a result of testing are 1 in 400.

Another procedure, ultrasound (or sonography), uses high-frequency sound waves to determine the size and position of the fetus. Ultrasound can also detect defects in the central nervous system and digestive system of the fetus. Knowing the position of the fetus assists practitioners in performing amniocentesis and in delivering the child.

A third procedure, chorionic villus sampling (CVS), involves snipping tissue from the developing fetal sac. CVS can be used at 10 to 12 weeks of pregnancy with the results available in 12 to 48 hours. This test is an attractive option for couples at high risk for having a baby with Down syndrome or a debilitating hereditary disease.

Parents are usually referred for genetic counselling before such tests, so they will understand the test and the potential significance of the results beforehand and have a chance to ask questions and understand their options, particularly should the test reveal a serious birth defect.

what do you **THINK?**

What are the most important concerns you have for choosing a health practitioner for your or your partner's pregnancy? What behaviours might you have to change if you found out that you or your partner was pregnant? In what ways would your life change if you had a child born with a birth defect? What type of prenatal tests would you consider before the birth of your child?

CHILDBIRTH

Where to Have Your Baby

Today's prospective mothers have many delivery options. These range from hospital birth supervised by a physician to home birth with a midwife, with a number of options in between. When considering birthing alternatives, parental values are important. Many couples, for instance, feel that the modern medical establishment has dehumanized the birth process; thus they choose to deliver at home or at a birthing centre, a homelike setting outside a hospital where women can give birth and receive postdelivery care from a

Dilation and effacement of the cervix

Transition

Pushing

Birth of the baby

Delivery of the placenta

FIGURE 8.8
The Birth Process

team of professional practitioners, including midwives or physicians and registered nurses.

Labour and Delivery

The birth process has three stages. The exact mechanisms that signal the mother's body that the baby is ready to be born are unknown. During the few weeks preceding delivery, the baby normally shifts and turns to a head-down position, and the cervix begins to dilate (open up). The junction of the pubic bones also loosens to permit expansion of the pelvic girdle during birth (see Figure 8.8).

In the first stage of labour, the amniotic sac breaks, causing a rush of fluid from the vagina (commonly referred to as "breaking of the waters"). Contractions (initially similar to what cramps feel like when a woman has her menstrual cycle) in the abdomen and lower back also signal the beginning of labour. Early contractions push the baby downward, putting pressure on the cervix and thereby causing it to dilate further. The first stage of labour may last from a couple of hours to more than a day for a first birth, and is usually much shorter during subsequent births.

The end of the first stage of labour, called **transition**, is the part of the process when the cervix becomes fully dilated and the baby's head begins to move into the vagina, or the birth canal. Contractions, these ones much stronger, intense and forceful, usually come quickly during transition. Transition usually lasts 30 minutes or less.

The second stage of labour follows transition when the cervix has become fully dilated. Contractions become rhythmic, stronger, and more painful as the uterus works to push the baby through the birth canal. The second stage of labour (called the expulsion stage) may last between one and four hours (though it can also be shorter for some women) and concludes when the infant is finally pushed out of the mother's body.

After delivery, the attending practitioner cleans the baby's mucus-filled breathing passages, and the baby takes its first breath, generally accompanied by a loud wail. (The traditional "slap" on the baby's buttocks, often romanticized in movies, is no longer a common practice.) In the meantime, the mother continues into the third stage of labour, during which the placenta, or afterbirth, is expelled from the womb. This stage is usually completed within 30 minutes of delivery. The umbilical cord is then tied and severed. The stump of cord attached to the baby's navel dries up and drops off within a few days.

Amniotic sac: The protective pouch surrounding the baby.

Transition: The process during which the cervix becomes nearly fully dilated and the head of the fetus moves into the birth canal.

Prenatal Education

In terms of facilities and professionals, expectant parents in Canada can receive a variety of services for prenatal education in the community where they live. Most prenatal programs inform parents of what to expect during labour and delivery, encourage them to participate in the planning and decision-making around labour and delivery (where to have the birth, who will be at the birth, choice of pain control methods, and so on), and include instruction in a range of comfort measures including breathing techniques.

Drugs in the Delivery Room

Because painkilling drugs given to the mother during labour can cause sluggish responses in the newborn, many women choose drug-free labours and deliveries. Drug-free labour involves the use of physical activity, massage, and controlled rhythmic breathing to control pain. Many women who choose "natural" childbirth mistakenly believe that the activities taught in their classes will make their labour and delivery painless. When it comes time to give birth, they may feel inadequate because they experience the normal pain associated with childbirth. Pain is to be expected, and if it becomes too intense, the mother has the option of receiving medication to provide some relief.

This is an issue that the mother should discuss with her practitioner before the birth of her baby. It is important to know your practitioner's position on the use of painkilling drugs during delivery and to understand if it is in keeping with your own. A woman's partner should know her wishes beforehand so that he or she can advocate for her during the labour. Women should also understand that they may change their mind about pain control during labour and that this is okay.

Breastfeeding and the Postpartum Period

Although the new mother's milk will not begin to flow for two or more days following delivery, her breasts secrete a yellowish substance called colostrum. Because this fluid contains vital antibodies to help fight infection, it is wise to allow the newborn to suckle. Given the overwhelmingly supportive research, it is strongly recommended that full-term newborns be breastfed. This recommendation does not mean that breast milk is the only adequate method of nourishing a baby. Prepared formulas also provide nourishment that allows a baby to grow and thrive.

In addition to being perfectly suited to a baby's nutritional needs, there are other advantages to breastfeeding. Babies who are breastfed have fewer illnesses and a much lower hospitalization rate because breast milk contains maternal antibodies and immunological cells that stimulate the infant's immune system. When breastfed babies do get sick, they recover more quickly. They are also less likely to become obese than babies fed formulas, and they have fewer allergies.

For some mothers and babies, breastfeeding is established easily but for others it is difficult at first and may require support from a lactation consultant or breastfeeding clinic. This is normal and mothers who want to breastfeed but are having problems should not hesitate to ask for help.

When deciding whether to breast- or bottle-feed, mothers need to consider their own desires and preferences. Both feeding methods can supply the physical and emotional closeness so essential to the parent–child relationship.

The postpartum period typically lasts four to six weeks after delivery. During this time, the mother's reproductive organs revert to a nonpregnant state. Many women experience energy depletion, anxiety, mood swings, and depression during this period. This experience, known as **postpartum depression**, appears to be a normal end-product of the birth process. For most women, the symptoms gradually

Breastfeeding enhances the development of intimate bonds between mother and child.

disappear as their bodies return to normal. For others, the symptoms, coupled with the stresses of managing a new family, can lead to more severe depression that lasts for several months.

what do you THINK?

What are the advantages and disadvantages of breastfeeding? How does society view breastfeeding? Why? Do we effectively enable women to breastfeed? Why or why not?

Complications

Problems and complications can occur during labour and delivery, even following a successful pregnancy. Such possibilities should be discussed with the practitioner prior to labour so the mother understands what medical procedures may be necessary for her safety and for that of her child.

Caesarean Section (C-Section)

If labour lasts too long, if a baby is presenting incorrectly (about to exit the uterus anything but head first), or if the baby is in distress, a **Caesarean section (C-section)** may be necessary. This surgical procedure involves making an incision across the mother's abdomen and through the uterus to remove the baby. This operation is also performed in cases in which labour is extremely difficult, maternal blood pressure falls rapidly, the placenta separates from the uterus too soon, the mother has diabetes, or other problems occur.

A Caesarean section can be traumatic for the mother if she is not prepared. Risks to the mother are the same as for any major abdominal surgery, and recovery from birth takes considerably longer. Although a C-section may be necessary in certain cases, some physicians and critics feel that the option has been used too frequently in Canada. The 1986 National Conference on Aspects of Caesarean Birth recommended guidelines to deal with rising Caesarean rates. Overall rates of C-section subsequently dropped from 20 percent in 1987 to 15 percent in 1993. The guidelines dealt with three scenarios: breech presentation, prolonged labour, and previous Caesarean section. The adage was formerly "Once a Caesarean, always a Caesarean." Now, however, surgical techniques allow many women who had a C-section to deliver subsequent children vaginally. Repeat Caesareans decreased from 39 percent in the mid-1980s to 34 percent in 1993.[17]

Miscarriage

One in ten pregnancies does not end in delivery. Loss of the fetus before it is viable is called a **miscarriage** (also referred to as spontaneous abortion). An estimated 70 to 90 percent of women who miscarry eventually become pregnant again. Reasons for miscarriage vary. In some cases, the fertilized egg fails to divide correctly. In others, genetic abnormalities, maternal illness, or infections are responsible. Maternal hormonal imbalance, a weak cervix or toxic chemicals in the environment may also cause a miscarriage. In most cases, the cause is not known.

A blood incompatibility between mother and father can cause **Rh factor** problems, and sometimes miscarriage. Rh is a blood protein. Rh problems occur when the mother is Rh-negative and the fetus is Rh-positive. During a first birth, some of the baby's blood passes into the mother's bloodstream. An Rh-negative mother may manufacture antibodies to destroy the Rh-positive blood introduced into her bloodstream at the time of birth. Her first baby will be unaffected, but subsequent babies with positive Rh factor will be at risk for a severe anemia called hemolytic disease because the mother's Rh antibodies will attack the fetus's red blood cells.

Medical advances now offer prevention and treatment for this condition. The mother and fetus can be tested, and if Rh incompatibility is found, intrauterine transfusions can be given or an early delivery by C-section can be performed, depending upon the individual case. Prevention of the problem is preferable to treatment. All women with Rh-negative blood should be injected with a medication called RhoGAM within 72 hours of any birth, miscarriage, or abortion. This injection will prevent them from developing the Rh antibodies.

Another cause of miscarriage is **ectopic pregnancy**, or implantation of a fertilized egg outside the uterus. A fertilized egg may implant itself in the fallopian tube

---

Postpartum depression: The experience of energy depletion, anxiety, mood swings, and depression that women may feel during the postpartum period.

Caesarean section (C-section): A surgical procedure in which a baby is removed through an incision made in the mother's abdominal and uterine walls.

Miscarriage: Loss of the fetus before it is viable; also called spontaneous abortion.

Rh factor: A blood protein related to the production of antibodies. If an Rh-negative mother is pregnant with an Rh-positive fetus, the mother will manufacture antibodies that can kill the fetus.

Ectopic pregnancy: Implantation of a fertilized egg outside the uterus, usually in a fallopian tube.

or, occasionally, in the pelvic cavity. Because these structures are not capable of expanding and nourishing a developing fetus, the pregnancy cannot continue. Such pregnancies are surgically terminated. Most often, the affected fallopian tube is also removed.

Ectopic pregnancy is generally accompanied by pain in the lower abdomen or an aching feeling in the shoulders as the blood flows toward the diaphragm. If bleeding is significant, blood pressure drops and the woman can go into shock. If an ectopic pregnancy goes undiagnosed and untreated, the fallopian tube ruptures, and the woman is then at significant risk of hemorrhage, peritonitis (infection in the abdomen), and death.

The incidence rate of ectopic pregnancy has escalated in Canada in recent years and no one really understands why. We do know that ectopic pregnancy is a potential side effect of pelvic inflammatory disease (PID), which has become increasingly common in recent years, because the scarring or blockage of the fallopian tubes characteristic of this disease prevents the fertilized egg from passing to the uterus. About 50 percent of women who have had an ectopic pregnancy conceive again, although they are at a higher risk of another.

No matter what the cause of a miscarriage (even if the pregnancy was unwanted) it can be an emotional experience, and the woman may need support for some time afterwards.

Stillbirth

Stillbirth is one of the most traumatic events a couple can face. A stillborn baby is one that is born dead, often for no apparent reason. The grief experienced following a stillbirth is usually devastating and can last for years. In many cases, no amount of reassurance from the attending physician, relatives, or friends can assuage the grief or guilt. In Canada, 8494 (or a rate of 1.0 per 1000 live births) were stillbirths in 2005.[18] The highest rates of stillbirth occur in women ages 25 to 29 (2.0) and 30 to 34 (2.0).

Sudden Infant Death Syndrome

The sudden death of an infant under one year of age for no apparent reason is called sudden infant death syndrome (SIDS). SIDS is the leading cause of death for Canadian infants between 28 days and one year of age. On average, three infants die per week in Canada of SIDS.[19] Although this rate has decreased over the years, it remains a public health concern, particularly given that Aboriginal infants have a higher risk than non-Aboriginal infants.[20] SIDS, also referred to

as "crib death," is not a disease itself but rather is designated the cause of death after all other possibilities are ruled out. A SIDS death is sudden and silent; the death occurs quickly, often associated with sleep and with no signs of suffering.

Because SIDS is a diagnosis of exclusion, doctors do not know what causes it. However, several risk factors have been identified:[21]

- Risk is greater in males.
- Risk is greater in infants 2 to 4 months.
- Risk is greater in infants from families of lower socioeconomic status.
- Risk is greater when infants sleep on their front rather than their back; there may also be an increased risk when infants sleep on their sides.
- Risk is greater with maternal smoking during pregnancy.
- Risk is greater when the infant is exposed to secondhand smoke in the home.
- Risk is greater if the infant's head is covered during sleep.
- Risk is greater with overheating.
- Risk may be greater when the infant shares a bed with his or her parents.
- Risk appears to be reduced through breastfeeding.

Given these risk factors, the Public Health Agency of Canada[22] makes several recommendations:

1. For sleep, normal healthy infants should be placed on their backs.
2. All infants should be cared for in a smoke- and drug-free environment.
3. All infants should be dressed and covered in a manner to prevent overheating, even during illness.
4. All women should be encouraged and helped to breastfeed their babies.
5. Firm, flat bedding should be used for normal, healthy infants, with sheets and light blankets as needed, and without products to maintain the sleeping position.

The death of an infant—whether a result of a known cause or not—is traumatic for parents, family, and friends. The lack of a discernible cause, the suddenness of the tragedy, and the involvement of the legal system make a SIDS death especially difficult, leaving a great sense of loss and a need for understanding. Some communities have support groups to help parents and other family members through this grieving process. On a more positive note, infant mortality rates in Canada have been declining over the past 35 years.[23] In 1995, the infant mortality rate was 6.2 per 1000, compared to 27.3 per 1000 in 1960.

INFERTILITY

An estimated one in six Canadian couples experiences **infertility**, or difficulties in conceiving. The reasons for this phenomenon include the trend toward delaying childbirth (as a woman gets older, she is less likely to conceive), the use of IUDs, and the rise in the incidence of pelvic inflammatory disease.

Causes in Women

As noted, one cause of infertility in women is **pelvic inflammatory disease (PID)**, a serious infection that scars the fallopian tubes and blocks sperm migration. Women often develop PID as a result of a gonorrhea or chlamydia infection that progresses to the fallopian tubes and the ovaries. The risk of infertility after one bout of PID is 12 percent. After two bouts, it doubles to nearly 25 percent, and following three bouts, it increases to higher than 50 percent.[24]

Endometriosis is a major cause of infertility. In this disorder, parts of the endometrial lining of the uterus implant themselves outside the uterus—in the fallopian tubes, lungs, intestines, outer uterine walls, ovarian walls, or on the ligaments that support the uterus. The disorder can be treated surgically or with hormonal preparations. Success rates vary. Approximately 35 percent of women diagnosed with endometriosis are infertile.

Polycystic ovary syndrome, an endocrine disorder that affects about 5 percent of women, regardless of ethnicity, is a leading cause of infertility.[25] A Canadian study found that a 12-week exercise intervention, combined with nutritional counselling, was effective in improving hormonal profile in the women who participated.[26] Further research is needed to confirm this exploratory research.

Causes in Men

Among men, the single largest fertility problem is low sperm count. Although only one viable sperm is needed for fertilization, research indicates that the other sperm in the ejaculate aid in the fertilization process. There are normally 60 to 80 million sperm per millilitre of semen. When the count drops below 20 million, fertility declines. Low sperm count may be attributable to environmental factors, such as exposure of the scrotum to intense heat or cold, radiation,

or altitude, or even to wearing excessively tight underwear or outerwear. The mumps virus damages the cells that make sperm. Varicose veins above one or both testicles can also render men infertile. Male infertility problems account for approximately 40 percent of infertility cases.

Treatment

For the couple desperately wishing to conceive, the road to parenthood may be long and frustrating. Fortunately, medical treatment can identify the cause of infertility in about 90 percent of affected couples. The chances of becoming pregnant range from 30 to 70 percent, depending on the specific cause of the infertility. The countless tests and the invasion of privacy that characterize some couples' efforts to conceive can put stress on an otherwise strong, healthy relationship. Before starting fertility tests, the wise couple will reassess their priorities. Some will choose to undergo counselling to clarify their feelings about the fertility process. A good physician or fertility team will take the time to ascertain the couple's level of motivation.

Fertility tests for men include a sperm count, sperm motility, and analysis of any disease processes present. Women are thoroughly examined by an obstetrician/gynecologist for the composition of cervical mucus, the presence and extent of tubal scarring, and evidence of endometriosis. Complete fertility testing may take four to five months and can be emotionally stressful. In some cases, surgery can correct structural problems such as tubal scarring. In others, administering hormones can improve the health and number of ova and sperm. Sometimes pregnancy can be achieved by collecting the male's sperm from several ejaculations and inseminating the female at a later time. Many couples also seek "alternative" methods of improving fertility, such as acupuncture, naturopathy, and "fertility yoga."

When all surgical and hormonal attempts to restore a couple's natural fertility fail, there are still some techniques available that may allow them to have a child. **Fertility drugs** can be used to stimulate ovulation in women. Ninety percent of women who use these drugs will begin to ovulate, and half will conceive. Fertility

Stillbirth: The birth of a dead baby.

Infertility: Difficulties in conceiving.

Pelvic inflammatory disease (PID): An infection that scars the fallopian tubes and consequently blocks sperm migration, leading to infertility.

Endometriosis: A disorder in which uterine lining tissue establishes itself outside the uterus.

Fertility drugs: Hormones that stimulate ovulation in women not ovulating.

drugs are associated with a number of side effects, including headaches, irritability, restlessness, depression, fatigue, edema (fluid retention), abnormal uterine bleeding, breast tenderness, vasomotor flushes (hot flashes), and visual difficulties. Women using fertility drugs are also at increased risk of multiple ovarian cysts (fluid-filled growths) and liver damage. The drugs sometimes trigger the release of more than one egg. Thus, a woman treated with one of these drugs has a 1 in 10 chance of having multiple births. Most multiple births are twins, but triplets and even quadruplets are not uncommon.

Alternative insemination of a woman with her partner's sperm (as mentioned above) is another treatment option. If this procedure fails, the couple may choose insemination by an anonymous donor from a "sperm bank." Many men donate their sperm to such banks. The sperm are classified according to the physical characteristics of the donor (for example, blond hair, blue eyes), and then frozen for future use. Sperm can survive in this frozen state for up to five years. The woman being inseminated usually chooses sperm from a man whose physical characteristics resemble those of her partner or match her own personal preferences. Given the concern about the possibility of transmitting the AIDS virus and other diseases through alternative insemination, all donors are routinely screened for diseases before they donate.

In vitro fertilization, often referred to as "test tube" fertilization, involves collecting a viable ovum from the prospective mother and transferring it to a nutrient medium in a laboratory, where it is fertilized with sperm from the woman's partner or a donor. After a few days, the embryo is transplanted into the mother's uterus, where, it is hoped, it will develop normally.

In **gamete intrafallopian transfer (GIFT)**, the egg is "harvested" from the woman's ovary and placed in the fallopian tube with her partner's or a donor's sperm. Less expensive and time-consuming than in vitro fertilization, GIFT mimics nature by allowing the egg to be fertilized in the fallopian tube and to migrate to the uterus according to the normal timetable. The success rate for this procedure is approximately 20 percent.

In **nonsurgical embryo transfer**, a donor egg is fertilized by the man's sperm and then implanted in the woman's uterus. This procedure may also be used in cases involving the transfer of an already-fertilized ovum into the uterus of another woman.

Embryo transfer is another treatment for infertility. In this procedure, an ovum from a donor's body is artificially inseminated by the man's sperm, allowed to stay in the donor's body for a time, and then transplanted into the prospective mother's body. Some laboratories are experimenting with **embryo freezing**,

in which a fertilized embryo is suspended in a solution of liquid nitrogen. When desired, it is gradually thawed and implanted into the prospective mother. The first birth of a frozen embryo in the United States was reported in June 1986. In the future, this technique may make it possible for young couples to produce an embryo and save it for later implantation when they are ready to have a child, thus reducing the risks of fertilization of older eggs.

Surrogate Motherhood

Between 60 and 70 percent of infertile couples are able to conceive after treatment. The rest decide to live without children, adopt, or attempt surrogate motherhood. Surrogate motherhood is also a consideration for male homosexual couples. In this option, the couple arranges for a woman to be alternatively inseminated by one of the partners' sperm. The surrogate then carries the baby to term and surrenders it at birth to the couple. Although it is illegal in Canada to pay a surrogate mother for having a child, she can be compensated for the expenses involved. It has been estimated that legal and medical expenses can run as high as $30 000. Couples considering surrogate motherhood are advised to consult a lawyer regarding contracts between the involved parties.

---

what do you THINK?

What option would you most likely select if you found that you and your partner had fertility problems? Why?

Alternative insemination: Fertilization accomplished by depositing a partner's or a donor's semen into a woman's vagina.

In vitro fertilization: Fertilization of an egg in a nutrient medium and subsequent transfer back to the mother's body.

Gamete intrafallopian transfer (GIFT): The harvesting of an egg from the female partner's ovary, which is then placed with the male partner's sperm in her fallopian tube, where it is fertilized and then migrates to the uterus for implantation.

Nonsurgical embryo transfer: In vitro fertilization of a donor egg by the male partner's (or a donor's) sperm and subsequent transfer to the female partner's or another woman's uterus.

Embryo transfer: Alternative insemination of a donor with the male partner's sperm; after a time, the embryo is transferred from the donor to the female partner's body.

Embryo freezing: The freezing of an embryo for later implantation.

PEARSON
myhealthlab

Go to MyHealthLab at **www.pearsoned.ca/myhealthlab.** Here you will find self-assessments, case studies, links to health on the net, and much more.

DISCUSSION QUESTIONS

1. Create a list of the five most effective contraceptive methods. What are the pros and cons for their use? Which would you choose and why?

2. When planning a pregnancy, what sort of planning should take place? What aspects of maternal and paternal health should be considered?

3. What are some of the most important decisions that your parents made about raising you? How would you raise your child differently? The same?

4. Describe the growth of the fetus through the three trimesters. What medical checkups or tests should be done during each trimester?

5. Identify the decisions parents face when thinking about childbirth, including where to have the child and whether to use medication for pain during delivery. How does the first-time parent decide what to do?

6. If you and your spouse were having difficulty getting pregnant, what would be your options? If you were infertile, what would your options be then?

APPLICATION EXERCISE

Reread the "Consider This . . ." scenario at the beginning of the chapter and answer the following questions:

1. What concerns you most about Jamila and Karim's relationship? Is it realistic that two people can date for several months and never discuss sex? What would you have done differently from Jamila and Karim? Why?

2. If you could tell incoming first-year students three personal rules about using birth control and protection from sexually transmitted infections, what would they be?

MYSEARCHLAB EXERCISE

1. Log on to www.MySearchLab.com.

2. Retrieve the following two articles:

   a. Article AN 22306521 " A Conceptual Model of Women's Condom Use Intentions: Integrating Intrapersonal and Relationship Factors" by S. Marie Harvey, Linda J. Beckman, Mary A. Gerend, Sheryl Thorburn Bird, Sam Posner, Heather C. Huszti, and Christine Galavotti.

   b. Article AN 22306508 " Condoms + Pleasure = Safer Sex? A Missing Addend in the Safer Sex Message" by L. A. J. Scott-Sheldon, K. L. Marsh, B. T. Johnson, and D. E. Glasford.

3. Respond to the following:

   a. In what way do women and men approach condom use differently? The same? What about teenagers?

   b. How should condom use be promoted for heterosexual men? Women? Gay men? Teenagers?

   c. Consider your own sexual activities and what you currently use to prevent pregnancy and STIs. Are your efforts effective? What can/should you do differently?

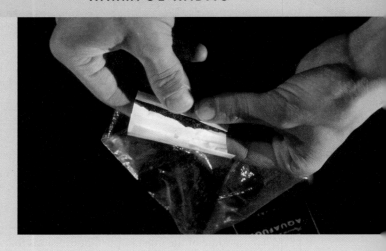

CHAPTER 9

LICIT AND ILLICIT DRUG USE

Understanding Addictions

CONSIDER THIS . . .

Tracey is a student-athlete on the varsity basketball team. Overall, she is a dedicated student-athlete who likes to live life to the fullest and is willing to experience life outside the box. As a result, she infrequently smokes a little pot when she does not have a game on the next day or two. At National Championships one year, Tracey is randomly selected for drug testing. Although Tracey did not smoke up the night before, she tests positive for marijuana.

What would happen to a student-athlete in Tracey's situation at your university/college? What would happen to a student caught smoking pot? Is the treatment/reaction to these situations the same among students, faculty, administration, and the community? Why or why not? How does infrequent marijuana use influence an athlete's ability to train and/or compete? How does infrequent marijuana use influence a student's academic ability?

CHAPTER OBJECTIVES

- Define drug use, misuse, abuse, and addiction.
- Describe the addiction process for a drug or behaviour.
- Identify drug interactions.
- Identify general precautions when taking over-the-counter drugs.
- Describe the use, misuse, and abuse of controlled substances in Canada, including frequency, financial impact, arrests for drug offences, and the impact on life.

There is no doubt that substance and behavioural dependency challenge the health of Canadians. Further, the effect of these dependencies goes beyond the individual users/participants and extends to their families, friends, and communities. In recent years, it has also become increasingly clear that chemical dependency represents only one part of Canada's health issues with addiction. Indeed, many Canadians struggle with compulsive and harmful behaviours that not only are conventional but also enhance the lives of people who can engage in them moderately. For example, some people become addicted to shopping or exercise, while others engage in these behaviours without personal, social, or financial harm.

✳ DRUG USE, MISUSE, AND ABUSE

Many people fail to take the time and effort needed to make intelligent decisions regarding their use of drugs. Although drug abuse is usually defined in connection with illicit psychoactive drugs, many people abuse and misuse prescription and over-the-counter drugs as well as legal drugs such as caffeine, tobacco, and alcohol. While **drug use** is considered taking a drug for the reason it was intended, **drug misuse** is considered the use of a drug for a purpose for which it was not intended. For example, taking an over-the-counter pain reliever when you have a headache is an example of drug use, while taking a friend's prescription painkiller for your headache is misuse (because it was not prescribed for you). Drug misuse also includes not taking prescription or over-the-counter drugs according to the directions and not completing the full dose of a prescription, among other things. **Drug abuse** is defined as the excessive use of any drug. Excessive use, however, is difficult to quantify, partly because what is excessive use for one person may not be for another.

There are risks and benefits to the use of any chemical substance. Intelligent decision making requires a clear-headed evaluation of these risks and benefits and the realization that unforeseeable reactions or problems could arise. In order to compare risks to benefits, you may want to create a profile for each drug you use or are considering using. A drug profile identifies the active ingredients in the drug, receptor sites that will be affected, main effects, side effects, and any potential adverse reactions. You should then consider your rationale for considering taking the drug.

Individual Response to Drugs: Set and Setting

Individuals differ in how they respond to drugs. Set and setting are two factors that can influence the main side effects of drugs. **Set** is the total internal environment, or mindset, of a person at the time a drug is taken. Physical, emotional, and social factors interact to influence the drug's effect on that particular person. Expectations of what the drug will or will not do are also part of the set. For example, a person who reads two pages of reported side effects for a particular drug may experience more side effects when taking that drug than someone who chose not to read this information. In other cases, set may be related to the user's mood. A person who is "pumped" for the party and plans to get drunk is likely to feel the effects of alcohol faster than when he or she is not as much in the mood to party. The elderly are particularly susceptible to their set.

Whereas *set* refers to the drug user's internal environment, **setting** refers to the drug user's total external environment. It encompasses the physical and social aspects of that environment at the time the person takes the drug. If the user is surrounded by wild colours, heavy-metal rock music, and a noisy crowd of people, the drug will generally produce a different effect than when it is taken in a quiet place with soft music, soothing colours, and relaxed company.

what do you THINK?

What expectations do university or college students have when taking drugs? In what ways are these students susceptible to set and setting? What can be done to reduce or enhance the influence of set and setting? For what reasons would you want to reduce or enhance your set and setting?

Drug use: Taking a drug in a way for which it was intended.

Drug misuse: Taking a drug not prescribed for you or for a purpose for which it was not intended or in a way for which it was not intended.

Drug abuse: The excessive use of a drug.

Set: The total internal environment, or mindset, of a person at the time a drug is taken.

Setting: The total external environment of a person at the time a drug is taken.

DEFINING ADDICTION

Addiction is defined as "a persistent, compulsive dependence on a behaviour or substance."[1] In the past, addiction was used only to describe dependence on a substance. Now the definition has been extended to include mood-altering behaviours or activities. Generally, when a person is addicted to a substance or behaviour, his or her academic performance or work suffers, relationships deteriorate, economic hardships develop, and there are negative effects on physical and mental health. A person with an addiction generally exhibits at least three of the following behaviours:

- makes excessive use of a substance or behaviour—that is, uses a greater quantity or over a longer period than intended

- expresses a persistent desire, or makes unsuccessful efforts, to cut down or control use of the substance or engagement in the activity

- spends a great deal of time getting or using the substance or engaging in the behaviour or recovering from its effects and after-effects

- is frequently too intoxicated or incapacitated by the after-effects to fulfill major obligations

- gives up regular activities to use the substance or engage in the behaviour

- continues to use the substance or participate in the activity despite problems with it

- develops a physical tolerance to the substance (therefore needs more to get the same effect)

- exhibits withdrawal when not using the substance or engaging in the behaviour

- uses the substance or engages in the behaviour to relieve or avoid withdrawal symptoms

Physiologic dependence is only one indicator of addiction. Psychological dynamics play an important role, which explains why behaviours not related to the use of chemicals—gambling, for example—can also be addictive. In fact, psychological and physiologic dependence are so intertwined that it is not possible to separate the two. For every psychological state, there is a corresponding physiological state. In other words, everything you feel is tied to a chemical process occurring in your body.[2]

Chemicals are responsible for the most profound addictions, not only because they produce dramatic mood changes, but also because they cause cellular changes to which the body adapts so well that it eventually requires the chemical in order to function normally. Thus, for a particular behaviour to be addictive, it must have the potential to produce a positive mood state—which results in a chemical change in the body.

Since behaviours such as gambling, spending/shopping, working, exercise, and sex also create changes at the cellular level along with positive mood changes, a person can become addicted to them. Although the mechanism is not well understood, all forms of addiction likely reflect a dysfunction of certain biochemical systems in the brain.[3]

✳ The Physiology of Addiction

Virtually all mental, emotional, and behavioural functions occur as a result of biochemical interactions between nerve cells in the body. Biochemical messengers, called neurotransmitters, exert their influence at specific receptor sites on nerve cells. Drug use and chronic stress can alter these receptor sites and cause the production and breakdown of neurotransmitters.

Mood-altering chemicals, for example, fill up the receptor sites for the body's natural "feel-good" neurotransmitters (endorphins) so that nerve cells are fooled into believing they have enough neurotransmitters and therefore shut down production of these substances temporarily. When the drug use is stopped, those receptor sites become emptied, resulting in uncomfortable feelings that remain until the body resumes neurotransmitter production or more of the drug is consumed. Some people's bodies always produce insufficient quantities of these neurotransmitters, so they naturally seek chemicals like alcohol as substitutes, or they pursue behaviours like vigorous physical activities/exercise or thrill-seeking activities such as sky diving or riding a rollercoaster that increase natural production. Thus we may be "wired" to seek substances or experiences that increase pleasure or reduce discomfort.

Generally when a drug is consumed regularly or a behaviour engaged in frequently, tolerance develops. **Tolerance** is a phenomenon in which progressively larger doses of a drug or more intense involvement in an experience is needed to obtain the desired effects. All of us develop some degree of tolerance to drugs and mood-altering behaviours. The difference between those who do and do not become addicted usually relates to the quantity of use and the negative effects as a result of the use.

Withdrawal is another phenomenon associated with drugs and mood-altering experiences. The drug or activity replaces or causes an effect that the body normally creates on its own. If the experience is repeated often enough or the substance ingested frequently enough, the body makes an adjustment: and as a result requires the drug or experience to obtain the effect it previously produced itself. Stopping the behaviour or no longer ingesting the drug will therefore result in withdrawal. Withdrawal symptoms of

Early Spirituality Deters Alcohol Abuse

Teens who have an active spiritual life are 50 percent less likely to become addicted to drugs or alcohol or even to try illegal drugs than those with no religious beliefs or training, a new study reports.

"Alcoholism, in addition to being a biological disorder, is a spiritual disorder," lead author Dr. Lisa Miller told Reuters Health. "Adolescents who claim to have a personal relationship with the divine are only half as likely to become alcoholics or drug addicts, or for that matter even to try contraband drugs (marijuana and cocaine). This is particularly important because onset of alcoholism and drug addiction usually occurs in adolescents."

To determine the relationship between the religiosity and substance use of 676 adolescents aged 15 to 19, Miller and colleagues conducted a study using self-report survey data. This was the first study to show that personal spirituality strongly protected against developing alcoholism or drug abuse.

SPIRITUAL, NOT RELIGIOUS

"The findings show that a personal sense of spirituality helps adolescents avoid alcohol and drug use and abuse," Miller told Reuters. "Unlike adults in [Alcoholics Anonymous], adolescents in this study were shown not to be helped by a rigid or forced adherence to religion."

In other words, "religion" forced upon adolescents by their parents or others had little effect, but if teens have made a personal choice to pursue a spiritual life, they were much less likely to drink or take drugs.

"Spirituality . . . is the most central bearing in an adolescent's life," Miller emphasized. "It cannot be ignored by parents, or the adolescent will go 'shopping' for meaning, communion and transcendence," she said.

The authors of this study concluded that adolescents at high risk might be protected from addiction or drug abuse if they engaged with a higher power or became involved in a religious community.

The survey questioned teens about their personal devotion, personal conservatism, and institutional conservatism, defined as "representing an active personal relationship with the divine, representing a personal choice to teach and adhere closely to creed, in some cases initiated through a 'born-again' experience, and as the degree of fundamentalism in a religious denomination."

The study was published in the September 2000 issue of the *Journal of the American Academy of Child and Adolescent Psychiatry.*

chemical dependencies are generally the opposite of the effects of the drug taken. For example, withdrawal from cocaine includes a characteristic "crash" (depression and lethargy), while withdrawal from barbiturates involves trembling, irritability, and convulsions. Withdrawal symptoms for addictive behaviours are usually less dramatic. They usually involve discomforts such as anxiety, depression, irritability, guilt, anger, and frustration, with an underlying preoccupation with or craving for another experience. Withdrawal syndromes range from mild to severe. The severest form of withdrawal syndrome is delirium tremens (DTs), which occurs in approximately 5 percent of individuals withdrawing from alcohol.

The Addictive Process

Addiction is a process that evolves over time. It begins when a person repeatedly seeks the illusion of relief to avoid unpleasant feelings or situations. This pattern is known as **nurturing through avoidance** and is a maladaptive way of taking care of emotional needs.[4] As a person becomes increasingly dependent on the addictive behaviours/drug, there is a corresponding deterioration in relationships with family, friends, and co-workers, in performance at work or school, and in personal life. Eventually, these individuals do not find the addictive behaviours or drug pleasurable but still consider it preferable to the unhappy realities they seek to escape.

Addiction: A persistent, compulsive dependence on a behaviour or substance.

Tolerance: Phenomenon in which a progressively larger dose of a drug or more intense involvement in a behaviour is needed to produce the desired effects.

Withdrawal: Experienced by individuals addicted to a drug or behaviour when the drug is not consumed or behaviour not engaged in. Generally the symptoms are opposite to the effects experienced when engaging in the substance or behaviour.

Nurturing through avoidance: Repeatedly seeking the illusion of relief to avoid unpleasant feelings or situations.

Signs of Addiction

Although different opinions exist as to the cause, most experts agree that there are universal signs of addiction. Addictions are characterized by four common symptoms: (1) **compulsion**, which is described by obsession, or excessive preoccupation, with the behaviours or drug and an overwhelming need to engage in it; (2) **loss of control**, or the inability to predict reliably whether any isolated occurrence of the behaviours or use of a drug will be healthy or damaging; (3) **negative consequences**, such as physical damage, legal trouble, financial problems, academic failure, relationship difficulties, and family dissolution, which do not occur with healthy involvement in any behaviours or drug use; and (4) **denial**, or the inability to perceive that the behaviours or drug use are self-destructive. These four components are present in all addictions, whether chemical or behavioural.

Traditionally, diagnosis of an addiction was limited to drug addiction and based on three criteria: (1) the presence of an abstinence syndrome, or withdrawal; (2) an associated pattern of pathologic behaviours (deterioration in work or academic performance, relationships, and social interaction); and (3) **relapse**, the tendency to return to the addictive behaviours or drug after a period of abstinence. Furthermore, until recently, health professionals were unwilling to diagnose an addiction until medical symptoms appeared in the patient. Now we know that although withdrawal, pathological behaviours, relapse, and medical symptoms are valid indicators of addiction, they do not characterize all addictive behaviours.

---

what do you THINK?

Since the path to addiction is often gradual and not defined by amount or frequency, how can you monitor your behaviours and/or drug use to avoid addiction? In other words, how much is too much and how frequent is too frequent?

ADDICTIVE BEHAVIOURS

Most people have no difficulty understanding addiction to drugs because a chemical is ingested. More difficult to understand is addiction to behaviours, particularly when the behaviour is essential to healthy living (for instance, exercise or eating) or a normal part of life (for instance, sex or shopping). Although there are a number of behaviours that we can become addicted to, two common behaviours are profiled here: gambling and shopping.

Gambling

Gambling is a form of recreation and entertainment for many Canadians. Most who gamble do so casually and moderately. For some, however, it is not just a fun and exciting recreational activity but rather a compulsive or pathological behaviour. Pathological gambling is considered a mental disorder by the American Psychiatric Association. Ten characteristics are listed, including

- preoccupation with gambling
- unsuccessful attempts to cut back or quit
- using gambling to escape problems
- lying to family members to conceal gambling

A Canadian study of the characteristics of problem gambling indicated that the profile of the Canadian gambler is somewhat different from the American gambler.[5] Specifically, lying to family members or friends and trying to recover previous gambling losses were more frequently reported than relationship breakups and job losses. It was also noted that video lottery terminals play a major role in gambling problems in Canada.[6]

People addicted to gambling or drugs describe similar cravings and highs. Research shows that individuals addicted to gambling have decreased blood flow to a key section of the brain's reward system.[7] As with people addicted to drugs, it is thought that individuals addicted to gambling compensate for this deficiency by overdoing it and then getting hooked. Most gambling addicts gamble for the excitement, not the money, placing increasingly larger bets to achieve the desired level of excitement.

Men are more likely to gamble than women, as are individuals who are divorced, of lower income, of African Canadian heritage, older, and living within 100 kilometres of a casino.[8] Gambling among college or university students is increasing in prevalence, which is perhaps not a surprise given the number of online sources teaching individuals how to gamble more effectively. Further, students may have easier access to opportunities to gamble given the advent of online gambling the growing number of casinos, scratch tickets, lotteries, and sports betting networks. Poker, in particular, has increased in popularity amongst students. Access to poker on the internet and televised poker tournaments is likely a factor in the large number of young people now spending an unhealthy amount of time and money playing poker.

Young people are two to three times more likely than adults to develop gambling problems.[9] And just as in off-campus life, male students are more likely to gamble than female students are. Other common characteristics include spending more time watching TV, using computers for non-academic purposes, spending less time studying, earning lower grades, participating in intercollegiate athletics, and engaging in heavy, episodic drinking and using illicit drugs in the past year.[10]

Whereas people who gamble casually—that is, for entertainment—can stop any time they wish and are able to see the importance of quitting, individuals addicted to gambling are not able to control their urge to gamble even when faced with devastating consequences: high debt, legal problems, and the loss of most things meaningful, including homes, families, jobs, health, and even their lives. Negative effects of gambling on health include increased risk of cardiovascular problems as well as an increase rate of suicide.

Shopping and Borrowing

Although compulsive spending has been a pervasive problem for some time in Canada, a more insidious form of addiction lurks in the new "plastic generation." Credit card companies entice people, even students, to have it all right now—whether or not you can afford it.

Credit card companies are succeeding, with millions of MasterCards and VISAs in existence. Add to that the ease offered by cable shopping stations, catalogue shopping, and shopping over the internet, and the opportunity to overspend is greater than ever before. The resulting debt is phenomenal. Although most people manage debt with careful planning, some spend money to meet emotional needs not fulfilled elsewhere. Anxiety, self-doubt, and anger lead to spending as a way of coping with daily stressors. College and university students may be particularly vulnerable to spending problems because advertisers and credit card companies target them heavily.

Compulsive gambling and shopping frequently lead to compulsive borrowing to support the addiction. Irresponsible investments and purchases lead to debts that the individual who is addicted tries to repay by borrowing more. Compulsive debtors borrow money repeatedly from family, friends, or institutions despite the problems this causes. Whereas most people incur overwhelming debt through a combination of hardship and ignorance about financial management, compulsive debtors incur debt primarily as result of buying or gambling behaviours in which they have engaged for the pleasurable feelings that result and/or to relieve painful feelings of withdrawal.

DRUG DYNAMICS

Have you ever walked into a drugstore looking for some cough syrup or a pain reliever and become overwhelmed by the options available? Although there are literally tens of thousands of drugs at our disposal, choices among them should not be made lightly. All drugs are chemical substances that have the potential to alter the structure and function of our bodies. Quite simply, all drug use involves risks. You can minimize these risks by asking appropriate questions of health providers and by being a critical consumer of all drugs.

Drugs work because they physically resemble the chemicals produced naturally within the body (see Figure 9.1). For example, many painkillers resemble the endorphins (literally "morphine within") manufactured in the body. Most bodily processes result from chemical reactions or changes in electrical charge. Because drugs possess an electrical charge and a chemical structure similar to chemicals that occur naturally in the body, they can affect physiological and psychological functions in many different ways.

A current explanation of drug actions is the receptor site theory, which states that drugs attach themselves to specific **receptor sites** in the body. These sites are specialized cells to which a drug is able to attach because of its size, shape, electrical charge, and chemical properties. Most drugs can attach at multiple receptor sites located throughout the body in such places as the heart and blood system, the lungs, liver, kidneys, brain, and gonads (testicles or ovaries). The physiology of drug activity and its effect on human behaviours is very complex.

Compulsion: Obsessive preoccupation with a behaviour or substance and an overwhelming need to engage in it.

Loss of control: Inability to predict reliably whether any isolated involvement with the addictive substance or behaviour will be healthy or damaging.

Negative consequences: Difficulties such as physical damage, legal trouble, financial ruin, academic failure, relationship difficulties, family dissolution, and others as a result of continued engagement in a substance or behaviour.

Denial: Inability to perceive or accurately interpret the effects of drug use or engaging in a behaviour.

Relapse: The tendency to return to the addictive behaviours or drug after a period of abstinence.

Receptor sites: Specialized cells to which drugs can attach themselves.

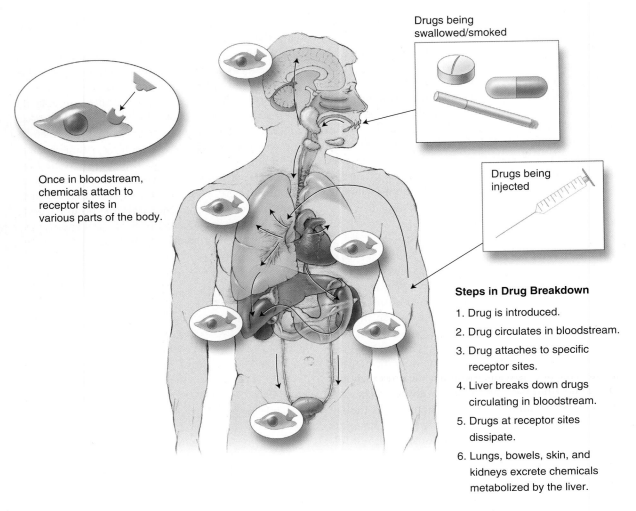

Once in bloodstream, chemicals attach to receptor sites in various parts of the body.

Drugs being swallowed/smoked

Drugs being injected

Steps in Drug Breakdown

1. Drug is introduced.
2. Drug circulates in bloodstream.
3. Drug attaches to specific receptor sites.
4. Liver breaks down drugs circulating in bloodstream.
5. Drugs at receptor sites dissipate.
6. Lungs, bowels, skin, and kidneys excrete chemicals metabolized by the liver.

FIGURE 9.1
How the Body Metabolizes Drugs

TYPES OF DRUGS

Drugs are divided into six categories: prescription drugs, recreational drugs, over-the-counter (OTC) drugs, herbal preparations, illicit drugs, and commercial drugs. Each category includes drugs that stimulate the body, depress body functions, produce hallucinations, or have the potential to alter a person's mood or behaviours (that is, **psychoactive drugs**).

- **Prescription drugs** can be obtained only with a written prescription from a licensed physician. In 2005 the total expenditure in Canada on drugs (including prescription and non-prescription drugs) was $23.3 billion and is forecasted to reach 26.9 billion in 2007.[11] Prescribed drug expenditure is forecasted to increase to $20.9 billion in 2006 and to $22.5 billion in 2007, accounting for 83.3 and 83.6 percent, respectively, of total drug expenditure in Canada.[12]

- **Recreational drugs** belong to a vague category, with boundaries dependent upon how recreation is defined. Generally, these drugs contain chemicals that people use to help them relax or socialize. These drugs are legal even though they are psychoactive. Alcohol, tobacco, and caffeine are included in this category.

- **Over-the-counter (OTC) drugs** can be purchased without a physician's prescription. Expenditures specifically on OTC products (which are not usually covered by health care) were forecasted to reach $4.4 billion in 2006 and $4.6 billion in 2007.[13]

- **Herbal preparations** form another vague category that includes approximately 750 substances such as herbal teas and other products of botanical origin believed to have medicinal properties.

- **Illicit (illegal) drugs** are the most notorious substances. Although laws governing their use, possession, cultivation, manufacture, and sale differ from country to country, illicit drugs are generally recognized as harmful. These drugs are psychoactive.

- **Commercial preparations** are the most universally used yet least commonly recognized as products with a drug action. More than 1000 of these substances exist, including seemingly benign items such as perfumes, cosmetics, household cleansers, paints, glues, inks, dyes, gardening chemicals, pesticides, and industrial by-products.

Routes of Administration of Drugs

Route of administration refers to the way in which a drug is taken into the body. Common routes include oral ingestion, injection, inhalation, inunction, and suppository.

Oral ingestion is the most common method for taking drugs and includes tablets, capsules, and liquids that we swallow. Oral ingestion generally results in relatively slow absorption because the drug must pass through the stomach, where it is acted on by digestive juices, and then move on to the small intestine before it enters the bloodstream. Alcohol is the one exception to this rule since the majority of it is absorbed into the bloodstream without digestion.

Many oral preparations are coated to keep them from being dissolved by corrosive stomach acids before they reach the intestine and to protect the stomach lining from irritation. If your stomach contains food, absorption is slower than if your stomach is empty. Some drugs should not be taken with certain foods because they inhibit the drug's action. Others must be taken with food to prevent stomach irritation.

Injection, another common method of taking a drug, involves the use of a hypodermic syringe. This method usually results in rapid absorption, depending on the type of injection. **Intravenous injection**, or injection directly into a vein, puts the drug in its most concentrated form directly into the bloodstream. Effects will be felt within three minutes, making this route extremely effective, particularly in medical emergencies. However, there is risk of serious or even fatal reactions as a result of this effective and efficient administration of a drug. When illicit drugs are injected, the risk of overdose is particularly high.[14] In addition, some serious diseases, such as hepatitis and HIV infection, can be transmitted in this way. For this reason, intravenous injection is also one of the most dangerous routes of administration. **Intramuscular injection** results in much slower absorption of the drug than intravenous injection. This type of injection places the hypodermic needle into muscular tissue, usually in the buttocks or in the triceps on the back of the upper arm. Normally used to administer antibiotics and vaccinations, this route of administration ensures a slow and consistent dispersion of the drug into the body tissues. **Subcutaneous injection** puts the drug into the layer of fat directly beneath the skin. Its common medical uses are for administration of local anesthetics and for insulin replacement therapy. A drug injected subcutaneously will circulate even more slowly than an intramuscularly injected drug because it takes longer to be absorbed into the bloodstream.

Inhalation refers to the ingestion of drugs through the nostrils. This method transfers the drug rapidly into the bloodstream through the alveoli (air sacs) in the lungs. Some examples of inhalation include nasal sprays, cocaine snorting, and the inhalation of aerosol sprays, gases, or fumes from solvents. The drug effects are usually felt immediately after inhalation and do not last long because only small amounts can be absorbed and metabolized in the lungs.

Inunction introduces drugs into the body through the skin. Common examples include the small adhesive patches used to alleviate motion sickness or nicotine patches used to assist individuals when they stop smoking. These patches slowly release their chemicals for a consistent dispersal.

Psychoactive drugs: Drugs that have the potential to alter mood or behaviours.

Prescription drugs: Drugs that can be obtained only with a written prescription from a licensed physician.

Recreational drugs: Legal drugs that people use to relax or socialize.

Over-the-counter (OTC) drugs: Drugs that can be purchased without a physician's prescription.

Herbal preparations: Substances of plant origin believed to have medicinal properties.

Illicit drugs: Drugs whose use, possession, cultivation, manufacture, and/or sale are illegal.

Commercial preparations: Commonly used chemical substances with a drug action, such as cosmetics, household cleaning products, and industrial by-products.

Route of administration: The manner in which a drug is taken into the body.

Oral ingestion: Intake of drugs through the mouth.

Injection: The introduction of drugs into the body via a hypodermic needle.

Intravenous injection: The introduction of drugs directly into a vein.

Intramuscular injection: The introduction of drugs into muscles.

Subcutaneous injection: The introduction of drugs into the layer of fat directly beneath the skin.

Inhalation: The introduction of drugs through the nostrils.

Inunction: The introduction of drugs through the skin.

Whenever you take more than one drug at a time, you should consider how they will interact. For example, women who take oral contraceptives should strictly follow the dosage instructions and be aware that medicines such as penicillin may alter the contraceptive's effectiveness. Asking a pharmacist is a good way to learn about drug interactions.

Suppositories are drugs mixed with a waxy medium that are designed to melt at body temperature. Most suppositories are inserted into the anus past the rectal sphincter muscles. As the wax melts, the drug is released and absorbed through the rectal walls into the bloodstream. Since there are many blood vessels here, the effects of the drug are usually felt within 15 minutes. Other suppositories are inserted in the vagina. These suppositories often involve antifungal agents that treat problems in the vagina itself as opposed to drugs meant to travel in the bloodstream.

✳ DRUG INTERACTIONS

Most people are aware that sharing medications, using outdated prescriptions, taking higher doses than recommended, or using drugs as a substitute for dealing with personal problems may result in serious health consequences. However, many are not aware of the risks of taking several drugs simultaneously. The most dangerous interactions are synergism, antagonism, inhibition, and intolerance. Other negative interactions may occur between drugs and nutrients when consumed together.

Synergism, also known as potentiation, is an interaction of two or more drugs in which the effects of the individual drugs are multiplied beyond what is normally expected. Synergism can be expressed mathematically as $2 + 2 = 10$. A synergistic interaction is most likely to occur when central nervous system depressants such as alcohol, opiates (morphine, heroin), antihistamines (cold remedies), sedative hypnotics (Quaaludes), minor tranquillizers (Valium, Librium, and Xanax), and barbiturates are combined.

The worst possible combination is alcohol and barbiturates (sleeping preparations such as Seconal and phenobarbital) because the combination leads to a slowdown of the brain centres that normally control vital functions. Respiration, heart rate, and blood pressure can drop to the point of inducing coma or death.

Prescription drugs carry special labels warning the user of potential drug interactions. Many OTC preparations carry similar warning labels. Because the dangers associated with synergism are so great, you should always check for possible drug interactions before using a prescribed or OTC drug. You should also consider synergistic actions when consuming recreational drugs with or without prescription and/or OTC drugs. Pharmacists, physicians, drug information centres, or community drug education centres can answer your questions. Even if one of the drugs in question is an illegal substance, you should still try to determine the dangers involved in combining it with other drugs. Health-care professionals are legally bound to maintain confidentiality even when they know that a client is using illegal substances. The Building Communication Skills box suggests questions you should ask before taking any prescription or OTC drug. These can be adapted to include recreational and illegal drugs.

what do you THINK?

What types of drugs do you typically use? How do you usually take them? Are you aware of the risks and benefits of their administration?

Asking the Right Questions

At one time or another you will use prescription or OTC drugs to restore or maintain your health. How can you be certain that you need a medication in the first place, that you are taking the right medication for you, and that your medication is not robbing you of vital nutrients or being rendered ineffective by other drugs you are taking or foods you are ingesting? Only by asking the right questions of the right people can you be sure. Listed below are questions to pose to your physician, your pharmacist, or yourself before you take any drug.

1. What is your diagnosis?

2. Is your physician or pharmacist aware of all the other drugs you take, including prescription drugs (don't forget, birth control pills are drugs), OTCs, recreational drugs, and others?

3. Do you know the name of the medication you are taking? Is it the chemical name, a generic name, or a brand name?

4. Are you certain of how often you should take the medication, for how long you should take it, and in what dosage?

5. Do you know when your medication should be taken in relation to food intake?

6. Do you know if you can drink alcohol while on your medication?

7. What are the known side effects of the medication? What should you do if you experience any of the side effects?

8. Can you stop taking your medication when you start feeling better, or do you continue to take the drug until the prescription is finished?

9. Do you know what you should do if you forget to take your medication at the scheduled time?

10. Do you know what signs and symptoms signal that you are allergic to the medication?

11. Do you know how and where to store your medication?

12. Are there any drug–nutrient interactions that you should be aware of?

13. Are there any potential drug interactions that you should be aware of?

14. Are there any adverse consequences of long-term use of the medication?

Antagonism, although not usually as serious as synergism, can produce unwanted and unpleasant effects. In an antagonistic reaction, one drug blocks the action of the other at the receptor site. The "blocking" drug occupies the receptor site, preventing the second drug from attaching, and this alters its absorption and action.

Inhibition is a type of interaction in which the effects of one drug are eliminated or reduced by the presence of another drug, again with the interaction occurring at the receptor site. A common inhibitory reaction occurs between antacid tablets and Aspirin. Antacids inhibit the absorption of Aspirin, resulting in a less effective pain reliever. Other inhibitory reactions occur between alcohol and contraceptive pills and between antibiotics and contraceptive pills. Specifically, alcohol and antibiotics diminish the effectiveness of birth control pills in some women.

Intolerance occurs when drugs combine in the body, resulting in extremely uncomfortable reactions. The drug Antabuse, used to help individuals addicted to alcohol to give it up, works using this type of interaction. It binds liver enzymes (the chemicals the liver produces to break down alcohol), making it impossible for the body to metabolize alcohol. As a result, the user of Antabuse who drinks alcohol experiences nausea, vomiting, and, occasionally, fever.

Cross-tolerance occurs when a person develops a physiological tolerance to one drug and, as a result, a similar tolerance to other drugs with similar effects. For example, cross-tolerance can develop between alcohol and barbiturates, two depressant drugs.

PRESCRIPTION DRUGS

Even though prescription drugs are administered under medical supervision, the critical consumer should still take precautions. Complications and

Suppositories: Mixtures of drugs and a waxy medium designed to melt at body temperature; usually inserted into the anus or vagina.

Synergism: An interaction of two or more drugs in which the effects of the individual drugs are magnified beyond what is expected of their individual contribution.

Antagonism: A type of interaction in which one drug blocks the action of another at the receptor site.

Inhibition: A type of interaction in which the effects of one drug are eliminated or reduced by the presence of another drug at the receptor site.

Intolerance: A type of interaction in which two or more drugs taken together produce extremely uncomfortable reactions.

Cross-tolerance: The development of a tolerance to one drug that carries over to another similar drug.

serious negative health consequences arising from the use of prescription drugs are common. Responsible decision making about prescription drug use requires the consumer to acquire basic drug knowledge.

Types of Prescription Drugs

Antibiotics are drugs used to fight bacterial infection. Bacterial infections continue to be among the most common serious diseases in the world, with the vast majority cured by antibiotics. There are almost 100 different antibiotics available and dispensed by intramuscular injection or in tablet or capsule form. Some, called broad-spectrum antibiotics, are designed to control diseases caused by a number of bacterial species. These medications may also kill off helpful bacteria in the body, thus triggering secondary infections. For example, some vaginal infections are related to long-term use of antibiotics. Further, it is believed that the misuse of antibiotics has led to an increase in drug-resistant bacteria.

Sedatives are central nervous system depressants that induce sleep and relieve anxiety. Used heavily in the 1950s and 1960s in the form of phenobarbital or Seconal, they gradually fell out of favour because of the risks involved, including a high potential for addiction. Detoxification can be life-threatening and must be medically supervised.

what do you THINK?

What is the difference between drug use, misuse, and abuse? Give examples of each. Are drug abuse and addiction the same thing? Why or why not? Is it possible to use illicit drugs without becoming addicted to them?

Tranquillizers are another form of central nervous system depressant. They are classified either as major or minor tranquillizers. The most powerful tranquillizers are used in the treatment of major psychiatric illnesses. When used appropriately, these strong sedatives are capable of reducing violent aggressiveness and self-destructive impulses. About 5 percent of Canadians aged 15 and older report using sleeping pills, and 5 percent report using tranquillizers.[15] Women and older Canadians are more likely to report using these medications.[16]

Antidepressants are powerful substances used to treat clinically diagnosed cases of depression. These drugs inhibit the release of certain neurotransmitters in the brain, thereby moderating the user's mood.

Amphetamines are stimulants prescribed less commonly now than in the past. Like other psychoactive drugs, they can be purchased legally and illegally. Amphetamines suppress appetite and elevate respiration, blood pressure, and pulse rate. Tolerance to these powerful stimulants develops rapidly, and the user trying to cut down or quit may experience unpleasant **rebound effects**. These severe withdrawal symptoms, peculiar to stimulants, include depression, irritability, violent behaviours, headaches, nausea, and deep fatigue.

Use of Generic Drugs

Generic drugs are sold under a chemical name rather than a brand name. These alternatives to more expensive brand-name drugs contain the same active ingredients. There is, however, some controversy about the effectiveness of some generic drugs. Differences in minor ingredients can affect the way the drug is absorbed, which may cause discomfort or an allergic reaction in some users. If you experience any allergic reactions to a prescribed generic drug, tell your pharmacist or doctor, who can recommend an alternative drug. A list of medicines that can be interchanged has been approved in Canada. If your doctor or pharmacist fails to offer you the option of using a generic drug, you should ask if such a substitute exists and if it would be safe for you to use it.

OVER-THE-COUNTER (OTC) DRUGS

Over-the-counter (OTC) drugs are non-prescription drugs used in self-diagnosis and self-medication. Canadians spend many millions yearly on OTC preparations for relief of everything from runny noses to ingrown toenails. Most OTC drugs are manufactured from a basic group of 1000 chemicals. Combinations of as few as 2 and as many as 10 of these chemicals result in the many different OTC drugs available today. Perhaps because of the common belief that OTC products are safe and effective, indiscriminate use, misuse, and abuse often occurs. OTC drugs, like any other drugs, have the potential to produce dependency, tolerance, and addiction, as well as adverse toxic reactions.

Types of OTC Drugs

Analgesics are pain relievers. The earliest pain relievers were made of derivatives manufactured from the opium poppy. Today, pain relievers ranging from Aspirin to morphine are among the most commonly

OxyContin

OxyContin is the trade name for the long-lasting form of the prescription opioid (pain reliever) oxycodone. Oxycodone is also an ingredient in Percocet and Percodan. OxyContin contains much higher doses, at 10 to 80 mg. OxyContin is specially formulated for slow release and as such is intended to provide relief from moderate to severe pain for up to 12 hours. Individuals prescribed OxyContin swallow one tablet twice daily. Although most users take this medication appropriately, they should be monitored closely because of their high risk of dependency.

How is OxyContin abused? OxyContin is formulated to be swallowed whole to provide the slow release into the blood stream; however, when it is chewed or crushed, the slow release properties are destroyed. Thus, when users chew or crush tablets the oxycodone effects occur very rapidly causing a high or euphoria which is described as similar to the high from heroin.

Oxycodone is a potent opioid. When large amounts of oxycodone are released into the body all at once (whether chewed, snorted, or injected), there is a high risk of overdose and death similar to a heroin overdose. Symptoms of overdose include laboured or slow breathing, extreme somnolence progressing to coma, cardiac arrest, and death.

OxyContin users who inject the drug have the additional risks associated with sharing needles (that is, hepatitis, HIV).

Addiction is also a problem, with the user requiring larger and larger doses to achieve the desired effect because tolerance quickly develops. Eventually the drug is needed to simply prevent feeling sick. Withdrawal symptoms include muscle aches, nausea, diarrhea, loss of appetite, restlessness, insomnia, runny nose, teary eyes, and sweating.

Source: Centre for Addiction and Mental Health, "What Is OxyContin," 2004. Retrieved March 2, 2006, from www.camh.net/About_Addiction_Mental_Health/ Drug_and_Addiction_Information/oxycontin.

used drugs. In fact, most Canadians when surveyed said they had taken pain relievers in the past month.[17] Although pain relievers come in several forms, the most common are Aspirin, acetaminophen (Tylenol, Pamprin, Pandol), ibuprofen (Advil, Motrin, Nuprin), and ibuprofen-like drugs such as naproxen sodium (Aleve, Anaprox) and ketoprofen (Orudis).

Most pain relievers work at the receptor sites by interrupting pain signals. Some are categorized as non-steroidal anti-inflammatory drugs (NSAIDS), also called **prostaglandin inhibitors**. Prostaglandins are chemicals that resemble hormones and are released by the body in response to pain. Scientists believe that the additional pain caused by the release of prostaglandins signals the body to begin the healing process. Prostaglandin inhibitors restrain the release of prostaglandins, thereby reducing the pain. Common NSAIDS include ibuprofen, naproxen sodium, and Aspirin.

Acetylsalicylic acid (ASA), commonly known as Aspirin, relieves pain by inhibiting the body's production of prostaglandins. It brings down fever by increasing the flow of blood to the skin's surface, which causes sweating and therefore cooling of the body. ASA is also commonly used to reduce the inflammation and swelling of arthritis. Furthermore, ASA's anticoagulant (interference with blood clotting) effects make it a useful daily medication for reducing the risk of heart attacks.

Acetaminophen is the active ingredient found in Tylenol and related medications. Like ASA, acetaminophen is an effective analgesic and antipyretic (fever-reducing) drug. It does not, however, provide relief from inflamed or swollen joints. The side effects associated with acetaminophen are generally minimal, though overdose can cause liver damage.

Most analgesics have side effects, the most common of which is drowsiness due to the depression of the central nervous system. Label warnings are important to read. Some warnings caution specifically against

Antibiotics: Prescription drugs designed to fight bacterial infection.

Sedatives: Central nervous system depressants that induce sleep and relieve anxiety.

Tranquillizers: Drugs taken to relax the body and relieve anxiety.

Antidepressants: Drugs used to treat clinically diagnosed depression.

Amphetamines: Drugs that suppress appetite and increase breathing rate, blood pressure, and heart rate.

Rebound effects: Severe withdrawal effects, including depression, nausea, and violent behaviours.

Generic drugs: Drugs marketed by their chemical name rather than a brand name.

Analgesics: Pain relievers.

Prostaglandin inhibitors: Drugs that inhibit the production and release of prostaglandins (released by the body in response to pain).

driving or operating heavy machinery when using analgesics, and most state they should not be taken with alcohol. Specific to ASA, possible side effects include allergic reactions, ringing in the ears, stomach bleeding, and ulcers. Since research has linked ASA to the potentially fatal condition Reye's syndrome, children, teenagers, and young adults (up to age 25) who are at risk for developing this syndrome are recommended to use an alternative analgesic.

Cold, Cough, Allergy, and Asthma Relievers

These substances are popular OTC drugs intended to provide relief of the symptoms of coughs, colds, allergy, and asthma that affect millions of sufferers. The operative word in their titles is *reliever*. Most of these drugs are designed to alleviate or reduce some or all of the discomforting symptoms associated with upper-respiratory-tract maladies. Unfortunately, no drug exists to actually cure these conditions. The drugs available provide temporary relief until the sufferer's immune system prevails. Aspirin or acetaminophen are often included in cold preparations. The basic types of OTC cold, cough, and allergy relievers are

- Expectorants. These drugs are formulated to loosen phlegm, allowing the user to cough and clear congested respiratory passages.

- Antitussives. These drugs are designed to calm or curtail the cough reflex. They are most effective when the cough is "dry," and does not produce phlegm (for which an expectorant is required).

- Antihistamines. These drugs are central nervous system depressants that dry runny noses, clear postnasal drip, clear sinus congestion, and reduce tears.

- Decongestants. These drugs are designed to reduce nasal stuffiness due to colds.

- Anticholinergics. These drugs are often added to cold preparations to reduce nasal secretions and tears.

It is important to read the labels of cough, cold, allergy, and asthma relievers for a number of reasons. First, some cold compounds contain alcohol in concentrations that may exceed 40 percent, while others contain a lot of sugar. Equally important to consider are the various drug ingredients included and the potential interactions as a result. In fact, many cough and cold medications contain expectorants and antitussives, which means conflicting actions could be caused in the body (that is, phlegm loosened to be coughed and cleared combined with a curtailed or reduced cough reflex).

Stimulants

Non-prescription stimulants are sometimes used by students in college or university in the last minute panic to complete assignments or in "all-nighter" study sessions. The active ingredient in most OTC stimulants is caffeine. Although caffeine heightens wakefulness, increases alertness, and relieves fatigue, it also can result in increased nervousness, irritability, anxiety, and involuntary muscle twitches (see Chapter 10).

Sleeping Aids and Relaxants

These drugs are often used to induce the drowsy feelings that precede sleep. The principal ingredient is an antihistamine called pyrilamine maleate. Chronic reliance on sleeping aids may lead to addiction.

Dieting Aids

Some people use **laxatives** or **diuretics** ("water pills") to achieve weight loss. Since laxatives were designed to relieve constipation, their use to reduce body weight is considered drug misuse. There are health risks for both laxatives and diuretics. Frequent use of laxatives disrupts the body's natural elimination process and may result in constipation or even obstipation (inability to have a bowel movement). In addition to being inefficient in producing weight loss, laxatives deplete the body of needed fluids, salts, and minerals. Further, the user gains the lost weight back upon drinking fluids, and may have created dangerous chemical imbalances with the elimination of potassium and sodium, which have important roles in maintaining electrolyte balance. Depletion of these vital minerals may cause weakness, dizziness, fatigue, and sometimes death.

ILLICIT DRUGS

Illicit drug use is a problem in our society, and though we may not be users ourselves, we are bound to be influenced by them in one way or another. It is important to understand how these drugs work and why people use them. In this section, we focus our attention on illicit drugs—drugs that are illegal to possess, produce, or sell.

On June 19, 1996, the Senate passed Bill C-8, the Controlled Drugs and Substances Act. The Act came into force on May 14, 1997. It replaced Canada's main laws on illicit drugs—the Narcotic Control Act and parts of the Food and Drugs Act. The Controlled Drugs and Substances Act significantly expanded the reach of Canada's drug laws and continued Canada's heavy reliance on a failed policy of criminal prohibition.[18]

Illicit drug users come from all walks of life. Most illicit drug use occurs in places other than dilapidated crack houses, and few users fit the stereotype of the crazed junkie. The reasons we have for using drugs vary from one situation to another and from one person to another. Age, sex, genetic background, culture, education, physiology, personality, life experiences, and expectations are factors that play a role in a person's choice to use illicit drugs.

Health Canada and the Canadian Executive Council on Addictions sponsored the Canadian Addiction Survey 2004 (CAS), which included a random sample of almost 14 000 Canadians aged 15 or older interviewed by telephone.[19] In this survey, 39.2 percent of Canadian women reported use of marijuana (cannabis) in their lifetime, with 10.2 percent indicating use in the past year. Lifetime use of marijuana was 50.1 percent for men and past-year use 18.2 percent. Typical age of initiation was 17 years for both men and women. Illicit drug use varies with age, province, marital status, education and income.[20] Women report a 12.2 percent lifetime use of illicit drugs, while men report a 21.1 percent lifetime use. In 2002, between 1455 and 1695 deaths in Canada were attributed to illicit drugs. Acute care hospital days were estimated to be 318 000 to 352 000.[21]

It is estimated that 185 million people worldwide—or 4.3 percent of the population aged 15 and older—used illicit drugs in the late 1990s.[22] Globally, 0.4 percent of deaths and 0.8 percent of "disability adjusted life years" (that is, the time a person lives with a physical or mental disability) were attributed to illicit drug use.[23] Further, the World Health Organization suggested that "illicit drugs account for the highest proportion of disease burden among low mortality, industrialized countries in the Americas, Eastern Mediterranean, and European regions [and that the] economic reliance on the drug trade, and drug dependence leaves many individuals open to exploitation by criminals and criminal organizations; threatening the health of men, women and children, the rule of law, and ultimately, the vitality and strength of all our communities."[24]

Why do Canadians choose to use illicit drugs? There is no clear answer. Economic despair, issues related to the family or community, a general sense of hopelessness, or a need to relieve boredom may be powerful engines leading to use. These factors, combined with increased availability and diversity of drugs, attitudes and beliefs that illicit drug use is common, and potentially liberal parental attitudes may explain the use of illicit drugs for some.

Social policy also affects drug use, although its effects are extremely hard to evaluate. However, illicit drug use declined significantly during the first five years of Canada's Drug Strategy, when the focus was on the general public. It started rising again during Phase II, when the focus shifted to street youth and high-risk groups. The resurgence of drug use we currently witness is led largely by mainstream youth. Ultimately, we must aim our prevention messages at all youth. According to the Canadian Centre on Substance Abuse, all young people—dropouts and A+ students alike—are vulnerable to drug use and should be viewed as an at-risk population.[25]

Anti-drug programs have been developed to deal with the problems of illegal drug use. The major drawback of most of these programs is their failure to take a multi-dimensional approach. The tendency has been to focus on only one aspect of drug use rather than the many interrelated factors that contribute to the problem. For example, many programs consider the drugs themselves the culprits. Others oversimplify the drug use by exhorting potential users to "just say no," ignoring the fact that drugs are an integral part of many people's social or cultural lives. The pressures to take drugs are often tremendous, and the reasons for using them complex.

People who develop drug problems usually think they can control their use when they start. Initially, their drug use is viewed as a fun and controllable pastime. Peer influence is a strong motivator for drug use, especially among adolescents. Typically, teens and young adults believe that drug use in others is much greater than what it really is. Some people use drugs to cope with feelings of worthlessness and despair, others to battle depression and anxiety. Some view drugs as the quick answer to life's difficulties. Since the majority of illegal drugs produce physiological and psychological dependence, the idea that a person can use these substances regularly without becoming addicted is foolish. To find out if you are controlled by drugs or by a drug user, complete the questionnaires in the Rate Yourself box.

---

what do you THINK?

Do you think you can control your use of drugs? How do you know? Are the current laws in Canada effective at controlling illicit drug use? Why or why not?

Laxatives: Drugs used to soften stool and relieve constipation.

Diuretics: Drugs that increase the excretion of urine from the body.

Recognizing a Drug Problem

PEARSON
myhealthlab

ARE YOU CONTROLLED BY DRUGS?

How do you know if you are dependent on the drugs you use? Persons dependent on drugs cannot stop using them; their use hurts themselves and those around them.

Take the following assessment. The more times you respond "yes," the more likely you are controlled by the drugs you use.

	Yes	No
1. Do you use drugs to handle stress or escape from life's problems?	❑	❑
2. Have you unsuccessfully tried to cut down or quit using your drug?	❑	❑
3. Have you ever been in trouble with the law or arrested because of your drug use?	❑	❑
4. Do you think a party or social gathering is not fun unless drugs are available?	❑	❑
5. Do you avoid people or places that do not support your drug use?	❑	❑
6. Do you neglect your responsibilities because you would rather use your drug?	❑	❑
7. Have your friends, family, professors, or employer expressed concern about your drug use?	❑	❑
8. Do you do things under the influence of drugs that you would not normally do?	❑	❑
9. Have you seriously thought that you might have a drug problem?	❑	❑

ARE YOU CONTROLLED BY A DRUG USER?

Is your life controlled by a drug user? Your love and care (codependency) may actually enable the drug user to continue his or her use, hurting you, him- or herself, and others.

Take this assessment; the more "yes" checks you make, the more likely that you are being controlled by a drug user.

	Yes	No
1. Do you often have to lie or cover up for the drug user?	❑	❑
2. Do you spend time counselling the person about problems related to his or her drug use?	❑	❑
3. Have you taken on additional financial or family responsibilities to cover this person's drug use?	❑	❑
4. Do you feel that you have to control the drug user's behaviour?	❑	❑
5. At the office or in classes, have you done work/completed assignments or attended meetings for the user?	❑	❑
6. Do you often put your own needs and desires after the user's?	❑	❑
7. Do you spend time each day worrying about your situation?	❑	❑
8. Do you analyze your behaviour to find clues to how it might affect the drug user?	❑	❑
9. Do you feel powerless and at your wits' end about the user's drug use?	❑	❑

Source: Reprinted by permission of Krames Communications, 1100 Grundy Lane, San Bruno, CA 94066–3030.

CONTROLLED SUBSTANCES

Cocaine

Cocaine is a crystalline white alkaloid powder derived from the leaves of the South American coca shrub (not related to cocoa plants).[26] These leaves have been chewed for thousands of years by people in Peru and Bolivia to lessen hunger and fatigue. Pure cocaine was isolated in 1860 by a German pharmacology graduate student. In the 1880s, Freud praised the powerful stimulant effects of cocaine as the treatment for a variety of illnesses, including depression, as well as for alcohol and opioid addiction. Cocaine use then increased and it was widely and legally available in Canada in medicine and soft drinks. With increased use, the risks of cocaine became clear, and in 1911 Canada passed laws restricting its importation, manufacture, sale, and possession.

Cocaine is generally sold on the street as a hydrochloride salt—a fine, white crystalline powder known as "blow," "C," "coke," "crack," "flake," "freebase," "rock," or "snow," among other names.[27] Street dealers often dilute it with inert (non-psychoactive) but similar-looking substances such as cornstarch, talcum powder, and sugar, or with active drugs such as procaine and benzocaine (used as local anesthetics), or other central nervous system stimulants such as amphetamines.

According to the most recent Canadian Addiction Survey, lifetime cocaine use ranged from 9.4 to 11.8 percent for women ages 15 to 44 years. For men, lifetime cocaine use was greatest in men between the ages of 35 and 44 years at 21.4 percent.[28]

Cocaine affects mood, judgment, and motor skill coordination. Cocaine has its most dramatic effects on vision, as it may cause a higher sensitivity to light, the perception of halos around bright objects, and difficulty focusing. Users have also reported blurred vision, glare problems, and hallucinations, particularly "snow lights"—weak flashes or movements of light in the peripheral field of vision, which tend to make drivers swerve toward or away from the lights. Some users have also reported auditory hallucinations (for example, ringing bells) and olfactory hallucinations (for example, the smell of smoke or gasoline).

Cocaine also heightens feelings such as irritability, excitability, and startle response. Users reported that sudden sounds, such as horns or sirens, caused them severe anxiety coupled with rapid steering or braking reactions, even when the source of the sound was not in the immediate vicinity of their vehicles. Suspiciousness, distrust, and paranoia—other reactions to cocaine—have prompted users to flee in their cars or drive evasively. Further, users report attention lapses while driving, reckless driving, and ignoring relevant stimuli such as changes in traffic signals.[29]

Although cocaine use has declined from its peak in the 1980s, it continues to be a commonly used and abused illicit drug today.

Methods of Cocaine Use

Cocaine can be taken in several ways. The powdered form of the drug is "snorted" through the nose. Smoking (freebasing) and intravenous injections are more dangerous means of using cocaine. When cocaine is snorted, it can cause damage to the mucous membranes in the nose and sinusitis. Further, snorting cocaine can damage the user's sense of smell, and occasionally it creates a hole in the septum. Smoking, or "freebasing," cocaine can result in lung and liver damage. Freebasing is more popular than injecting cocaine because of the risk of contracting diseases such as AIDS and hepatitis by sharing needles. A major risk of freebasing relates to the volatile mixes it requires and the risk of explosion; some users have been killed or seriously burned.

Many cocaine users still occasionally "shoot up." Injecting allows the user to introduce large amounts of cocaine rapidly into the body. Within seconds, there is an incredible sense of euphoria. This intense high lasts only 15 to 20 minutes, and then the user heads into a "crash." To prevent the unpleasant effects of the crash, users often shoot up frequently, which can severely damage their veins. Besides AIDS and hepatitis, users who inject themselves are at risk for skin infections, inflammation of the arteries, and infection of the lining of the heart.

Physical Effects of Cocaine

The effects of cocaine are felt rapidly. Snorted cocaine enters the bloodstream through the lungs in less than one minute and reaches the brain in less than three minutes. When cocaine binds at its receptor sites in the central nervous system, it produces intense pleasure. The euphoria quickly abates and the desire to regain the pleasurable feelings makes the user want more.

Cocaine is an anesthetic and a central nervous system stimulant. In tiny doses, it can slow heart rate. In larger doses, the physical effects are dramatic: increased heart rate and blood pressure, loss of appetite that can lead to dramatic weight loss, convulsions, muscle twitching, irregular heartbeat, even death due to overdose. Other effects of cocaine include temporary relief of depression, decreased fatigue, talkativeness, increased alertness, and heightened self-confidence. Again, however, as the dose increases, users become irritable and apprehensive and their behaviours may turn paranoid or violent.

Cocaine: A powerful stimulant drug with strong psychological effects.

Cocaine-Affected Babies

Because cocaine easily crosses the placenta (as virtually all drugs do), the fetus is vulnerable when a pregnant women uses the drug. The most threatening problem during pregnancy is the increased risk of a miscarriage. Should the pregnant user reach full term, her baby is usually born with brain damage, heart defects, kidney problems, and malformed heads, arms, and fingers. These babies tend to show signs of withdrawal at birth, including irritability, jitteriness, and the inability to eat or sleep properly. They seem to be unable to respond or to relate to people the way normal babies do, and are difficult to console and comfort. Because it is so difficult for adults to interact with them, their social and emotional development is negatively affected. Cocaine is also transmitted from a mother who uses to her breast-fed baby. The baby is then exposed to all the physical and mental effects of cocaine use.[30]

Freebase Cocaine

Freebase is a form of cocaine more powerful and costly than the powder or chip (crack) form. Street cocaine (cocaine hydrochloride) is converted to pure base by removing the hydrochloride salt and many of the "cutting agents." The end product, freebase, is smoked through a water pipe. Because freebase cocaine reaches the brain within seconds, it is more dangerous than cocaine that is snorted. It produces a quick, intense high that disappears quickly, leaving an intense craving for more. Freebasers typically increase the amount and frequency of the dose. They often become severely addicted and experience serious health problems and financial ruin.[31] Side effects of freebasing include weight loss, increased heart rate and blood pressure, depression, paranoia, and hallucinations. Freebase is an extremely dangerous drug and is responsible for a large number of cocaine-related hospital emergency-room visits and deaths.

Crack

Crack is the street name given to freebase cocaine processed from cocaine hydrochloride using ammonia or sodium bicarbonate (baking soda) and water, then heating the substance to remove the hydrochloride. Crack can also be processed with ether, but this is much riskier because ether is a flammable solvent. The mixture (90-percent-pure cocaine) is then dried. The soapy-looking substance that results can be broken up into "rocks" and smoked. These rocks are approximately five times as strong as cocaine. Crack gets its name from the popping noises it makes when burned. A crack user may quickly become addicted to the drug.

Addiction is accelerated by the speed at which crack is absorbed through the lungs (it hits the brain within seconds after use) and by the intensity of the high.

> ## what do you THINK?
>
> What makes cocaine use attractive? In what circumstances would you consider using cocaine? What are the risks and benefits of its use?

Amphetamines

Amphetamines include a large and varied group of synthetic agents that stimulate the central nervous system. Small doses of amphetamines act like adrenaline (a hormone that naturally stimulates the body) and improve alertness, lessen fatigue, and generally elevate mood.[32] With repeated use, physiological and psychological dependence develops. Sleep patterns are affected (insomnia); heart rate, breathing rate, and blood pressure increase; restlessness, anxiety, appetite suppression, and vision problems are common. High doses over long time periods can produce hallucinations, delusions, and disorganized behaviours. Abusers become paranoid, fearing everything and everyone. Some become very aggressive or antisocial.

Amphetamines are sold under a variety of names. "Bennies" (amphetamine/Benzedrine), "dex" (dextroamphetamine/Dexedrine), and "meth" or "speed" (methamphetamine/Methedrine) are some of the most common. Other street terms for amphetamines are "cross tops," "crank," "uppers," "wake-ups," "lid poppers," "cartwheels," and "blackies." Amphetamines do have therapeutic uses in the treatment of attention deficit hyperactivity disorder in children (Ritalin®, Cylert) and of obesity (Pondimin).

Methamphetamine

An increasingly common form of amphetamine, **methamphetamine** (meth) is a potent, long-acting, addictive drug that strongly activates the brain's reward centre by producing a sense of euphoria.[33] "Crystal meth" can cause brain damage, resulting in impaired motor skills and cognitive functions, psychosis, and increased risk for heart attack and stroke. Methamphetamine can be snorted, smoked, injected, or orally ingested. Depending on the method of use, the drug will affect the user in different ways. Users often experience tolerance immediately, making meth a highly addictive drug from the very first time it is used. When snorted, the effects can be felt in three to five minutes; if orally ingested, the user will experience effects within 15 to 20 minutes. The pleasurable effects of meth are typically an intense rush lasting only a few minutes when snorted or a high lasting over eight hours when smoked.

Physical Effects of Methamphetamine

Smaller doses of methamphetamine produce increased physical activity, alertness, and a decreased appetite. However, the drug's effects quickly wear off, and the user seeks more. Long-term use of meth can cause severe dependence, psychosis, paranoia, aggression, weight loss, and stroke. Abusers often do not sleep or eat for days, as they continually inject up to 1 gram of the drug every two to three hours. A high state of irritability and agitation has been associated with violent behaviours among some users. Use of meth is an increasingly serious problem. A possible contributing factor to the increasing rate of meth use is that it is relatively easy to make. Meth is produced by "cookers," using recipes that often include common OTC ingredients such as ephedrine and pseudoephedrine, found in cold and allergy medication, as well as lethal ingredients such as drain cleaner, battery acid, and others.

Ice is a potent form of methamphetamine created in Canada and imported primarily from Asia, particularly South Korea and Taiwan. When smoked, ice is odourless, and its effects can last for more than 12 hours. Like other methamphetamines, the "down" side of this drug is devastating. Prolonged use can cause fatal lung and kidney damage, as well as long-lasting psychological damage. In some instances, major psychological dysfunction can persist as long as two and a half years after last use.

✔ Marijuana

Although archaeological evidence documents the use of **marijuana** (also known as "grass," "weed," "pot," "dope," and "ganja," among other names[34]) as far back as 6000 years, the drug did not become popular in North America until the 1960s. Marijuana remains by far the most extensively used illicit drug, with 44.5 percent of Canadians over the age of 15 years reporting use in their lifetime and 14.1 percent indicating use in the past 12 months.[35]

Physical Effects of Marijuana

Marijuana is derived from either the *cannabis sativa* or *cannabis indica* (hemp) plants. Today's top-grade cannabis produces reactions similar to hashish. **Tetrahydrocannabinol (THC)** is the psychoactive substance in marijuana and the key to determining how powerful a high the marijuana will produce. Two decades ago, marijuana ranged in potency from 1 to 5 percent THC, while today's crop averages 8 to 15 percent.

Hashish, a potent cannabis preparation derived mainly from the thick, sticky resin of the plant, contains high concentrations of THC. Hash oil, a substance produced by percolating a solvent such as ether through dried marijuana to extract the THC, is a tarry liquid that may contain up to 70 percent THC.

Marijuana can be brewed and drunk in tea or baked into quick breads or brownies. THC concentrations in such products are impossible to estimate. Most of the time, however, marijuana is rolled into cigarettes (joints) or packed firmly into a pipe. Some people smoke marijuana through water pipes called "bongs." Effects are generally felt within 10 to 30 minutes and wear off within three hours.

The most noticeable effect of THC is the dilation of the eyes' blood vessels, which produces the characteristic bloodshot eyes. Smokers of the drug also exhibit coughing, dry mouth and throat ("cotton mouth"), increased thirst and appetite, lowered blood pressure, and mild muscular weakness, primarily exhibited in drooping eyelids. Users who take a high dose in an unfamiliar or uncomfortable setting are more likely to experience anxiety and the paranoid belief that their companions are ridiculing or threatening them.

Effects of Chronic Marijuana Use

Potential long-term effects of heavy or regular marijuana use include (1) an increased risk of cancer because of the tar and other known cancer-causing agents in cannabis, (2) irritation to the respiratory system (in fact, smoking three to four joints per day has an effect similar to that of smoking 20 cigarettes), (3) reduced motivation for work and study, (4) schizophrenia, and (5) impaired attention, memory, and

Freebase: The most powerful distillate of cocaine.

Crack: A distillate of powdered cocaine that comes in small, hard "chips" or "rocks."

Amphetamines: A large and varied group of synthetic agents that stimulate the central nervous system.

Methamphetamine (meth): A powerfully addictive drug that strongly activates certain areas of the brain and affects the central nervous system.

Ice: A potent, inexpensive stimulant with long-lasting effects.

Marijuana: A psychoactive stimulant that intensifies reactions to environmental stimuli.

Tetrahydrocannabinol (THC): The chemical name for the active ingredient in marijuana.

Hashish: The sticky resin of the cannabis plant, high in THC.

ability to process complex information.[36] Other risks associated with marijuana include suppression of the immune system and blood pressure changes. Research suggests that pregnant women who smoke marijuana are at a higher risk for stillbirth or miscarriage and for delivering low-birthweight babies and babies with abnormalities of the nervous system. Babies born to women who use marijuana during pregnancy are five times more likely to have features similar to those exhibited by children with fetal alcohol spectrum disorders.

Debates concerning the effects of marijuana on the reproductive system have yet to be resolved. Studies conducted in the mid-1970s suggested that marijuana inhibited testosterone (and thus sperm) production in males and caused chromosomal breakage in ova and sperm. Subsequent research in these areas was inconclusive. The question of whether the high-level THC plants currently available will increase the risks associated with this drug is, as yet, unanswered.

Marijuana and Medicine

Although recognized as a dangerous drug by the Canadian government, marijuana also has several medical purposes. It helps to control side effects such as the severe nausea and vomiting produced by chemotherapy, the chemical treatment for cancer. It also improves appetite and forestalls the loss of lean muscle mass associated with AIDS-wasting syndrome. Marijuana reduces the muscle pain and spasticity caused by diseases such as multiple sclerosis. It also temporarily relieves the eye pressure of glaucoma (a progressive disease characterized by increased fluid pressure in the eyeball).

Marijuana and Driving

Marijuana use presents clear hazards for drivers of motor vehicles as well as for others on the road. The drug substantially reduces a driver's ability to react and to make quick decisions. Studies reveal that 60 to 80 percent of marijuana users sometimes drive while high.[37] One Canadian study of cannabis users and driving reported common physical effects of heightened nervousness, greater alertness, and poorer concentration, resulting in reduced driving ability.[38] Studies of automobile accident victims show that 6 to 12 percent of nonfatally injured drivers and 4 to 16 percent of fatally injured drivers had THC in their bloodstreams. Perceptual and other performance deficits resulting from marijuana use may persist for some time after the high subsides. Users who attempt to drive, fly, or operate heavy machinery often fail to recognize their impairment.

Opiates

Opiates are among the oldest analgesics known. These drugs cause drowsiness, relieve pain, and induce euphoria. Also called **narcotics**, they are derived from the parent drug **opium**, a dark, resinous substance made from the milky juice of the opium poppy. Other opiates include morphine, codeine, heroin, and black tar heroin.

The word *narcotic* comes from the Greek word for "stupor" and is generally used to describe sleep-inducing substances. For many years, opiates were widely used by the medical community to relieve pain, induce sleep, curb nausea and vomiting, stop diarrhea, and sedate psychiatric patients. During the late 19th and early 20th centuries, many patent medicines contained opiates. Suppliers advertised these concoctions as cures for everything from menstrual cramps to teething pains.

Among the opiates widely used by medical practitioners was **morphine**. First manufactured in the early nineteenth century, morphine was named after Morpheus, the Greek god of sleep, and is more powerful than opium. **Codeine**, a less powerful analgesic, is derived from morphine.

All opiates are highly addictive. Growing concern about addiction led to government controls of narcotic use. Subsequent legislation required physicians prescribing opiates to keep careful records. Physicians are still subject to audits of their prescriptions of these agents. Some opiates are still used today for medical purposes. Morphine is sometimes prescribed by doctors in hospital settings for relief of severe pain. Codeine is found in prescription cough syrups and in other painkillers. Several prescription drugs, including Percodan, Demerol, and Dilaudid, contain synthetic opiates. All opiate use is strictly regulated.

Physical Effects of Opiates

Opiates are powerful central nervous system depressants. In addition to relieving pain, these drugs lower heart rate, respiration, and blood pressure. Side effects include weakness, dizziness, nausea, vomiting, euphoria, decreased sex drive, visual disturbances, and lack of coordination. Of all the opiates, heroin is the most notorious. Because all opiate addiction follows a similar progression, we will use heroin as a model for narcotic abuse in the following paragraphs.

Heroin Addiction

Heroin and black tar heroin are powerful opiates. Heroin is a white powder derived from morphine. Black tar heroin is a sticky, dark brown, foul-smelling substance, also made from morphine. Heroin is a depressant. It produces a dreamy, mentally slow feeling and drowsiness in the user. It also can cause drastic mood swings of euphoric highs followed by depressive lows. Heroin also slows respiration and urinary output and constricts the pupils of the eyes (hence the image of the stereotypical drug user hiding his eyes behind a pair of dark sunglasses). Symptoms of tolerance and withdrawal can appear within three weeks of first use.

The most common route of administration for heroin addicts is "mainlining"—intravenous injection of powdered heroin mixed in a solution—though fear of HIV and hepatitis infection has resulted in some users avoiding needles. Many users describe the "rush" they feel when injecting themselves as intensely pleasurable, whereas others report unpredictable and unpleasant effects. The temporary nature of the rush contributes to the drug's high potential for addiction—many addicts shoot up four or five times a day. Mainlining causes veins to scar, and if this practice is frequent enough the veins collapse. Once a vein has collapsed, it can no longer be used to inject heroin into the bloodstream. Addicts become expert at locating new veins to use: in the feet, the legs, and the temples. When they do not want their needle tracks (scars) to show, they inject themselves under the tongue, in the groin, or other places that are less visible to others.

Treatment for Heroin Addiction

Most programs designed to help individuals addicted to heroin have not been successful. The rate of recidivism (tendency to return to previous behaviours) is high. Some individuals resume their drug use even after years of drug-free living because the craving for the injection rush is still so strong. It takes a great deal of discipline to seek alternative, non-drug highs. Individuals addicted to heroin experience a distinct pattern of withdrawal. They begin to crave another dose four to six hours after their last dose. Symptoms of withdrawal include an intense desire for the drug, yawning, a runny nose, sweating, and crying. About 12 hours after the last dose, addicts experience sleep disturbance, dilated pupils, loss of appetite, irritability, goosebumps, and muscle tremors. The most difficult time in the withdrawal process occurs 24 to 72 hours after last use. All the preceding symptoms continue along with nausea, abdominal cramps, restlessness, insomnia, vomiting, diarrhea, extreme anxiety, hot and cold flashes, elevated blood pressure, and rapid heartbeat and respiration. Once the peak of withdrawal has passed, these symptoms begin to subside. Still, the recovering addict has many hurdles to jump.

Methadone maintenance is one type of treatment available for people addicted to heroin or other opiates. Methadone is a synthetic narcotic that blocks the effects of opiate withdrawal. It is chemically similar enough to opiates to control the tremors, chills, vomiting, diarrhea, and severe abdominal pains of withdrawal. The methadone dose is decreased over a period of time until the individual is weaned off the drug.

Methadone maintenance is controversial because of its potential for addiction. Critics contend that the program merely substitutes one drug for another, with the addiction remaining. Proponents argue that people on methadone maintenance are less likely than those still using heroin to engage in criminal activities to support their addictions. For this reason, many methadone maintenance programs are government financed and available to clients free of charge or at reduced costs.

Psychedelics

Psychedelics are a group of drugs whose primary pharmacological effect is to alter feelings, perceptions, and thoughts in the user. The major receptor sites for most of these drugs are in the part of the brain responsible for interpreting outside stimuli before allowing these signals to travel to other parts of the brain. This area is called the **reticular formation** and is located in the brain stem at the upper end of the spinal cord. When a psychedelic drug is present at a reticular formation receptor site, messages become scrambled and the user may see wavy walls instead of straight ones or smell colours or hear tastes. This mixing of sensory messages is known as synesthesia.

In addition to synesthetic effects, users may recall events long buried in the subconscious mind or become less inhibited than when in a non-drug state. Some psychedelic drugs are erroneously labelled "hallucinogens." Hallucinogens are substances capable of

Narcotics: Drugs that induce sleep and relieve pain; primarily the opiates.

Opium: The parent drug of the opiates; made from the milky juice of the opium poppy.

Morphine: A derivative of opium; sometimes used by medical practitioners to relieve pain.

Codeine: A drug derived from morphine; used in cough syrups and some painkillers.

Heroin: A derivative of morphine, usually injected into the bloodstream.

Methadone maintenance: A treatment for people addicted to opiates in which methadone, a synthetic narcotic, is used to block the withdrawal symptoms.

Psychedelics: Drugs that distort the processing of sensory information in the brain.

Reticular formation: An area in the brain stem responsible for relaying messages to other areas in the brain.

Battling Addictions

Recognizing that a problem exists is one of the most difficult steps in the process of battling addictions, due to individual levels of denial. "Intervention" is a planned process of confrontation by significant others to break down the denial compassionately so that the individual can see the destructive nature of his or her addiction. The individual must learn that the addiction is destructive and requires treatment. Once this has been accomplished, treatment and recovery can begin.

Treatment and recovery for any addiction begin with abstinence—refraining from the addictive behaviours. But abstinence does little to change the personality and psychological dynamics or the biological and environmental influences behind the addictive behaviours. Recovery involves learning new ways of looking at oneself, others, and the world. It may require exploration of a traumatic past so that psychological wounds can be healed. It requires new ways of taking care of oneself, physically and emotionally. It involves developing communication skills and new ways of having fun. Recovery programs are the fuel that gives addicts the energy to resist relapsing. For a large number of addicts, recovery begins with a period of formal treatment. A good treatment program should have the following characteristics:

- professional staff familiar with the specific addictive disorder for which help is being sought
- a flexible schedule of inpatient and outpatient services
- access to medical personnel who can assess the addict's medical status and provide treatment for all medical concerns as needed
- medical supervision of addicts at high risk for a complicated detoxification
- a team approach to treatment of the addictive disorders (for example, medical personnel, counsellors, psychotherapists, social workers, clergy, educators, dietitians, fitness counsellors, and family members)
- group and individual therapy options
- integration of peer-led support groups and encouragement to continue involvement after treatment ends
- structured after-care and relapse-prevention programs
- a clean and attractive environment
- a cordial and helping staff

Highly structured treatment programs help their clients get started on a lifetime program of personal recovery. They include wellness programs to teach critical self-care skills, educational programs to formulate a deep understanding of the addiction, self-help groups to provide a foundation of support after treatment, and several forms of therapy, including those listed below.

- **Individual therapy.** Addicts can identify and experience feelings they have been chronically medicating with their addictive behaviours. During sessions, addicts begin to deal with issues related to their addiction.
- **Group therapy.** The group provides an opportunity for developing communication skills and offers an environment where addicts learn how to be honest with themselves and others. The standard care in a treatment program is to combine group therapy with individual therapy.
- **Family therapy.** Family therapy helps all members of the family to recover from their potentially codependent roles.
- **12-step programs.** One of the most common types of peer support groups is a 12-step program, patterned after Alcoholics Anonymous. These programs are designed to keep individuals free of their addictions through honest acknowledgment of their shortcomings and through the mutual support of others who had similar experiences. There are 12-step programs for every addiction, including Narcotics Anonymous and Sex and Love Addicts Anonymous, as well as for families and others who have a relationship with the person who is addicted to the drug.
- **Alternatives to 12-step programs.** Because 12-step programs adhere to a spiritual basis in the recovery process, some individuals for whom a spiritual approach is uncongenial have sought or started alternative groups.

creating auditory or visual **hallucinations**, or images that are perceived but not real. Not all psychedelic drugs are capable of producing hallucinations. The most widely recognized psychedelics are LSD, mescaline, psilocybin, and psilocin.

LSD

Of all the psychedelics, **lysergic acid diethylamide (LSD)** has the most notoriety. This chemical was first synthesized in the late 1930s by the Swiss chemist Albert Hoffman. It resulted from experiments aimed at deriving medically useful drugs from the ergot fungus found on rye and other cereal grains. Psychiatrists initially felt it could be beneficial to patients unable to remember and recognize suppressed traumas, and the drug was used for such purposes from 1950 through 1968. Known on the street as "acid," LSD continues to be widely available.

An odourless, tasteless, white crystalline powder, LSD is most frequently dissolved in water to make a solution that can then be used to manufacture the street forms of the drug: tablets, blotter acid, and "windowpane." What the LSD consumer usually buys is blotter acid—small squares of blotter-like paper that have been impregnated with the liquid. The blotter is swallowed or chewed briefly. LSD also comes in tiny thin squares of gelatin called "windowpane" and in tablets called "microdots," which are less than 3 millimetres across (it would take 10 or more of these to add up to the size of an ASA tablet).

LSD is one of the most powerful drugs known, producing strong effects in doses as low as 20 micrograms (equivalent in size to the average-sized postage stamp). The potency of the typical dose of LSD currently ranges from 20 to 80 micrograms, compared to the 150 to 300 micrograms commonly used in the 1960s.

Despite its reputation for being primarily a psychedelic, LSD produces a large number of physical effects, including slightly increased heart rate, elevated blood pressure and temperature, goose flesh (roughened skin), increased reflex speeds, muscle tremors and twitches, perspiration, increased salivation, chills, headaches, and mild nausea. Since the drug also stimulates uterine muscle contractions, it can lead to premature labour and miscarriage in pregnant women. Research into the effects of long-term LSD use remains inconclusive. As with any illegally purchased drug, users are also exposed to the risks associated with the purchase an impure product.

The psychological effects of LSD vary from person to person. The set and setting in which the drug is used are strong influential factors. Euphoria is the common psychological state produced by the drug, but dysphoria (a sense of evil and foreboding) may also be experienced. The drug also shortens attention span, causing the mind to wander. Thoughts may be interposed and juxtaposed as well. The user may thus be able to experience several different thoughts simultaneously. Synesthesia occurs occasionally. Users become introspective, and suppressed memories may surface, often taking on bizarre symbolism. Many more effects are possible, including decreased aggressiveness and enhanced sensory experiences.

While there is no evidence of physiological dependence with LSD use, psychological dependence is likely. Many LSD users become depressed for one or two days following a trip and use the drug to relieve this depression. The result is a cycle of LSD use to relieve post-LSD depression, which often leads to psychological addiction.

what do you THINK?

Why do many drugs, including LSD and cocaine, have histories in the medical field? Why are these drugs no longer used for medicinal purposes? Are there any circumstances for which their use may be acceptable? Why or why not?

Mescaline

Mescaline is one of hundreds of chemicals derived from the **peyote** cactus. This small, button-like cactus grows in the southwestern United States and parts of Latin America. Natives of these regions have long used the dried peyote buttons during religious ceremonies. In fact, members of the Native American Church (a religion practised by thousands of North American First Nations peoples) have been granted special permission to use the drug during ceremonies in some US states.

Users normally swallow 10 to 12 dried peyote buttons. These buttons taste bitter and generally induce immediate nausea or vomiting. Long-time users claim that the nausea becomes less noticeable. Those who are able to keep the drug down begin to feel the effects within 30 to 90 minutes, when mescaline reaches maximum concentration in the brain. The effects may persist for up to 9 or 10 hours. Mescaline is a powerful hallucinogen. It is also a central nervous system stimulant.

Products sold on the street as mescaline are likely synthetic chemical relatives of the true drug. Street names of these products include DOM, STP, TMA, and MMDA. These drugs can be toxic in small quantities.

Psilocybin

Psilocybin and psilocin are the active chemicals in a group of mushrooms sometimes called "magic mushrooms." Psilocybe mushrooms, which grow throughout the world, can be cultivated from spores or can be harvested wild. Because many mushrooms resemble the psilocybe variety, people who use wild mushrooms for any purpose should be certain of what they are

Hallucination: An image (auditory or visual) that is perceived but not real.

Lysergic acid diethylamide (LSD): Psychedelic drug causing sensory disruptions; also called "acid."

Mescaline: A hallucinogenic drug derived from the peyote cactus.

Peyote: A cactus with small "buttons" that, when ingested, produce hallucinogenic effects.

Psilocybin: The active chemical found in psilocybe mushrooms; it produces hallucinations.

doing. Mushroom varieties can easily be misidentified, and mistakes can be fatal. Psilocybin is similar to LSD in its physical effects, which wear off in four to six hours. The exact chemical content is difficult to determine and varies in each mushroom; therefore the effects can vary tremendously.

Deliriants

Delirium is an agitated mental state characterized by confusion and disorientation. Almost all psychoactive drugs will produce delirium at high doses, with **deliriants** producing this effect at relatively low (subtoxic) levels.

PCP

Phencyclidine (PCP) is one of the best-known deliriants. It is a synthetic substance that became a black-market drug in the early 1970s. PCP was originally developed as a "disassociative anesthetic," which means that patients given this drug could keep their eyes open, apparently remain conscious, and feel no pain during a medical procedure. Patients would afterward experience amnesia for the time the drug was in their system. Such a drug had obvious advantages as an anesthetic during surgery, but its unpredictability and drastic effects (post-operative delirium, confusion, and agitation) resulted in a discontinuation of its use, and it was withdrawn from the legal market.

On the illegal market, PCP is a white, crystalline powder that users often sprinkle onto marijuana cigarettes. It is dangerous and unpredictable regardless of how it is administered. Common street names for PCP are "angel dust" for the crystalline powdered form and "peace pill" and "horse tranquillizer" for the tablet form.

The effects of PCP depend on the dosage. As little as five milligrams produces effects similar to strong central nervous system depressants. These effects include slurred speech, impaired coordination, reduced sensitivity to pain, and reduced heart and respiratory rates. Doses between 5 and 10 milligrams cause fever, salivation, nausea, vomiting, and total loss of sensitivity to pain. Doses greater than 10 milligrams result in a dramatic drop in blood pressure, coma, muscular rigidity, violent outbursts, and possible convulsions and death.

Psychologically, PCP may produce either euphoria or dysphoria. It is also known to produce hallucinations as well as delusions and overall delirium. Some users experience a prolonged state of "nothingness." The long-term effects of PCP use are unknown.

Designer Drugs

Designer drugs are structural analogues (drugs that produce similar effects) of more familiar illicit drugs.

These illegal drugs are manufactured by underground chemists to mimic the psychoactive effects of controlled drugs. At present, at least three types of synthetic drugs are available on the illegal drug market: analogues of phencyclidine (PCP), fentanyl and meperidine (both synthetic narcotic analgesics), and amphetamine and methamphetamine, which have hallucinogenic and stimulant properties.[39]

Although PCP analogues have been identified in street samples of drugs, they are less frequently used today than other forms of designer drugs. Analogues of fentanyl are much more common; the pharmacological properties are similar to those of heroin or morphine. These analogues, known as "synthetic heroin" or "new heroin," may be addictive and carry the risk of overdose.

Amphetamine and methamphetamine analogues are the most common forms of designer drugs on campuses today. These analogues often cause hallucinations and euphoria. Ecstasy is one example; it is actually a chemical called methylene dioxymethylamphetamine, or MDMA, and is similar to the hallucinogen MMDA. In small to moderate doses, ecstasy can produce feelings of energy, confidence, pleasure, well-being, increased sociability, and closeness to others. Larger doses do not enhance these desired effects. In fact, large doses of ecstasy are associated with grinding of teeth, jaw pain, sweating, increased blood pressure and heart rate, anxiety, panic attacks, blurred vision, nausea, vomiting, and convulsions.[40]

Inhalants

Inhalants are chemicals that produce vapours that, when inhaled, cause hallucinations as well as intoxicating and euphoric effects. Inhalants are not commonly recognized as drugs. They are legal to purchase and universally available and potentially dangerous when used incorrectly. These drugs and the high that results from their use appeal to those who cannot afford illicit substances.

Included in this category are organic solvents resulting from the distillation of petroleum products (rubber cement, model glue, paint thinner, lighter fluid, varnish, wax, spot removers, and gasoline). Most of these substances are sniffed by users. Because they are inhaled, the volatile chemicals in these products reach the bloodstream within seconds. An inhaled substance is not diluted or buffered by stomach acids or other body fluids and thus is more potent and dangerous than the same substance would be if swallowed. This characteristic, along with the fact that dosages are extremely difficult to control because everyone has unique lung and breathing capacities, makes inhalants particularly dangerous. An overdose of fumes can result in unconsciousness. If the user's oxygen intake is reduced during the inhaling process, death can result within five minutes.

Amyl Nitrite

Sometimes called "poppers" or "rush," **amyl nitrite** is often prescribed to alleviate chest pain in heart patients. It is packaged in small, cloth-covered glass capsules that can be crushed to release the active chemical. The drug relieves chest pains because it causes rapid dilation of the small blood vessels and reduces blood pressure. That same dilation of blood vessels in the genital area is thought to enhance sensations or perceptions of orgasm. It also produces fainting, dizziness, warmth, and skin flushing.

Nitrous Oxide

Laughing gas" is the popular term for **nitrous oxide**. It is sometimes used as an adjunct to dental anesthesia or minor surgical anesthesia. It is also used as a propellant chemical in aerosol products such as whipped toppings. Users experience a state of euphoria, floating sensations, and illusions. Effects also include pain relief and a "silly" feeling, demonstrated by laughing and giggling (hence the term "laughing gas"). Regulating dosages of this drug can be difficult. Sustained inhalation can lead to unconsciousness, coma, and death.

Steroids

Public awareness of **anabolic steroids** is heightened by media stories about their use in amateur and professional athletes, particularly since the Olympics in Seoul when Ben Johnson lost the gold medal he had won for Canada in the 100 metre race when he tested positive for their use. Anabolic steroids are artificial forms of the male hormone testosterone that promote muscle growth and strength. Although these **ergogenic drugs**—that is, substances used to enhance athletic performance—are used primarily by young men to increase their strength, power, bulk (weight), and speed and thus improve their athletic performance, others not involved in athletics use steroids for the intimidation factor of increased muscle size or simply to improve their physique.

Most steroids are obtained through black-market sources. Steroids are available in two forms: injectable solution and pills.[41] Anabolic steroids produce a state of euphoria, diminished fatigue, and increased bulk and power in both sexes. These qualities give steroids an addictive quality. When users stop, they appear to undergo psychological withdrawal, mainly caused by the disappearance of the physique they have become

Steroid acne.

accustomed to. Steroids cause several adverse effects in men and women. These drugs cause mood swings (aggression and violence, sometimes known as "roid rage") acne, liver tumours, elevated cholesterol levels, hypertension, kidney disease, and immune system disturbances. There is also a danger of HIV transmission through shared needles. In women, large doses of anabolic steroids trigger masculine changes, including lowered voice, increased facial and body hair, male pattern baldness, enlarged clitoris, decreased breast

Delirium: An agitated mental state characterized by confusion and disorientation produced by psychoactive drugs.

Deliriant: Any substance that produces delirium at relatively low doses, including PCP and some herbal substances.

Phencyclidine (PCP): A deliriant commonly called "angel dust."

Designer drug: A synthetic analogue (creates effects similar to the drug it mimics) of an existing illicit drug.

Inhalants: Products sniffed or inhaled in order to produce highs.

Amyl nitrite: A drug that dilates blood vessels; used normally to relieve chest pain.

Nitrous oxide: The chemical name for "laughing gas," a substance used for surgical or dental anesthesia.

Anabolic steroids: Artificial forms of the hormone testosterone that promote muscle growth and strength.

Ergogenic drug: Substance that enhances athletic performance.

New Legislation Protects Children Exposed to Drug Manufacturing and Trafficking: First in Canada to Address Emerging Social Issue

by Jody Korchinski, Alberta Children's Services

Edmonton—Children exposed to serious drug activity, such as manufacturing and trafficking, will benefit from additional protection under a new law introduced in the Alberta Legislature by Children's Services Minister Heather Forsyth. Bill 2, the Drug-Endangered Children Act (DECA), was passed on November 1, 2006, and is the first legislation of its kind in Canada.

"Drug manufacturing and trafficking have enormous implications on the well-being and safety of our children," said Forsyth. "We need to keep ahead of this emerging social issue."

The legislation deals with specific drug activity such as manufacturing, particularly crystal methamphetamine labs and indoor marijuana grow operations, and trafficking. It identifies who is a drug-endangered child and makes it clear that a child exposed to a parent or guardian's drug activity is a victim of abuse and requires intervention.

This legislation is an excellent tool to help caseworkers and police rescue children endangered by an adult's involvement in serious drug activity. It raises awareness of the plight of drug-endangered children and lets Albertans know the province is committed to taking action. The government expects this will result in an increase in the number of people who report this type of abuse.

"Exposing a child to this type of drug activity is abuse, and it won't be tolerated in Alberta," said Forsyth. "We have a responsibility to take action to protect these children, and that is what this legislation aims to do."

Source: Alberta Children's Services news release, February 23, 2006. Retrieved August 25, 2009, from www.alberta.ca/acn/200602/1947798C6A2FC-B956-53FB-AB44F17ADEDDB1CF.html.

---

size, and changes in or absence of menstruation. When taken by healthy males, anabolic steroids shut down the body's production of testosterone, causing men's breasts to grow and testicles to shrink.

A new and alarming trend is the use of other drugs to achieve the "performance-enhancing" effects of steroids. These steroid alternatives are sought in order to avoid the penalties (such as being banned from sports) for illicit use of anabolic steroids. The two most common steroid alternatives are gamma hydroxybutyrate (GHB) and Clenbuterol. GHB is a deadly, illegal drug that is a primary ingredient in many of these "performance-enhancing" formulas. GHB does not produce a high. It does, however, cause headaches, nausea, vomiting, diarrhea, seizures and other central nervous system disorders, and possibly death. Another steroid alternative, Nandrolone, has turned up in drug tests, and yet another, Clenbuterol, has become an extremely popular item on the black market. Canada conducts around 2000 doping control tests per year on premier athletes. Most (70 percent) are random. Excluding body building, power lifting, and junior football (which have a 25-percent positive test result), there is about a 3-percent violation rate. For Olympic sports, the rate is 1 percent.[42]

what do you THINK?

How do reports in the media about the use of steroids by athletes affect the popularity or use of these drugs? Would you consider using steroids to improve your appearance? Your athletic performance?

SOLUTIONS TO THE PROBLEM

In 2000, a 9-percent increase in cannabis offences in Canada contributed to the 9-percent increase in the overall rate of drug offences, continuing the upward trend that began in 1994. Cannabis offences accounted for three-quarters of all drug-related incidents. More than two-thirds of these were for possession. Increases were also seen in the rate of cocaine offences (+6 percent) and other drug offences (+12 percent). Heroin offences dropped by 8 percent.[43]

In general, researchers in the field of drug education agree that a multimodal approach to drug education is best. Students should be taught about the use, misuse,

Managing Drug Use Behaviour

After reading this chapter, you should know that addictions produce devastating effects not only on the user but also on the user's family and friends. Addictions usually, but not always, progress gradually, and it is difficult to know when a person crosses the line from habit to addiction. Keep in mind that drug use is problematic when it results in negative personal, social, financial, work- or study-related consequences. If a person continues to use a drug despite negative consequences, chances are that he or she is addicted to it.

MAKING DECISIONS FOR YOU

When you have a medical problem (even a minor one such as a headache), you need to decide how best to treat it. What are the symptoms that you need to relieve? What questions should you ask your pharmacist or physician? What drugs (legal or illegal) are you currently using that could cause interactions? What are the pros and cons of each alternative? Which alternative is the best solution for you?

CHECKLIST FOR CHANGE: MAKING PERSONAL CHOICES

* Do you know the key questions to ask to create a drug profile for the drugs you currently use and for those you are considering using?
* Do you read the warning labels on the prescribed and OTC drugs that you take?
* Do you take prescribed and OTC drugs only for the problem for which it is being prescribed?
* Do you ask your doctor or pharmacist if you should avoid alcohol—or any foods, beverages such as coffee or caffeinated soft drinks, or other drugs—while taking an OTC or prescribed medication?
* If taking oral contraceptives, do you ask about prescribed drugs and their influence on the effectiveness of your oral contraceptive?
* Do you purchase generic drugs instead of brand-name products?
* Do you know what resources exist in the community (and/or at your university or college) to help people answer questions about drugs?
* What illicit drugs are you familiar with? How did you become familiar with them? What drugs are most popular among your peers? What is it about these drugs that make them popular?
* How do you and your peers feel about illicit drug use? Is it condoned or condemned? What influences these thoughts? What has led to these feelings?

* Have you thought of alternatives for your drug consumption?
* Are you prepared for the challenge of refusing to use illicit drugs when offered and for the consequences of that decision?
* Do you practise assertiveness? Do you practise voicing your opinion regardless of the subject?

CHECKLIST FOR CHANGE: MAKING COMMUNITY CHOICES

* Do you know what comprises the current drug problems on your campus and in your community?
* Would you be willing to assist a friend in combatting his or her substance abuse problem? Would you accompany him or her to support groups?
* Would you be willing to be a role model in community programs such as Big Brothers or Big Sisters?
* Do you volunteer your time for campus or community organizations that provide opportunities for high-risk youth?
* Would you be willing to volunteer to help at an addiction hotline or community centre?

CRITICAL THINKING

You have a major term paper due in three days, and you have just completed the reading for it. You are worried about how you will get it done, and realize you may have to pull an all-nighter. If you don't get at least a B, you will lose your academic scholarship and be forced to leave school. A friend tells you that last semester she took a few lines of cocaine; it not only helped her stay awake, but also stimulated her thinking. She got an A– on the paper and experienced no side effects. She suggests you try it, too.

Using the DECIDE model described in Chapter 1, decide how you will keep yourself awake to finish your paper. What is the best approach for you to handle this situation?

and abuse of licit and illicit drugs. Factual information free from scare tactics must be presented; moralizing about drug use does not work. Critical to these teachings is expanding students' decision-making and critical thinking skills. Further, the realities of drug use must be presented. As mentioned previously, many young people assume that drug use among their peers is higher than it really is. Programs that teach people to control drugs, as opposed to allowing drugs to control them, are needed, as are interventions that teach about the influence of set and setting. Reinforcing self-esteem is mandatory. It is not enough to urge people to "just say no"; alternatives to drug use should also be included.

All drug abuse prevention approaches probably help a bit, but neither alone nor in combination do they offer a total solution to the problem. Drug use has been a part of human behaviours for thousands of years, and it is not likely to disappear in the near future. For this reason, we need to educate ourselves and develop the self-discipline necessary to avoid dangerous drug use including kinds of drug use that lead to dependencies.

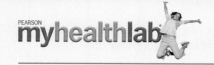

Go to MyHealthLab at **www.pearsoned.ca/myhealthlab.** Here you will find self-assessments, case studies, links to health on the net, and much more.

DISCUSSION QUESTIONS

1. How does an addiction develop? Is it possible to gauge your drug use (quantity and frequency) to prevent becoming addicted?
2. How does the set and setting influence a person's response to drugs?
3. What environmental factors influence the main effects and side-effects of psychoactive drugs?
4. How do analgesics work?
5. What general precautions should OTC drug users consider?
6. Create three drug misuse and abuse prevention programs aimed at primary, junior, or secondary school children. Think about what messages would have reached you at those particular age levels.
7. Design a pamphlet that clearly describes drug use, misuse, and abuse for students in your community.
8. Discuss the physiological and psychological effects of an illicit drug. How does this compare to a licit drug like alcohol?
9. List non-drug alternative behaviours to drug use. Are these realistic? What could make them more enticing?

APPLICATION EXERCISE

Reread the "Consider This . . ." scenario at the beginning of the chapter and answer the following questions.

1. Do you think that university and college athletes should be tested for all illicit drugs? Why or why not? What about recreational drugs like tobacco, caffeine, and alcohol?
2. In what way(s) are university and college athletes held to a higher standard than other students regarding their attitudes and behaviours? Is this fair? Why or why not?
3. How would you feel about random drug testing of students?

MYSEARCHLAB EXERCISE

1. Log on to www.MySearchLab.com.

2. Choose the Psychology, Sociology, or Education database and "drugs" as your keyword. How many articles do you find?

3. Add "illegal" or "illicit" to your search. Now how many articles do you find?

4. Skim the articles. What themes do you find in the titles?

5. Choose one article that interests you.

   a. Read it.
   b. Create a one-page summary or five-slide presentation to share with your class.
   c. Share the summary or presentation with your class. Respond to questions from your classmates.

CHAPTER 10

ALCOHOL, TOBACCO, AND CAFFEINE

Unacknowledged Drugs with Risk for Addictions

WARNING
CIGARETTES ARE
HIGHLY ADDICTI
Studies have shown that tobacco car
harder to quit than heroin or cocai

Health Canada

CONSIDER THIS . . .

Teresa is a waitress at a local restaurant. In the entry-way there is a large warning sign about the dangers of drinking alcohol while pregnant. While taking a drink order from a woman, Teresa notices that the woman is in maternity clothes and in the advanced stages of pregnancy. Teresa takes the order and tells the restaurant manager that she feels uneasy serving alcohol to a pregnant woman. The manager says, "Mind your own business," and tells her to take the woman the drink. Teresa delivers the drink. During the course of the evening, she takes several more drinks to the same woman.

Should Teresa refuse to serve the pregnant woman? Why or why not? What are Teresa's moral or ethical obligations? If the baby is born with alcohol-related problems, should the mother be sued for endangering her child?

CHAPTER OBJECTIVES

- Describe the alcohol-use patterns of post-secondary students as well as the physiological and behavioural effects of alcohol consumption.

- Explain the symptoms, causes, and treatments of alcoholism, its cost to society, and its effects on the family.

- Identify the social issues involved in tobacco use, including those surrounding smokeless tobacco.

- Explain the physiological short- and long-term effects of smoking.

- Compare the benefits and risks of caffeine consumption.

When you hear references to the dangers of drugs, what comes to mind? Usually the term *drugs* conjures images of people using cocaine, heroin, marijuana, LSD, PCP, and other illegal substances. Although people use the word *drugs* to refer to one set of dangerous substances, they often refuse to categorize alcohol as a drug, primarily because its consumption is socially accepted and alcohol sales are booming. Similarly, tobacco and caffeine are seldom considered drugs, also likely because of their legality and acceptable use. In the fiscal year ending March 31, 2007, Canada's beer and liquor sales were $18.0 billion, an increase of 4.9 percent from the years before and an amount equivalent to almost 218.7 million litres of alcoholic beverages.[1]

Although beer continues to be the alcoholic drink of choice for most Canadians in terms of volume and dollar value, more consumers are turning to wine, where sales now capture 28 percent of the market (compared to 21 percent 10 years previously).[2]

Most of us think of alcohol the way it is portrayed in ads or in the movies: a way of having fun with company and an important adjunct to a romantic dinner or a cozy evening in front of the fireplace. And moderate use of alcohol can be part of celebrations or special times without health risk. In fact, research shows that low levels of use may actually reduce some health risks. Still, alcohol is a drug that affects your physical and mental behaviours. Further, the tragedies associated with alcohol receive far less attention than cocaine-related deaths, drug busts, and efforts to eradicate marijuana crops. Nevertheless, they are far more common—with potentially devastating effects on people of all ages.

ALCOHOL: AN OVERVIEW

Although 79.3 percent of Canadians reported alcohol consumption in the past year, only 44 percent reported drinking weekly.[3] Males are more likely than females to report drinking in the past year (82.0 versus 76.8 percent), and the highest past-year drinking rates (90.8 percent) are found in the 18- to 19-year-old age group.[4] In the Canadian Addiction Survey, a light infrequent drinker is classified as someone who reported drinking alcohol less than once a week, with fewer than five drinks consumed; in contrast, a light frequent drinker consumes fewer than five drinks per occasion more than once a week.[5] A heavy infrequent drinker is someone who consumes five or more drinks at a time less than once a week, while a heavy frequent drinker consumes five or more drinks more than once per week.[6] Using these definitions, 36.0 and 62.0 percent of Canadian males and females aged 15 or older, respectively were classified as light infrequent drinkers,

40.9 and 29.2 percent were light frequent drinkers, 9.0 and 5.1 percent were heavy infrequent drinkers, and 14.2 and 3.7 percent were heavy frequent drinkers.[7] Clearly, males are more likely to drink than females, more frequently and in greater quantity.

In terms of alcohol sales, beer remains the most popular choice, capturing 47 percent of sales.[8] The market share of spirits is 25 percent and of wine is 28 percent.[9] Reports from 2004 indicated that when total sales were considered, consumers in Quebec and Newfoundland and Labrador purchased the most (115 litres per capita per year), while consumers in Saskatchewan purchased the least (94.4 litres).[10] Per capita purchases of beer were also highest in Quebec and Newfoundland and Labrador and lowest in British Columbia.[11] Consumers in Newfoundland and Labrador also bought the most spirits. The greatest wine purchasers came from Quebec, Alberta, and British Columbia.[12]

Alcohol can benefit and harm an individual. Most scientific evidence about the benefit as well as the harm comes from industrialized countries such as Canada, cultures where alcohol consumption is largely accepted and where dietary intake and inactive lifestyles lend themselves to heart diseases. Moderate alcohol consumption reduces, in certain age groups, the risk of coronary heart disease and ischemic stroke. Low-risk drinking guidelines suggest consuming no more than 14 standard drinks for men or 9 standard drinks for women per week.[13] Despite this individual benefit, the harm associated with the misuse and abuse of alcohol still constitutes a major public health problem in developed and developing countries. In fact, in Canada 22.6 percent (30.2 percent men; 15.1 percent women) of the population reporting exceeding these low-risk guidelines over the past year.[14]

Almost 10 percent of current drinkers report some sort of harm to themselves as a result of their drinking in the past year.[15] Of these, 3 percent report negative effects on friendships and social life and 5.4 percent report negative effects to their physical health. More alarming is that 32.7 percent of the respondents to the Canadian Addiction Survey reported being harmed the past year because of someone else's drinking.[16] Of these, 10 percent indicated family or marriage difficulties, 22.1 percent reported being insulted or humiliated, 15.5 percent indicated serious arguments or quarrels, 15.8 percent reported verbal abuse, 10.8 percent were pushed or shoved, and 3.2 percent were physically assaulted. Alcohol is a significant factor in hospital admissions, road deaths, industrial accidents, accidental drowning, homicide, and suicide.[17] It is estimated that 6507 Canadians lost their lives as a result of alcohol consumption in 1995, with the largest number of deaths stemming from impaired driving accidents, and that 82 014 Canadians were hospitalized due to alcohol misuse.[18] Total costs of alcohol

While alcohol has long been seen as a "social lubricant" by post-secondary students, alcohol abuse and associated behaviours continue to be serious problems on many campuses.

abuse in 2002 (the latest data available) when measured in terms of health care, law enforcement, loss of productivity in the work place and home, and premature death or disability were estimated to be $14.6 billion or 36.6 percent of the total costs for substance abuse (also includes tobacco and illicit drugs).[19]

✔• Alcohol and the Post-Secondary Student

Alcohol is the most widely used, misused, and abused recreational drug in our society. It is also the most popular drug on campuses, where approximately 94.5 percent of students consume alcoholic beverages. The Addiction Research Foundation estimates that one-third of Ontario students consume more than 15 drinks per week: a level that puts them at health risk. A greater number of alcohol users live in residence (41 percent), are between 17 and 22 years of age (65 percent), and have lower grades (49.5 percent D students, 22.6 percent A students).[20]

what do you THINK?
Are binge drinking and alcohol abuse the same thing? Why or why not? If you drink to get drunk does that indicate a problem? Why or why not?

University or college is a critical time to become conscious of and responsible about your drinking. A number of social factors are involved in campus drinking. There is little doubt that alcohol is a part of campus culture and tradition. It is used to relieve tensions and to celebrate. Its ability to lower inhibitions makes it the "social lubricant" of choice for many students, giving them an easy way to initiate conversations, create friendships, and find a date and/or companion for the evening.

How do students view the drinking patterns of themselves and their peers? Students consistently report that their friends drink much more than they do. Further, actual consumption is higher than self-reports. Such misinformation may promote or be used to excuse excessive drinking practices among post-secondary students.

Binge drinking on campuses continues to be a big problem. **Binge drinking** is defined as the consumption of five drinks in a row by men or four in a row by women on a single occasion. The express purpose of binge drinking is to become intoxicated.

Although everyone is at risk for alcoholism and alcohol-related problems, post-secondary students are particularly vulnerable for the following reasons:

- Alcohol exacerbates their already high risk for suicide, automobile accidents, and falls.

- Many university and college customs, norms, traditions, and mores encourage several dangerous practices and patterns of alcohol use, misuse, and abuse.

- Campuses are heavily targeted by advertising and promotions from the alcohol industry, including the employment of liquor representatives and distributors on most campuses.

- It is more common for post-secondary students than their peers to drink excessively in a variety of drinking games and other dangerous drinking practices.

- Post-secondary students are particularly vulnerable to peer influences and have a strong need to be accepted by their peers.

In an effort to prevent alcohol abuse, many universities and colleges institute strong policies against excessive consumption. Furthermore, help is made available to students with drinking problems. Today, individual and group counselling are offered on most campuses, and more attention is directed toward the prevention of alcohol abuse. Several student organizations also promote responsible drinking and responsible party hosting. Many campuses also provide "safe" rides home.

✸ Rights versus Responsibilities

Most of us recognize the dangers associated with alcohol consumption in general, yet we tend to deny that such things could happen to us. We are aware of the relationship between alcohol and traffic accidents, spouse battering and child abuse, violent crimes, unprotected sexual activity, and family disruption, but we also like to believe that these tragedies happen only to other people. Many students refuse to acknowledge that alcohol is a drug simply because they do not wish to see themselves as drug users. Our society condones, approves, and often encourages the consumption of alcoholic beverages. It also informs how to drink responsibly, yet the reality is that seldom do a person's words match their actions, particularly in the university or college environment, where excessive consumption of alcohol is often the norm, not the exception.

If you make the choice to drink, you should do so judiciously, with complete information about the risks. The physiological and psychological reactions of the human body to alcohol are strong. For this reason, you should approach the drug carefully be and well informed. To avoid the devastating effects of alcohol abuse, you must adhere to the same principles of prevention that apply to any potentially harmful substance. The Canadian Centre for Substance Abuse and the Centre for Addiction and Mental Health recommend fewer than 14 standard drinks per week for men, fewer than 9 standard drinks per week for women, and not more than 2 standard drinks on any one day.[21]

PHYSIOLOGICAL AND BEHAVIOURAL EFFECTS OF ALCOHOL

The intoxicating substance found in beer, wine, liquor, and liqueurs is **ethyl alcohol**, or **ethanol**. It is

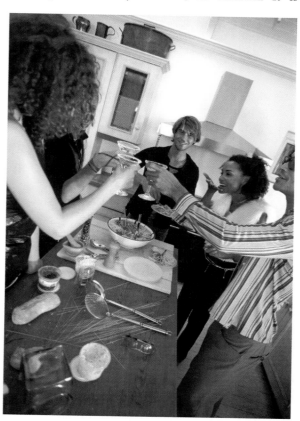

When drinking alcohol, it is important to choose beverages containing a lower percentage of alcohol such as wine or beer, as well as to eat prior to and while drinking to reduce blood alcohol content.

Binge drinking: Drinking to become intoxicated; five drinks in a single sitting for men and four drinks for women.

Ethyl alcohol (ethanol): A drug produced by fermentation and found in many beverages.

Contributing Factors to Alcohol Abuse and Related Problems on Campus

Many students are not aware of the reality of alcohol use, misuse, and abuse on their campuses. The following statistics provide a brief glimpse into the issues.

- Alcohol kills more people under the legal drinking age than cocaine, marijuana, and heroin combined.
- Half a million students aged 15 to 24 are unintentionally injured each year while intoxicated.
- One night of heavy drinking can impair the ability to think abstractly for up to 30 days, limiting a student's ability to understand a professor's lecture, think through a football play, write a paper, or take an exam.
- College and university administrators estimate that alcohol is a factor in 29 percent of dropouts, 38 percent of academic failure, and 64 percent of violent behaviours.
- Over the past decade, there has been a threefold increase in the number of college and university women who report having been drunk on 10 or more occasions in the previous month.
- Areas of a campus offering cheap beer prices have more crime, including trouble between students and police or other campus authorities, arguments, physical fighting, property damage, false fire alarms, and sexual misconduct.
- Alcohol is involved in more than two-thirds of suicides among post-secondary students, 90 percent of sexual assaults, and 95 percent of violent crime on campus.
- The likelihood that a woman will be raped is far greater on campuses with a high rate of binge drinking.
- Each year, more than 100 000 students aged 18 to 24 reported being too intoxicated to know if they had consented to having sex.
- College and university binge drinking occurs more often among male students, students who reside on campus, varsity athletes, and members of fraternities and sororities. Approximately 40 percent of fraternity and sorority members report being frequent binge drinkers, and college or university athletes are 50 percent more likely to binge drink than non-athletes.
- Rates of binge drinking among high-risk students (younger, white males) are lower on more diverse campuses.
- Post-secondary students under the legal drinking age are more prone to binge drinking and pay less for their alcohol than their older classmates. Though underage students drink less often, they consume more per occasion than older students.
- One risk of binge drinking and excessive alcohol consumption is "passing out." During this time, the drinker who passed out could vomit, choke on his or her own vomit, and die. If someone passes out at a party or later at home, it is important to place him or her in the recovery position (that is, on his or her side, upper arm extended with the lower arm bent such that the hand is under his or her cheek) and stay with them until they have "slept it off."

Sources: Data were compiled from the numerous studies cited throughout this chapter and from M. Mohler-Kuo et al., "College Rapes Linked to Binge-Drinking Rates," *Journal of Studies on Alcohol* 65.1 (2004); H. Wechsler, "Watering Down the Drinks: The Moderating Effect of College Demographics on Alcohol Use in High Risk Groups," *American Journal of Public Health* 93.11 (2003): 1929–1933; T. F. Nelson et al., "Alcohol and Collegiate Sports Fans," *Addictive Behaviors* 28.1 (2003): 1–11; R. W. Hingson et al., "Magnitude of Alcohol-Related Mortality and Morbidity among U.S. College Students Aged 18–24," *Journal of Studies on Alcohol* 63.2 (2002): 136–144.

produced during a process called **fermentation**, whereby plant sugars are broken down by yeast organisms, yielding ethanol and carbon dioxide. Fermentation continues until the solution of plant sugars (called mash) reaches a concentration of 14 percent alcohol. At this point, the alcohol kills the yeast and halts the chemical reactions that produce it.

Manufacturers then add other ingredients that dilute the alcohol content of the beverage, such as in beer and wine. Other alcoholic beverages are produced through further processing called **distillation**, during which alcohol vapours are released from the mash at high temperatures. The vapours are then condensed and mixed with water to make the final product, such as in fortified wines and spirits.

The **proof** of an alcoholic drink is a measure of the percentage of alcohol in the beverage. The word *proof* comes from "gunpowder proof," a reference to the gunpowder test, whereby potential buyers tested the distiller's product by pouring it on gunpowder and attempting to light it. If the alcohol content was at least 50 percent, the gunpowder would burn; otherwise the water in the product would put out the flame. Thus, alcohol percentage is 50 percent of the given proof. For example, 80-proof whiskey or scotch is 40-percent alcohol by volume. The proof of a beverage

TABLE 10.1

Psychological and Physiological Effects of Various Blood Alcohol Concentration Levels

Number of Drinks†	Blood Alcohol Concentration*	Psychological and Physiological Effects
1	0.02%–0.03%	No overt effects, slight mood elevation
2	0.05%–0.06%	Feeling of relaxation, warmth; slight decrease in reaction time and in fine-muscle coordination
3	0.08%–0.09%	Balance, speech, vision, and hearing slightly impaired; feelings of euphoria, increased confidence; loss of motor coordination
4	0.11%–0.12%	Coordination and balance becoming difficult; distinct impairment of mental faculties, judgment
5	0.14%–0.15%	Major impairment of mental and physical control; slurred speech, blurred vision, lack of motor skills
7	0.20%	Loss of motor control—needs help moving about; mental confusion
10	0.30%	Severe intoxication; minimum conscious control of mind and body
14	0.40%	Unconsciousness, threshold of coma
17	0.50%	Deep coma
20	0.60%	Death from respiratory failure

†One drink = one beer (4–5% alcohol, 375 mL), one highball (31 mL whiskey), or one glass table wine (157 mL).
*For each hour elapsed since the last drink, subtract 0.015% blood alcohol concentration, or approximately one drink.

Source: Modified from data given in Ohio State Police Driver Information Seminars and the National Clearinghouse for Alcohol and Alcoholism Information, Rockville, MD.

provides an indication of its strength. Therefore, consuming the same amount (that is, volume) of lower-proof drinks will produce fewer alcohol effects than higher-proof drinks. Most spirits are 40 percent alcohol, wines are between 12 and 15 percent alcohol, and ales are between 6 and 8 percent. The alcoholic content of most beers is between 2 and 6 percent, varying according to the type of beer.

Behavioural Effects

Behaviour changes caused by alcohol vary with the setting and with the individual. Alcohol may allow shy people to be less inhibited and more willing to talk to others. It may also cause a depressed person to become even more depressed. In people reluctant to share emotions, it may bring out violence and aggression. In many cases, alcohol will do for the drinker what the drinker expects and wants it to do, making it possible for the user to blame his or her inappropriate behaviours on the alcohol. It is because of this expected effect, combined with reduced inhibitions, that a person who normally does not dance well tears a strip off the dance floor. In other words, a person who normally inhibits dancing behaviours may actually dance

better after a drink or two, simply because his or her inhibitions have been reduced.

Blood alcohol concentration (BAC) is the ratio of alcohol to total blood volume. It is the factor used to measure the physiological and behaviour effects of alcohol. Despite individual differences, alcohol produces some general behaviour effects based on BAC (see Table 10.1). At a BAC of 0.02, a person feels slightly relaxed and his or her mood—whatever that may be—is generally enhanced. At a BAC of 0.05, relaxation increases, there is some motor impairment, and a willingness to talk becomes apparent. At a BAC of 0.08, the person feels euphoric and there is further motor impairment. At a BAC of 0.10, the depressant effects of

Fermentation: The process whereby yeast organisms break down plant sugars to yield ethanol.

Distillation: The process whereby mash is subjected to high temperatures to release alcohol vapours, which are then condensed and mixed with water to make the final product.

Proof: A measure of the percentage of alcohol in a beverage.

Blood alcohol concentration (BAC): The ratio of alcohol to total blood volume; the factor used to measure the physiological and behaviour effects of alcohol

alcohol become apparent, drowsiness sets in, and motor skills are further impaired, followed by a loss of judgment. Thus, a driver may not be able to estimate distances or speed, and some drinkers lose their ability to make value-related decisions and may do things they would not do when sober. As BAC increases, the drinker suffers increased physiological and psychological effects. All these changes are negative; that is, physical and mental functions are impaired not enhanced.

People can acquire physiological and psychological tolerance to the effects of alcohol through regular use. The nervous system adapts over time, so greater quantities of alcohol are required to produce the same physiological and psychological effects. Furthermore, some people learn to modify their behaviours so that they appear to be sober even when their BAC is quite high. This ability is called **learned behavioural tolerance**.

Absorption and Metabolism

Alcohol is rapidly absorbed into the bloodstream from the small intestine, and less rapidly from the stomach and colon. In proportion to its concentration in the bloodstream, alcohol decreases activity in parts of the brain and spinal cord. The drinker's blood alcohol concentration depends on

- the amount consumed in a given time
- the drinker's size, sex, body build, and metabolism
- the type and amount of food in the stomach

Once alcohol has passed into the bloodstream, you cannot slow its absorption by eating or drinking. Mood also influences the rate of absorption, since emotions affect how long it takes for the contents of the stomach to empty into the intestine. Powerful moods, such as stress and tension, are likely to cause the stomach to "dump" its contents into the small intestine. That is why alcohol is absorbed much more rapidly when people are tense than when they are relaxed.

Consuming fruit sugar may shorten the duration of alcohol's effect by increasing the rate of elimination from the blood (that is, metabolism). In the average adult, the rate of metabolism is about 8.5 grams (that is, about two-thirds of a drink) of alcohol per hour. This rate varies dramatically among individuals, however, depending on the user's drinking history, physique, sex, liver size, and genetic factors.[22]

what do you THINK?

Have you or someone you know ever chosen specifically to alter conditions so as to increase BAC (that is, to get drunk quicker)? Are these wise practices? Why or why not?

Alcohol is metabolized in the liver, where it is converted by the enzyme alcohol dehydrogenase to acetaldehyde. It is then rapidly oxidized to acetate, converted to carbon dioxide and water, and eventually excreted from the body. Acetaldehyde is a toxic chemical that can cause immediate symptoms such as nausea and vomiting as well as long-term effects such as liver damage.

Like food, alcohol contains calories. Proteins and carbohydrates (starches and sugars) each contain 4 kilocalories per gram while fat contains 9 kilocalories per gram. Alcohol, although similar in structure to carbohydrates, contains 7 kilocalories per gram. Although a source of energy—and therefore considered a food—alcohol is not considered a nutrient because it is not essential to our body, nor does it perform any necessary function.[23]

A drinker's BAC depends on his or her weight and body fat, the water content in the body tissues, the concentration of alcohol in the beverage consumed, the rate of consumption, and the volume of alcohol consumed. Heavier people have larger body surfaces through which to diffuse alcohol; therefore, they have lower concentrations of alcohol in their blood than thin people after drinking the same amount. Because alcohol does not diffuse as rapidly into body fat as into water, alcohol concentration is higher in a person with more body fat. Because a woman is likely to have more body fat and less water in her body tissues than a man of the same weight, she will have a higher BAC than a man after drinking the same amount of alcohol. (See Table 10.2.)

Women and Alcohol

Body fat is not the only contributor to the differences in alcohol's effects on men and women. Compared to men, women have half as much alcohol hydrogenase, the enzyme that breaks down alcohol in the stomach before it has a chance to get to the bloodstream and the brain. Therefore, if a man and a woman drink the same amount of alcohol, the woman's BAC will be approximately 30 percent higher than the man's, leaving her more vulnerable to slurred speech, careless driving, and other drinking-related impairments. Table 10.2 compares blood-alcohol levels by sex, weight, and consumption. Although this table provides an estimate of probable BAC levels, many additional factors may cause considerable variation. For this reason, you should always err on the side of caution when gauging your BAC.

Breathalyzer and Other Tests

The breathalyzer tests used by law enforcement officers are designed to determine BAC based on the amount of alcohol exhaled in the breath. Urinalysis yields a BAC based on the concentration of unmetabolized alcohol in

TABLE 10.2
Calculation of Estimated Blood Alcohol (BAC) for Men and Women

Body Weight (kg)	Number of Drinks: Males									
	1	2	3	4	5	6	7	8	9	10
45.4	0.043	0.087	0.130	0.174	0.217	0.261	0.304	0.348	0.391	0.435
56.8	0.034	0.069	0.103	0.139	0.173	0.209	0.242	0.278	0.312	0.346
68.2	0.029	0.058	0.087	0.116	0.145	0.174	0.203	0.232	0.261	0.290
79.5	0.025	0.050	0.075	0.100	0.125	0.150	0.175	0.200	0.225	0.250
90.9	0.022	0.043	0.065	0.087	0.108	0.130	0.152	0.174	0.195	0.217
102.3	0.022	0.045	0.068	0.091	0.113	0.136	0.159	0.182	0.204	0.227
113.6	0.020	0.041	0.061	0.082	0.101	0.122	0.142	0.162	0.182	0.202

Body Weight (kg)	Number of Drinks: Females									
	1	2	3	4	5	6	7	8	9	10
45.4	0.050	0.101	0.152	0.203	0.253	0.304	0.355	0.406	0.456	0.507
56.8	0.040	0.080	0.120	0.162	0.202	0.244	0.282	0.324	0.364	0.404
68.2	0.034	0.068	0.101	0.135	0.169	0.203	0.237	0.271	0.304	0.338
79.5	0.029	0.058	0.087	0.117	0.146	0.175	0.204	0.233	0.262	0.292
90.9	0.026	0.050	0.076	0.101	0.126	0.152	0.177	0.203	0.227	0.253
102.3	0.022	0.045	0.068	0.091	0.113	0.136	0.159	0.182	0.204	0.227
113.6	0.020	0.041	0.061	0.082	0.101	0.122	0.142	0.162	0.182	0.202

Body weight: Calculations are for people who have a normal body weight for their height, who are free of drugs or other affecting medications, and who are neither unusually thin nor obese.

Drink equivalents:
1 drink = 43 mL (1.5 oz) of rum, rye, scotch, brandy, gin, vodka, etc.
1 drink = 341-mL (12-oz) bottle of normal-strength (5%) beer
1 drink = 85 mL (3 oz) of fortified wine
1 drink = 142 mL (5 oz) of table wine

Using the chart: Find the appropriate figure using the proper chart (male or female), body weight, and number of drinks consumed. Then subtract the time factor (see Time Factor Table, below) from the figure on the chart to obtain the approximate BAC. For example, for a 68-kg man who has had 4 drinks in 2 hours, take the figure 0.116 (from the chart for males) and subtract 0.030 (from the Time Factor Table) to obtain a BAC of 0.086 percent.

Time Factor Table

Hours since first drink	1	2	3	4	5	6
Subtract from BAC	0.015	0.030	0.045	0.60	0.075	0.090

Source: Copyright © 1991 by Glen Evans and Robert O'Brien. Reprinted with permission of Facts On file, Inc., an imprint of Infobase Publishing, Inc.

the urine. Breath analysis, urinalysis, and blood tests are used to determine whether a driver is over the legal limit, with blood tests providing the most accurate measures.

Learned behavioural tolerance: The ability of drinkers to modify their behaviours so that they appear sober even when they have high BAC levels.

Immediate Effects

Alcohol is a central nervous system (CNS) depressant. The primary action of ethanol is to reduce the frequency of nerve transmissions and impulses at synaptic junctions. This reduction of nerve transmissions causes a significant reduction in CNS functions, with resulting decreases in respiratory rate, pulse rate, and blood pressure. As CNS depression deepens, vital functions become noticeably reduced. In extreme cases, coma and death can result (see also Table 10.1).

Alcohol is a diuretic that increases urinary output. Although this effect might be expected to lead to automatic **dehydration** (loss of water), the body actually retains water, most of it in the muscles or in the cerebral tissues. This is because water is usually pulled out of the **cerebrospinal fluid** (fluid within the brain and spinal cord) instead, leading to what is known as mitochondrial dehydration at the cellular level within the nervous system. Mitochondria are miniature organs within cells responsible for specific functions. They rely heavily on fluid balance. When mitochondrial dehydration occurs from drinking, the mitochondria cannot carry out their normal functions, resulting in symptoms that include the "morning-after" headaches suffered by some drinkers.

---

what do you THINK?

Think about the last time you consumed alcohol. How much did you consume? Over how long? Calculate your blood alcohol content using the information presented in Table 10.2. How long did it take until your BAC was reduced to 0?

Alcohol is also an irritant to the gastrointestinal system and may cause indigestion and heartburn if consumed on an empty stomach. Long-term use of alcohol causes repeated irritation that has been linked to cancers of the esophagus and stomach. In addition, people who engage in brief drinking sprees during which they consume unusually high amounts of alcohol put themselves at risk for irregular heartbeat or even total loss of heart rhythm, which can cause disruption in blood flow and possible damage to the heart muscle.

A **hangover** is sometimes experienced the morning after consuming alcohol. The symptoms of a hangover are familiar to those who drink: headache, upset stomach, anxiety, depression, thirst, and, in severe cases, an almost overwhelming desire to crawl back into bed. People who get hangovers often also stay up too late or engage in other behaviours likely to leave them feeling unwell the next day. The causes of hangovers are not well known, but the effects of congeners are suspected. **Congeners** are toxic forms of alcohol metabolized more slowly than ethanol. Your body metabolizes the congeners after the ethanol is gone from your system, and their toxic by-products are thought to contribute to the hangover. It usually takes 12 hours to recover from a hangover. Bed rest, plenty of fluids, solid food, and a pain reliever may reduce the discomforts of a hangover; however, nothing cures it but time.

Drug Interactions

When you use any drug (and alcohol is a drug), you need to be aware of the possible interactions with prescription drugs, over-the-counter drugs, or other drugs you are taking or considering taking. Table 10.3 summarizes possible interactions. (See also Chapter 9).

Long-Term Effects
Effects on the Nervous System

Since alcohol is a CNS depressant, the nervous system is especially sensitive to it. Even people who drink moderately experience a decrease in brain size and weight accompanied by a slight loss of intellectual ability. The damage that results from alcohol use is localized primarily in the left side of the brain, which is responsible for written and spoken language, logic, and mathematical skills. The degree of shrinkage appears to be directly related to the amount of alcohol consumed. In terms of memory loss, the evidence suggests that having one drink every day is less likely to result in damage than saving up for a binge and consuming seven or eight drinks in a night.

Cardiovascular Effects

The cardiovascular system is affected by alcohol in a number of ways. Evidence suggests that the effect of alcohol on the heart is not all bad. Some studies suggest that moderate drinkers suffer fewer heart attacks, have less cholesterol buildup, and are less likely to die of heart disease than either nondrinkers or heavy drinkers.[24] However, drinking is not recommended as a preventive measure against heart disease because the benefits do not outweigh the risks. Alcohol contributes to high blood pressure and a slightly increased heart rate and cardiac output. Those who report drinking three to five drinks a day, regardless of ethnicity or sex,

TABLE 10.3

Drugs and Alcohol: Actions and Interactions

Drug Class/Name(s)	Effects with Alcohol
Anti-alcohol: Antabuse	Severe reactions to even small amounts: headache, nausea, blurred vision, convulsions, coma, possible death.
Antibiotics: Penicillin, Cyantin	Reduces therapeutic effectiveness of antibiotics.
Antidepressants: Elavil, Sinequan, Tofranil, Nardil	Increased central nervous system (CNS) depression, blood pressure changes. Combined use of alcohol and MAO inhibitors, a specific type of antidepressant, can trigger massive increases in blood pressure, even brain hemorrhage and death.
Antihistamines: Allerest, Dristan	Drowsiness and CNS depression. Impairs driving ability.
ASA: Aspirin, Anacin, Excedrin, Bayer	Irritates stomach lining. May cause gastrointestinal pain, bleeding.
Depressants: Valium, Ativan, Placidyl	Dangerous CNS depression, loss of coordination, coma. High risk of overdose and death.
Narcotics: Heroin, Codeine, Darvon	Serious CNS depression. Possible respiratory arrest and death.
Stimulants: Caffeine, Cocaine	Masks depressant action of alcohol. May increase blood pressure, physical tension.
Tylenol, Acetaminophen	Risk of liver damage, particularly with heavy alcohol consumption and maximum recommended doses of acetaminophen.

Source: Adapted by permission from *Drugs and Alcohol: Simple Facts about Alcohol and Drug Combinations* (Phoenix: DIN Publications, 1988), No. 121.

have higher blood pressure than those who drink less, or not at all.

People who engage in brief drinking sprees, during which they consume unusually large amounts of alcohol, also suffer some risks, including irregular heartbeat or total loss of heart rhythm. This condition has been called "holiday heart syndrome" because it typically occurs around holidays such as Thanksgiving, Christmas, and New Year's Eve—occasions when drinkers are likely to overindulge. It can cause disruption in blood flow and possible damage to the heart muscle. Prolonged drinking can also lead to deterioration of the heart muscle, a condition called cardiomyopathy.

Liver Disease

One of the most common diseases related to alcohol abuse is **cirrhosis** of the liver. It is among the top 10 causes of death in Canada. One result of heavy drinking is that the liver begins to store fat—a condition known as "fatty liver." If there is insufficient time between drinking episodes, this fat cannot be transported to storage sites and the fat-filled liver cells stop functioning. Continued drinking causes a further

stage of liver deterioration called fibrosis, in which the damaged area of the liver develops fibrous scar tissue. Cell function can be partially restored at this stage with proper nutrition and abstinence from alcohol. However, if the person continues to drink, cirrhosis results: liver cells die and the damage is permanent. **Alcoholic hepatitis** is a serious condition resulting from prolonged use of alcohol. A chronic inflammation of the liver develops, which may be fatal in itself or progress to cirrhosis.

Dehydration: Loss of fluids from body tissues.

Cerebrospinal fluid: Fluid within and surrounding the brain and spinal cord tissues.

Hangover: The physiological reaction to excessive drinking, including such symptoms as headache, upset stomach, anxiety, depression, diarrhea, and thirst.

Congeners: Forms of alcohol metabolized more slowly than ethanol that produce toxic by-products.

Cirrhosis: The last stage of liver disease associated with chronic heavy use of alcohol, during which liver cells die and damage is permanent.

Alcoholic hepatitis: Condition resulting from prolonged use of alcohol in which the liver is inflamed. It can result in death.

Cancer

Heavy drinkers (more than 5 drinks per day, more than 12 times per year) are at higher risk for certain types of cancer, particularly those of the gastrointestinal tract. The repeated irritation caused by long-term use of alcohol has been linked to cancers of the esophagus, stomach, mouth, tongue, and liver. Research also indicates a link between breast cancer and moderate consumption in women. A landmark study found that women between the ages of 34 and 59 who consumed between three and nine drinks a week were 30 percent more likely than nondrinkers to develop breast cancer.[25] It is unclear how alcohol exerts its carcinogenic effects, though it is thought that it inhibits the absorption of carcinogenic substances, permitting them to be taken to sensitive organs.

Other Effects

An irritant to the gastrointestinal system, alcohol may cause indigestion and heartburn if consumed on an empty stomach. It also damages the mucous membranes and leads to inflammation of the esophagus, chronic stomach irritation, problems with intestinal absorption, and chronic diarrhea. Alcohol abuse is a major cause of chronic inflammation of the pancreas, the organ that produces digestive enzymes and insulin. Chronic abuse of alcohol inhibits enzyme production, which further inhibits the absorption of nutrients. Drinking alcohol can block the absorption of calcium, a nutrient that strengthens bones. This should be of particular concern to women, because as women age their risk for osteoporosis (bone thinning and calcium loss) increases. Heavy consumption of alcohol worsens this condition.

Evidence also suggests that alcohol impairs the body's ability to recognize and fight foreign bodies such as bacteria and viruses. Thus, individuals become more susceptible to colds and flues.

Fetal Alcohol Spectrum Disorders

Alcohol consumed by the mother has harmful effects on fetal development. Alcohol consumed during the first trimester of pregnancy poses the greatest threat to organ development, while exposure during the last trimester, when the brain is developing rapidly, is most likely to affect CNS development.

A series of disorders collectively called **fetal alcohol spectrum disorder (FASD)** is caused by prenatal exposure to alcohol and leads to lifelong developmental and cognitive disabilities among Canadian children.[26] FASD occurs when alcohol ingested by the mother passes through the placenta into the fetus's bloodstream. Because the fetus is so small, its BAC will be much higher than that of the mother. Thus, consumption of alcohol during pregnancy affects the fetus far more seriously than the mother.

FASD is the leading cause of developmental delay in Canada and North America, with an incidence estimated at 1 to 6 in 1000 live births.[27] FASD includes the following disorders related to alcohol consumption during pregnancy: **fetal alcohol syndrome (FAS)**, **fetal alcohol effects (FAE)**, partial fetal alcohol effects, alcohol-related neurodevelopmental disorders, and neurobehavioural disorder–alcohol exposed. FAS is characterized by retarded growth prenatally and postnatally, facial anomalies, CNS dysfunction as noted by intellectual impairment, structural abnormalities, developmental delay, and complex behavioural problems.[28] One-fifth of FAS children have difficulty sleeping and are hyperactive. Many have severe learning disabilities and are dyslexic. Congenital heart problems are more common than in normal babies, as are genitor-urinary problems. There is an increased incidence of spina bifida, hip dislocation, and delayed skeletal maturation. FAE is used to describe children with prenatal exposure to alcohol but only some FAS characteristics.

As there is no definitive information regarding a safe quantity of alcohol during pregnancy, women who are or wish to become pregnant should abstain from alcohol. Health professionals should reassure women who have consumed small amounts of alcohol occasionally during pregnancy that the risk is likely minimal. Pregnant women should also know that not drinking at any time during a pregnancy will benefit themselves and their babies.

In June 1992, the Standing Committee on Health and Welfare, Social Affairs, Seniors, and the Status of Women released its report *Fetal Alcohol Syndrome: A Preventable Tragedy*. Since then, Health Canada has worked with health-care professionals to identify and implement prevention strategies; produced pamphlets and videos on FAS; and, with the Association of Canadian Distillers and the Brewers' Association of Canada, sponsors a national information service resource centre providing links to support groups, prevention projects, and experts on FASD (1-800-559-4514).

---

what do you THINK?

Why do we hear so little about FASD given that it is the leading cause of developmental delay in North America? If you or your partner were pregnant, would you drink? Why or why not? How would you handle the societal pressures to consume alcohol?

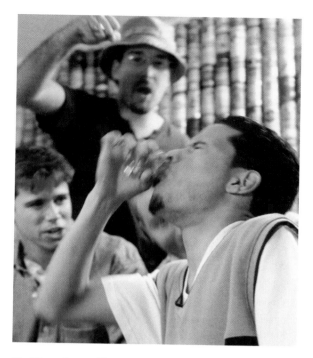

Deciding when and how much to drink is no simple matter. Irresponsible consumption of alcohol can easily result in disaster.

Drinking and Driving

The leading cause of death for all age groups from 5 to 34 years old (including university and college students) is traffic accidents. Young people between 15 and 29 years old account for 38 percent of motor vehicle fatalities. The rate is highest for 20- to 24-year-olds, at 14.7 percent.[29] Impaired driving is a major cause of death, killing about 1350 Canadians each year and injuring many more.[30]

✳ ALCOHOLISM

Alcohol use becomes **alcohol abuse** or **alcoholism** when there is excessive consumption or a level of consumption that interferes with work, school, or social and family relationships. Alcoholism is one of many addictions or dependencies on substances or behaviours that have mood-altering consequences.

As noted previously, 8.8 percent of Canadians between the ages of 15 and 65 reported harm to self in the past year as a result of their drinking. Of the past-year drinkers, 6.2 percent indicated heavy drinking (five or more drinks for males and four or more drinks for women on a single occasion) at least once per week, with men between the ages of 18 and 24 years the most likely to report heavy drinking. Further, 22.6 percent of past-year drinkers exceeded the low-risk drinking guidelines (that is, consuming no more than 14 standard drinks for men or 9 standard drinks for women per week). Again, men between the ages of 18 and 24 were most likely to exceed these guidelines.

As previously noted, the most common areas affected by excessive drinking are physical health (5.4 percent), financial position (4.7 percent), and social health (3.0 percent). Almost one-third (32.7 percent) of Canadians say they have had problems from other people's drinking, such as being disturbed by loud parties (23.8 percent), being insulted or humiliated (22.1 percent), having a serious argument (15.5 percent), being physically abused (14.0 percent), and experiencing marital difficulties (10.0 percent). There were 8103 deaths and 1 587 054 acute care hospital days attributed to alcohol in Canada in 2002.[31] Motor vehicle accidents accounted for the largest number of alcohol-related deaths, while accidental falls and alcohol dependence syndrome accounted for the largest number of alcohol-related hospitalizations.

How, Why, Whom?

As with other addictions, tolerance, psychological dependence, and withdrawal symptoms must be present to qualify a person as addicted to alcohol. Addiction usually results from chronic use over a period of time that may vary from person to person. People who have problems with alcohol, including irresponsible users, are not necessarily people who are addicted to it. The stereotype of the person on skid row addicted to alcohol applies to only 5 percent of those who are affected. The remaining 95 percent of individuals addicted to alcohol live in some type of extended family unit. They can be found at all socioeconomic levels and in all professions, ethnic groups, geographic locations, and religions. You have a 1 in 10 chance or risk of becoming addicted to alcohol. Individuals addicted to alcohol tend to have a

Fetal alcohol spectrum disorder (FASD): A broad category of disorders relating to consumption of alcohol during pregnancy; includes fetal alcohol syndrome, fetal alcohol effects, partial fetal alcohol effects, alcohol-related neurodevelopmental disorders, and neurobehavioural disorder–alcohol exposed.

Fetal alcohol syndrome (FAS): A disorder that may result in the fetus if a mother regularly consumes alcohol during pregnancy. Among its effects are mental retardation, small head, tremors, and abnormalities of the face, limbs, heart, and brain.

Fetal alcohol effects (FAE): A syndrome describing children with a history of prenatal alcohol exposure but without all the physical or behavioural symptoms of FAS. Among its symptoms are low birthweight, irritability, and possible permanent mental impairment.

Alcohol abuse (alcoholism): Use of alcohol that interferes with work, school, or personal relationships or that entails violations of the law.

The Public Rates Drinking and Driving as One of Canada's Most Serious Social Issues

According to the 2002 Road Safety Monitor, an annual national opinion poll conducted by the Traffic Injury Research Foundation (TIRF), most Canadians believe that drinking and driving is a priority social issue, and the most important road safety issue that they face.

Drinking and driving occurrence in Canada:

- 86 percent of Canadians rated drinking and driving as a serious problem.
- 16.1 percent of drivers reported driving within two hours of consuming alcohol in the 30-day period prior to the survey.
- 7.9 percent of drivers admitted to driving when they thought they were over the legal limit at some point in 2002.
- It is estimated that, during 2002, there were more than 8 million trips in which the driver was impaired.

A relatively small group of individuals makes our roads particularly dangerous:

- Fewer than 3 percent of drivers account for more than 80 percent of all impaired driving trips.
- Young drivers (aged 16 to 18) and older drivers (aged 65 and over) are least likely to drive after drinking.

- Canadians aged 18 to 34 are most likely to report driving after drinking.

Canadian drivers support the following initiatives aimed at decreasing the incidence of drinking and driving:

- Requiring drivers suspected of drinking to perform sobriety tests
- Mandatory breath testing of drivers involved in collisions
- Alcohol ignition interlocks
- Immediate impoundment of vehicles driven by impaired drivers
- A zero blood alcohol content restriction for convicted offenders
- Greater use of police spot checks

Source: Adapted from the Traffic Safety Research Foundation, 2002 Road Safety Monitor.

number of attitudes behaviours in common. People who recognize in themselves any of these attitudes and behaviours discussed in the following paragraphs should seek professional help to determine whether alcohol has become a controlling factor in their lives.

Women are the fastest-growing component of the population becoming addicted to alcohol. They tend to become addicted at a later age and after fewer years of heavy drinking than men. Women at highest risk for alcohol-related problems are those living common law in their 20s or early 30s, or who have a husband or partner who drinks heavily.

The Causes of Alcoholism

We know that alcoholism is a disease with biologic, psychological, and social/environmental components, but we do not know what role—or how much of a role—each of these components plays.

Biologic and Family Factors

Research into the hereditary and environmental causes of alcoholism has found higher rates of alcoholism among family members of individuals addicted to alcohol. In fact, according to researchers, alcoholism is four to five times more common among the children of those who are addicted to alcohol than in the general population.

Individuals categorized with type 1 alcoholism are individuals who had at least one parent who was a problem drinker and grew up in an environment that encouraged heavy drinking. Their drinking is reinforced by family and social events that include heavy drinking. These individuals share certain personality characteristics; they avoid novelty and harmful situations and are concerned about the thoughts and feelings of others. Individuals classified with type 2 alcoholism are typically males only. These men are the biological sons of fathers who in addition to being alcoholics have a history of violence and drug use. These men display the opposite characteristics of individuals considered type 1 alcoholics; they do not seek social approval, they lack inhibition, and they are prone to novelty-seeking behaviours.[32]

Scientists are on the trail of an "alcohol gene," but so far they have not found one. In 1990, it appeared that a

The Emotional Trauma of Losing a Loved One to Impaired Driving

The loss of someone you love is always devastating. When the death is sudden and violent, it can be even more traumatic. Hurt, anger, sadness, and frustration are some of the emotions a senseless and violent death causes. The loss of a loved one because of an impaired driving crash brings an abrupt end to that person's life, his or her future dreams and aspirations. There is no chance to say good-bye, no time to say thank you or I am sorry. There are loose ends that will never be tied. In particular, someone who has lost a child or a partner often feels guilty that he or she could not protect them.

The violence of auto accidents often leaves the victims unrecognizable. The hospital or funeral home may not permit viewing of the body, which can lead families into painful fantasies about how their loved one looked; or they may doubt that the person actually died. For many families, seeing the body gives them closure that the person they loved is really gone.

Central to the trauma that families and friends experience after a crash is the senselessness of the death. The fact that the death could have been prevented and is clearly someone's fault is one of the most painful parts of grieving. Knowing that someone chose to be negligent is hard to understand. Many people report feelings of intense anger, even rage, at the offender.

Anger can be central to the grieving process. There is anger not only at the offender but also "the system" and at other family members. Because people experience the sudden loss differently, some may feel anger at the way other family members appear to be moving on or not moving on. Even anger toward the person who has died—due to feelings of abandonment—is not unusual. Anger covers up the underlying sadness that may be more difficult to endure.

Anxiety and fear are also common. Suddenly families realize their vulnerability, a concept that may not have been fully understood before. Often people hold on to the belief that bad things do not happen to good people. When that idea is destroyed, it may be replaced with fear and a sense of powerlessness that is overwhelming.

The emotional aftermath of losing a loved one to impaired driving is filled with feelings and experiences not even touched upon in this short discussion. The road to feeling better is often blocked; many people feel they will not be happy again. While it is true that life will never be the same, families do survive the ordeal. Many manage to gain strength and find happiness again. Ultimately, what people are left with is sorrow. Sorrow encompasses the knowledge that you will always feel sadness over the tragic loss of your loved one; however, it is also a step away from being overwhelmed by grief.

Source: Mothers Against Drunk Driving (MADD) Canada. Retrieved August 26, 2009 from the Transport Canada website: www.tc.gc.ca/roadsafety/safedrivers/impaireddriving/smashed.

specific gene linked to alcoholism had been discovered. It turned out, however, that not only was the gene not found consistently in every person addicted to alcohol studied, it also existed in some individuals who were not alcoholics.[33]

Because the effects of heredity and environment are so difficult to separate, some researchers have chosen to examine this issue through twin and adoption studies. So far, these studies have produced inconclusive results. However, a slightly higher rate of similar drinking behaviours has been demonstrated among identical twins. Further, sons living away from their biologic parents who are alcoholics tend to more closely resemble them in drinking behaviours than they do their adoptive or foster parents.

Social and Cultural Factors

There are numerous factors that may mitigate or exacerbate problems with alcohol. Many individuals begin to drink because of peer pressure—because everyone else is doing it. Others may begin drinking as a way to dull the pain of an acute loss or an emotional or social problem. For example, students may drink to escape the stress involved in university or college life, disappointment over unfulfilled expectations, difficulties in forming relationships, or the loss of the security of home, loved ones, and close friends. Unfortunately, the emotional discomfort that causes many people to turn to alcohol also ultimately causes them to become even more uncomfortable as the depressant effect of the drug begins to take its toll. Thus, the person who is already depressed may become even more depressed, antagonizing friends and other social supports until these supports turn away.

Family attitudes toward alcohol also influence whether or not a person will develop a drinking problem. It has been demonstrated that people raised in cultures in which drinking is a part of religious or ceremonial activities or in which alcohol is a traditional part of the family meal are less prone to alcohol dependency. In contrast, in societies in which alcohol purchase is carefully controlled and drinking is regarded as a rite of passage to adulthood, such as that found in Canada, the tendency for abuse appears to be greater.[34]

Certain social factors have been linked with alcoholism as well. These include urbanization, the weakening of links to the extended family and a general loosening of kinship ties, increased mobility, and changing religious and philosophic values. Apparently, then, some combination of heredity and environment plays a decisive role in the development of alcoholism.

Effects of Alcoholism on the Family

Recently, it has been recognized that not only the person addicted to alcohol but also his or her entire family suffers. Although most research focuses on family effects during the late stages of alcoholism, the family unit actually begins to react early on as the person starts to show symptoms of addiction to alcohol.

Many families affected by alcoholism have no idea what normal family life is like. Family members unconsciously adapt to the behaviours of the person who is addicted to alcohol by adjusting their own behaviours. To minimize their feelings about the addiction or out of love for him or her, family members take on various abnormal roles. These roles actually help keep the person drinking. Children in such dysfunctional families generally assume at least one of the following roles:

- Family hero: tries to divert attention from the problem by being really good, almost too good to be true
- Scapegoat: draws attention away from the family's primary problem through delinquency or misbehaviour
- Lost child: becomes passive and quietly withdraws from upsetting situations as well as family life
- Mascot: disrupts tense situations by providing comic relief

For children in alcoholic homes, life is a struggle. They have to deal with constant stress, anxiety, and embarrassment. Because the individual who is an alcoholic is often the centre of attention, the children's wants and needs are usually ignored. It is not uncommon for these children to be victims of violence, abuse, neglect, or incest. As previously noted, when such children grow up they have a greater tendency to become alcoholics themselves than do children from nonalcoholic families.

Over time, we have come to recognize the unique problems of adult children of individuals addicted to alcohol whose difficulties in life stem from a lack of parental nurturing during childhood. Among these problems are an inability to develop social attachments, a need to be in control of all emotions and situations, low self-esteem, and depression.

Fortunately, not all individuals who grew up in alcoholic families are doomed to have lifelong problems. Many of these people develop a resiliency in response to their family's problems and enter adulthood armed with positive strengths and valuable career-oriented skills, such as the ability to assume responsibility, strong organizational skills, and realistic expectations of their jobs and those of others.

Costs to Society

As previously noted, the alcohol industry in Canada registered sales of more than $18 billion in the fiscal year ending March 31, 2007, providing employment for more than 14 000 persons and generating significant revenue for provincial and federal governments. The average beverage sales per capita per year for Canadians was $667.[35]

The benefits of alcohol sales to the economy should be considered alongside the consequences of alcohol abuse and addiction. Wider society suffers the consequences of individuals' alcohol abuse. The figure of

$18.45 billion, or 2.7 percent of GDP, represents the most optimistic estimate of the cost of addiction to society. The actual number could be significantly higher. Of this amount, alcohol abuse accounts for $7.5 billion.[36]

Women and Alcoholism

In the past, women have consumed less alcohol and had fewer alcohol-related problems than men. Now, a greater percentage of women, especially college- and university-aged women, are choosing to drink and many are drinking more heavily.

Studies indicate that there are now almost as many women as men who become alcoholics. However, there appear to be differences between men and women when it comes to alcohol abuse:[37]

1. Women attribute the onset of problem drinking to a specific life stress or traumatic event more frequently than men.

2. Women's alcoholism starts later and progresses more quickly than men's; this phenomenon is called "telescoping."

3. Women tend to be prescribed mood-altering drugs more often than men; women thus face the risks of drug interaction or cross-tolerance more often.

4. Men not addicted to alcohol tend to divorce their spouses who are addicted nine times more often than they do their spouses without an alcohol addiction; women addicted to alcohol are thus not as likely to have a family support system to aid them in their recovery.

5. Women addicted to alcohol do not tend to receive as much social support as men in their treatment and recovery.

6. Unmarried, divorced, or single-parent women tend to have significant economic problems that may make entry into a treatment program especially difficult.

what do you THINK?

Think about your campus and the cultural norms surrounding alcohol use. Do women drink as frequently as men? Why or why not? Do women on campus drink heavily? Why or why not? Does the campus culture view men's and women's drinking in the same way? What supports are available on campus for individuals with a drinking problem? What supports are available in the local community?

RECOVERY

Most individuals addicted to alcohol and problem drinkers who seek help have experienced a turning point or dramatic occurrence, such as a failed relationship or confrontation at work. Regardless of the reasons for seeking help, it has finally been recognized that alcohol controls the person's life—this is a critical component of recovery. The first step on the road to recovery is to regain that control and to assume responsibility for personal actions.

The Family's Role

Family members of an individual addicted to alcohol sometimes take action before that person does. They may go to an organization or a treatment facility to seek help for themselves and their relative. An effective method of helping an individual addicted to alcohol confront the disease is a process called **intervention**. Essentially, an intervention is a planned confrontation with the person who is an alcoholic that involves several family members plus professional counsellors. The family members express their love and concern, telling the person who has the addiction that they will no longer refrain from acknowledging the problem and affirming their support for appropriate treatment. A family intervention is often the turning point for a growing number of individuals addicted to alcohol.

Treatment Programs

There are hundreds of residential care facilities in Canada for the treatment of alcohol and drug addiction, funded by a mix of municipal, provincial, and federal sources. There are also outpatient, detox, walk-in, and crisis centres. Treatment programs are based on various models and offered in many other languages in addition to French and English. Upon admission to a treatment facility, the individual is given a complete physical exam to determine whether there are underlying medical problems that will interfere with treatment. Individuals addicted to alcohol who quit drinking typically experience withdrawal symptoms, such as

• hyperexcitability

• confusion

• sleep disorders

Intervention: A planned confrontation with a person addicted to alcohol in which family members and/or friends express their concern about the drinking.

- convulsions
- agitation
- tremors of the hands
- brief hallucinations
- depression
- headache
- seizures

In a small percentage of individuals, alcohol withdrawal results in a severe syndrome known as **delirium tremens (DTs)**. Delirium tremens is characterized by confusion, delusions, agitated behaviours, and hallucinations.

Withdrawal from alcohol is very difficult and medically risky—more so than for many other addictive substances or behaviours. Thus, for any long-term addiction to alcohol, medical supervision is usually necessary. Detoxification, the process by which individuals addicted to alcohol end their dependence, is commonly carried out in a medical facility where they can be monitored to prevent fatal withdrawal reactions. Withdrawal usually takes 7 to 21 days. Shortly after detoxification, treatment begins for psychological addiction. Most treatment facilities keep their patients from three to six weeks. Treatment at private treatment centres costs several thousand dollars, but some insurance programs or employers will assume most of this expense.

Family Therapy, Individual Therapy, and Group Therapy

Various individual and group therapies are also available. In family therapy, the person and family members gradually examine the psychological reasons underlying the addiction. In individual and group therapy, individuals addicted to alcohol learn positive coping skills for use in situations that have regularly caused them to drink. On some campuses, the problems associated with alcohol abuse are so great that student health centres are offering their own treatment programs.

Other Types of Treatment

Two other treatments are drug and aversion therapy. For drug therapy, disulfiram (trade name Antabuse) is the drug of choice for treating individuals addicted to alcohol. If alcohol is consumed, the drug causes unpleasant intolerant effects such as headache, nausea, vomiting, drowsiness, and hangover. These symptoms discourage one from drinking. Aversion therapy is based on conditioning therapy. It works on the premise that the sight, smell, and taste of alcohol will acquire aversive properties if repeatedly paired with a

noxious stimulus. For a period of 10 days, the individual takes drugs that induce vomiting when combined with alcohol. These treatments work best in conjunction with counselling.

Alcoholics Anonymous (AA) is a private, nonprofit, self-help organization founded in 1935. The organization, which relies on group support to help people stop drinking, currently has more than one million members, with branches all over the world. People attending their first AA meeting will find that last names are never used. Neither is anyone forced to speak. Members are taught to believe that their alcoholism is a lifetime problem. They share their stories with the group and are asked to place their faith, and control of the habit, in the hands of a "higher power." The road to recovery is taken one step at a time. AA offers specialized meetings for individuals who are homosexual, atheist, HIV-positive, and professionals.

Alcoholics Anonymous also has auxiliary groups to help spouses or partners, friends, and children of individuals addicted to alcohol. Al-Anon is the group dedicated to helping adult relatives and friends of the person who is addicted understand the disease and learn how they can be part of the recovery process. The support gained from talking with others with similar problems is one of the greatest benefits derived from participation in Al-Anon. Many members learn how to exert greater control over their own lives. Some are able to rid themselves of the guilt they feel about their participation in their loved one's alcoholism.

Alateen, another AA-related organization, is designed to help adolescents live with a parent or parents who are alcoholics. Teens are taught that they are not at fault for their parents' problems with alcohol. They learn skills to develop their self-esteem so they can function better socially. Alateen also helps the children of people addicted to alcohol to overcome their guilt feelings.

✱ Relapse

Roughly 60 percent of individuals addicted to alcohol relapse (resume drinking) within the first three months of treatment. Why is the relapse rate so high? Treating an addiction requires more than getting the person who is addicted to stop using; it also requires getting the person to break a pattern of behaviours that has dominated his or her life—often for some time.

People seeking to regain a healthy lifestyle must not only confront their addiction, but also guard against the tendency to relapse. Individuals with compulsive personalities need to learn to understand themselves and take control. Others need to view treatment as a long-term process that takes a lot of effort beyond attending a weekly self-help group meeting. In order to work, a recovery program must offer the individual addicted to alcohol ways to increase self-esteem and resume personal growth.

✳ SMOKING

Health consequences of the tobacco epidemic in developed and developing countries are devastating. By 2020, tobacco use is expected to kill more people than any single disease. Since the middle of the twentieth century, tobacco products have killed more than 60 million people in developed countries alone.[38]

Canadians have been smoking less since 1966, when 54 percent of men and 28 percent of women were smokers. The Canadian Tobacco Use Monitoring Survey reported (from data collected between February and June 2008) that slightly more than 4.9 million Canadians were current smokers, representing 18 percent of the population 15 years of age and older.[39] More men than women smoke (20 versus 16 percent). Thirteen percent of Canadians report smoking daily and another 5 percent report occasional smoking. Daily smokers consume, on average, 15 cigarettes per day. In the 15- to 19-year-old group, 15 percent reported smoking; 8 percent reported smoking daily, with an average of 11.3 cigarettes. Seven percent of 15- to 19-year-olds were occasional smokers. In the 20- to 24-year-old group, 19 percent reported daily smoking, with another 9 percent reporting occasionally lighting up. In this age group, males who smoke daily consume more cigarettes per day than females (16.4 versus 9.6).[40]

Despite the reduced rate of smoking in the population, it remains the number one preventable cause of death in Canada. Every year, smoking kills five times more Canadians than car accidents, murder, suicide, and alcohol abuse combined. Deaths attributed to tobacco in 2002 totalled 37 209, or 16.6 percent of all deaths, while acute-care hospital days attributable to tobacco were 2 210 155, or 10.3 percent of all hospital days.[41]

inhaled, chewed, or placed against the gums. **Chewing tobacco**, also known as "smokeless tobacco," is placed between the gums and teeth for sucking or chewing.

The chemical stimulant nicotine is the major psychoactive substance in these products. In its natural form, **nicotine** is a colourless liquid that turns brown upon oxidation (exposure to oxygen). When tobacco leaves are burned in a cigarette, pipe, or cigar, nicotine is released and inhaled into the lungs. Sucking or chewing tobacco releases nicotine into the saliva, and is then absorbed through the mucous membranes in the mouth.

Smoking is the most common form of tobacco use. Smoking delivers a strong dose of nicotine to the user, along with an additional 5000 chemicals, 50 of which are known to cause cancer. Among these chemicals are various gases and vapours that carry particulate matter in concentrations that are 500 000 times as great as the most air-polluted cities in the world. Particulate matter condenses in the lungs to form a thick, brownish sludge called tar. **Tar** contains various carcinogenic (cancer-causing) agents such as benzopyrene and chemical irritants such as phenol. Phenol has the potential to combine with other chemicals to contribute to the development of lung cancer.

In healthy lungs, millions of tiny hairlike tissues called cilia sweep away foreign matter. Once the foreign material is swept up and collected by the cilia, it can be expelled from the lungs by coughing. Nicotine impairs the cleansing function of the cilia by paralyzing them for up to one hour following the smoking of a single cigarette. Tars and other solids in tobacco smoke are thus allowed to accumulate and irritate sensitive lung tissue.

Tar and nicotine are not the only harmful chemicals in cigarettes. In fact, tars account for only 8 percent of the components of tobacco smoke. The remaining 92 percent is made up of various gases, the most dangerous

what do you THINK?

What would it be like if Canada were smoke-free? Is your campus smoke-free? If not, what would it take to get it there? Has Canada and each of its provinces gone far enough to protect the rights of nonsmokers? Why or why not? What about smokers and their rights?

Tobacco and Its Effects

Tobacco is available in several forms. Cigarettes, cigars, and pipes are used for burning and inhaling tobacco. **Snuff** is a finely ground form of tobacco that can be

Delirium tremens (DTs): A state of confusion brought on by withdrawal from alcohol. Symptoms include hallucinations, anxiety, and trembling.

Alcoholics Anonymous (AA): An organization whose goal is to help individuals addicted to alcohol stop drinking; includes auxiliary branches such as Al-Anon and Alateen.

Snuff: A powdered form of tobacco sniffed and absorbed through the mucous membranes in the nose or placed inside the cheek and sucked.

Chewing tobacco: A stringy type of tobacco placed in the mouth and then sucked or chewed.

Nicotine: The stimulant chemical in tobacco products.

Tar: A thick, brownish substance condensed from particulate matter in smoked tobacco.

of which is **carbon monoxide**. In tobacco smoke, the concentration of carbon monoxide is 800 times higher than the level considered safe. In the human body, carbon monoxide reduces the oxygen-carrying capacity of the red blood cells by binding with the receptor sites for oxygen. Smoking thus diminishes the capacity of the circulatory system to carry oxygen, causing oxygen deprivation in many body tissues. The heat from tobacco smoke, which can reach 880°C, is also harmful to the smoker. Inhaling hot gases and vapours exposes sensitive mucous membranes to irritating chemicals that weaken the tissues and contribute to the development of cancers of the mouth, larynx, and throat.

Filtered cigarettes designed to reduce levels of gases such as hydrogen cyanide and hydrocarbons may actually deliver more hazardous carbon monoxide to the user than non-filtered brands. Some smokers use low-tar and nicotine products (that is, mild, special, or "lite") thinking these are safer forms of cigarettes. True, they contain 10 percent less carbon monoxide and 8 percent less nicotine, but they contain the same level of the other harmful chemicals. Furthermore, since there is less nicotine, smokers tend to inhale more deeply when smoking this kind of cigarette and actually inhale more of the dangerous chemicals than they would if they smoked regular cigarettes.

Clove cigarettes contain about 40 percent ground cloves (a spice) and about 60 percent tobacco. Many users mistakenly believe that these products are made entirely of ground cloves and that smoking them eliminates the risks associated with tobacco. In fact, clove cigarettes contain higher levels of tar, nicotine, and carbon monoxide than regular cigarettes. In addition, the numbing effect of eugenol, the active ingredient in cloves, allows smokers to inhale the smoke more deeply.

Nicotine is a powerful CNS stimulant that produces an aroused, alert mental state. Nicotine also stimulates the adrenal glands, increasing the production of adrenaline. The physical effects of nicotine stimulation include increased heart and respiratory rate, constriction of blood vessels, and subsequent increased blood pressure because the heart must work harder to pump blood through the narrowed vessels. Because smoking increases the "stickiness" of the blood, there is an increased risk of developing blood clots when you smoke. This risk is further elevated when smoking is combined with use of oral contraceptives.

Nicotine decreases the stomach contractions that signal hunger. It also decreases blood sugar levels. These factors, along with decreased sensation in the taste buds, reduce appetite. For this reason, many smokers eat less and weigh, on average, 3 kilograms less than nonsmokers. Beginning smokers usually feel the effects of nicotine with their first puff. These symptoms, called **nicotine poisoning**, include dizziness, lightheadedness, rapid, erratic pulse, clammy skin, nausea, vomiting, and diarrhea. The effects of nicotine poisoning cease when tolerance to the chemical develops. Medical research indicates that tolerance develops almost immediately in new users, perhaps after the second or third cigarette. In contrast, tolerance to most other drugs, such as alcohol, develops over a period of months or years.

❋ Smoking—A Learned Behaviour

Taking up smoking is a gradual process. It begins with forming a predisposition to smoking—that is, a perception that smoking is a normal behaviour accepted and pervasive in society or one's peer group. Smoking usually starts with an experimental stage when it happens repeatedly but irregularly; then regular use, followed by addiction. The transition from first experimenting with smoking to daily use usually takes an average of two to three years.

About 85 percent of smokers start before age 16. New smokers do not expect to become addicted, believing instead that they will be able to quit whenever they want to, discounting the prospect of addiction and the potential adverse health effects of that future addiction. Only 10 percent of smokers begin after the age of 18. It seems probable that the level of knowledge and experience acquired by age 18 relate to the decision not to start smoking.

Tobacco product promotions are intended to convey a positive brand image and convey as many "impressions" (exposures to the consumer) as possible in order to create and maintain the perception that tobacco use is desirable, socially acceptable, healthy, sexy, and more pervasive in society than it really is. These promotions are primarily directed to young people, particularly young women, partly because the tobacco companies know that most people make the decision as to whether or not to smoke by the age of 16.

This positive image of tobacco use is precisely the perception that people need in order to feel reassured about smoking. Promotion affects tobacco consumption in three interrelated ways:

- by influencing the smoking decision process among starters through helping to shape and reinforce their belief that it's okay to smoke

- by influencing the amount consumed by smokers

- by hindering the quitting decision process among those who are addicted by acting as a reassuring cue to smoke[42]

Smokeless Tobacco

Smokeless tobacco is just as addictive as cigarettes due to its nicotine content. Although there is nicotine in all tobacco products, smokeless tobacco contains more of the substance than cigarettes. An average-sized dip or chew held in your mouth for 30 minutes gives as much nicotine as smoking four cigarettes. Thus, a two-can-a-week snuff dipper gets as much nicotine as a one-and-a-half-pack-a-day smoker.

One of the major risks of chewing tobacco is **leukoplakia**, a condition characterized by leathery white patches inside the mouth produced by contact with irritants in tobacco juice. Smokeless tobacco also impairs the senses of taste and smell, causing the user to add salt and sugar to food, which may contribute to high blood pressure and obesity. Some smokeless tobacco products contain high levels of sodium (salt), which also contributes to high blood pressure. Another risk of using smokeless tobacco is caused by the addition of fibreglass to the tobacco, which helps cut the lining in the mouth to facilitate the uptake of nicotine by the bloodstream. In addition, dental problems are common among users: contact with tobacco juice causes receding gums, tooth decay, bad breath, and discoloured teeth. Damage to the teeth and jawbone can contribute to early loss of teeth. Users of all tobacco products may not be able to use the vitamins and other nutrients in food effectively. In some cases, vitamin supplements may be recommended by a physician.

This 25-year-old cancer survivor has undergone surgery to remove neck muscles, lymph nodes, and his tongue. He began using smokeless tobacco at age 13; by age 17, he was diagnosed with squamous cell carcinoma. He now speaks out about the dangers of smokeless tobacco.

what do you THINK?

Why do people use smokeless tobacco? Do you think the health risks of smokeless tobacco are well understood? Should smokeless tobacco be forbidden in public places just as cigarettes are banned? Why do you think chewing tobacco has attracted athletes? Do you think the use of smokeless tobacco should be banned in high school, college, and university athletics? Why or why not?

Environmental Tobacco Smoke

As the population of nonsmokers rises, so does the demand for the right to breathe clean air. As a result, smoking is banned in many public places, particularly those that are indoors.

Environmental tobacco smoke (ETS) is divided into two categories: mainstream smoke and second-hand smoke (also called sidestream smoke). **Mainstream smoke** refers to smoke drawn through tobacco while inhaling; **secondhand smoke** refers to smoke from the burning end of a cigarette and the smoke exhaled by a smoker. People who breathe smoke as a result of someone else's smoking are said to be involuntary or passive smokers.

Although involuntary smokers breathe less tobacco than active smokers, they still face risks from exposure to tobacco smoke. Secondhand smoke actually contains more carcinogenic substances than the smoke that a smoker inhales directly—about twice as much tar and nicotine, 5 times as much carbon monoxide, and 50 times as much ammonia. There is also evidence that secondhand smoke may pose an even greater risk for death due to heart disease than for

Carbon monoxide: A gas found in cigarette smoke that binds at oxygen receptor sites in the blood.

Nicotine poisoning: Symptoms often experienced by beginning smokers; they include dizziness; diarrhea; lightheadedness; rapid, erratic pulse; clammy skin; nausea; and vomiting.

Leukoplakia: A condition characterized by leathery white patches inside the mouth produced by contact with irritants in tobacco juice.

Environmental tobacco smoke (ETS): Smoke from tobacco products, including sidestream and mainstream smoke.

Mainstream smoke: Smoke drawn from a cigarette, cigar, or pipe while inhaling.

Secondhand smoke: Cigarette, pipe, or cigar smoke released into the air and inhaled by nonsmokers (as well as smokers).

Global anti-smoking efforts

Day by day, smoking is becoming a thing of the past in Canada. The number of smokers declines every year, in tandem with an increase in efforts by government and health activists to tighten up restrictions on the sale and use of tobacco.

Smoking has been banned from most offices for some time, but the bans have now extended to bars, restaurants and other public places. Some cities have banned indoor smoking outright, shutting down separate smoking rooms altogether.

Canada is considered to be at the forefront of anti-smoking legislation, but the rest of the world is beginning to catch up. Here's a sampler of homegrown and global anti-smoking measures:

Efforts in Canada

NEWFOUNDLAND AND LABRADOR

The province's Smoke-free Environment Act was amended on July 1, 2005, to ban smoking in all public places, including bars and bingo halls.

PRINCE EDWARD ISLAND

Without a specially ventilated smoking room, smokers are out of luck in public places and workplaces. Also, food can't be served in these rooms.

NOVA SCOTIA

Halifax regional council unanimously adopted a policy in October 2009 to restrict smoking at about 480 outdoor venues where children are present, such as parks, rinks and sports fields.

Smoking in public spaces was banned provincewide after Dec. 1, 2006, with a minimum fine of $2,000 for those who choose to light up. The only exceptions are designated rooms in nursing homes and long-term-care facilities.

Prominent displays of tobacco products in stores are also prohibited under the act.

Taxi cabs, bowling alleys, schoolyards and other public places were smoke-free as of Jan. 1, 2003. In bars and restaurants, smoking is restricted after 9 p.m. to an enclosed room that's separately ventilated and available only to adults. As well, tobacco can be seized from people under 19.

Nova Scotia has banned smoking in prison. In April 2008, the province also outlawed smoking in vehicles carrying children.

NEW BRUNSWICK

As of October 2004 there has been a provincewide ban on smoking in all public areas. Restaurants and bars can't have smoking sections or glassed-in smoking areas.

QUEBEC

All private designated smoking rooms were eliminated by May 30, 2008.

Restaurants, bars, clubs, bingo halls, casinos and shelters became smoke-free on May 31, 2006. Smoking is also forbidden within nine metres of any doorway leading to a health or social services institution, college, university or child-care facility.

A ban on smoking in all public places started in June 2006.

It's illegal to sell tobacco by mail order, over the internet, on school grounds or in health-care, social services or child-care facilities.

ONTARIO

Retail behind-counter displays of tobacco were banned after 2008. In 2009, Ontario also outlawed smoking in vehicles carrying children.

On June 1, 2006, the Smoke-Free Ontario Act prohibited smoking in all workplaces and enclosed spaces open to the public, except for private homes and hotel rooms.

In Toronto in 2004, all bars, pool halls, bingo halls, casinos, and racetracks became smoke-free, with fines ranging from $205 to $5,000. A plan to outlaw smoking rooms by 2005 was sent back to council for review.

The Northwestern (Ontario) Health Unit banned smoking in all public places and private businesses as of Jan. 1, 2003, with fines ranging from $5,000 to $25,000.

The City of Ottawa banned smoking in all workplaces and public spaces, with no allowance for designated smoking rooms, on Aug. 1, 2001.

It's illegal to sell tobacco at hospitals, psychiatric facilities, nursing homes, long-term-care facilities and charitable institutions.

MANITOBA

The Non-Smokers' Health Protection Act banned smoking in public areas, with the exception of group-living facilities and hotel rooms, as of October 2004. Restaurants and bars can't have smoking sections or glassed-in smoking areas.

As of January 2002, it became illegal to smoke in any indoor location in Winnipeg where minors are present. Some coffee shops and restaurants avoid this problem by banning children.

All public places in Winnipeg became smoke-free as of Sept. 1, 2003.

SASKATCHEWAN

Saskatchewan in 2009 outlawed in all enclosed places of employment, including offices, warehouses, vehicles and some mines.

On Jan. 19, 2005, the Supreme Court of Canada ruled the province could reinstate the "shower curtain law" that requires store owners to keep tobacco products out of sight.

As of January 2005, all public places, including outdoor areas and veterans' clubs, became smoke-free under the Tobacco Control Act, with fines of up to $10,000 for smokers who violate it.

Bingo parlours, bars, casinos, restaurants and bowling alleys after Dec. 31, 2002, were required to designate 40 per cent of their space as non-smoking. By 2004, this percentage increased to 60 per cent.

ALBERTA

The Smoke-free Places Act, effective January 2006, restricts smoking in public places and workplaces where minors are allowed. Casinos, bingo halls, and bars don't fall under these restrictions.

Some Albertan municipalities have enacted tougher bylaws, and Peace River, Stettler, Wainwright, Drumheller, Olds, Airdrie and Jasper are 100 per cent smoke-free in public places. Calgary banned all smoking in public places, including restaurants and bars, as of Jan. 1, 2007.

People under age 18 who are caught smoking or in possession of tobacco products after April 1, 2003, can be fined $100 and have their cigarettes seized.

In Edmonton, there has been no smoking in public places where children are served, except for lounges, since May 22, 2001.

BRITISH COLUMBIA

In 2009, British Columbia outlawed citizens from lighting a cigarette in a vehicle in the presence of a person under the age of 16. A province wide ban on smoking in public places began in 2008.

You can't smoke in public places like restaurants, bars, bingo halls, bowling alleys and casinos. Restaurant and bar owners may construct open smoking rooms where staff may volunteer to serve.

Victoria banned smoking in all workplaces and public spaces, with no allowance for designated smoking rooms, as of Aug. 1, 2001.

YUKON

In May 2008, the Yukon became the last of the provinces and territories to ban smoking in public places.

NORTHWEST TERRITORIES

In March 2006, legislation was passed confirming and enforcing the Workers Compensation ban on smoking in workplaces.

The Workers Compensation Board bans smoking in all enclosed businesses and work sites on May 1, 2004, including bars. Smoking rooms are only allowed in workplaces that are private residences.

NUNAVUT

Smoking was banned in all enclosed businesses and work sites on May 1, 2004, by the Workers Compensation Board. This includes bars. It also bans smoking within 15 metres of schools and three metres of entrances.

Source: CBC.CA

death due to lung cancer.[43] Secondhand smoke is estimated to cause more deaths per year than any other environmental pollutant.[44]

Lung cancer and heart disease are not the only risks involuntary smokers face. Children exposed to secondhand smoke also have a greater chance of developing other respiratory problems, such as cough, wheezing, asthma, and chest colds, along with a decrease in pulmonary performance. The greatest effects of secondhand smoke are seen in children under the age of five.

Cigarette, cigar, and pipe smoke in enclosed areas present other hazards to nonsmokers. The level of carbon monoxide from cigarette smoke contained in enclosed places is 4000 times higher than the standard recommended by the US Environmental Protection Agency for a definition of clean air. An estimated 10 to 15 percent of nonsmokers are extremely sensitive (hypersensitive) to cigarette smoke.[45] These people experience itchy eyes, difficulty breathing, painful headaches, nausea, and dizziness in response to minute amounts of smoke.

Efforts to reduce the hazards associated with passive smoking have been gaining momentum in recent years. As previously mentioned, smoking is now illegal in most public places, including government buildings, restaurants, cafés, coffee shops, shopping malls, schools, and universities. Hotels and motels, if not completely smoke-free, set aside rooms for nonsmokers, and car rental agencies designate certain vehicles for nonsmokers. Smoking has also been banned for some time on all domestic airline flights. Recently, some regions have declared vehicles containing children under the age of 18 years to be smoke-free as well. (See the Building Communication Skills box.)

QUITTING

From what we know about smoking cessation and the various programs that have developed to support people in their efforts, quitting is often a lengthy process involving several unsuccessful attempts before success is finally achieved. Even successful quitters suffer occasional slips, emphasizing the fact that quitting smoking is a dynamic process that may actually be never-ending.

Breaking the Nicotine Addiction

Nicotine addiction may be one of the toughest addictions to overcome. When smokers quit, **nicotine withdrawal** occurs; the symptoms of withdrawal include irritability, restlessness, nausea, vomiting, and intense cravings for tobacco. The person who quits has several options to manage the symptoms of withdrawal.

Nicotine Replacement Products

Non-tobacco products that put nicotine in the bloodstream have helped some people stop using tobacco. The two most common nicotine-replacement products are nicotine chewing gum and the nicotine patch, both available by prescription. Some individuals use a prescription chewing gum containing nicotine, called Nicorette, to help with the withdrawal symptoms by reducing their nicotine consumption gradually over time. Under the guidance of a physician, the individual chews between 12 and 24 pieces of gum per day for up to six months, with a plan for reducing consumption over time. Nicorette delivers about as much nicotine as a cigarette, but because it is absorbed through the mucous membrane of the mouth, it does not produce the same rush as the nicotine that is inhaled from a cigarette. As a result, the individual who stopped smoking does not experience withdrawal symptoms, and fewer cravings for nicotine are felt as the dosage is reduced until the person is completely weaned. There is some controversy surrounding the use of nicotine replacement gum. Opponents believe that it substitutes one addiction for another. Successful quitters counter that it is a valid way to help break a deadly habit without suffering the unpleasant withdrawal symptoms and cravings that often lead ex-smokers to resume smoking.

The nicotine patch, first marketed in 1991, is a popular method for those attempting to quit smoking. It is generally used in conjunction with a comprehensive smoking-behaviour cessation program. A small, thin patch is placed on the smoker's upper body to deliver a continuous flow of nicotine through the skin for 24-hours, helping to relieve the body's cravings for nicotine. The patch is worn for 8 to 12 weeks under the guidance of a physician. During this time, the dose of nicotine in the patch is gradually reduced until the smoker is fully weaned from nicotine. Occasional side-effects include mild skin irritation, insomnia, dry mouth, and nervousness. The patch is relatively inexpensive compared to the price of a pack of cigarettes, and some insurance plans will pay for it.

Breaking the Habit

For many smokers, the road to quitting includes some type of antismoking therapy. Among the more common therapy techniques are aversion therapy, operant conditioning, and self-control therapy. Prospective quitters must decide which method or combination of methods will work best for them.

Nicotine withdrawal: Symptoms, including nausea, headaches, and irritability, suffered by smokers who cease using tobacco.

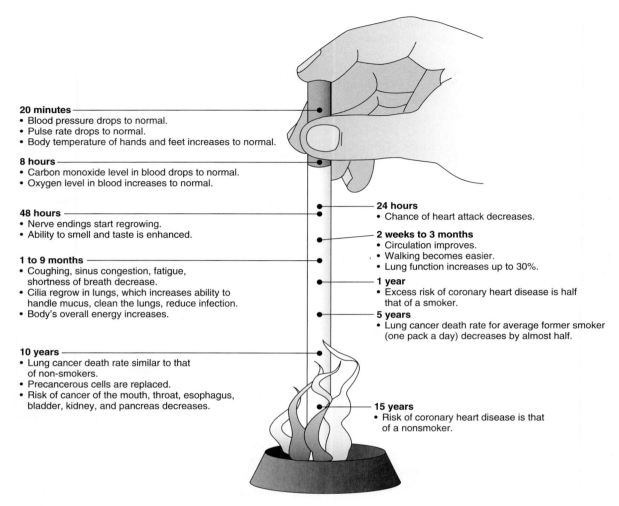

20 minutes
- Blood pressure drops to normal.
- Pulse rate drops to normal.
- Body temperature of hands and feet increases to normal.

8 hours
- Carbon monoxide level in blood drops to normal.
- Oxygen level in blood increases to normal.

48 hours
- Nerve endings start regrowing.
- Ability to smell and taste is enhanced.

1 to 9 months
- Coughing, sinus congestion, fatigue, shortness of breath decrease.
- Cilia regrow in lungs, which increases ability to handle mucus, clean the lungs, reduce infection.
- Body's overall energy increases.

10 years
- Lung cancer death rate similar to that of non-smokers.
- Precancerous cells are replaced.
- Risk of cancer of the mouth, throat, esophagus, bladder, kidney, and pancreas decreases.

24 hours
- Chance of heart attack decreases.

2 weeks to 3 months
- Circulation improves.
- Walking becomes easier.
- Lung function increases up to 30%.

1 year
- Excess risk of coronary heart disease is half that of a smoker.

5 years
- Lung cancer death rate for average former smoker (one pack a day) decreases by almost half.

15 years
- Risk of coronary heart disease is that of a nonsmoker.

FIGURE 10.1

When Smokers Quit

Within 20 minutes of smoking cessation, the body begins a series of changes that continues for years.

Source: G. Hanson and P. Venturelli, *Drugs and Society,* 5th ed. (Sudbury, MA: Jones and Bartlett, 1998), 320 © Jones and Bartlett, www.jbpub.com. Reprinted with permission.

Programs that combine several approaches have shown the most promise.

Benefits of Quitting

Many tissues damaged by smoking can repair themselves. As soon as smokers stop, their bodies begin the repair process. Within eight hours, carbon monoxide and oxygen levels return to normal, and "smoker's breath" disappears. Within a few days of quitting, the mucus clogging airways is broken up and eliminated. Circulation and the senses of taste and smell improve within weeks. Many ex-smokers who have kicked the cigarette habit say they have more energy, sleep better, and feel more alert. By the end of one year, the risk for lung cancer and stroke decreases. Within two years, the risk for heart attack drops to near-normal. At the end of 10 smoke-free years, the ex-smoker can expect to live out his or her normal life span. Figure 10.1 shows the health benefits of quitting smoking.

what do you THINK?

What could you do to help someone quit smoking? What are the most common barriers to quitting? When trying to stop smoking, why do people often interpret a relapse as a total failure? Alternatively, how could a relapse be viewed?

✱ CAFFEINE

Caffeine is the most popular and widely consumed drug in Canada. Almost half of Canadians drink coffee every day, and many others consume caffeine in some other form (tea, colas, chocolate), mainly for its well-known "wake-up" effect. Drinking coffee is legal and socially encouraged. Many people believe caffeine is not a drug and is not really addictive. Coffee and other caffeine-containing products seem harmless. If you share these attitudes, think again; research links caffeine to several health problems. **Caffeine** is a drug derived from the chemical family called **xanthines**. Two related chemicals, theophylline and theobromine, are found in tea and chocolate, respectively. Xanthines are mild CNS stimulants that enhance mental alertness and reduce feelings of fatigue. Other stimulant effects include increases in heart muscle contractions, oxygen consumption, metabolism, and urinary output. These effects are felt within 15 to 45 minutes of ingesting a product that contains caffeine.

Side effects of xanthines include wakefulness, insomnia, irregular heartbeat, dizziness, nausea, indigestion, and sometimes mild delirium. Some people also experience heartburn. As with other drugs, the user's psychological outlook and expectations will influence the effects. Different products contain different concentrations of caffeine. A 156-mL (5-ounce) cup of coffee contains 65 to 115 milligrams. Caffeine concentrations vary with the brand and strength of the brew. Small chocolate bars (28 grams) contain up to 15 milligrams of caffeine and theobromine. Table 10.4 outlines the caffeine content of various products.

✱ Caffeine Addiction

As the effects of caffeine wear off, users may feel let down—mentally or physically depressed, tired, and weak. To counteract this, people commonly choose to drink another cup of coffee. Habitually engaging in this practice leads to tolerance and psychological dependency. Until the mid-1970s, caffeine was not medically recognized as addictive. Chronic caffeine use and its attendant behaviours were called "coffee nerves." This syndrome is now recognized as caffeine intoxication, or **caffeinism**. Symptoms of caffeinism include chronic insomnia, jitters, irritability, nervousness, anxiety, and involuntary muscle twitches. Withdrawing the caffeine may compound the effects and produce severe headaches. (Some physicians ask their patients to take a simple test for caffeine addiction: do not consume anything containing caffeine, and if you get a severe headache within four hours, you are addicted and experiencing withdrawal symptoms.) Because caffeine meets the requirements for addiction—tolerance,

TABLE 10.4
Caffeine Content of Various Products

Product	Caffeine Content (average mg per serving)
Coffee (156-mL cup)	
Regular brewed	65–115
Decaffeinated brewed	3
Decaffeinated instant	2
Tea (175-mL cup)	
Hot steeped	36
Iced	31
Bottled (375 mL)	15
Soft drinks (375-mL serving)	
Jolt Cola	100
Dr. Pepper	61
Mountain Dew	54
Coca-Cola	46
Pepsi	36–38
Chocolate	
28 grams baking chocolate	25
28 grams chocolate candy bar	15
1/2 cup chocolate pudding	4–12
Over-the-counter drugs	
No Doz (2 tablets)	200
Excedrin (2 tablets)	130
Midol (2 tablets)	65
Anacin (2 tablets)	64

Source: Office of Department of Health and Welfare, October 2001.

Caffeine: A stimulant found in coffee, tea, chocolate, and some soft drinks.

Xanthines: The chemical family of stimulants to which caffeine belongs.

Caffeinism: Caffeine intoxication brought on by excessive caffeine use; symptoms include chronic insomnia, irritability, anxiety, muscle twitches, and headaches.

psychological dependency, and withdrawal symptoms—it can be classified as addictive. Although you would have to drink 67 to 100 cups of coffee in a day to produce a fatal overdose of caffeine, you may experience sensory disturbances after consuming only 10 cups of coffee within a 24-hour period. These symptoms include tinnitus (ringing in the ears), spots before the eyes, numbness in arms and legs, poor circulation, and visual hallucinations. Because 10 cups of coffee is not an extraordinary amount to drink in one day, caffeine use clearly poses health threats.

The Health Consequences of Long-Term Caffeine Use

Long-term caffeine use has been suspected of being linked to a number of serious health problems, ranging from heart disease and cancer to mental dysfunction and birth defects. Further, high consumption (more than six cups of coffee) of unfiltered coffees such as French press and boiled/perked coffee are linked to elevated low-density-lipoprotein concentrations.[46] However, no strong evidence exists to suggest that moderate caffeine use (less than 300 milligrams daily, approximately three cups of coffee) produces harmful effects in healthy, nonpregnant people. In fact, there may be some benefit to frequent moderate consumption of coffee—whether decaffeinated or caffeinated—in terms of reducing risk for type 2 diabetes, though more research is warranted to better understand the mechanisms providing this benefit.[47] Coffee and other products containing caffeine also have potential benefits as ergogenic aids, facilitating athletic performances and potentially positively altering carbohydrate and fat metabolism during exercise.[48]

It appears that caffeine does not cause long-term high blood pressure and is not linked to strokes; nor is there any evidence of a relationship between caffeine and heart disease. However, people who suffer from irregular heartbeat are cautioned against using caffeine because the resultant increase in heart rate might be life-threatening. Both decaffeinated and caffeinated coffee products contain ingredients that can irritate the stomach lining and be harmful to people with stomach ulcers. For years, caffeine consumption was linked with fibrocystic breast disease, a condition characterized by painful, noncancerous lumps in the breasts. Although these conclusions have been challenged, many clinicians advise patients with mammillary cysts to avoid or limit their caffeine use.

PEARSON
myhealthlab

Go to MyHealthLab at **www.pearsoned.ca/myhealthlab**. Here you will find self-assessments, case studies, links to health on the net, and much more.

DISCUSSION QUESTIONS

1. When it comes to drinking alcohol, how much is too much? How often is too often? How can you control your consumption of alcohol so that you do not drink too much or too often?

2. What factors may cause someone to progress from being a social drinker to becoming addicted to alcohol? What effect does alcoholism have on the family of the person who becomes addicted?

3. Describe your campus culture regarding alcohol. Create a video/commercial that portrays this culture and the risks associated with it.

4. Discuss the varied forms in which you can ingest tobacco. In each form, how do chemicals enter your system? What are the physiological effects of nicotine?

5. Discuss the risks of smokeless tobacco. Do you think that smokeless tobacco should be banned from all levels of sport? Why or why not?

6. People who smoke often claim they have the right to smoke in public places. From what you have learned about secondhand smoke, how would you argue against an individual's right to smoke in public?

7. Do you drink coffee or other beverages that contain caffeine? Do you limit your consumption of these beverages? Why or why not? Are you addicted to caffeine? How could you find out? What are the risks of caffeine addiction or excessive caffeine consumption?

8. Describe the health risks and potential benefits of coffee and caffeine consumption.

APPLICATION EXERCISE

Reread the "Consider This . . ." scenario at the beginning of the chapter and answer the following questions.

1. What responsibility do the restaurant owner and employees have for protecting the fetus?

2. What responsibility does the mother have for protecting her fetus?

3. If you were the waiter/waitress, what would you do?

MYSEARCHLAB EXERCISE

1. Log on to www.MySearchLab.com.

2. Retrieve article AN 36236940, "Factors That Predict Self-Perceived Problem Drinking among College Students," by E. E. Eshbaugh.

3. Respond to the following questions:

   a. Why do you think most students are not able to identify their own risky behaviours regarding alcohol consumption—that is, drinking more than four (for a female) or five (for a male) drinks on one occasion?

   b. What are the risks of binge drinking? Consider all components of health and wellness.

   c. How might students on your campus be convinced that a moderate consumption of alcohol should be the norm, not the exception?

CHAPTER 11

CARDIOVASCULAR DISEASE, DIABETES, AND CANCER

Reducing Your Risks

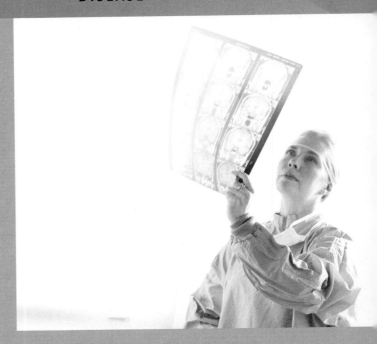

CONSIDER THIS . . .

Kassandra is an avid sunbather. She thinks the glow of a tan makes her look healthy and attractive. In fact, when she cannot get the tan she desires from the sun, she spends time in a tanning bed. This year, she has decided to get a jump on her tan and is studying for her final exams outside under the sun every minute she can. In her efforts to get tanned as quickly as possible, she has decided to not wear sunscreen.

How many others like Kassandra do you know? What is the risk of suntanning—under the sun or in tanning beds? What will it take to change the attitude that a suntan makes a person look healthy and attractive? What can a person do to reduce his or her risk of developing skin cancer? What do you know about sunscreen and how and when to apply it?

CHAPTER OBJECTIVES

- Describe the anatomy and physiology of the heart and the circulatory system.

- Identify the various types of heart disease and the risk factors for developing them.

- Describe the symptoms, causes, and risk factors of diabetes.

- Identify the various types of cancer and the risk factors for developing it.

- Explain the importance of lifestyle choices in preventing heart disease, type 2 diabetes, and cancer.

Heart disease and cancer continue to be the two leading causes of death in Canada. Increasing dramatically in prevalence is type 2 diabetes, with significant personal and societal consequences. Not surprisingly, the actions you take today have a significant impact on reducing your risk for these diseases now and in the future.

CARDIOVASCULAR DISEASES

Cardiovascular disease (CVD) is a class of diseases of the heart and blood vessels, which are the leading cause of death worldwide.[1] In Canada, CVD account for more than 32 percent of all deaths.[2] This mortality (that is, death) rate for CVD has decreased from 47 percent in 1979.

How do health experts account for this decline? There are no simple answers. Advances in medical techniques, earlier and better diagnostic procedures and treatments, better emergency medical assistance programs, and training of people in cardiopulmonary resuscitation (CPR) have greatly aided individuals with CVD. Refinements in surgical techniques and improvements in heart transplants and artificial heart devices have enabled many to live longer lives. Despite these medical advances in treatment of CVD, the onus remains on the individual for prevention, since 80 percent of premature deaths from CVD could be prevented through a healthy dietary intake, regular physical activity, and avoiding tobacco.[3] More specifically, you can reduce your risk for CVD by controlling high blood pressure and reducing your dietary intake of saturated fats and cholesterol. By maintaining your weight, decreasing your sodium intake, engaging in regular physical activity, and changing your lifestyle to reduce your stress response, you can lower your blood pressure. You can also monitor the levels of fat and cholesterol in your blood and adjust your dietary intake to prevent your arteries from becoming clogged. Understanding how your cardiovascular system works will help you to understand your risks for CVDs and what can be done to reduce these risks.

try it NOW!
Learn about your risk of developing CVD!

Right now, you can find out about your likelihood of developing CVD and take steps to modify your risk. The Heart and Stroke Foundation has a website with various online tools that identify individual risk. Visit: www.heartandstroke.com and click on "risk assessment."

UNDERSTANDING YOUR CARDIOVASCULAR SYSTEM

The **cardiovascular system** refers specifically to the network of elastic tubes through which blood flows as it carries oxygen and nutrients to all parts of the body. It includes the heart, lungs, arteries, arterioles (small arteries), and capillaries (minute blood vessels). It also includes venules (small veins) and veins, the blood vessels though which blood flows as it returns to the heart and lungs.[4]

Under normal circumstances, the human body contains approximately six litres of blood. This blood transports nutrients, oxygen, waste products, hormones, and enzymes throughout the body. It also regulates body temperature, cellular water levels, and acidity levels of body components, and aids in bodily defence against toxins and harmful microorganisms. An adequate blood supply is essential to health and well-being.

How does the heart ensure that blood is constantly recirculated to body parts? The four chambers of the heart work together to deliver oxygenated blood where it is needed and to remove carbon dioxide (see Figure 11.1).

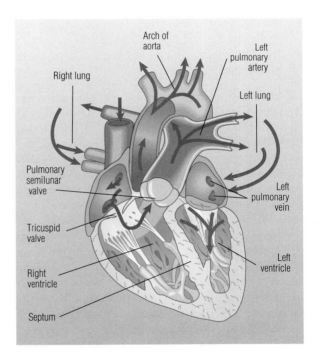

FIGURE 11.1
Anatomy of the Heart

Cardiovascular diseases (CVD): Diseases of the heart and blood vessels.

Cardiovascular system: A complex system comprising the heart and blood vessels that transports nutrients, oxygen, hormones, and enzymes throughout the body and regulates temperature, the water levels of cells, and the acidity levels of body components.

The two upper chambers of the heart, called **atria**, or auricles, are large collecting chambers that receive blood from the rest of the body. The two lower chambers, known as **ventricles**, pump the blood out again. Small valves regulate the steady, rhythmic flow of blood between chambers and prevent inappropriate backwash. The tricuspid valve, located between the right atrium and the right ventricle, the pulmonary (pulmonic) valve, between the right ventricle and the pulmonary artery, the mitral valve, between the left atrium and left ventricle, and the aortic valve, between the left ventricle and the aorta, allow blood to flow in only one direction.[5]

Heart activity depends on a complex interaction of biochemical, physiological, and neurological signals. The following is a simplified version of the steps involved:

1. Deoxygenated blood enters the right atrium after circulating through the body.

2. From the right atrium, blood moves to the right ventricle and is pumped through the pulmonary artery to the lungs, where it receives oxygen.

3. Oxygenated blood from the lungs then returns to the left atrium of the heart.

4. Blood from the left atrium is forced into the left ventricle.

5. The left ventricle pumps blood through the aorta to the body.

Different types of blood vessels are required for different parts of this process. **Arteries** carry blood away from the heart—except for pulmonary arteries, which carry deoxygenated blood to the lungs, where they pick up oxygen and drop off carbon dioxide. As they branch off from the heart, the arteries divide into smaller blood vessels called **arterioles**, and then into even smaller blood vessels called capillaries.

Capillaries have thin walls that permit the exchange of oxygen, carbon dioxide, nutrients, and waste products with body cells. Carbon dioxide and waste products are transported to the lungs and kidneys through **veins** and venules (small veins).

For the heart to function properly, the four chambers must beat in an organized manner. This is governed by an electrical impulse that directs the heart muscle to move when the impulse moves across it, resulting in a sequential contraction of the four chambers. This signal starts in a small bundle of highly specialized cells, the **sinoatrial node (SA node)**, located in the right atrium. The SA node serves as a form of natural pacemaker for the heart.[6] People with damaged or nonfunctional natural pacemaker activity have a mechanical pacemaker inserted to ensure the smooth passage of blood through the sequential phases of the heartbeat.

At rest, the average adult heart beats 70 to 80 times per minute. A woman's resting heart rate tends to be slightly higher than a man's. A person's heart with a high level of physical fitness beats about 50 to 60 times per minute (see Chapter 4). To supply the working muscles with the nutrients they need, the heart beats harder when engaged in physical activity. When the mind and body experience severe stress, the heart may beat over 200 times per minute, particularly in an individual who is overweight and/or with a low level of physical fitness. A healthy heart functions more efficiently and is better able to accommodate to overwork than an unhealthy one.

TYPES OF CARDIOVASCULAR DISEASES

Although most of us associate CVD with heart attacks, there are a number of different types. The four most common forms include:

*   atherosclerosis (characterized by deposits of plaque in the inner lining of the arteries)

*   coronary heart disease (a result of atherosclerotic plaque building up in the arteries such that coronary artery blood flow is reduced; when the blood flow is severely restricted or blocked a heart attack [myocardial infarction] results; when the blood flow is reduced [approximately 75 percent], but not blocked, chest pain [angina pectoris] often occurs)

*   stroke (cerebrovascular accident that occurs as a result of reduced blood supply to the brain)

*   hypertension (chronic high blood pressure)

Other less common forms of CVD include irregular heartbeat (arrhythmia), congestive heart failure, and congenital and rheumatic heart disease.

Irrespective of lifestyle behaviours, some individuals are at a greater risk than others for CVD.[7] Generally, risk increases with age; men are at a greater risk than women, and individuals of African, South Asian, and First Nations descent are at greater risk than other ethnicities. Others are at risk because of their lifestyle choices. These will be discussed later in this chapter.

Atherosclerosis

Atherosclerosis is a type of arteriosclerosis. **Arteriosclerosis** is a general term for the narrowing or "hardening" of the arteries. The end result of arteriosclerosis is reduced blood flow to vital organs. Atherosclerosis is characterized by deposits of fatty substances, cholesterol, cellular waste products, calcium, and fibrin (a clotting material in the blood) in the inner lining of an artery. The resulting build-up is referred to as atherosclerotic **plaque**.[8] Plaque may partially or totally block the blood's flow through an artery. When plaque develops, two things can happen: (1) bleeding (hemorrhage) into the plaque or (2) formation of a blood clot (thrombus) on the plaque's surface. If either of these occurs and an artery is blocked, the chances of a heart attack or stroke increase.[9]

Atherosclerosis does not suddenly occur. In fact, evidence suggests that atherosclerotic plaque begins to form in the womb, and worsens as the years pass. As such, atherosclerosis is not an all-or-nothing disease but occurs in varying degrees. Further, there are lifestyle choices individuals make in regard to physical activity and dietary intake that significantly influence the amount of plaque that develops. If the arteries are occluded (blocked with plaque) to about 75 percent in the heart, angina pectoris (chest pain) results. When the arteries are 90 to 95 percent occluded and a blood clot attempts to travel through them, a myocardial infarction (heart attack) or ischemic stroke (if the blood clot is in occluded arteries in the brain) occurs.

The process of plaque buildup begins when the protective inner lining of the artery (endothelium) becomes damaged, allowing fat, cholesterol, and other substances in the blood to affix to the arterial walls, eventually obstructing blood flow. The three major causes of such damage are (1) dramatic fluctuations in blood pressure, (2) elevated levels of cholesterol, triglycerides, and glucose in the blood, and (3) cigarette smoking. Viral infections may also be contributing factors. Cigarette smoke aggravates and speeds up the development of atherosclerosis, particularly in the coronary arteries, the aorta, and the arteries of the legs because of the damage caused to the inner arterial walls.[10]

what do you THINK?

Did you know that deposits of atherosclerotic plaque are likely forming in your arteries right now? Do you know your cholesterol and triglyceride levels? Do you know your blood pressure? Have your parents or grandparents been diagnosed with high cholesterol or high blood pressure? What actions should you take to reduce your risk for atherosclerosis?

Coronary Heart Disease

Coronary heart disease (CHD), also called coronary artery disease, is the major disease of the cardiovascular system. It is the result of atherosclerotic plaque accumulation such that a blockage occurs in one or more of the coronary arteries and blood flow is impeded. As previously mentioned, chest pain or angina pectoris results when the blockage is equivalent to 75 percent or more while complete blockage results in a heart attack.

A **heart attack**, or **myocardial infarction**, involves a blockage of the normal blood supply to an area of the heart. This condition is often brought on by a **coronary thrombosis**, or blood clot in the coronary artery. When blood does not flow readily, there is a corresponding decrease in oxygen flow. The most common symptoms of a heart attack include

- uncomfortable pressure or pain in chest lasting more than a few seconds
- mild to intense pain spreading to the shoulders, neck, or arms
- lightheadedness, fainting, sweating, nausea, or shortness of breath
- anxiety, nervousness, and/or cold, sweaty skin
- paleness or pallor
- increased or irregular heart rate
- feeling of impending doom

Atria: The two upper chambers of the heart, which receive blood.

Ventricles: The two lower chambers of the heart, which pump blood through the blood vessels.

Arteries: Vessels that carry blood away from the heart.

Arterioles: Small arteries.

Capillaries: Minute blood vessels that branch out from the arterioles; through which the exchange of oxygen, carbon dioxide, nutrients, and waste products happens.

Veins: Vessels that carry blood back to the heart.

Sinoatrial node (SA node): Node serving as a form of natural pacemaker for the heart.

Arteriosclerosis: Refers to narrowing and hardening of the arteries.

Atherosclerosis: A type of arteriosclerosis characterized by plaque deposits in the inner lining of arteries.

Plaque: Combination of fatty substances, cholesterol, cellular waste products, calcium, and fibrin.

Heart attack or **Myocardial infarction:** A blood clot that prevents blood from flowing through the heart.

Coronary thrombosis: A blood clot in a coronary artery.

Because 40 percent of heart attack victims die within the first two hours, immediate attention is vital to the patient's survival.

Since many women do not experience the symptoms above, in women the following may be indicative of a heart attack: unusual fatigue, shortness of breath, and sleep disturbances.

If the heart blockage is extremely minor, the otherwise healthy heart will adapt over time by using small unused or underused blood vessels to reroute the needed blood. This system, known as **collateral circulation**, is a form of self-preservation that allows a damaged heart muscle to heal itself. When heart blockage is more severe, the body is unable to adapt on its own and outside lifesaving support is critical. The two hours following a heart attack are believed to be the most critical period for treatment; more than 40 percent of heart attack victims die within this time.[11] Following this time period, 12 percent of Canadians who experience a heart attack die within 30 days. Long-term survival after 30 days reaches 91 to 93 percent.[12]

It is believed that normal nonatherosclerotic arteries can also go into spasm and cause circulatory impairment. Excessive calcium and potassium are among the suspected causes of these spasms.

As a result of atherosclerosis and other circulatory impairments, the heart's oxygen supply is often reduced, a condition known as ischemia. Individuals with **ischemia** often suffer from varying degrees of **angina pectoris** or chest pains. Many of these individuals experience short episodes of angina when they exert themselves physically. Symptoms of angina range from a slight feeling of indigestion to a feeling that the heart is being crushed. Generally, the more serious the oxygen deprivation, the more severe the pain.

Currently, several methods of treating angina are available. In mild cases, rest is critical. The most common treatments for more severe cases involve using drugs that affect (1) the supply of blood to the heart muscle or (2) the heart's demand for oxygen. Pain and discomfort are often relieved with nitroglycerin, a drug used to relax (dilate) veins, thereby reducing the amount of blood returning to the heart and thus lessening its workload. Patients whose angina is caused by spasms of the coronary arteries are often given drugs called calcium channel blockers. These drugs prevent calcium atoms from passing through coronary arteries and causing heart contractions. They also appear to reduce blood pressure and to slow heart rates. **Beta blockers** are another major type of drug used to treat angina. The chemical action of beta blockers serves to control potential overactivity of the heart muscle.

When a stroke occurs, the result is the death of brain cells. Consequences of a stroke include speech impairment, memory loss, and loss of motor control. Although some strokes affect parts of the brain that regulate heart and lung function and result in death within minutes, others are mild and result in temporary dizziness or slight weakness or numbness. Mild strokes are called **transient ischemic attacks** and often indicate an impending major stroke. The key to surviving a stroke is to obtain medical treatment within three hours of the first symptom.[13] Although almost three-quarters of Canadians recognize at least one warning sign of stroke, only half would call 9-1-1 if they or someone they knew was experiencing the warning sign.[14] The most common symptoms include

- sudden weakness or numbness of the face, arm, or leg on one side of the body

- sudden dimness or loss of vision, particularly in only one eye

- loss of speech, or trouble talking or understanding speech
- sudden, severe headache with no known cause
- unexplained dizziness, unsteadiness, or sudden fall, especially with any of the previous symptoms

Stroke

Like the heart muscle, brain cells must have a continuous and adequate supply of oxygen in order to survive. A **stroke** (also called a cerebrovascular accident) occurs when the blood supply to the brain is cut off. Strokes (see Figure 11.2) may be caused by a **thrombus** (blood clot), an **embolus** (a wandering clot), or an **aneurysm** (a weakening in a blood vessel that causes it to bulge and, in severe cases, burst).

Hypertension

Hypertension or chronic high blood pressure is unique because it is a CVD itself, and a risk factor for CHD and stroke. When blood pressure is chronically elevated, the workload on the heart is greater, which may damage the heart's ability to pump blood effectively throughout the body and result in heart muscle damage.[15] High blood pressure may also damage the interior walls of the arteries, which facilitates atherosclerotic plaque accumulation.[16]

Sustained high blood pressure, or **hypertension**, that cannot be attributed to any specific cause is known as **essential hypertension**. Approximately 90 percent of all cases of high blood pressure fit this category. **Secondary hypertension** refers to high blood pressure caused by specific factors, such as kidney disease, obesity, or tumours of the adrenal glands.

Blood pressure is measured in two parts and is expressed as two numbers separated by a slash—for example, 120/80, or 120 over 80. Both values are measured in millimetres of mercury (mmHg). The first number refers to **systolic pressure**, or the pressure on the walls of the arteries when the heart contracts, pumping blood to the rest of the body. The second value refers to **diastolic pressure**, or the pressure on the arterial walls during the heart's relaxation phase. During this phase, blood re-enters the chambers of the heart, preparing for the next heartbeat. As shown in Table 11.1, a blood pressure reading of 120 over 80 mmHg is generally considered normal. Systolic values between 120 and 139 mmHg or diastolic values of 80 to 89 mmHg are usually considered pre-hypertensive, and a blood pressure reading greater than 140 over 90 mmHg is classified as hypertensive.[17] Research indicates that risk for CVD doubles for each increase of 20/10 mmHg above 115/75.[18]

Collateral circulation: Following the complete occlusion of a coronary artery, rerouting of needed blood through unused or underused blood vessels.

Ischemia: Insufficient blood flow relative to the demand of the tissue which results in a decrease in oxygen

Angina pectoris: Severe chest pain occurring as a result of reduced oxygen flow to the heart.

Beta blockers: A type of drug used to treat angina; controls potential overactivity of the heart muscle.

Transient ischemic attacks: Mild form of stroke; often an indicator of impending major stroke.

Stroke: Results when the blood supply to the brain is severely reduced or cut off.

Thrombus: Blood clot.

Embolus: Blood clot forced through the circulatory system.

Aneurysm: A weakened blood vessel that may bulge under pressure and, in severe cases, burst.

Hypertension: Chronic high blood pressure; 140/80 mmHg or greater.

Essential hypertension: Hypertension as a result of unknown causes.

Secondary hypertension: Hypertension as a result of another condition such as kidney disease, obesity, or tumours of the adrenal glands.

Systolic pressure: The upper number in the blood pressure fraction, refers to the pressure on the walls of the arteries when the heart contracts.

Diastolic pressure: The lower number in the blood pressure fraction, refers to pressure on the walls of the arteries during the relaxation phase of heart activity.

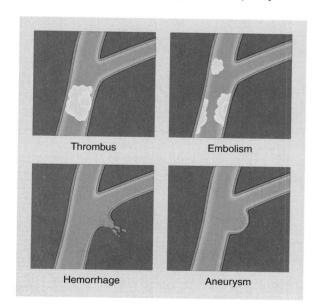

Thrombus

Embolism

Hemorrhage

Aneurysm

FIGURE 11.2
Common Blood Vessel Disorders

TABLE 11.1

Blood Pressure Classifications

Classification	Systolic Reading (mmHg)	Diastolic Reading (mmHg)
Normal	<120	<80
Prehypertension	120–139	80–89
Hypertension		
Stage 1	140–159	90–99
Stage 2	≥160	≥100

Note: If systolic and diastolic readings fall into different categories, treatment is determined by the highest category. Readings are based on the average of two or more properly measured, seated readings on each of two or more health care provider visits.

Source: National Heart, Lung, and Blood Institute, *The Seventh Report of the Joint National Committee on Prevention, Detection, Evaluation, and Treatment of High Blood Pressure* (NIH Publication No. 03-5233) (Bethesda, MD: National Institutes of Health, May 2003).

Arrhythmia, Congestive Heart Failure, and Congenital and Rheumatic Heart Disease

Arrhythmia refers to an irregular heartbeat. It may be suspected, for instance, when a person complains of a racing heart in the absence of physical activity or anxiety; *tachycardia* is the medical term for an abnormally fast heartbeat. On the other end of the continuum is *bradycardia*, or abnormally slow heartbeat. When a heart goes into **fibrillation**, it exhibits a sporadic, quivering pattern of beating resulting in extreme inefficiency in moving blood through the cardiovascular system. If untreated, this condition may be fatal. Not all arrhythmias are life-threatening. Excessive caffeine or nicotine consumption can trigger arrhythmia. For the most part, in the absence of other symptoms, arrhythmias are not serious. However, severe cases may require drug therapy or an external electrical stimulus to prevent further, more serious complications.

Congestive heart failure occurs when the heart muscle is damaged or overworked and lacks the strength to continue the blood circulating process. Individuals afflicted with rheumatic fever, pneumonia, or other cardiovascular problems in the past often have weakened heart muscles. In addition, the walls of the heart and the blood vessels may be damaged from previous radiation or chemotherapy treatments for cancer. These weakened muscles respond poorly when stressed; blood flow out of the heart is diminished, and the return flow of blood through the veins begins to back up, causing congestion in the tissues. This pooling of blood causes enlargement of the heart and decreases the amount of blood that can be circulated. Blood begins to accumulate in other body areas, such as in the vessels in the legs and ankles or the lungs, causing swelling or difficulty in breathing. If untreated, congestive heart failure results in death. Most cases respond well to diuretics (water pills) for relief of fluid accumulation, digitalis, a drug that increases the pumping action of the heart, and a vasodilator that expands blood vessels and decreases resistance, allowing blood to flow more easily, thus reducing the workload on the heart.

Approximately 1 out of every 125 children is born with some form of **congenital heart disease** (heart disease present at birth). These diseases range from slight murmurs caused by valve irregularities which some children outgrow, to serious complications in heart function that can only be corrected with surgery. The underlying causes of congenital heart diseases are unknown but believed to be related to hereditary factors; maternal diseases, such as German measles (rubella), occurring during fetal development; or chemical intake (particularly alcohol) by the mother during pregnancy. Due to advances in pediatric cardiology, the prognosis for children with congenital heart defects is better now than ever before.

Rheumatic heart disease is attributed to rheumatic fever, an inflammatory disease caused by an unresolved streptococcal infection of the throat ("strep throat") that may affect many connective tissues of the body, especially those of the heart, the joints, the brain, or the skin. In a small number of cases, the streptococcal infection can lead to an immune response in which antibodies attack the heart as well as the bacteria.

✳ CONTROLLING YOUR RISKS FOR CARDIOVASCULAR DISEASES

The four primary risk factors for CVD are high blood pressure (hypertension), high blood fats (hyperlipidemia), smoking, and physical inactivity. Secondary risk factors include, stress, obesity, and diabetes. These primary and secondary risk factors are primarily under your control. There are other risk factors, such as age, sex, ethnicity, and hereditary factors that you cannot control.

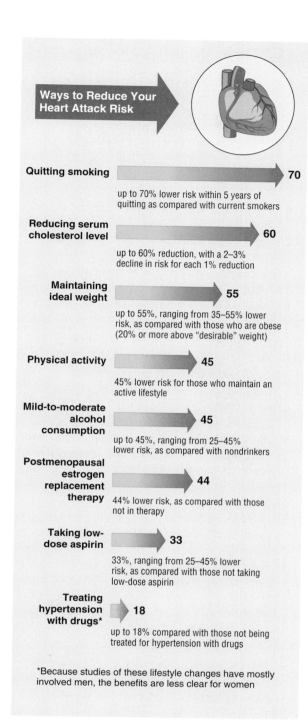

Ways to Reduce Your Heart Attack Risk

Quitting smoking — 70
up to 70% lower risk within 5 years of quitting as compared with current smokers

Reducing serum cholesterol level — 60
up to 60% reduction, with a 2–3% decline in risk for each 1% reduction

Maintaining ideal weight — 55
up to 55%, ranging from 35–55% lower risk, as compared with those who are obese (20% or more above "desirable" weight)

Physical activity — 45
45% lower risk for those who maintain an active lifestyle

Mild-to-moderate alcohol consumption — 45
up to 45%, ranging from 25–45% lower risk, as compared with nondrinkers

Postmenopausal estrogen replacement therapy — 44
44% lower risk, as compared with those not in therapy

Taking low-dose aspirin — 33
33%, ranging from 25–45% lower risk, as compared with those not taking low-dose aspirin

Treating hypertension with drugs* — 18
up to 18% compared with those not being treated for hypertension with drugs

Because studies of these lifestyle changes have mostly involved men, the benefits are less clear for women

FIGURE 11.3

Estimated Average Reduction in Risk for Heart Attack*

*Estimated risk reductions refer to the independent contribution of each risk factor to heart attack and do not address the wide range of known or hypothesized reactions among them.

Source: Adapted from information appearing in J. E. Mason, "Medical Progress: The Primary Prevention of Myocardial Infarction," *New England Journal of Medicine* 326 (May 21, 1992): 1406–1416.

Knowledge of the factors that contribute to CVD and how to make lifestyle changes that reduce your risk may motivate you to make the necessary health-promoting lifestyle changes. Figure 11.3 summarizes known ways to reduce your risk for heart attack. These risks have an elevated impact when combined. For example, if you have high blood pressure, high cholesterol, a family history of heart disease, and smoke cigarettes, you run a much greater risk of having a heart attack or other CVD than someone with only one risk. To assess your risks for heart disease, see the Rate Yourself box.

Risks You Can Control

✱ High Blood Pressure

As mentioned previously, high blood pressure (hypertension) is a unique risk factor for CHD because it is also a CVD itself. It is considered the leading risk for stroke and a major factor for heart disease.[19] In general, the higher your blood pressure, the greater your risk for CHD. High blood pressure is known as the "silent killer," because it usually has no symptoms. The latest data available from Statistics Canada (2005)[20] indicate that 14.9 percent of the population 12 years of age or older have been diagnosed by a health professional with high blood pressure. Overall, more women (15.7%) than men (14.1%) have been diagnosed, though this may relate to women living longer than men. Very few 12- to 19-year-olds (0.5 percent) or 20- to 34-year-olds (2.5 percent) have high blood pressure. In the 35- to 44-year-old age group, 6.6 percent have high blood pressure. Rates more than double in the 45- to 54-year-old age group, with 15.6 percent having high blood pressure. In the older age groups, rates of high blood pressure increase dramatically, with 29.8 percent of 55- to 64-year-olds, 42.3 percent of 65- to 74-year-olds and 46.6 percent of all individuals over the age of 75 having high blood pressure. After the age of 65, more females than males have high blood pressure, with the greatest difference noted in the over-75 group (50.8 versus 40.3 percent). Individuals of African and South Asian descent are not only three

Arrhythmia: An irregularity in heartbeat.

Fibrillation: A sporadic, quivering pattern of heartbeat resulting in inefficient moving of the blood.

Congestive heart failure: Occurs when the heart muscle is damaged or overworked and lacks the strength to maintain blood circulation.

Congenital heart disease: Heart disease present at birth.

Rheumatic heart disease: A heart disease caused by unresolved streptococcal infection of the throat.

Understanding Your Risk for CVD

Each of us has a unique level of risk for various diseases. Some of these risks you can take action to change; others are risks that you need to consider as you plan a lifelong strategy for overall risk reduction. Respond to each of the following, then total your points in each section. The higher your score, the greater your risk. If you answer "don't know" for any question, talk to your parents or other family members as soon as possible to find out if you have any unknown risks.

PART I: ASSESS YOUR FAMILY RISK FOR CVD

1. Do any of your primary relatives (mother, father, grand-parents, siblings) have a history of heart disease or stroke?

   Yes _____ (1 point) No_____ (0 points) Don't Know _____

2. Do any of your primary relatives (mother, father, grand-parents, siblings) have diabetes?

   Yes _____ (1 point) No_____ (0 points) Don't Know _____

3. Do any of your primary relatives (mother, father, grand-parents, siblings) have high blood pressure?

   Yes _____ (1 point) No_____ (0 points) Don't Know _____

4. Do any of your primary relatives (mother, father, grand-parents, siblings) have a history of high cholesterol?

   Yes _____ (1 point) No_____ (0 points) Don't Know _____

5. Would you say that your family consumed a high-fat diet (lots of red meat, dairy, butter/margarine) during your time spent at home?

   Yes _____ (1 point) No_____ (0 points) Don't Know _____

   Total _____

PART II: ASSESS YOUR LIFESTYLE RISK FOR CVD

1. Is your total cholesterol level higher than it should be?

   Yes _____ (1 point) No_____ (0 points) Don't Know _____

2. Do you have high blood pressure?

   Yes _____ (1 point) No_____ (0 points) Don't Know _____

3. Have you been diagnosed as prediabetic or diabetic?

   Yes _____ (1 point) No_____ (0 points) Don't Know _____

4. Do you smoke?

   Yes _____ (1 point) No_____ (0 points) Don't Know _____

5. Would you describe your life as being highly stressful?

   Yes _____ (1 point) No_____ (0 points) Don't Know _____

   Total _____

PART III: ASSESS YOUR ADDITIONAL RISKS FOR CVD

1. How would you best describe your current weight?

   a. Lower than what it should be for my height and weight (0 points)

   b. About what it should be for my height and weight (1 point)

   c. Higher than it should be for my height and weight (1 point)

2. How would you describe the level of exercise that you get each day?

   a. Less than what I should be exercising each day (1 point)

   b. About what I should be exercising each day (0 points)

   c. More than what I should be doing each day (0 points)

3. How would you describe your dietary behaviours?

   a. Eating only the recommended number of calories per day (0 points)

   b. Eating less than the recommended number of calories per day (0 points)

   c. Eating more than the recommended number of calories per day (1 point)

4. Which of the following best describes your typical dietary behaviours?

   a. I eat from the major food groups, trying hard to get the recommended amount of fruits and vegetables. (0 points)

   b. I eat too much red meat and consume too much saturated fat from meats and dairy products each day. (1 point)

   c. Whenever possible, I try to substitute olive oil or canola oil for other forms of dietary fat. (0 points)

5. Which of the following best describes you?

   a. I watch my sodium intake and try to reduce stress in my life. (0 points)

   b. I have a history of Chlamydia infection. (1 point)

   c. I try to eat 5 to 10 milligrams of soluble fibre each day and to substitute a soy product for an animal product in my diet at least once each week. (0 points)

   Total _____

Source: TOTAL FITNESS AND WELLNESS, 4th ed., by Scott K. Powers, Stephen L. Dodd and Virginia J. Noland. © 2006, pp. 277–278. Reprinted by permission of Pearson Education, Inc. Upper Saddle River, New Jersey.

Controlling the amount and type of fat you eat is one thing you can do to lower your risk for heart disease

times more likely to become hypertensive than the general population, but they are also more likely to develop the problem at younger ages.[21]

Normal blood pressure varies for different individuals, depending on weight, physical fitness, sex, and ethnicity. As previously mentioned, 120 over 80 mmHg is a normal blood pressure level and a blood pressure of 140/90 mmHg or greater is considered hypertensive. Recently, Canadian blood pressure guidelines suggested that a blood pressure of more than 135/85 measured at home may also indicate high blood pressure.[22] Further, these guidelines indicated that a blood pressure reading between 130/85 and 139/89 mmHg should be considered high-normal blood pressure. Currently it is estimated that more than 2.5 million Canadians have high-normal blood pressure and approximately 1 million of them will develop full-blown high blood pressure over the next four years.[23]

If your blood pressure exceeds 140 over 90, you should make lifestyle changes to lower it (engage in regular physical activity, eat healthily, manage your stress, and attain a healthy body weight). Regular aerobic exercise normally lowers blood pressure by 5 to 15 mmHg.[24] Controlling your sodium intake can also reduce your risk since it contributes to approximately 17 000 cases of stroke and heart disease in Canada each year.[25] Even though the average Canadian consumes more than 3100 mg of sodium per day, the adequate daily intake has been set at between 1200 and 1500 mg each day.[26] Since the majority of the sodium we consume comes from processed foods, reducing consumption of these would assist in lowering your intake. (See also Chapter 5.) If these lifestyle changes do not reduce your blood pressure to more normal values, you may need to take medication. Similarly, if your blood pressure is pre-hypertensive (that is, between 120/80 and 140/90), you should adjust your lifestyle in an attempt to lower your blood pressure to what is considered normal.

✳ Blood Fat and Cholesterol Levels

You do not actually consume LDLs or HDLs directly in your diet, rather a dietary intake high in saturated fats raises your LDL cholesterol levels. This sends the body's blood-clotting system into high gear, increasing the viscosity of the blood in just a few hours, which in turn increases risk for heart attack or stroke. A fatty diet also elevates the amount of cholesterol in the blood, contributing to atherosclerosis. Foods particularly high in saturated fat include coconut oil, palm kernel oil, butter, cream, whole milk, and beef. Regular physical activity, reducing saturated and trans fat intake, and increasing monounsaturated fat and omega-3 fat intakes can benefit your blood lipid profile and reduce risk for heart disease (see Chapter 5 for more details). A total cholesterol concentration of less than 5.2 millimoles per litre (mmol/L) or 200 milligrams per decilitre (mg/dL) indicates a low risk for heart disease, while values greater than 5.2 mmol/L (or 240 mg/dL) indicate high risk.[27] Values between 200 and 240 mg/dL are considered moderate risk.

Although risk values are established for total cholesterol, it is really the individual components that you need to be concerned about. **Low-density lipoproteins (LDLs)** are often referred to be "bad" cholesterol because they tend to build up or accumulate on artery walls. In contrast, **high-density lipoproteins (HDLs)** or "good" cholesterol remove cholesterol from artery walls, thus serving as a protector. In theory, if LDL levels get too high (greater than or equal to 3.4 mmol/L) or HDL levels too low (less than 0.9 mmol/L)—largely because of too much saturated fat in the diet, lack of physical activity, high stress, or genetic predisposition—cholesterol will accumulate on the arterial walls and lead to CVD. The goal then is to manage the ratio of HDL to total cholesterol by lowering LDLs or raising HDLs or both. Regular physical activity and a healthy dietary intake low in saturated and trans fat (see also Chapter 5 for more details) continue to be the best method for maintaining healthy ratios.

Triglycerides, the type of fat we normally consume, are also manufactured by our bodies. As people get older or fatter or both, their triglyceride and cholesterol levels tend to rise. According to the Heart and Stroke Foundation of Canada,[28] a triglyceride level greater than or equal to 2.3 mmol/L increases risk for CVD.

Low-density lipoproteins (LDLs): A combination of protein, triglycerides, and cholesterol in the blood that accumulate on arterial walls.

High-density lipoproteins (HDLs): A combination of protein, triglycerides, and cholesterol in the blood that facilitate the transport of LDLs to the liver for metabolism and elimination from the body.

Triglycerides: The most common form of fat in the body, consumed and manufactured in the body.

Obesity Link to Heart Disease Confirmed

Dr. Jean-Pierre Després, Director of Research Cardiology at Laval's University Hospital in Quebec, is a member of the International Day for Evaluation of Abdominal Obesity (IDEA) study, which examined the relationship of abdominal obesity to cardiovascular disease in 170 000 individuals in 63 countries. The results of this study confirmed that abdominal obesity, as measured by waist circumference in men and women, was associated with the presence of cardiovascular disease. More specifically, it was found that a 14- or 14.9-centimetre increase in waist circumference, in men and women respectively, increased the risk of cardiovascular disease from 21 to 40 percent. Furthermore, this study showed that a 16-year increase in age tripled the likelihood of an adult developing cardiovascular disease.

Dr. Després commented, "this is the first time a study of this magnitude has been conducted worldwide in a primary care population," and "these figures show that patients do not feel that having their waist measured is intrusive. The importance and the clinical significance of these results will stimulate initiation of additional studies that will aid us in identifying patients most at risk and help us to evaluate the impact that new treatments will have on the overall cardiometabolic risk of these patients."

Source: "Obesity Link to Heart Disease Confirmed," report by Jennifer Tryon, *Global National*, March 14, 2006: www.canada.com/nationalpost/news/story. html?id=5ee25c66-9c9b-4fe7-a05a-be485d60cddc$k=95067.

Cigarette Smoking

The link between cigarette smoking and heart disease has been firmly established. The risk for CVD is 70 percent greater for smokers than for nonsmokers. Further, the more a person smokes, the greater his or her risk of developing heart disease. Smokers who have a heart attack are more likely to die suddenly (within one hour) than non-smokers. Evidence also indicates that chronic exposure to environmental tobacco smoke (passive smoking or secondhand smoke) also increases risk of heart disease.[29] If the effects of smoking are combined with other risk factors, the danger is greater than the sum of the added effects.

Cigarette smoking increases the risk of heart disease in several ways. First, the drug nicotine, a central nervous system stimulant, increases heart rate, heart output, blood pressure, and oxygen use by heart muscles. In other words, nicotine causes the heart to work harder. Second, the carbon monoxide in cigarette smoke displaces oxygen in heart tissue, resulting in the heart being forced to work harder to get enough oxygen to the working tissues. Third, nicotine can lead to irregular heart rates (that is, arrhythmias) that may result in sudden death. Finally, cigarette smoke damages the lining of the arteries, allowing plaque to accumulate more easily. This additional accumulation constricts the vessels, increasing blood pressure and forcing the heart to work harder.

Physical Inactivity

Inactivity is another primary risk factor for CVD. The good news is that you don't have to be an exercise fanatic to reduce your risk for CVD. Even moderate levels of low-intensity physical activity are beneficial if done regularly and on a long-term basis. Such activities include walking for pleasure, gardening, housework, and dancing. See also Chapter 4 for more appropriate physical activity suggestions.

Engaging in physical activity on a regular basis reduces risk for heart disease in a number of ways. First, physical activity of a sufficient intensity strengthens the heart, improves circulation, and improves your blood profile by increasing HDLs. Because of the increases in HDL, there is a reduced level of atherosclerotic plaque development. Third, physical activity plays an important role in reducing hypertension, maintaining body weight, and managing and preventing the stress response.

Obesity

Obesity also may increase risk for CVD. A body with excessive fat causes strain to the heart in its efforts to push blood through the many kilometres of capillaries that supply each kilogram of fat with needed nutrients. As such, people who are overweight or obese and sedentary are more likely to develop heart disease and stroke even if they have no other risk factors. Moreover, evidence indicates that where fat accumulates or is distributed on the body may affect a person's risk for CHD. Specifically, if excess fat accumulates around your upper body and waist (apple-shaped), you are at a greater risk than if your excess fat accumulates around your hips and thighs (pear-shaped). A waist girth greater than 102 centimetres for men and 88 centimetres for women significantly relates to elevated triglyceride levels, low HDL concentrations, and hypertension.[30]

Diabetes

Individuals with diabetes, particularly those who have taken insulin for a number of years (that is, individuals with type 1 diabetes), have an increased risk for CVD. In fact, heart disease is the leading cause of death among individuals with diabetes. Because people who are obese have a higher risk for diabetes, distinguishing between the effects of the two conditions is difficult. Individuals with diabetes also tend to have elevated blood fat levels, increased atherosclerosis, and a tendency toward deterioration of small blood vessels, particularly in the eyes and extremities. Through a prescribed regimen of diet, physical activity, and medication, individuals with diabetes can control much of their increased risk for heart disease.

Individual Response to Stress

Some people react to stress on a daily basis. These stress reactions occur because of or in reaction to normal, usual daily activities. Consequently, these people typically have inconsistent, yet high, blood pressure when it is taken in an "unrested" state. However, when these people are asked to lie down and stay in a "rested" state for 10 minutes or more, their blood pressure often normalizes.[31] In one study, one out of five people had an extreme cardiovascular reaction to stressful stimulation (see Chapter 3).[32] These people experience alarm and resistance so strongly that, when under stress, their bodies produce large amounts of stress chemicals, which in turn lead to tremendous strain for the cardiovascular system. These people are called "hot reactors." Although their blood pressure may be normal when they are not under stress—for example, in a doctor's office—it increases dramatically in response to even small amounts of everyday tension. "Cold reactors" are those who are able to experience stress without harmful cardiovascular responses. Cold reactors may internalize stress, but their self-talk and perceptions about the stressful events lead them to a non-response state in which their cardiovascular system remains virtually unaffected. Other research investigating the relationship of personality to heart disease suggests that personality plays a role in effective coping of the stress response. See Chapter 3 for tips on managing your stress response that are effective for cold, hot, and more neutral reactors.

✔ Risks You Cannot Control

There are some risk factors for CVD that you cannot prevent or control. These include

- Heredity: Having a family history of heart disease increases risk significantly.

- Age: Eighty percent of all fatal heart attacks occur in people over the age of 65. The risk for CVD increases with age for both sexes.[33]

- Sex: Men are at a greater risk for CVD until older age. Women under 35 years of age generally have a fairly low risk for CVD. (For a more detailed discussion, see the next section.)

- Ethnicity: First Nations and Inuit people have three times the rate of heart problems of Canadians in general.[34] Also at greater risk for heart disease are individuals of African and South Asian descent.[35]

WOMEN AND CARDIOVASCULAR DISEASE

Many more women die from heart disease and stroke than from breast cancer. Currently, two in three women have one or more of the major risk factors for heart disease.[36] While men have more heart attacks and have them earlier in life, women have a much lower chance of survival. Although we understand the mechanisms that cause heart disease in men and women, their experiences in the health-care system, their reactions to life-threatening diseases, and a host of other technological and environmental factors may play a role in their survival rates.

Risk Factors for Heart Disease in Women

Premenopausal women are unlikely to have a heart attack unless they also have diabetes, high blood pressure, kidney disease, or a genetic predisposition to high cholesterol levels. Family history, oral contraceptive use, and smoking also increase the risk for heart disease in premenopausal women.

Once her estrogen production drops with menopause, a woman's chance of developing heart disease rises rapidly. In fact, a 60-year-old woman has the same heart attack risk as a 50-year-old man, and by her late 70s, a woman has the same heart attack risk as a man her age.

Cholesterol is another factor to consider in women's increased risk for heart disease as they age. Although women aged 25 and over tend to have lower cholesterol levels than men of the same age, when they reach 45 years things change. Most men's cholesterol levels become more stable, while LDL and total cholesterol levels in women rise, with the gap widening after the age of 55. Studies of men indicate that for every 1-percent drop in cholesterol, there is a 2-percent decrease in CVD risk. If this holds true for women, prevention efforts focusing on dietary interventions and physical activity may significantly help postmenopausal women reduce their risk for CVD.

When data from seven cycles of the National Population Health Survey from 1994/1995 to 2006/2007 were examined in a longitudinal format, results indicated that women's risk of heart disease was significantly elevated if she also had depression—even after adjusting for other risk factors (for example, marital status, income, high blood pressure, diabetes, BMI, smoking, leisure-time physical activity, alcohol consumption, and use of hormone replacement therapy).[37] This same relationship was not found in men.

Recognizing Heart Disease in Postmenopausal Women

Postmenopausal women often do not display the same recognizable symptoms of heart disease as men. The first sign of heart disease in men is generally a myocardial infarction. In women, the first sign is usually uncomplicated angina pectoris. Because chest discomfort rather than pain is the common manifestation of angina in women, and because angina has a much more favourable prognosis in women than in men, many physicians ignore the condition in their female patients or treat it too casually.

A heart attack also causes different symptoms in women than in men. In men, a heart attack usually manifests itself as crushing chest pain radiating to the shoulders, arms, neck, jaw, or back as well as dizziness, paleness, difficulty breathing, sweating, nausea, vomiting, or anxiety.[38] In women, a heart attack results in much more vague symptoms such as pain in the neck, jaw, or arms; heaviness in the shoulders, back, or the pit of the stomach; and feeling out of breath, tired, sweating, nausea, or vomiting.[39] If these symptoms are experienced for two minutes or longer, it is critical to seek help immediately (call 9-1-1) or get to the nearest hospital that offers emergency cardiac care.

In the past decade, three main reasons why signs of heart disease in women may be overlooked have been postulated: (1) physicians may often be sex-biased in their delivery of health care, tending to concentrate on women's reproductive organs rather than on the whole body; (2) physicians tend to view heart disease in men as a more severe problem because they traditionally have a higher incidence of the disease; and (3) women decline major procedures more often than men. Other explanations for diagnostic and therapeutic difficulties encountered by women with heart disease include[40]

- Delay in diagnosing a possible heart attack, due to the complexity of interpreting chest pain in women because symptoms of heart attack are vague and much different than in men.

- Typically less aggressive treatment of women who have had a heart attack.

- Their older age, on average, and frequency of other health problems.

- Women's coronary arteries are often smaller than men's, making surgical or diagnostic procedures more difficult technically.

- Their increased incidence of post-infarction angina or heart failure.

what do you THINK?

How do men and women differ in their experiences with heart disease? How might women play a role in the under-diagnosis of their heart disease? What actions do you think individuals can take to help improve this situation for women? What actions can communities and medical practitioners take?

NEW WEAPONS AGAINST HEART DISEASE

The victim of a heart attack today has a variety of options not available a generation ago. Medications can strengthen heartbeat, control arrhythmias, remove fluids in cases of congestive heart failure, and relieve pain. Further, bypass surgery and angioplasty have become relatively commonplace procedures in hospitals throughout the nation.

Techniques of Diagnosing Heart Disease

Several techniques can be used to diagnose heart disease, including electrocardiogram, angiography, and positron emission tomography scans. An **electrocardiogram** is a record of the electrical activity of the heart measured during a stress test. Patients walk or run on treadmills while their hearts' functions are monitored. Another method of testing for heart disease is **angiography** (often referred to as "cardiac catheterization"), in which a needle-thin tube called a catheter is threaded through blocked heart arteries, a dye is injected, and an X-ray is taken to discover which areas are blocked. A more recent and even more effective method of measuring heart activity is **positron emission tomography**, also called a **PET scan**, which produces three-dimensional images of the heart as blood flows through it. During a PET scan, a patient receives an intravenous injection of a radioactive tracer. As the tracer decays, it emits positrons that are picked up by the scanner and transformed by a computer into colour images of the heart.

Other tests include the following:

- Radionuclide imaging (includes such tests as thallium test, multinucleated gated angiography scan, and acute infarct scintigraphy). In these procedures, substances called radionuclides are injected into the bloodstream. Computer-generated pictures can then show them in the heart. These tests can show how well the heart muscle is supplied with blood, how well the heart's chambers are functioning, and which part of the heart has been damaged.

- Magnetic resonance imaging (MRI). This test uses powerful magnets to look inside the body. Computer-generated pictures can show the heart muscle, identify damage from a heart attack, diagnose certain congenital heart defects, and evaluate disease of larger blood vessels such as the aorta.

- Ultrafast computed tomography (CT). This is an especially fast form of X-ray of the heart designed to evaluate bypass grafts, diagnose ventricular function, and measure calcium deposits.

- Digital cardiac angiography. This modified form of computer-aided imaging records pictures of the heart and its blood vessels.

Angioplasty versus Bypass Surgery

During the 1980s, **coronary bypass surgery** seemed to be the ultimate technique for treating patients who had coronary blockages or suffered heart attacks. In coronary bypass surgery, a blood vessel taken from another site in the patient's body (usually the saphenous vein in the leg or the internal mammary artery) is implanted to transport blood by bypassing blocked arteries. The effectiveness of bypass operations, particularly for elderly people, has been questioned, particularly with less invasive treatment options now available.

A procedure called **angioplasty** (also called balloon angioplasty) has fewer risks and is believed by many to be more effective than bypass surgery in selected cardiovascular cases. This procedure is similar to angiography. A needle-thin catheter is threaded through blocked heart arteries. The catheter has a balloon at the tip,

which is inflated to flatten fatty deposits against the artery walls, allowing blood to flow more freely. Angioplasty patients are generally awake but sedated during the procedure and spend only one or two days in the hospital after treatment. Most people can return to work within five days. Only about 1 percent of all angioplasty patients die during or soon after the procedure. Risks of this procedure include spontaneous collapse of the vessel worked on in 3 to 7 percent of cases, and in about 30 percent of all angioplasty operations, the treated arteries become clogged again within six months. Some patients may undergo the procedure as many as three times within a five-year period. Some surgeons argue that given angioplasty's high rate of recurrence, bypass may still be a more effective method of treatment.

Other research suggests that in many instances, drug treatments may be as effective in prolonging life as invasive surgical techniques, but it is critical that doctors follow an aggressive drug treatment program and more important that patients comply. Among the most effective treatments are beta blockers and calcium channel blockers, used to reduce high blood pressure and treat other symptoms. Cholesterol-lowering medications are also effective.

Research indicates that low doses of Aspirin (80 milligrams daily or every other day) are beneficial to heart patients because of their blood-thinning properties. It should be pointed out that higher doses do not provide additional protection. Aspirin is even recommended as a preventive strategy for individuals without current heart disease symptoms. However, given the additional risks from emergency surgery or accidental bleeding, Aspirin should be taken as a preventive measure only if your physician recommends it.

Thrombolysis

Whenever a heart attack occurs, prompt action is the key factor in the patient's eventual prognosis. When a

Electrocardiogram: A record of the electrical activity of the heart measured during a stress test.

Angiography: A technique for examining blockages in heart arteries. A catheter is inserted into the arteries, a dye injected, and an X-ray taken to find the blocked areas.

Positron emission tomography (PET scan): Method for measuring heart activity by injecting a patient with a radioactive tracer scanned electronically to produce a three-dimensional image of the heart and arteries.

Coronary bypass surgery: A surgical technique in which one or more blood vessels are implanted to bypass one or more clogged coronary arteries.

Angioplasty: A technique in which a catheter with a balloon at the tip is inserted into a clogged artery; the balloon is inflated to flatten fatty deposits against artery walls, allowing blood to flow more freely.

coronary artery gets blocked, the heart muscle doesn't die immediately, but time determines how much damage occurs. If a victim gets to an emergency room and is diagnosed fast enough (within two hours), a form of reperfusion therapy called **thrombolysis** can sometimes be performed. Thrombolysis involves injecting an agent such as TPA (tissue plasminogen activator) to dissolve the clot and restore some blood flow, thereby reducing the amount of tissue that dies from ischemia. These drugs must be used within one to three hours of a heart attack for best results, and once again, the importance of dialling 9-1-1 when the symptoms of a heart attack are first noticed cannot be over-emphasized.

what do you THINK?

With all the new diagnostic procedures and treatments for prevention and intervention of CVD, how can a health consumer ensure that he or she will get the best treatment when needed? Where can one go for information? Why might women, members of certain minority groups, and the elderly need a "health advocate" who can help them get through the system?

DIABETES: INCIDENCE AND MORTALITY

Diabetes is a serious, widespread, and costly chronic disease. It is characterized by high blood sugar (glucose) levels. Untreated diabetes results in numerous health problems, including blindness, amputation, and kidney dysfunction. From 1996/1997 to 2005 (the most recent data available), the number of Canadians 12 years and older diagnosed with diabetes almost doubled.[41] These estimates indicate that 4.9 percent of the Canadian population has diabetes. At all ages except for 15 to 19 years and 20 to 35 years, males are more likely to have diabetes than females. Further, diagnoses increase with age, particularly after the age of 54 years, with 10.1 percent of people between the ages of 55 to 64 years and 14.6 of all individuals over the age of 65 years having a positive diagnosis.

What causes diabetes? In healthy people, the pancreas, a powerful enzyme-producing organ, produces the hormone insulin in sufficient quantities to allow the body to use or store glucose. When the pancreas fails to produce enough insulin to regulate sugar metabolism or when the body fails to use insulin effectively, diabetes develops. Individuals with diabetes exhibit hyperglycemia, or elevated blood sugar levels, and high glucose levels in their urine. Other symptoms include excessive thirst, frequent urination, hunger, a tendency to tire easily, wounds that heal slowly, numbness or tingling in the extremities, changes in vision, skin eruptions, and in women, a tendency toward vaginal yeast infections.

Type 1 diabetes, also called insulin-dependent diabetes and formerly referred to as juvenile-onset diabetes, is an autoimmune disease in which the immune system destroys the insulin-making beta cells. It most often appears in childhood or adolescence, with rare cases diagnosed in early to mid-adult years. People with type 1 diabetes typically depend on insulin injections or oral medications because their body does not produce the insulin it needs.

In type 2 diabetes, also called non-insulin dependent diabetes and formerly called adult-onset diabetes, insulin production is deficient or the body is unable to utilize all available insulin. Type 2 diabetes accounts for 90 to 95 percent of all diabetes cases and in the past did not appear until after the age of 40 years—hence the term "adult-onset." Currently, type 2 diabetes is diagnosed across the age spectrum, including children and adolescents, and because of the frequency of diagnoses in younger individuals (reflective of current Canadian lifestyle), it can no longer be considered an adult-onset disease. Specifically, type 2 diabetes is linked to obesity and physical inactivity, both of which can be modified to control and prevent diabetes and improve health. Further, if people with type 2 diabetes change their lifestyle (that is, become more physically active, eat well, lose weight), they may be able to avoid the need for oral medications or insulin indefinitely.

A third type of diabetes, gestational diabetes, can develop in women during pregnancy. Although once believed to be only a transient event that disappeared after pregnancy, today experts realize that women with gestational diabetes have an increased risk of developing type 2 diabetes within 5 to 10 years of giving birth.[42] This is particularly true for women who do not lose the weight they gained during pregnancy and for those with subsequent pregnancies and weight gain with each one.

Understanding Risk Factors

Diabetes tends to run in families.[43] As previously mentioned, being obese, coupled with low levels of physical activity, dramatically increases risk of type 2 diabetes. This, too, often runs in families—not because of a genetic link, but rather an environmental or lifestyle link. Older persons and mothers of babies weighing more than 4 kilograms at birth are also at increased risk. About 80 percent of all individuals with type 2 diabetes are obese at the time of diagnosis. Weight loss, better nutrition, control of blood glucose levels, and regular physical activity are important factors in lowering blood sugar and improving the efficiency of cellular use of insulin. These lifestyle improvements can also help to prevent overwork of the pancreas and the development of diabetes. In fact, recent findings indicate that regular, moderate intensity physical activity and a healthy diet can reduce one's risk of type 2 diabetes significantly.[44] Individuals of African Canadian descent and First Nations and Inuit Canadians have much higher rates of type 2 diabetes than others, which is most likely related to lifestyle factors such as low levels of physical activity and poor dietary intakes.

Controlling Diabetes

Most physicians attempt to control type 1 and latter stages of type 2 diabetes with a variety of insulin drugs. Most drugs are taken orally, although self-administered hypodermic injections are prescribed when other treatments are inadequate. Recent breakthroughs in individual monitoring, implantable insulin monitors and pumps, and insulin inhalers have given many people with diabetes the opportunity to lead more normal lives. Some people with type 2 diabetes can manage their diagnoses effectively by losing weight, engaging in regular physical activity, and eating foods rich in complex carbohydrates, low in sodium, and high in fibre.

Physical activity, particularly walking, is often prescribed to assist with the management of type 2 diabetes.[45] These recommendations should be individualized and should specifically identify the quantity and quality of walking required. More than 10 000 steps may be needed, as well as a walking speed that elicits improvements in cardiorespiratory fitness.[46]

Complications Associated with Diabetes

Depending on the type and severity of the disease, diabetes results in many complications and increases the severity of existing conditions, including

- CVD. Heart disease and stroke cause about 65 percent of deaths among people with diabetes. More than 70 percent of people with diabetes have hypertension.

- Eye disease and blindness. Diabetes is the leading cause of blindness.

- Kidney disease. The kidneys in many people with diabetes often fail. Dialysis is a common treatment for these individuals.

- Amputations. More than 60 percent of nontraumatic amputations of lower limbs are a result of diabetes. Foot care programs that include regular exams and patient education could prevent as many as 85 percent of these amputations.

- Pregnancy complications. Poorly controlled diabetes can cause major birth defects in 5 to 10 percent of all pregnancies and accounts for 15 to 20 percent of spontaneous abortions.

- Flu- and pneumonia-related deaths. People with diabetes have a threefold increase of dying as a result of complications from the flu or pneumonia compared to people without diabetes.

CANCER INCIDENCE AND MORTALITY

An estimated 171 000 new cases of cancer and 75 300 deaths from cancer will occur in Canada in 2009.[47] It is projected that 40 percent of women and 45 percent of men will develop cancer in their lifetime and that one of every four Canadians will die of cancer (24 percent of women; 29 percent of men). The greater number of new cases of cancer is primarily due to an aging population. Mortality from cancer is declining for males of all ages, for women under the age of 70, and most rapidly in children and adolescents.

Lung cancer continues to be the leading cause of premature death due to cancer, accounting for 28.3 percent of all cancer deaths in men and 26.3 percent in women.[48] It is expected that 23 400 new cases (12 800 for males and 10 700 for females) of lung cancer will be diagnosed in 2009.[49] It should be pointed out that although lung cancer is the number one cancer killer of men and women, it is only the second highest for new cases. In men there are more new cases of prostate cancer (25 500) expected in 2009, while in women more new cases of breast cancer (22 700) are expected. The third-highest expected cancer incidence for 2009 for men and women is colorectal cancer, with 12 100 and 9900 new cases, respectively.

Not everyone is equally at risk for all types of cancers. Cancer incidence and mortality vary greatly by age, sex, ethnicity, and socioeconomic status. Because cancer risk is strongly associated with lifestyle and behaviours, differences in ethnic and cultural groups can provide clues to factors involved in its development. Culturally influenced values and belief systems can also affect whether or not a person seeks care, participates in screenings, or follows recommended treatment options. In Canada, cancer incidence and mortality are higher in the Atlantic provinces and Quebec and lowest in British Columbia.[50]

Thrombolysis: Injection of an agent to dissolve clots and restore some blood flow, thereby reducing the amount of tissue that dies from ischemia.

What Is Cancer?

Cancer is the name given to a large group of diseases characterized by the uncontrolled growth and spread of abnormal cells. It may be hard to understand how normal, healthy cells become cancerous, but if you think of a cell as a small computer, programmed to operate in a particular fashion, the process may become clearer. Under normal conditions, healthy cells are protected by the immune system as they perform their daily functions of growing, replicating, and repairing body organs. When something interrupts normal cell programming, uncontrolled growth and abnormal cellular development result in a new growth of tissue. This new tissue serves no physiological function and is called a **neoplasm**. When this neoplasmic mass forms a clump of cells it is known as a **tumour**.

Not all tumours are **malignant** (cancerous); in fact, most are **benign** (non-cancerous). Benign tumours are generally harmless unless they grow to obstruct or crowd out normal tissues or organs. A benign tumour of the brain, for instance, is life-threatening when it grows and causes blood restriction resulting in a stroke. The only way to determine whether a given tumour or mass is benign or malignant is through **biopsy**, or microscopic examination of cell development.

Benign and malignant tumours differ in several key ways. Benign tumours are generally composed of ordinary-looking cells enclosed in a fibrous shell or capsule that prevents their spreading to other body areas. Malignant tumours are usually not enclosed in a protective capsule and can therefore spread to other organs. This process, known as **metastasis**, makes some forms of cancer particularly aggressive in their ability to overcome bodily defences. By the time they are diagnosed, malignant tumours have frequently metastasized throughout the body, making treatment extremely difficult. Unlike benign tumours, which merely expand to take over a given space, malignant cells invade surrounding tissue, emitting clawlike protrusions that disrupt chemical processes within healthy cells. More specifically, malignant cells disturb the ribonucleic acid (RNA) and deoxyribonucleic acid (DNA) within the normal cells. Tampering with these substances that control cellular metabolism and reproduction produces mutant cells that differ in form, quality, and function from normal cells.

What Causes Cancer?

After decades of research, most cancer epidemiologists believe that the majority of cancers are preventable and can be avoided by healthier choices in lifestyle and environment.[51] In fact, the recently released "Policy and Action for Cancer Prevention Food Nutrition, and Physical Activity: A Global Perspective," by the World Cancer Research Fund in conjunction with the American Institute for Cancer Research, clearly stated that two-thirds of all cancers could be prevented based on lifestyle changes.[52] One-third could be prevented by not using tobacco and another one-third could be prevented by being physically active and eating well. Many specific causes of cancer are well documented, the most important of which are smoking, obesity, and a few organic viruses. Most research supports the idea that cancer is caused by external (chemicals, radiation, viruses, and lifestyle) and internal (hormones, immune conditions, and inherited mutations) factors. These causal factors may act together or in sequence to promote cancer development. We do not know why some people have malignant cells in their body and never develop cancer while others may take 10 years or more to develop the disease. Many factors are believed to cause cancer, and a combination of these factors can dramatically increase one's risk of the disease.

One theory proposes that cancer results from spontaneous errors during cell reproduction. Perhaps cells that are overworked or aged are more likely to break down, causing genetic errors that result in mutant cells. Another theory suggests that cancer is caused by some external agent or agents that enter a normal cell and initiate the cancerous process. Numerous environmental factors, such as radiation, chemicals, hormonal drugs, immunosuppressant drugs (drugs that suppress the normal activity of the immune system), and other toxins are considered possible **carcinogens** (cancer-causing agents) (see Figure 11.4); perhaps the most common carcinogen is the tar found in cigarettes. The greater the dose or exposure to environmental hazards, the greater the degree of risk. Thus, people forced to work, live, and pass through areas that have high levels of environmental toxins may be at greater risk of cancer.

A third theory came out of research on certain viruses believed to cause tumours in animals. This research led to the discovery of **oncogenes**, suspected cancer-causing genes present on chromosomes. Although oncogenes are typically dormant, scientists theorize that certain conditions, such as age, stress, and exposure to carcinogens, viruses, and radiation may activate these oncogenes. Once activated, they begin to grow and reproduce in an out-of-control manner. Scientists are uncertain whether only people who develop cancer have oncogenes or whether we all have **proto-oncogenes**, genes that can become oncogenes under certain conditions. Many **oncologists** (physicians who specialize in the treatment of malignancies) believe that the oncogene theory may lead to a greater understanding of how individual cells function and may bring us closer to developing an effective treatment for cancer.

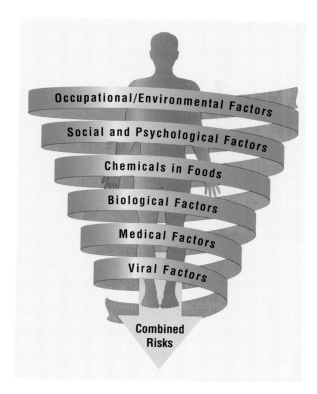

FIGURE 11.4
Suspected Causes of Cancer

stress, and other lifestyle factors seem to play a role. Further confirming this theory is that colon and rectal cancer occur more frequently among persons with a high-fat, low-fibre dietary intake, in those who don't eat enough fruits and vegetables, and in those who are physically inactive.

Keep in mind that a high relative risk does not guarantee cause and effect. It merely indicates the likelihood of a particular risk factor being related to a particular outcome. In other words you can modify your lifestyle behaviours to reduce your risk.

Smoking

Of all the potential risk factors for cancer, smoking is among the greatest; it is the leading cause of preventable death in the world today. In developing countries, smoking is responsible for 80 percent of all deaths from lung cancer.[55] In Canada, tobacco is responsible for nearly one in five deaths annually. Recent declines in smoking have likely had a direct effect on the overall decrease in lung cancer rates; however, as previously noted, lung cancer remains the leading cause of cancer death in men and women.

Researchers once believed that cigarettes caused only cancers of the lung, pancreas, bladder, and kidney, and (synergistically with alcohol) the larynx, mouth, pharynx, and esophagus. However, recent evidence indicates that several other types of cancer are also related to tobacco use. Most notably, cancers of the stomach, liver, and cervix are directly related to long-term smoking.

Risks for Cancer

✳ Lifestyle

Anyone can develop cancer; however, most cases affect adults beginning in middle age. In fact, nearly 80 percent of cancers are diagnosed at ages 55 and over. Cancer researchers refer to one's cancer risk when they assess risk factors. *Lifetime risk* refers to the probability that an individual, over the course of a lifetime, will develop cancer or die from it. In 2009, as noted previously, 45 percent of men and 40 percent of women have a lifetime risk of developing cancer.[53]

Relative risk is a measure of the strength of the relationship between risk factors and a particular cancer. Basically, relative risk compares your risk if you engage in certain known risk behaviours with that of someone who does not engage in such behaviours. For example, if you smoke, you have a 20-fold relative risk of developing lung cancer compared to a nonsmoker. In other words, the chances of getting lung cancer are about 20 times greater in a smoker than in a nonsmoker.[54]

Over the years, researchers have found that certain behaviours result in a higher incidence of cancer. In particular, dietary intake, sedentary lifestyle (and resultant obesity), consumption of alcohol or cigarettes,

Cancer: A large group of diseases characterized by the uncontrolled growth and spread of abnormal cells.

Neoplasm: A new growth of tissue that serves no physiologic function, resulting from uncontrolled, abnormal cellular development.

Tumour: A neoplasmic mass that grows more rapidly than surrounding tissues.

Malignant: Very dangerous or harmful; refers to a cancerous tumour.

Benign: Harmless; refers to a non-cancerous tumour.

Biopsy: Microscopic examination of tissue to determine if a cancer is present.

Metastasis: Process by which cancer spreads from one area to different areas of the body.

Carcinogens: Cancer-causing agents.

Oncogenes: Suspected cancer-causing genes present on chromosomes.

Proto-oncogenes: Genes that can become oncogenes under certain conditions.

Oncologists: Physicians who specialize in the treatment of malignancies.

Obesity

It is difficult to sort through the volumes of evidence about the role of nutrients, obesity, sedentary lifestyle, and related variables in the development of cancer. That said, cancer is more common among people who are obese, and risk increases as level of obesity increases. A study of more than 900 000 adults indicates a significant relationship between a high body mass index (BMI) and death rates for cancers such as that of the esophagus, colon, rectum, liver, kidney, and pancreas.[56] Women with a high BMI have a higher mortality rate from breast, uterine, cervical, and ovarian cancers; men with a high BMI have higher death rates from prostate and stomach cancers. In this study, 34 percent of all cancer deaths were attributable to overweight and obesity. Other findings relevant to the obesity–cancer link are as follows:

- The relative risk of breast cancer in postmenopausal women is 50 percent higher for women who are obese.
- The relative risk of colon cancer in men is 40 percent higher for men who are obese.
- The relative risks of gallbladder and endometrial cancer are five times higher in individuals who are obese compared to those at a healthy weight.

Biologic Factors

Some early cancer theorists believed that we inherit a genetic predisposition toward certain forms of cancer.[57] Cancers of the breast, stomach, colon, prostate, uterus, ovaries, and lungs do appear to have a heredity link. Specifically, a woman has a much higher risk of developing breast cancer if her mother, sisters, or daughters (i.e., primary relatives) had the disease, particularly if they had it at a young age. Hodgkin's disease and certain leukemias also show familial patterns. Whether these familial patterns are attributable to genetic susceptibility or to the fact that people in the same families experience similar environmental risks remains uncertain.

Sex also affects the likelihood of developing certain forms of cancer. For example, breast cancer occurs primarily among females, although men occasionally get breast cancer. Of the 22 900 new cases expected in 2009, 180 will be in males.[58] Obviously, factors other than heredity and familial relationships affect which sex develops a particular cancer. In the 1950s and 1960s, for example, women rarely contracted lung cancer. But with increases in the number of women who smoked and the length of time they smoked, lung cancer became a leading cause of cancer deaths for Canadian women in the 1980s. Although sex plays a role in certain cases, other variables, such as lifestyle, are probably more significant in other cases.

Occupation and Environment Factors

Various occupational hazards are known to cause cancer when exposure levels are high or exposure is prolonged. Overall, however, workplace hazards account for only a small percentage of all cancers. One of the most common occupational carcinogens is asbestos, a fibrous substance once widely used in the construction, insulation, and automobile industries. Nickel, chromate, and chemicals such as benzene, arsenic, and vinyl chloride have been shown to be carcinogens for humans. Also, people who routinely work with certain dyes and radioactive substances may have increased risks for cancer. Working with coal tars, as in the mining profession, or working near inhalants, as in the auto-painting business, is also hazardous. Those who work with herbicides and pesticides also appear to be at higher risk, although the evidence is inconclusive to date for low-dose exposures.

Because people are sometimes forced to work near hazardous substances, it is imperative that worksites enact policies and procedures designed to minimize or eliminate toxic exposure.

Ionizing radiation—radiation from X-rays, radon, cosmic rays, and ultraviolet radiation (primarily UV-B radiation)—is the only form of radiation linked to cancer. (See the section on skin cancer.)

While reports about cancer-case clusters in communities around nuclear power facilities have raised public concerns, studies show that clusters do not occur more often near nuclear power plants than they do by chance in wider geographical areas.[59]

Social and Psychological Factors

Although orthodox medical personnel are skeptical of overly simplistic prevention centres that focus on humour and laughter as the way to prevent cancer, we cannot rule out the possibility that negative emotional states contribute to disease development. People who are lonely, depressed, and lack social support are more susceptible to cancer than their mentally and emotionally healthy counterparts. Similarly, people under chronic stress and those with poor nutrition or sleep habits develop cancer at a slightly higher rate than the general population. Experts believe that severe depression or prolonged stress may reduce the activity of the body's immune system, thereby wearing down bodily resistance to cancer.

Chemicals in Foods

Among the food additives suspected of causing cancer is sodium nitrate, a chemical used to preserve and give colour to red meat. Research indicates that the actual carcinogen is not sodium nitrate but nitrosamines,

Canadian Cancer Statistics 2006: Cancer Screening in Canada Not Realizing Full Potential

TORONTO—Fewer Canadians would die from cancer if cancer screening in Canada was enhanced and expanded, according to a special report in *Canadian Cancer Statistics 2006* released by the Canadian Cancer Society.

The report also states that some screening tests can help prevent cancer (for example, cervical and colorectal cancers) as they detect pre-cancerous conditions, which can then be treated or removed.

"We have solid scientific evidence that screening through an organized program can reduce cancer deaths and, in some cases, even the incidence of certain cancers," says Heather Logan, Director, Cancer Control Policy, Canadian Cancer Society. "Existing cancer screening has helped reduce the cancer toll in Canada. However, we need to do more to make the most of this opportunity, which has the potential to significantly reduce the cancer burden in this country."

The special report—*Progress in Cancer Control: Screening*—says that cancer screening in Canada is not reaching its full potential because:

- participation in existing cervical and breast cancer screening programs needs to be enhanced. Barriers have to be identified so that effective methods to reach out to women can be developed.

- an organized colorectal cancer screening program has not been implemented in any province or territory in Canada, despite scientific evidence showing it would be an effective way to reduce both incidence [of] and death [from] this common cancer.

In addition, the special report states more research is needed to identify effective screening tests for prostate, lung, and ovarian cancers.

Screening is the early detection of cancer by testing or checking for disease in people who don't show any symptoms of the disease. Detecting cancer early usually improves the likelihood of successful treatment, which leads to fewer Canadians dying from the disease. Screening can also help prevent some cancers by detecting pre-cancerous stages of the disease.

BREAST CANCER

Current evidence suggests that breast cancer deaths could be reduced by as much as one-quarter if 70 percent of women in the target age group (50–69 years) participated in organized screening programs. Every province and territory (except Nunavut) had an organized breast-screening program by 2003. However, none of the organized programs have achieved the nationally established target of 70 percent participation.

"While it's encouraging that the proportion of women in organized breast cancer screening programs has increased

over time, in 2003 participation was only 34 percent nationally," says Logan.

The special report also says that about 61 percent of Canadian women reported having a screening mammogram within two years. This is likely because mammography is also available through centres not affiliated with organized programs.

"The percentage of women who have been screened is probably somewhere between 34 and 61 percent, and this is too low," says Logan. "However, breast cancer death rates have been declining and screening is one reason for this downward trend."

The Canadian Cancer Society recommends that women between the ages of 50 and 69 have a screening mammogram and a clinical breast exam every two years.

Women report that barriers to screening include not having a regular doctor or living in rural areas. "It's important to understand the barriers so that effective methods to reach out to women can be developed. For example, for women living in rural areas, a portable mammography unit may encourage women to get screened," says Logan.

COLORECTAL CANCER

In Canada, scientific evidence shows that colorectal cancer deaths could be reduced by 17 percent if 70 percent of Canadians between the ages of 50 and 74 had a fecal occult blood test (FOBT) every two years.

"This is a potentially significant drop in deaths from colorectal cancer," says Logan. "Although some informal screening is taking place, there is no organized colorectal screening program in Canada."

In addition, FOBT screening could have an impact on incidence of colorectal cancer as this test can detect blood in the stool from pre-cancerous polyps. Once identified, these polyps can be removed by colonoscopy or sigmoidoscopy before they become cancerous.

CERVICAL CANCER

Largely as a result of "ad-hoc" (not organized) screening for cervical cancer with the Pap test, incidence rates have declined by 50 percent and death rates by 60 percent since 1977. The Pap test can identify pre-cancerous lesions that can then be treated, and can identify cancer at an early stage when treatment is most effective.

"Because of the long history of high-quality cervical cancer screening in Canada, the benefit achieved so far may be close to the maximum," says Logan. "However, it might be possible to see even further reductions in both incidence and death for this cancer if all elements of an organized screening program are incorporated, which would include identifying opportunities to increase participation."

The special report says that screening in Canada could be enhanced and improved if:

- Canada's capacity to review scientific evidence about screening was strengthened so that appropriate health policy recommendations could be developed in a timely fashion;

- adequate funding and support was provided for screening programs that scientific evidence shows are effective at reducing cancer death rates;

- more research was done to identify screening tests for those cancers for which there is not yet sufficient evidence to support an organized cancer screening program (for example, the prostate specific antigen [PSA] test for prostate cancer and CT scans for those at high risk of lung cancer).

"Many Canadians have been touched personally by cancer, and millions more have supported friends and family members in their fight against this devastating disease," says the Honourable Tony Clement, Minister of Health. "This is why the Government of Canada is committed to implementing a five-year Canadian Strategy for Cancer Control.

"We recognize the enormous contribution the Canadian Cancer Society and others in the cancer community have made," he adds. "We are proud to again partner with them in developing this report, and we are pleased to continue our work with the provinces and territories on national quality standards and targets for cancer screening programs."

If funding is allocated from provincial governments, implementing organized cancer screening programs is the responsibility of provincial cancer agencies (not every province has a cancer agency). The federal government is supportive of the development of screening policies and guidelines.

"Achieving maximum benefit from cancer screening across Canada requires continued work by all levels of government, cancer organizations, experts and Canadians," says Logan. "The Canadian Strategy for Cancer Control provides an effective mechanism to bring these groups together so this important issue can be dealt with in a coordinated and collaborative way. By working together we can identify gaps, develop ways to provide more opportunity for people to get screened, and target funding to areas with the most need.

"The Canadian Cancer Society is looking forward to working with the government to implement this important health initiative for Canadians."

For individual Canadians, Logan urges them to take full advantage of current cancer screening programs. "Talk to your doctors about what cancer screening tests are best for you," says Logan. "It could save your life."

Logan adds that the Society will continue its work in developing screening recommendations, getting this information to Canadians, and advocating governments to ensure appropriate screening programs are implemented.

Screening is delivered in two ways in Canada—through organized programs or through what is called "ad-hoc" screening. Screening is most effective and cost-efficient when offered through an organized screening program. There are defined elements for an organized program, which include follow-up guidelines, recruitment strategies, and monitoring and evaluation. Ad-hoc screening may include some of these elements, but not all.

Source: Canadian Cancer Society. Media Release, April 11, 2006. Retrieved August 28, 2009, from www.cancer.ca/ccs/internet/mediareleaselist/ 0,,3172_615815452_943322260_langId-en,00.html. Used with permission of the Canadian Cancer Society/National Cancer Institute of Canada: *Canadian Cancer Statistics 2006*, Toronto, Canada, 2006.

substances formed when the body digests sodium nitrates. Sodium nitrate has not been banned, primarily because it kills the bacterium *Clostridium botulinum,* which is the cause of the highly virulent food-borne disease called botulism. It should also be noted that the bacteria found in the human intestinal tract may contain more nitrates than a person could ever take in when eating cured meats or other nitrate-containing food products. Nonetheless, concern about the carcinogenic properties of nitrates has led to the introduction of meats that are nitrate-free or contain reduced nitrates.

There is also concern about the possible harm caused by pesticide and herbicide residues. While some of these chemicals cause cancer at high doses in experimental animals, the very low concentrations found in some foods are well within government-established safety levels. Continued research regarding pesticide and herbicide use is essential for maximum

food safety and the continuous monitoring of agricultural practices is necessary to ensure a safe food supply. It is important to find a balance between chemical use and the production of quality food products. Policies protecting consumer health and ensuring the continued improvement in food production through development of alternative, low-chemical pest and herbicide control and reduced environmental pollution should be the goal of prevention efforts.

Infectious Diseases

According to recent estimates, 17 percent of new cancers worldwide will be attributable to infections.[60] Infections are thought to influence cancer development in several ways, most commonly through chronic inflammation, suppression of the immune system, or chronic stimulation.

HBV, HCV, and Liver Cancer

Viruses such as hepatitis B (HBV) and C (HCV) are believed to stimulate cancer cells in the liver because they are chronic diseases that cause inflammation of liver tissue. This may prime the liver for cancer or make it more hospitable for cancer development. Global increases in HBV and HCV rates and concurrent increases in liver cancer rates provide evidence of such an association.

HPV and Cervical Cancer

Nearly 100 percent of women with cervical cancer have evidence of human papilloma virus (HPV) infection, believed to be a major cause of cervical cancer. HPV is a group of more than 100 different types of viruses, of which 40 are transmitted through sexual activity.[61] In fact, it is estimated that at least 75 percent of sexually active men and women in Canada will have at least one HPV infection in their lifetime. HPV types 16 and 18 are responsible for 70 percent of all cervical cancers while HPV types 6 and 11 are responsible for 90 percent of genital warts.[62] A vaccine that protects against these HPV types is available for young women in Canada and should be viewed as a complement to cervical cancer screening (that is, the Pap test), not a replacement.[63]

what do you THINK?

Given what you've read and heard about the immunization available to reduce your risk of developing cervical cancer, would you take it? Why or why not? If you have the immunization, what lifestyle behaviours will you still have to incorporate to (1) further reduce your risk for and/or ensure early detection of cervical cancer, and (2) to prevent the transmission of other sexually transmitted infections?

Medical Factors

Some medical treatments increase a person's risk for cancer. One famous example is the widespread use of the prescription drug diethylstilbestrol (DES), widely used from 1940 to 1960 to control problems with bleeding during pregnancy and to reduce the risk of miscarriage. It was not until the 1970s that the dangers of this drug became apparent in daughters of mothers who took it during their pregnancy, as they were found to have an increased risk for cancers of the reproductive organs. Another example is the use of estrogen replacement therapy for postmenopausal women because of the potential risk of increased uterine cancer. Ironically, chemotherapy, which is used to treat cancer, may also increase risk for other forms of cancer.

TYPES OF CANCER

As noted previously, the term *cancer* refers to hundreds of different diseases. Four broad classifications are made according to the type of tissue from which the cancer arises.

- Carcinomas—Epithelial tissues (tissues covering body surfaces and lining most body cavities) are the most common sites for cancers. Carcinoma of the breast, lung, intestines, skin, and mouth are examples. These cancers affect the outer layer of the skin and mouth as well as the mucous membranes. They metastasize through the circulatory or lymphatic system initially and form solid tumours.

- Sarcomas—Sarcomas occur in the mesodermal, or middle, layers of tissue—for example, in bones, muscles, and general connective tissue. They metastasize primarily via the blood in the early stages. These cancers are less common but generally more virulent than carcinomas. They also form solid tumours.

- Lymphomas—Lymphomas develop in the lymphatic system—the infection-fighting regions of the body—and metastasize through the lymph system. Hodgkin's disease is one type of lymphoma. Lymphomas also form solid tumours.

- Leukemia—Cancer of the blood-forming parts of the body, particularly the bone marrow and spleen, is called leukemia. A non-solid tumour, leukemia is characterized by an abnormal increase in the number of white blood cells.

The seriousness and general prognosis of a particular cancer are determined through careful diagnosis by trained oncologists. Once laboratory results and clinical observations have been made, cancers are rated by level and stage of development. Those diagnosed as "carcinoma in situ" are localized and are often curable. Cancers given higher level or stage ratings have spread farther and are less likely to be cured.

Lung Cancer

Symptoms of lung cancer include a persistent cough, blood-streaked sputum, chest pain, and recurrent attacks of pneumonia or bronchitis. Treatment depends on the type and stage of the cancer. Surgery, radiation therapy, and chemotherapy are treatment options. If the cancer is localized, surgery is usually the treatment of choice. If the cancer has spread, surgery is used in combination with radiation and chemotherapy. Despite advances in medical technology, survival rates for lung cancer have improved only slightly in recent years. Just 15 percent of people with lung cancer

(13 percent for men; 18 percent for women) live five or more years after diagnosis.[64]

Prevention

Smokers, especially those who smoked for more than 20 years, and people exposed to certain industrial substances such as arsenic and asbestos or to radiation from occupational, medical, or environmental sources, are at the highest risk for lung cancer.[65] Exposure to secondhand cigarette smoke increases the risk for nonsmokers. Some researchers have theorized that as many as 90 percent of all lung cancers could be prevented if people did not smoke. Quitting smoking—or not starting—are the best measures you can take to prevent lung cancer. Any time is a good time to quit smoking, with health improvements noted almost immediately (see Chapter 10 for more details).

Breast Cancer

About one in nine women will develop breast cancer at some time in their lives and one in 27 will die as a result of it.[66] Although this oft-repeated ratio has frightened many women, it represents a woman's lifetime risk. Thus, not until the age of 80 does a woman's risk of breast cancer rise to one in nine.[67] Risks at earlier ages include:

- Age 50: 1 in 50
- Age 60: 1 in 24
- Age 70: 1 in 14

Breast cancer incidence among women rose steadily over the past three decades—although the rate of increase is declining somewhat—whereas mortality rates for breast cancer declined slightly since 1986 and particularly since 1990. This pattern of divergent trends is consistent with benefits achieved through screening programs and improved treatments.[68]

Breast cancer can and does occur in men too. About 1 percent of all estimated breast cancer cases will occur in men.[69] Men and women share the same risk factors for breast cancer and the same warning signs.[70] Warning signs of breast cancer include persistent breast changes such as a lump, thickening, swelling, dimpling, skin irritation, distortion, retraction or scaliness of the nipple, nipple discharge, pain, or tenderness. Risk factors for breast cancer may vary considerably.[71] Typically, risk factors include being over the age of 40, having a primary relative (a mother, sister, or daughter) who had breast cancer, never having had children or never having breastfed, having your first child after age 30, early menarche, a late age of menopause, obesity after menopause, consuming two or more drinks of alcohol per day, and a higher education and socioeconomic

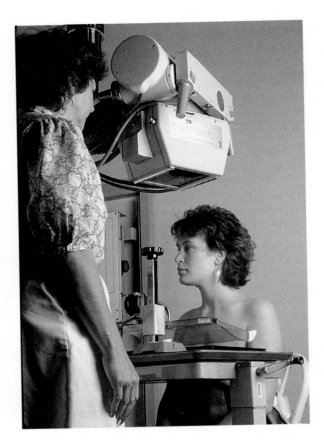

Mammography and other early detection techniques greatly increase a woman's chance of surviving breast cancer.

status. Other potential risk factors include a dietary intake high in saturated fats; exposure to pesticides and other chemicals; weight gain, particularly after menopause; physical inactivity; and a genetic predisposition.

Although risk factors are useful tools, they do not always adequately predict individual susceptibility. However, because of increased awareness, better diagnostic techniques, and improved treatments, individuals with breast cancer have a better chance of surviving today. A key factor in survival rests with individual recognition of early symptoms.[72]

Prevention

Research on the role of physical activity in reducing the risk for breast cancer has generated excitement in the scientific and lay communities. In one study of more than 1000 women aged 40 or younger (545 with breast cancer, 545 without), physical activity patterns were examined. The women who averaged four hours of physical activity per week since menstruating had a 58 percent lower risk. Researchers speculated that physical activity may protect women by altering the production of the ovarian hormones estrogen and progesterone during menstrual cycles.[73]

Regular self-examination (see Figure 11.5) and mammography offer the best hope for early detection of breast cancer. Although breast cancer screening with mammography and clinical breast exam could reduce mortality by nearly one-third in most women aged 50 to 69 years if they were regularly screened, only 34 percent participate in organized screening in Canada.[74] All women, regardless of age, should become familiar with their breasts, how they feel, and what is normal for them (see the Taking Charge box on page 304 for more details). Despite the controversy over the cost-effectiveness and usefulness of a mammogram before the age of 40, many health professionals recommend that if you have any of the risk factors listed above, are prone to fibrous breasts, and are worried about your condition, a mammogram may be warranted. Consult with your physician if you are in doubt, as it is generally best to be a proactive health consumer.

Treatment

Today, people with breast cancer (similar to any other type of cancer) have many treatment options. Fortunately, there are services available to help you get the best information, even if you live in a fairly remote area of the country. The important thing to remember is that, in most instances, taking the time to thoroughly check your physician's track record and his or her philosophy on the best treatment is always a good idea. Often, cancer support groups can give you invaluable information and advice. Treatments range from the simple lumpectomy to radical mastectomy to various combinations of radiation or chemotherapy. Figure 11.5 reviews these options. Remember that it is always a good idea to seek more than one opinion before making a decision.

Lumpectomy
Performed when tumor is in earliest localized stages. Prognosis for recovery is better than 95 percent. Only tumor itself is removed. Some physicians may also remove normal tissue in surrounding area.

Simple mastectomy
Removal of breast and underlying tissue. Prognosis for full recovery better than 80 percent.

Modified radical mastectomy
Breast and lymph nodes in immediate area removed. Prognosis for full recovery dependent on level of spread.

Radical mastectomy
Removal of breast, lymph nodes, pectoral muscles, all fat and underlying tissue. Prognosis for recovery may be as low as 60 percent dependent on level of spread.

FIGURE 11.5

Selected Surgical Procedures for Diagnosed Breast Cancer

Colorectal Cancers

Although colorectal cancers are the second leading cause of cancer deaths in men and women, many people are unaware of their potential risk. Bleeding from the rectum, blood in the stool, and changes in bowel habits are the major warning signals. People over the age of 40, with a family history of colorectal cancer, a personal or family history of polyps (benign growths) in the colon or rectum, or inflammatory bowel problems such as colitis have an increased risk. Canadian and international researchers discovered four new genes related to colorectal cancer.[75] This adds to the previous six already identified, and together these genes indicate an up to six-fold increase in lifetime risk of developing colorectal cancer. Further, a dietary intake high in fats or low in fibre may also increase risk.[76]

Because colorectal cancer tends to spread slowly, the prognosis is quite good if it is caught in the early stages. Treatment often consists of radiation or surgery. Chemotherapy, although not used extensively in the past, is a possibility today. A permanent colostomy, the creation of an abdominal opening for

Know Your Breasts

No matter what your age, breast health starts with knowing your breasts. You should be aware of what is normal for your breasts even if you are having regular screening tests. Many women discover their own breast cancer through changes in the look and feel of their breasts.

Breast tissue covers an area larger than just the breast. It extends up to the collarbone and from the armpit across to the breastbone in the centre of the chest. The breasts sit on the chest muscles that cover the ribs.

Become familiar with your breast tissue by looking at and feeling your breasts. In the past experts suggested that this should be done by following a particular method every month. Research has shown that this isn't necessary. There really isn't a right or wrong way to check your breasts, as long as you get to know the whole area of your breast tissue—up to your collarbone, under your armpits and including your nipples—well enough to notice changes. So get to know your breasts and what is normal for you, any way that works best for you.

It may be normal for your breasts to be lumpy or tender before your period. Breast tissue changes with age, too. Understanding what is normal for you will help you recognize changes and know what to report to your doctor.

WHAT TO LOOK FOR

Remember, lumps in the breast are very common, especially just before your period. Most lumps are not breast cancer.

Most often breast cancer is first noticed as a painless lump in the breast or armpit. You or your partner may discover the lump, or your doctor may find it during a routine physical exam or screening mammogram.

Other signs might include:

- lump or swelling in the armpit
- changes in breast size or shape

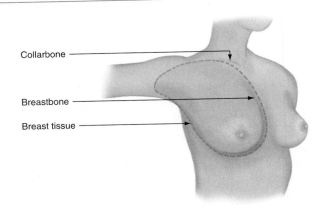

Collarbone

Breastbone

Breast tissue

- dimpling or puckering of the skin—thickening and dimpling skin is sometimes called orange peel
- redness, swelling, and increased warmth in the affected breast
- inverted nipple—nipple turns inwards
- crusting or scaling on the nipple

Often, these symptoms are not caused by cancer. Other health problems can cause them. Testing is necessary to make a diagnosis.

Source: "Know Your Breasts," and "Signs and Symptoms of Breast Cancer," 2008 Canadian Cancer Society.

---

the elimination of body wastes, is seldom required for people with colorectal cancer.[77]

Prostate Cancer

Cancer of the prostate continues to be the most frequently occurring cancer for men. It is the third leading cause of cancer deaths in males. In 2009, it is estimated that 24 700 Canadian men will be diagnosed with prostate cancer and about 4300 will die of the disease.[78] Beginning in 1994, the incidence of prostate cancer began to decline after increasing rapidly for several years. It was noted in 2008 that mortality rates due to prostate cancer continued to decline.[79]

Most signs and symptoms of prostate cancer are nonspecific—that is, they mimic the signs of infection or enlarged prostate. Symptoms include weak or interrupted urine flow or difficulty starting or stopping the urine flow; the need to urinate frequently; pain or difficulty in urinating; blood in the urine; and pain in the lower back, pelvis, or upper thighs. Many males mistake these symptoms for other nonspecific conditions, such as infections, and delay treatment.

Prevention of skin cancer includes keeping a careful watch for any new pigmented growths and for changes to any moles. Melanoma symptoms, as shown in the left photo, include scalloped edges, asymmetrical shapes, discolouration, and an increase in size. Basal cell carcinoma and squamous cell carcinoma (middle and right photos) should be brought to your physician's attention but are not as deadly as melanoma.

Fortunately, even with so many generalized symptoms, most prostate cancers are detected while they are still localized and have not progressed. Men with prostate cancer have an average five-year survival rate of 95 percent.[80] Because the incidence of prostate cancer increases with age, every man over the age of 40 should have an annual prostate examination.[81]

Skin Cancer

Skin cancer may be one of the most underrated of all cancers, particularly among young people. Although it is true that most people do not die of the common, highly curable basal or squamous cell skin cancers, many people do not know that another, highly virulent form of skin cancer known as **malignant melanoma** has become a major killer of young women. Rates for men over 50 are also increasing. Estimates for 2009 indicated that 5000 Canadians will be diagnosed with melanoma (2700 men; 2300 women), with 940 deaths expected.[82] Yet many people still bask unprotected on beaches, apparently not making the connection between death from melanoma and sunlight overexposure. The perception that health and a well-tanned body go together couldn't be farther from the truth.

Symptoms

Many people do not have any idea what to look for when considering skin cancer. Any unusual skin condition, especially a change in the size or colour of a mole or other darkly pigmented growth or spot, should be considered suspect. Scaliness, oozing, bleeding, the appearance of a bump or nodule, the spread of pigment beyond the border, change in sensation, itchiness, tenderness, and pain are all warning signs of the basal and squamous cell skin cancers. However, melanoma symptoms are slightly different. Often there is a sudden or progressive change in a mole's appearance from a small, mole-like growth to a

large, ulcerated, and easily-prone-to-bleeding growth. A simple ABCDE rule outlines the warning signals of melanoma:

- **A** is for *asymmetry*. One half of the mole does not match the other half.
- **B** is for *border irregularity*. The edges are ragged, notched, or blurred.
- **C** is for *colour*. The pigmentation is not uniform.
- **D** is for *diameter* greater than 6 millimetres.
- **E** is for *evolving*. The skin condition evolves/changes over time.

Any one of these symptoms should cause you to visit a physician.[83]

Testicular Cancer

Testicular cancer is currently one of the most common types found in young adult men. Men between the ages of 17 and 34 are at greatest risk. There has been a steady increase in diagnoses over the past several years in this age group. It is estimated that 900 new cases of testicular cancer will be found in 2009 and 30 men will die as a result of it.[84]

try it NOW!

Get in the habit of doing self exams. The survival rate for individuals with testicular cancer increases with early detection and treatment. Make a commitment to perform a testicular exam once per month (see Figure 11.6 for the best method to do so). It is by taking a proactive role in your health that you can be involved in cancer prevention.

Malignant melanoma: A virulent cancer of the melanin (pigment-producing portion) of the skin.

Follow the instructions in the diagram carefully and examine your testes immediately after your next hot bath or shower. Heat causes the testicles to descend and the scrotal skin to relax, making it easier to find unusual lumps.

Examine each testicle by placing the index and middle fingers of both hands on the underside of the testicle and the thumbs on the top. Gently roll the testicle between your thumb and fingers, feeling for small lumps.

Changes or anything abnormal will appear at the front or side of your testicle. Did you find any unusual lumps? Are there any unusual signs of any kind? Are there any markings or lumps at any site?

Keep in mind that not all lumps are a sign of testicular cancer. Unusual lumps at any location, however, should be checked by a physician. Early detection greatly increases your chances of a complete cure. Repeat the examination every month and record your findings.

FIGURE 11.6
Testicular Self-Exam

Although the exact cause of testicular cancer is unknown, several possible risk factors have been identified. Men with undescended testicles appear to be at greatest risk. In addition, some studies indicate that there may be a genetic influence. In general, testicular tumours are first noticed as a painless enlargement of the testis or as an apparent thickening in testicular tissue. Because this enlargement is often painless, it is extremely important that all men, particularly those between the ages of 17 and 34 years, practice regular testicular self-examination (see Figure 11.6). If a suspicious lump or thickening is found, medical follow-up should be sought immediately.

Ovarian Cancer

Current estimates are that 2500 new cases of ovarian cancer will be diagnosed in 2009, with 1750 women succumbing to the disease.[85] Ovarian cancer is often silent, showing no obvious signs or symptoms until late in its development. The most common sign is enlargement of the abdomen (or a feeling of bloating) in women over the age of 40. Other symptoms include vague digestive disturbances, such as gas and stomach aches that persist without explanation.[86]

The risk for ovarian cancer increases with age, with the highest rates found in women in their 60s. Women who never had children are twice as likely to develop ovarian cancer as those who have. The main risk factor appears to be exposure to the reproductive hormone estrogen. Women who have multiple pregnancies or use oral contraceptives, which inhibit estrogen, are at lower risk. In addition, having one or more primary relatives (mother, sisters, grandmothers) who had the disease increases individual risk. With the exception of Japan, the highest incidence rates are reported in industrialized countries.[87]

Prevention

One study indicated that dietary intake may play a role in ovarian cancer.[88] Researchers found that when comparing 450 Canadian women newly diagnosed with ovarian cancer with 564 demographically similar, healthy women, the women without ovarian cancer had a dietary intake lower in saturated fat. Such results, particularly when combined with cardiovascular risks and other health risks, may provide yet another reason to reduce your overall intake of saturated fats.

The best way to protect yourself from ovarian cancer is with annual, thorough pelvic examinations. **Pap tests,** part of a pelvic exam, although useful in detecting cervical cancer, do not reveal ovarian cancer. Women over the age of 40 should have a cancer-related checkup every year. If you have any of the symptoms of ovarian cancer and they persist, see your doctor.

Uterine Cancer

Most cervical and endometrial (that is, uterine) cancers develop in the body of the uterus, usually in the endometrium (lining). The rest develop in the cervix, located at the base of the uterus. The overall incidence of early-stage uterine cancer—that is, cervical cancer—has decreased 50 percent since 1977, although it is estimated that 4400 new cases will still be diagnosed in 2009.[89] Further, invasive, later-stage forms of the disease appear to be decreasing, and mortality rates from cervical cancer have declined by 60 percent since 1977. Much of this apparent trend may be due to more effective regular screenings of younger women using the Pap test, a procedure in which cells taken from the cervical region are examined for abnormal cellular activity. Although these tests are very effective for detecting early-stage cervical cancer, they are less effective for detecting cancers of the uterine lining and not at all effective for detecting cancers of the fallopian tubes or ovaries.[90]

Risk factors for cervical cancer include early age of first vaginal intercourse, multiple sex partners, cigarette smoking, and sexually transmitted infections such as the herpes virus and HPV (the cause of genital warts). For endometrial cancer, a history of infertility, failure to ovulate, obesity, and treatment with tamoxifen or unopposed estrogen therapy are major risk factors.[91] Early warning signs of uterine cancer include bleeding outside the normal menstrual period or after menopause or persistent unusual vaginal discharge. These symptoms should be checked by a physician immediately.[92]

Leukemia

Leukemia is a cancer of the blood-forming tissues that leads to proliferation of millions of immature white blood cells. These abnormal cells crowd out normal white blood cells (which fight infection), platelets (which control hemorrhaging), and red blood cells (which prevent anemia). As a result, symptoms such as fatigue, paleness, weight loss, easy bruising, repeated infections, nosebleeds, and other forms of hemorrhaging occur. In children, these symptoms can appear suddenly.[93]

Leukemia can be acute or chronic in nature and can strike both sexes and all age groups. Chronic leukemia can develop over several months and have few symptoms. Although many people believe that leukemia is a childhood disease, leukemia strikes more adults than children.[94] Estimates for 2009 are that 4700 new cases of leukemia will be diagnosed (2700 in men; 1950 in women).[95] Further 2500 deaths are expected in 2009 from leukemia even though there has been a dramatic increase in the survival rate of patients with acute lymphocytic leukemia since the 1970s.

Oral Cancer

Cancer may develop in any part of the oral cavity. Most often it is found on the lips, the lining of the cheeks, the gums, and the floor of the mouth. The tongue, the pharynx, and the tonsils are other common sites. Current estimates (from 2009) are that there will be 3400 new cases (2200 in men; 1150 in women) of oral cancer diagnose in Canada with 1150 deaths forecasted.[96] Tobacco use—smoking, chewing, or dipping—is the most common risk factor for oral cancer.

---

what do you THINK?

What types of cancers are you and your friends at greatest risk for right now? What part(s) of your lifestyle put you most at risk? What are you willing to change?

FACING CANCER

As previously mentioned, 45 percent of men and 40 percent of women are likely to develop cancer in their lifetime, with approximately one in four Canadians dying as a result. At the current rates, cancer mortality will soon surpass mortality from CVD. Many factors have contributed to the rise in cancer mortality—one being simply longer life expectancies—but the increase in the incidence of lung cancer is probably the most important reason. However, recent advances in diagnosis and treatment have reduced much of the fear and mystery that surround cancer. Further, research continues with

---

Pap test: A procedure in which cells taken from the cervical region are examined for abnormal cellular activity.

various studies, including a large, population-based prospective study in Alberta, called The Tomorrow Project.[97]

Detecting Cancer

The earlier a person is diagnosed with cancer, the better his or her prospect for survival. Various high-tech diagnostic techniques exist to detect cancer. New high-technology diagnostic imaging techniques have replaced exploratory surgery for some cancer patients. **Magnetic resonance imaging (MRI)** is one example of such technology. In MRI, a huge electromagnet is used to detect hidden tumours by mapping the vibrations of the various atoms in the body on a computer screen. **Computerized axial tomography scanning (CAT scan)** uses X-rays to examine parts of the body. In both of these painless, noninvasive procedures, cross-section pictures can show a tumour's shape and location more accurately than conventional X-rays.

These medical techniques, along with regular self-examinations and checkups, play an important role in the early detection and secondary prevention of cancer. See the Building Communication Skills text box for recommendations regarding regular cancer screening. Familiarize yourself with the Seven Warning Signals of cancer, as shown in Figure 11.7. If you notice any of these signs, and they do not appear to be related to anything else, you should see a doctor immediately. Make sure that appropriate diagnostic tests are completed whenever any warning signs

appear. Also make a realistic assessment of your individual risk factors and try to avoid those you have control over.

New Hope in Cancer Treatments

Although cancer treatments have changed dramatically over the last 25 years, surgery, in which the tumour and surrounding tissue are removed, is still most common. Today's surgeons tend to remove less surrounding tissue than previously and to combine surgery with either **radiotherapy** (the use of radiation) or **chemotherapy** (the use of drugs) to kill cancerous cells.

Radiation works by destroying malignant cells or stopping cell growth. It is most effective in treating localized cancer masses. In the process of destroying malignant cells, radiotherapy also destroys healthy cells.

When cancer has spread throughout the body, it is necessary to use some form of chemotherapy. Similar to radiation therapy, chemotherapy attacks and kills cancerous and healthy cells. Ongoing research will result in new, less toxic drugs more effective at attacking cancerous cells only.

Whether used alone or in combination, radiotherapy and chemotherapy have possible side effects, including extreme nausea, nutritional deficiencies, hair loss, and general fatigue. Long-term damage to the cardiovascular system and many other systems of the body can be significant. It is important that you discuss these matters fully with your doctor.

Psychosocial and behavioural research has become increasingly important as health professionals seek answers to questions concerning complex lifestyle factors that appear to influence risks for cancer, as well as the survivability of patients with particular psychological and mental health profiles. Also, healthcare practitioners have become more aware of the psychological needs of patients and families and have begun to tailor treatment programs to meet the diverse needs of different people. In particular, individuals with cancer indicate higher levels of satisfaction and obtain better health outcomes when they are able to discuss their experience with health professionals.[98] Research by Bender et al.[99] indicates that women with breast cancer have many questions about the pain they will experience as a result of their treatment and of the cancer itself.

Cancer's Seven Warning Signals

1 Changes in bowel or bladder habits.

2 A sore that does not heal.

3 Unusual bleeding or discharge.

4 Thickening or lump in breast or elsewhere.

5 Indigestion or difficulty in swallowing.

6 Obvious change in a wart or mole.

7 Nagging cough or hoarseness.

If you have a warning signal,
see your doctor.

FIGURE 11.7
Cancer's Seven Warning Signs

Life after Cancer

Heightened public awareness and an improved prognosis for people with cancer has made the cancer experience less threatening and isolating than it once

Screening Guidelines for the Early Detection of Cancer in Asymptomatic People

CANCER-RELATED CHECKUP

For individuals undergoing periodic health examinations, a cancer related checkup should include health counselling and, depending on a person's age, might include examination for cancers of the thyroid, oral cavity, skin, lymph nodes, testes, and ovaries, as well as for some nonmalignant diseases.

BREAST

Women 40 and older should have an annual mammogram and an annual clinical breast exam (CBE) performed by a health care professional and should perform monthly breast self-examination (BSE). Ideally, the CBE should occur before the scheduled mammogram.

Women aged 20–39 should have a clinical breast exam performed by a health care professional every three years.

Women should know how their breasts normally feel and report any breast change promptly to their health care providers. Breast self-exam is an option for women starting in their twenties.

Women at increased risk (for instance, those with a family history, genetic tendency, or past breast cancer) should talk with their doctors about the benefits and limitations of starting mammography screening earlier, having additional tests (that is, breast ultrasound and MRI), or having more frequent exams.

COLON AND RECTUM

Beginning at age 50, men and women should follow one of the examination schedules below:

- A fecal occult blood test (FOBT) every year, or a flexible sigmoidoscopy (FSIG) every five years, or both annual fecal occult blood test and flexible sigmoidoscopy every five years*

- A double contrast barium enema every 5 to 10 years

- A colonoscopy every 10 years

*Combined testing is preferred over either annual FOBT or FSIG every five years alone. People who are at moderate or high risk for colorectal cancer should talk with a doctor about a different testing schedule.

PROSTATE

The American Cancer Society recommends that both the prostate-specific antigen (PSA) blood test and the digital rectal examination be offered annually, beginning at age 50, to men who have a life expectancy of at least 10 more years.

Men at high risk (African Canadian men and men with a strong family history of one or more first-degree relatives diagnosed with prostate cancer at an early age) should begin testing at age 45. Information should be provided to patients about what is known and what is uncertain about the benefits and limitations of early detection and treatment of prostate cancer so that they can make an informed decision.

UTERUS

- **Cervix:** Screening should begin approximately three years after a woman begins having vaginal intercourse but no later than 21 years of age. Screening should be done every year with Pap tests or every two years using liquid-based tests. At or after age 30, women who have had three normal tests in a row may get screened every two to three years, unless they have certain risk factors, such as HIV infection or a weak immune system. Screening after total hysterectomy (with removal of the cervix) is not necessary unless the surgery was done as a treatment for cervical cancer.

- **Endometrium:** The American Cancer Society recommends that all women be informed about the risks and symptoms of endometrial cancer and be strongly encouraged to report any unexpected bleeding or spotting to their physicians. Annual screening for endometrial cancer with endometrial biopsy beginning at age 35 should be offered to women with or at risk for hereditary nonpolyposis colon cancer (HNPCC).

Source: From *Cancer Facts and Figures 2007.* Copyright © 2007, American Cancer Society. Used with permission from American Cancer Society, Atlanta, GA.

---

was. Assistance for individuals with cancer is more readily available than ever before. Cancer support groups, cancer information workshops, and medical consultation are just a few of the forms of assistance now offered in many communities. Increasing efforts in cancer research, improvements in diagnostic equipment, and advances in treatment provide hope for the future.

Magnetic resonance imaging (MRI): A device that uses magnetic fields, radio waves, and computers to generate an image of internal tissues of the body for diagnostic purposes without the use of radiation.

Computerized axial tomography (CAT scan): A machine that uses radiation to view internal organs not normally visible on X-rays.

Radiotherapy: The use of radiation to kill cancerous cells.

Chemotherapy: The use of drugs to kill cancerous cells.

Managing Your Health

Although it is easy to read through a chapter like this and learn what we should be doing to keep ourselves healthy, few of us ever really think about what it takes to prevent serious illness. Relationships, financial worries, grades, time for fun, and other issues often take precedence over our long-term commitments to wellness.

MAKING DECISIONS FOR YOU

List the five things that matter to you most right now. Is appearance part of your list? Is being able to get through a day without feeling tired or unusually fatigued important? Are you motivated to change your health behaviours and take action to reduce your heart disease, diabetes, and cancer risks by engaging in more physical activity, reducing stress, and eating well? Was there anything about this chapter that made you think you should make a change now? Why is this important? What actions do you plan to take?

CHECKLIST FOR CHANGE: MAKING PERSONAL CHOICES

- Determine your hereditary risks. If they are high, outline the steps that you can take to reduce your overall risk, focusing on lifestyle and the factors you can control.
- Learn about the normal CVD risk changes that occur with age. Take the extra steps needed to minimize these risks.
- If you smoke, quit. If you don't smoke, don't start. Avoid secondhand smoke.
- If you chew, dip, or use snuff, quit. If you don't, don't start.
- Find out your cholesterol levels, including HDL and LDL levels.
- Reduce saturated and trans fat in your diet and take steps to reduce your triglyceride and cholesterol levels.
- Get out and do some physical activity. Every day. Even a relaxing walk every day is effective at reducing risk. Nobody says you have to run until you drop. Take it easy, but keep it up.
- Control your blood pressure. Monitor it regularly and see your doctor if you have high blood pressure.
- Manage your weight. Obesity is a significant risk factor for CVD, diabetes, and cancer.
- Manage your stress.
- Avoid excessive sunlight. When in the sun, wear sunscreen that contains at least SPF 15.
- Avoid excessive alcohol consumption.
- Monitor estrogen use—in the form of oral contraceptives or hormone replacement therapy, for instance—carefully.
- Avoid occupational exposures to carcinogens. Exposure to several different industrial agents (nickel, chromate, asbestos, vinyl chloride, and so on) increases risk for various cancers.
- Eat your vegetables and fruits. Eat at least seven or eight servings of fruits and vegetables every day to reduce your risk for lung, colon, pancreatic, stomach, bladder, esophageal, mouth, and throat cancer.
- Be happy; take care of your spiritual self.

CHECKLIST FOR CHANGE: MAKING COMMUNITY CHOICES

- Take a class in CPR. Your local Red Cross likely offers them; courses may also be available on campus. Be prepared to offer bystander CPR.
- Consider becoming an emergency medical technician (EMT). You don't have to make a career of it. But you could be prepared to save people in your dorm, your office building, and your community.
- Does your community have any major sources of carcinogens (toxic waste dumps, chemical factories, and so on)? What precautions are taken to ensure that any environmental risks are reduced?
- Does the Canadian Cancer Society have a local office at which you could volunteer some time?
- Does your community have cancer support groups that you could join if you were found to have cancer? Where would you find out about such support groups?

CRITICAL THINKING

You've been good friends with one of your 30-something neighbours for some time. Recently, after spending a good deal of time working on a community project together, you start to date. After a few terrific dates, during which you really hit it off socially, you find out that your friend had cancer two years ago, and that there is a 50-percent chance it will return within five years. You love this person, but wonder what to do. What if you commit yourself to this relationship and the cancer returns? You've always wanted to have children, but are concerned about what would happen if your partner died of cancer while your children are young. On the other hand, there is a 50-percent chance that the cancer will not return.

Using the DECIDE model described in Chapter 1, decide whether or not you would continue the relationship. Does it make any difference to you whether the person who survived cancer is male or female? Explain why or why not.

Gilda's Club: A Support Community for Thousands Living with Cancer

Gilda's Club is named in honour of the late comedian Gilda Radner, who, when describing the emotional and social support she received when she had cancer, called for such places of participation, education, hope, and friendship to be made available for people with cancer and their families and friends everywhere.

WHAT IS GILDA'S CLUB?

A free, non-residential, emotional and social support community for men, women, and children living with cancer. It includes not only people affected with cancer, but their families, caregivers, significant others and friends—because cancer affects everyone, not only the person with the physical disease. Unlike a social service agency, Gilda's Club is a community centre that is driven by its membership. It is open to all, without referral and at no cost. Funding is solicited from private individuals, corporations, and foundations.

THE UNIQUE VISION OF GILDA'S CLUB

Gilda's Club provides a meeting place where people with cancer can come together to learn how to live with cancer and celebrate the challenges and opportunities of everyday life. Its philosophy is premised on the belief that people gather strength and knowledge from support groups and social interaction in a cancer support community.

The first Gilda's Club, including a worldwide training centre, opened its signature red door in New York City in 1995. Many affiliates are open or under development in different parts of the world. Canada has one in Toronto and one in Montreal. Since 1995, thousands of members now attest to the fact that Gilda's Club has helped change their lives by restoring control and enabling them to plan their own emotional and social support, thus strengthening and enriching the entire family.

Source: Retrieved on March 21, 2006 from www.gildasclubtoronto.org.

Go to MyHealthLab at **www.pearsoned.ca/myhealthlab**. Here you will find self-assessments, case studies, links to health on the net, and much more.

✱ DISCUSSION QUESTIONS

1. List the different types of cardiovascular diseases. Compare and contrast their symptoms, risk factors, prevention, and treatment.
2. Discuss why age is such an important factor in women's risk for CVD. What can be done to lower women's risks in later life?
3. Describe the role of healthy eating in preventing CVD.
4. Describe the unique role of physical activity in preventing and treating CVD.
5. What is diabetes? Why are more people currently being diagnosed with type 2 diabetes?
6. What is cancer? What is the difference between a benign and a malignant tumour?
7. Describe the general risks for developing cancer. Which of these factors relate to you? What can you do to reduce this risk?
8. Why are breast and testicular self-exams important?
9. What symptoms signal that you have cancer instead of a minor illness? How soon should you seek treatment for any of the seven warning signs?

APPLICATION EXERCISE

Reread the "Consider This . . ." scenario at the beginning of the chapter and answer the following questions.

1. Consider Kassandra's case in the chapter opener. Why do you think so many young Canadians deny their risk for skin cancer?
2. As a friend of Kassandra's, what advice might you give her?
3. Think about close friends or people in your family who also are at risk for developing skin cancer or any other form of cancer. What could you do to help them become aware of their risks without preaching to them about their lifestyle choices and turning them off?
4. What kinds of community efforts are needed to change the perceptions that a "healthy glow" results from suntanning?

MYSEARCHLAB EXERCISE

1. Log on to www.MySearchLab.com.
2. Find an article to share with the class that discusses risk factors for cardiovascular diseases, type 2 diabetes, or cancer. Share what you learn with your group or class. With your group, make suggestions to reduce these particular risks. Share these suggestions with the class and create a master list for the class to learn to live by.

CHAPTER 12

INFECTIOUS AND NONINFECTIOUS CONDITIONS

Risks and Responsibilities

CONSIDER THIS . . .

Chandra and Tony have been seeing each other for a year. Their relationship is sexually active. Both had been sexually active prior to this relationship. Chandra is concerned and goes to the Health Unit for a sexual health checkup. She learns she has a sexually transmitted infection (STI). She can tell Tony herself, the Health Unit staff can arrange a confidential meeting and tell Tony for her, or she can ask her family doctor to talk with Tony. She is afraid of Tony's reaction and does not know if she is the carrier or became infected by Tony.

What do you think Chandra should do? What would you do? Why is Chandra worried about Tony's reaction? Is that a normal response? Why or why not? How would you react if your partner told you he or she had an STI?

CHAPTER OBJECTIVES

- Identify the risk factors for infectious diseases, including those you can and cannot control.

- Explain how the immune system works, as well as the role of vaccinations in fighting disease.

- Discuss the various sexually transmitted infections, including HIV, their means of transmission, and actions that prevent their spread.

- Identify common chronic diseases, including neurological disorders, sex disorders, diseases of the digestive system, and the varied musculoskeletal diseases.

Every moment of every day you are in contact with microscopic organisms that have the ability to make you sick. These disease-causing agents, or **pathogens**, are found in the air you breathe, in the foods you eat, and on nearly every person or object that you come into contact with. Most deaths from infectious diseases—almost 90 percent—are caused by only a handful of diseases. And most of these diseases have plagued humankind throughout history, often ravaging populations more effectively than wars.[1] There is fossil evidence that infections, cancer, heart disease, and a host of other ailments afflicted the earliest human beings. At times, infectious diseases wiped out whole groups of people through **epidemics** such as the Black Death or bubonic plague, which killed up to one-third of the population of Europe in the 1300s. A pandemic, or global epidemic, of influenza killed more than 20 million people in 1918, while strains of tuberculosis and cholera continue to cause premature death throughout the world.

In spite of our best efforts to eradicate them, these diseases continue to be a menace. But the news is not all bad; even though we are bombarded by potential pathogenic threats, our immune systems are remarkably adept at protecting us. Endogenous microorganisms are those that live in peaceful coexistence with their human host most of the time. For people in good health, and whose immune systems are functioning well, endogenous organisms are usually harmless; but, in sick people or those with a compromised immune system, these normally harmless pathogenic organisms can cause serious health problems.

Exogenous microorganisms are organisms that do not normally inhabit the body. When they do, however, they are apt to produce an infection or illness. The more easily these pathogens can gain a foothold in the body and sustain themselves, the more **virulent** or aggressive the organism, the higher the probability that it will overcome your body defences and cause disease. However, if your immune system is strong and your internal capacity to ward off disease is substantial, you should be able to fight even the most virulent attacker. Just because you inhale a flu virus does not mean that you will get the flu. Just because your hands are teeming with bacteria does not mean that you will get a bacterial infection. Several factors influence your susceptibility to these diseases.

Infectious diseases in Canada are controlled through ongoing vigilance by public health networks operating at local, regional, provincial, and national levels. Clean food and water, immunizations, and an excellent health-care system have maintained Canadians' health. Good nutrition and engaging in a physically active lifestyle are also factors in overall good health that help us as individuals combat infectious diseases. Nutritional status has been found to have an effect on resistance to infectious diseases in certain population groups such as infants, young children, and the elderly. Nutritional status can also affect the course of an infectious disease, as has been shown with individuals who are HIV-positive.[2] And regular physical activity of moderate intensity is also thought to boost immune system functioning.

INFECTIOUS DISEASE RISK FACTORS

At one time, it was believed that most diseases were caused by a single factor, but today we recognize that most diseases are **multifactorial**, or caused by the interaction of several factors from inside and outside the person. For a disease to occur, the host must be susceptible, meaning that the immune system must be in a weakened condition; an agent capable of transmitting a disease must be present; and the environment must be hospitable to the pathogen in terms of temperature, light, moisture, and other requirements. Other factors also increase or decrease levels of susceptibility.

Risk Factors You Cannot Control

Uncontrollable risk factors are those that increase your susceptibility to a disease and that you may have little or no control over. Some of the most common factors are examined below.

Heredity

Perhaps the single greatest factor influencing your longevity is your parents' longevity. Being born into a family in which heart disease, cancer, or other illnesses are prevalent increases your risk. Some people with a close relative who has diabetes develop diabetes themselves even though they take precautions, manage their weight, engage in regular physical activity, and eat a diet that follows the guidelines identified in Eating Well with Canada's Food Guide. Some diseases are a result of chromosomal inheritance. **Sickle cell anemia**, an inherited blood disease that primarily affects individuals of African descent, is often transmitted to the fetus when both parents carry the sickle cell trait. It remains unclear whether hereditary diseases are a result of chromosomal abnormalities or deficiencies in immune system functioning.

Aging

After the age of 40, we become more vulnerable to chronic diseases. Moreover, as we age, our immune systems respond less efficiently to invading organisms, increasing our risk for infection and illness. The same flu that produces an afternoon of nausea and diarrhea in a younger person may cause days of illness or even death in an older person. The very young are also at risk for many diseases, particularly if not vaccinated against them.

Environmental Conditions

Unsanitary conditions and the presence of drugs, chemicals, and hazardous pollutants and wastes in our food and water have a significant effect on our immune systems. Th weakening of **immunological competence**—the body's ability to defend itself against pathogens—in such situations has been well documented.[3]

what do you **THINK?**

Examine the risk factors you can and cannot control. What is your risk of contracting an infection from an invading pathogen? How is your risk affected by hereditary factors?

Risk Factors You Can Control

On a positive note, we have some degree of personal control over many risk factors for disease. Too much stress, an inadequate dietary intake, inactivity, lack of sleep, misuse or abuse of legal and illegal drugs, poor personal hygiene, high-risk behaviours, and other variables significantly increase our risk for a number of diseases. Factors we can control—at least partly—through lifestyle choices include vigour of immune response; pre-existing level of immunity; pre-existing disease; use of substances such as cigarettes, chew, dip, alcohol, and drugs; and psychological factors such as stress, depression, and anxiety.[4]

THE PATHOGENS: ROUTES OF INVASION

Pathogens enter the body in several ways. They may be transmitted by direct contact between infected persons, such as during sexual relations, kissing, or touching, or by indirect contact, such as by touching an object an infected person has contacted. The hands are probably the greatest source of transmission. You may also **autoinoculate** yourself, or transmit a pathogen from one part of your body to another. For example, you may touch a sore on your lip teeming with viral herpes and then transmit the virus to your eye when you scratch your itchy eyelid.

Pathogens are also transmitted by airborne contact, either through inhaling the droplet spray from a sneeze or through breathing air that carries a particular pathogen. You may become the victim of food-borne infection if you eat something contaminated by microorganisms. The *E. coli* bacteria and other virulent pathogens are responsible for a variety of diseases that pose significant threats to humans. Examples of these are found in Table 12.1.

Your "best friend" may be the source of animal-borne pathogens. Dogs—as well as cats, livestock, and wild animals—can spread numerous diseases through their bites, feces, or by carrying infected insects into your living areas. For example, ticks in some regions carry Lyme disease. Water-borne diseases are transmitted directly from drinking water and indirectly from foods washed or sprayed with water containing their pathogens. These pathogens can also invade your body if you wade or swim in contaminated streams, lakes, rivers, and reservoirs.

what do you **THINK?**

What are the most common pathogens you are currently exposed to? How can you best protect yourself against them?

Pathogen: A disease-causing agent.

Epidemic: Disease outbreak that affects many people in a community or region at the same time.

Virulent: Strong enough to overcome host resistance and cause disease.

Multifactorial disease: Disease caused by interactions of several factors.

Sickle cell anemia: Genetic disease resulting from chromosomal abnormalities commonly found among individuals of African descent.

Immunological competence: Ability of the immune system to defend the body from pathogens.

Autoinoculation: Transmission of a pathogen from one part of your body to another.

TABLE 12.1

Emerging Diseases: Challenges to Public Health

Over the past few decades, more than 30 diseases have been identified in humans for the first time. More than two-thirds of these diseases are known to have originated from animals—both wild and domestic species.

Disease/Cause Agent	Description
Avian influenza [Type A (H5N1)]	Previously thought to infect only birds (to whom it can be deadly), avian influenza first jumped to humans in 1997 in Hong Kong. Initial symptoms include fever, cough, and chills; most influenza infections cause only self-limited illness that does not require hospitalization. Symptoms after infection with the H5N1 strain can be severe in all age groups.
Ebola virus	A deadly disease concentrated in portions of Africa, Ebola can be transferred only by direct contact with infected blood, organs, secretions, semen, or contaminated needles. Transmission is enhanced by unsanitary, overcrowded conditions and poor preventive practices. No treatment or vaccine is available and 50 to 90 percent of those contracting the disease die.
Dengue fever	More than 200 000 cases of dengue fever occurred in Latin America alone during 1994, of which 5000 were dengue hemorrhagic fever (DHF), a severe form of the disease that causes high mortality. The type of mosquito that carries the disease is establishing new habitats in the Americas and parts of Africa and Asia. Over the past 40 or so years the number of cases has increased at least 20-fold.
E. coli bacteria	Illness caused by the Escherichia coli bacteria as a result of eating unwashed or poorly washed vegetables and undercooked meat.
Flesh-eating strep	A rare disease caused by a strain of Group A streptococcus bacterium that produces materials that dissolve tissue. Early diagnosis and treatment with antibiotics stops the disease.
Cholera	A bacterial disease affecting the intestinal tract of individuals who eat or drink food or water contaminated by fecal waste of an infected person. In 1992, a new strain of cholera was detected in the Bay of Bengal and spread to 10 other countries.
Tuberculosis	A pulmonary disease once thought to be almost eliminated from North America. Depressed social conditions and improper use of antibiotics have revived this airborne disease, which is particularly threatening to people with weakened immune systems. Strict adherence to drug therapy for several months can cure the disease.
West Nile virus	A flavivirus commonly found in Africa, West Asia, and the Middle East that can infect mosquitoes, birds, horses, humans, and some other mammals. Increasingly common in North America, most people experience only a mild case, characterized by flu-like symptoms that last for a few days. However, more extreme forms of this disease can cause encephalitis (inflammation of the brain) and meningitis (inflammation of the membrane around the brain and spinal cord), which can prove to be fatal.

Bacteria

Bacteria are single-celled organisms that are plantlike in nature but lack chlorophyll (the pigment that gives plants their green colouring). There are three major types of bacteria: cocci, bacilli, and spirilla. Bacteria may be viewed under a standard light microscope. Although there are several thousand species of bacteria, only approximately 100 cause diseases in humans. In many cases, it is not the bacteria themselves that cause disease but rather the poisonous substances, called **toxins**, that they produce. Some of these toxins are extremely powerful. Bacterial infections can take many forms, with the following being the most common.

Staphylococcal Infections

One of the most common forms of bacterial infection is the staph infection. **Staphylococci** are normally present on our skin at all times and seldom cause problems. But when there is a cut or break in the **epidermis**, or outer layer of the skin, staphylococci may enter and cause a localized infection. If you have ever had acne, boils, styes (infections of the eyelids), or infected cuts, you probably had a staph infection too.

At least one staph-caused disorder, **toxic shock syndrome**, is potentially fatal. Media reports in the early 1980s indicated that this disorder was exclusive to menstruating women, particularly those who used high-absorbency tampons for extended periods of time. Although tampons are strongly implicated, the actual mechanisms that produce this disease remain uncertain. Even though most cases of toxic shock syndrome occurred in menstruating women, the disease was first reported in 1978 in a group of children and continues to be reported in men, children, and nonmenstruating women. Most cases not related to menstruation occur in individuals recovering from wounds, surgery, and similar incidents.

To reduce the likelihood of contracting toxic shock syndrome, women should take the following precautions

- avoid superabsorbent tampons except during the heaviest menstrual flow;
- change tampons frequently, at least every four hours;
- use pads at night instead of tampons.

Call your doctor immediately if you have any of the following symptoms during menstruation: high fever, headache, vomiting, diarrhea and the chills, stomach pains, or shock-like symptoms such as faintness, rapid pulse, pallor (which can be caused by a drop in blood pressure), or a sunburn-like rash, particularly on fingers and toes.

Streptococcal Infections

Another common form of bacterial infection is caused by microorganisms called **streptococci**. A "strep throat" (severe sore throat characterized by white or yellow pustules at the back of the throat) is the typical streptococcal problem. Scarlet fever (characterized by acute fever, sore throat, and rash) and rheumatic fever (said to "lick the joints and bite the heart") are serious streptococcal infections.

Pneumonia

Pneumonia at one point was one of the leading causes of death in North America and across the world. This disease is characterized by chronic cough, chest pain, chills, high fever, fluid accumulation, and eventual respiratory failure. One of the most common forms of pneumonia is caused by bacterial infection and responds readily to antibiotic treatment. Other forms are caused by the presence of viruses, chemicals, or other substances in the lungs. In these types of pneumonia, treatment may be more difficult.

Legionnaire's Disease

Legionnaire's disease gained widespread publicity in 1976, when several legionnaires at the American Legion convention in Philadelphia contracted the disease and died before the invading organism was isolated and effective treatment devised. The symptoms are similar to those for pneumonia, which sometimes makes diagnosis difficult. In people whose immunity is compromised, particularly the elderly, delayed identification can have serious consequences, since Legionnaire's must be treated with erythromycin; **penicillin**, usually given for pneumonia is ineffective on Legionnaire's disease.

Tuberculosis

One of the leading fatal diseases in Europe and North America in the early 1900s, **tuberculosis (TB)** was largely controlled by the mid-1900s through improved sanitation, isolation of infected persons, and treatment

Bacteria: Single-celled organisms that may cause diseases in humans.

Toxins: Poisonous substances produced by certain microorganisms that cause various diseases.

Staphylococci: Found normally on our skin, only cause infection when there is a break in the skin.

Epidermis: The outermost layer of the skin.

Toxic shock syndrome: A potentially life-threatening bacterial infection most common in menstruating women.

Streptococci: A bacteria that can cause strep throat or scarlet fever.

Pneumonia: Disease of the lungs, usually caused by bacteria.

Penicillin: Antibiotic used to fight a variety of bacterially caused ailments.

Tuberculosis (TB): A disease caused by bacterial infiltration of the respiratory system.

with drugs such as rifampin or isoniazid. Although treatable with antibiotics, TB continues to be a worldwide problem, killing almost two million people each year.[5]

Several factors contribute to the resurgence of TB, including the phasing-out of surveillance and control programs, the emergence of multiple-antibiotic-resistant TB (MAR-TB), large-scale migration, social and natural disasters, and infection with the human immunodeficiency virus (HIV). The risk of developing clinical TB in tuberculin-positive individuals is very high in HIV-seropositive patients.[6] For most Canadians, the risk of developing TB is low, although there are approximately 1600 new cases reported each year.[7]

Tuberculosis is caused by bacterial infiltration of the respiratory system. It is transmitted by breathing infected air from an infected person's coughing or sneezing. Many people infected with TB are contagious without actually showing symptoms themselves. Symptoms include persistent coughing, weight loss, fever, and spitting up blood. Fortunately, the average healthy person is not at high risk; however, those who may be fighting other diseases, such as some of the HIV-related diseases, may be at increased risk. A quick test can usually detect TB. If you do have it, you can usually be treated and made noncontagious within two weeks and cured within six months.

Periodontal Diseases

Diseases of the tissue around the teeth, called **periodontal diseases**, affect three out of four adults over the age of 35. Improper home tooth care, including lack of flossing and poor brushing habits, and the failure to obtain regular professional dental care lead to increased bacterial growth, caries (tooth decay), and gum infections. If left untreated, permanent tooth loss may result. Further, untreated periodontal disease increases the risk for several systemic diseases, including coronary heart disease and type 2 diabetes.

✔• Viruses

Viruses are the smallest pathogens, approximately 1/500 the size of bacteria. Because of their tiny size, they are visible only under an electron microscope and were therefore not identified until the twentieth century. At present, more than 150 viruses are known to cause diseases in humans.

A virus consists of a protein structure that contains either ribonucleic acid (RNA) or deoxyribonucleic acid (DNA). It is incapable of carrying out the normal cell functions of respiration and metabolism. It cannot reproduce on its own and exists only in a parasitic relationship with the cell it invades.

Treatment of viral diseases is difficult because many viruses can withstand heat, formaldehyde, and large doses of radiation with little effect on their structure. In addition, some viruses may have **incubation periods** (the length of time required to develop fully and cause symptoms in their hosts) measured in years rather than hours or days. Termed **slow-acting viruses**, these viruses infect the host and remain in a semidormant state for years, causing a slowly developing illness. HIV is an example of a slow-acting virus.

Drug treatment for viral infections is limited. Drugs powerful enough to kill viruses tend to kill the host cells too, although some drugs are available that block stages in viral reproduction without damaging the host cells. We have another form of virus protection within our bodies. When exposed to certain viruses, the body begins to produce a protein substance known as **interferon**. Interferon does not destroy the invading microorganisms but sets up a protective mechanism to aid healthy cells in their struggle against the invaders. Although interferon research is promising, it should be noted that not all viruses stimulate interferon production.

The Common Cold

Caused by any number of viruses (some experts claim there may be more than 100 different viruses responsible for the common cold), colds are **endemic** among peoples throughout the world. Current research indicates that otherwise healthy people carry cold viruses in their noses and throats most of the time. These viruses are held in check until the host's resistance is lowered. In the true sense of the word, it is possible to "catch" a cold—from the airborne droplets of another person's sneeze or from skin-to-skin or mucous membrane contact—though recent studies indicate that the hands may be the greatest source of cold and other viral transmission.

Although numerous ideas exist concerning how to prevent or cure the common cold, including taking megadoses of vitamin C, little hard evidence supports them. The best rule of thumb for preventing the common cold is to keep your resistance level high. Eating well (see Chapter 5), getting adequate rest (six to nine hours each night), managing your stress (see Chapter 3), and engaging in regular physical activity (see Chapter 4) is your best approach to fighting off possible infection. Also, limit contact with people with newly developed colds since colds appear to be most contagious during the first 24 hours. Once you contract a cold, bed rest, plenty of fluids, and a pain reliever are

Hands may be the greatest source of viral transmission, so washing them often and well may help prevent you from catching or transmitting the common cold.

the tried-and-true remedies for adults. Continue to eat well and be physically active at a light or moderate intensity. Keep in mind that children should not be given Aspirin for colds or the flu because of the possibility of Reye's syndrome. Several over-the-counter preparations are available to alleviate various cold symptoms (see also Chapter 9).

Influenza

In otherwise healthy people—that is people without a compromised immune system—**influenza**, or flu, is usually not serious. Symptoms, including aches and pains, nausea, diarrhea, fever, and coldlike ailments, generally pass quickly. However, in combination with other disorders, or among the elderly (people 65+), those with respiratory or heart disease, or the very young (children under the age of five), the flu can be very serious.

To date, three major varieties of flu virus have been discovered, with many different strains existing within each variety. The "A" form of the virus is generally the most virulent, followed by the "B" and "C" varieties. If you contract one form of influenza you may develop immunity to it, but you may not necessarily be immune to other forms of the disease. There is little that can be done to treat individuals with the flu once the infection has become established. Similar to when you contract a cold, bed rest is recommended, as well as drinking plenty of fluids and trying to eat well. Physical activity should be limited or restricted until the fever has passed.

Some vaccines have proven effective for preventing certain strains of flu virus, but are totally ineffective against others. Flu vaccination is recommended for those with a compromised immune system, including adults and children with chronic pulmonary disorders, people of any age who are residents of nursing homes, people 65 years of age or over, and people with diabetes and other metabolic diseases—as well as people in health services. In many jurisdictions, vaccination for these most vulnerable groups is provided free of charge. Vaccination for people not in essential health services is also recommended, but the person bears the cost, generally a fee of $10 or $15. Because flu shots take anywhere from two to three weeks to become effective, you should get these shots in the fall, before the flu season begins.

Infectious Mononucleosis

This affliction of college- and university-aged people is often jokingly referred to as the "kissing disease." The symptoms of mononucleosis, or "mono," include

Periodontal diseases: Diseases of the tissue around the teeth.

Viruses: Minute parasitic microbes that cause disease.

Incubation period: The time between exposure to a disease and the appearance of the symptoms.

Slow-acting viruses: Viruses having long incubation periods, causing slowly progressive symptoms.

Interferon: A protein substance produced by the body that aids the immune system by protecting healthy cells.

Endemic: Continued prevalence of a specific infection or disease in a specific population or area.

Influenza: A common viral disease of the respiratory tract.

TABLE 12.2

Forms of Hepatitis: A Comparison

Disease	Incubation Period	Acute Infectious (% symptomatic)	Outcome
Hepatitis B	45–180 days	< 10% of childhood infections; 50% of adult infections	1% develop fulminant hepatitis; 1–10% of adults become chronic carriers; > 90% perinatal or early childhood infections become carriers
Hepatitis A	15–45 days	< 10% of childhood infections; 50% of adult infections	No chronic carriers
Hepatitis C	14–168 days	More often asymptomatic	50% become chronic carriers

Source: Health Canada, 2009©. Adapted and Reproduced with the permission of the Minister of Public Works and Government Services Canada, 2009.

sore throat, fever, headache, nausea, chills, and a pervasive weakness or tiredness in the initial stages. As the disease progresses, lymph nodes may continue to enlarge, and jaundice, spleen enlargement, aching joints, and body rashes may develop.

Theories on the transmission and treatment of mononucleosis are highly controversial. Caused by the Epstein-Barr virus, mononucleosis is readily detected through a monospot test, a blood test that measures the percentage of specific forms of white blood cells. Because many viruses are spread by transmission of body fluids, people once believed that young people passed the disease on when kissing. Although this is still considered a possible route of transmission, mononucleosis is not believed to be highly contagious. In fact, it does not appear to be easily contracted through normal, everyday personal contact. Multiple cases among family members are rare, as are cases between intimate partners.

Treatment of mononucleosis is often a lengthy process that involves bed rest, a healthy dietary intake that follows Eating Well with Canada's Food Guide, and medications to control the symptoms of the disease. Gradually, the body develops a form of immunity to the disease and the person gets well again.

Hepatitis

One of the most highly publicized viral diseases is **hepatitis**. The incidence of hepatitis is rising in Canada, with various educational programs implemented in the hopes of preventing further outbreaks. Hepatitis is generally defined as a virally caused inflammation of the liver, characterized by symptoms such as fever, headache, nausea, loss of appetite, skin rashes, pain in the upper right abdomen, dark yellow (with a brownish tinge) urine, and the possibility of jaundice. In fact, hepatitis is often "the disease your

friends diagnose" because of the yellowing of the whites of the eyes and the skin.

Treatment of all the forms of viral hepatitis (see Table 12.2) is somewhat limited. A healthy dietary intake, bed rest, and antibiotics to combat bacterial infections that may cause additional problems are recommended. Vaccines for hepatitis are available through a series of injections, although costs are high. Many provinces are beginning to require vaccinations against hepatitis B for health-care workers and others who may be exposed to blood-borne pathogens. Vaccination for hepatitis is also recommended when travelling outside Canada and the United States.

Mumps

Until 1969, mumps was a common viral disorder among children, with an average of 30 000 cases per year. That year, a vaccine become available and the disease seemed to be largely under control, with reported cases declining to between 1.2 and 3.5 per 100 000 from 1986 to 1995.[8] Approximately one-half of all mumps infections are not apparent because they produce only minor symptoms. Typically, there is an incubation period of 16 to 18 days, followed by symptoms caused by the lodging of the virus in the glands of the neck. The most common symptom is the swelling of the parotid (salivary) glands. One of the greatest dangers associated with mumps is the potential for sterility in men who contract the disease in young adulthood. Also, transient deafness may occur in fewer than one to five cases per 100 000, and may be permanent in some.[9]

Chicken Pox

Caused by the varicella-zoster virus, which also causes shingles (see below), chicken pox produces the characteristic symptoms of fever and tiredness 13 to 17 days after exposure, followed by skin eruptions that itch, blister, and produce a clear fluid. The virus is present in these blisters for approximately one week. Symptoms are generally mild, and immunity to subsequent infection appears to be lifelong. A chicken pox vaccine for use in children aged 12 months and older has been available in Canada since 2000. However, many unvaccinated children still contract the disease, and a small percentage of those vaccinated may as well. Scientists believe that after the initial infection, the virus goes into permanent hibernation and, for most people, there are no further complications. For a small segment of the population, however, the zoster virus may become reactivated. Blisters will develop, usually on only one side of the body and tending to stop abruptly at the midline. Cases in which the disease covers both sides of the body are far more serious. This disease, known as shingles, affects slightly more than 5 percent of the population each year, most often in individuals over 50 years of age.

Measles

Measles is the most contagious disease known to humans. Although there has been a 74 percent decrease in the disease, measles remains a major killer, accounting for about 200 000 deaths a year.[10] The **measles** virus may ultimately be responsible for more child deaths than any other single microbe, due to complications from pneumonia, diarrhea, and malnutrition.[11] Technically referred to as rubeola, measles is a viral disorder that often affects young children. Symptoms, appearing about 10 days after exposure, include an itchy rash and a high fever. The significant decrease in measles deaths is a result of an intensified vaccination campaign.[12]

Rubella (or **German measles**), is a milder viral infection believed to be transmitted by inhalation, after which the virus multiplies in the upper respiratory tract and passes into the bloodstream. German measles causes a rash, especially on the upper extremities. It is not generally a serious health threat and usually runs its course in three to four days. The major exceptions to this rule are newborns and pregnant women. Rubella can damage a fetus, particularly during the first trimester, creating a condition known as congenital rubella, in which the infant may be born blind, deaf, cognitively impaired, or with heart defects. Immunization has greatly reduced the incidence of measles and German measles. Infections in children not immunized against measles can lead to fever-induced problems such as rheumatic heart disease, kidney damage, and neurological disorders.

YOUR BODY'S DEFENCES: KEEPING YOU WELL

Physical and Chemical Defences

try it NOW!

Wash your hands to prevent infection. How can you clean your hands properly? Wet your hands with warm water and lather them with soap; scrub your hands for about 20 seconds—try counting to 20, say the alphabet, or sing "Happy Birthday." Rinse well and then dry your hands. Wash your hands whenever you use the bathroom, eat or prepare food, blow your nose, cough, or sneeze. It is preferable to use soap and water, though in a pinch, alcohol-based rubs can be used. These products, however, should not be used regularly as they kill both helpful and harmful bacteria and may contribute to antibacterial resistance.

Perhaps our single most critical early defence system is the skin. Layered to provide an intricate web of barriers, the skin allows few pathogens to enter. **Enzymes**, complex proteins manufactured by the body that appear in body secretions such as sweat, provide additional protection, destroying microorganisms on skin surfaces by producing inhospitable pH levels. Normal body pH is 7.0, but enzymatic or biochemical changes may cause the body chemistry to become more acidic (pH of less than 7.0), or more alkaline (pH of more than 7.0). In either case, microorganisms that flourish at a selected pH will be weakened or destroyed as these changes occur. A third protection is our frequent slight elevations in body temperature, which also create an inhospitable environment for many pathogens. Further, only when there are cracks or breaks such as that found in cuts, in the skin can pathogens gain easy access to the body.

The linings of the body provide yet another protection against pathogens. Mucous membranes in the respiratory tract and other linings of the body trap

Hepatitis: A virally caused disease in which the liver becomes inflamed, resulting in fever, headache, and jaundice.

Measles: A viral disease that produces symptoms including an itchy rash and a high fever.

Rubella (German measles): A milder form of measles that causes a rash and mild fever in children and may cause damage to a fetus or a newborn baby.

Enzymes: Organic substances that cause bodily changes and destruction of microorganisms.

and engulf invading organisms. Cilia, hairlike projections in the lungs and respiratory tract, sweep unwanted invaders toward body openings, where they are expelled. Tears, nasal secretions, ear wax, and other secretions found at body entrances contain enzymes designed to destroy or neutralize invading pathogens. Finally, any invading organism that manages to breach these initial lines of defence faces a formidable specialized network of defences from the immune system.

The Immune System: Your Body Fights Back

Immunity is the condition of being able to resist a particular disease by counteracting the substance that produces the disease. Any substance capable of triggering an immune response is called an **antigen**. An antigen can be a virus, a bacterium, a fungus, a parasite, or a tissue or cell from another individual. When invaded by an antigen, the body responds by forming substances called antibodies. **Antibodies** belong to a mass of large molecules known as immunoglobulins, a group of nine chemically distinct protein substances, each of which plays a role in neutralizing, setting up for destruction, or actually destroying antigens. Once an antigen breaches the body's initial defences, the body begins a careful process of antigen analysis. It considers the size and shape of the invader, verifies that the antigen is not part of the body itself, and then begins to produce a specific antibody to destroy or weaken the antigen. This process, which is much more complex than described here, is part of a system called humoral immune responses. Humoral immunity is the body's major defence against bacteria and bacterial toxins.

Cell-mediated immunity is characterized by the formation of a population of lymphocytes that can attack and destroy the foreign invader. These lymphocytes constitute the body's main defence against viruses, fungi, parasites, and some bacteria. Key players in this immune response are specialized groups of white blood cells known as macrophages (a type of phagocytic, or cell-eating, cell) and lymphocytes, other white blood cells in the blood, lymph nodes, bone marrow, and certain glands.

Two forms of lymphocytes in particular, the B-lymphocytes (B-cells) and T-lymphocytes (T-cells), are involved in the immune response. There are different types of B-cells, named according to the area of the body in which they develop. Most are manufactured in the soft tissue of the hollow shafts of the long bones. T-cells, in contrast, develop and multiply in the thymus, a multi-lobed organ that lies behind the breast-

bone. T-cells assist your immune system in several ways. Regulatory T-cells help direct the activities of the immune system and assist other cells, particularly B-cells, to produce antibodies. Dubbed "helper Ts," these cells are essential for activating B-cells, other T-cells, and macrophages. Another form of T-cell, known as the "killer Ts" or "cytotoxic Ts," directly attacks infected or malignant cells. Killer Ts enable the body to rid itself of cells infected by viruses or transformed by cancer; they are also responsible for the rejection of tissue and organ grafts. The third type of T-cells, "suppressor Ts," turns off or suppresses the activity of B-cells, killer Ts, and macrophages. Suppressor Ts circulate in the bloodstream and lymphatic system, neutralizing or destroying antigens, enhancing the effects of the immune response, and helping to return the activated immune system to normal levels. After a successful attack on a pathogen, some of the attacker T- and B-cells are preserved as memory T- and B-cells, enabling the body to quickly recognize and respond to subsequent attacks by the same kind of organism at a later time. Thus macrophages, T- and B-cells, and antibodies are the key factors in mounting an immune response.

Once people have survived certain infectious diseases, they become immune to them, meaning that in all probability they will not develop those particular diseases again. When the disease-causing microorganism next attacks them, their memory T- and B-cells are quickly activated to come to their defence. Immunization works on the same principle. Vaccines containing an attenuated (weakened) or killed version of the disease-causing microorganism or an antigen similar to but not as dangerous as the disease antigen are administered to stimulate the immune system to produce antibodies to build immunity from the disease.

Autoimmune Diseases

Although white blood cells and the antigen–antibody response generally work in our favour, the body sometimes makes a mistake and targets its own tissue as the enemy, builds up antibodies against that tissue, and attempts to destroy it. This is known as autoimmune disease (auto means "self"). Common examples of this type of disease are rheumatoid arthritis, lupus erythematosus, and myasthenia gravis.

In some cases, the antigen–antibody response completely fails to function. The result is a form of immune deficiency syndrome. Perhaps the most dramatic case of this syndrome was the "bubble boy," who died in 1984 after living his short life inside a sealed-off environment designed to protect him from all antigens. A much more common immune system disorder is acquired immune deficiency syndrome (AIDS), discussed later in this chapter.

Fever

If an infection is localized, pus formation, redness, swelling, and irritation often occur. These symptoms indicate a systematic response against the invading organisms. Another indication is the development of a fever, or a rise in body temperature above the norm of 37°C. Fever is frequently caused by toxins secreted by pathogens that interfere with the control of body temperature. Although this elevated temperature is often harmful to the body, it is also believed to act as a form of protection. A one- or two-degree elevation in temperature creates an environment that destroys some types of disease-causing organisms. Also, as body temperature rises, the body is stimulated to produce more white blood cells, which also destroy more invaders.

Pain

Although pain is not usually thought of as a defence mechanism, it plays a valuable role in the body's response to invasion. Pain is generally a response to injury. Pain may be either direct, caused by the stimulation of nerve endings in an affected area, or referred, meaning it is present in one place while the source is elsewhere. An example of referred pain is the pain in the arm or jaw often experienced by someone having a heart attack. Regardless of the cause of pain, most pain responses are accompanied by inflammation. Pain tends to be the earliest sign that an injury occurred and often causes the person to slow down or stop the activity, thereby protecting against further damage. Because it is often one of the first warnings of disease, persistent pain should not be overlooked, ignored, or masked with short-term pain relievers.

Vaccines: Bolstering Your Immunity

The body's natural defence mechanisms are our strongest allies in the battle against disease from birth until death. There are periods in our life, however, when either invading organisms are too strong or our natural immunity is too weak to protect us from catching a particular disease. It is at such times that we need outside assistance in developing immunity to an invading organism. Such assistance can be provided through a **vaccination**. Vaccines are given orally or by injection, and this form of artificial immunity is

termed *acquired immunity*, in contrast to *natural immunity*, which a mother passes to her fetus via their shared blood supply.

Today, depending on the virulence of the organism, vaccines containing live, weakened, or dead organisms are given to people for a variety of diseases. In some instances, if a person is already weakened by other diseases, vaccination may provoke an actual case of the disease. This happened with the smallpox vaccinations administered routinely in the 1960s. It was believed that the risk of contracting smallpox from the vaccine was actually greater than the chance of contracting the disease in an environment where it had essentially been eradicated. For this reason, routine smallpox inoculations were eliminated in the late 1960s. See Tables 12.3, 12.4, and 12.5 for the current recommendations in Canada for vaccines for children and adults.

✳ SEXUALLY TRANSMITTED INFECTIONS

There are more than 20 different types of **sexually transmitted infections** (STIs, formerly called STDs, or sexually transmitted diseases). These infections were once referred to as venereal diseases, this newer classification is believed to be broader in scope and reflective of the numbers and types of communicable infections, which are sometimes asymptomatic.[13] In Canada the incidence of STIs is rising, particularly among young people—with the majority of new infections attributed to those between the ages of 15 and 24 years.[14] Young people today generally become sexually active sooner and marry later and as a result have a greater number of partners, which increases their risk of acquiring an STI. Further, with the increase in the number of divorces, people are once again more likely to have multiple sexual partners during their life and increase their risk of developing an STI.

In many, the early symptoms of an STI are not serious. They range from mild discomfort to annoying

Antigen: Substance capable of triggering an immune response.

Antibodies: Substances produced by the body to destroy or weaken specific antigens.

Vaccination: Inoculation with killed or weakened pathogens or similar, less dangerous antigens in order to prevent or lessen the effects of some disease.

Sexually transmitted infections (STIs): Infectious diseases transmitted via vaginal, anal, and oral sexual contact.

TABLE 12.3

Recommended Childhood Immunization Schedule

Age	Immunization Against
2 months	Diphtheria, pertussis, tetanus, poliomyelitis, *haemophilus influenzae* b,[*] pneumococcal conjugate vaccine, meningococcal C conjugate vaccine
4 months	Diphtheria, pertussis, tetanus, poliomyelitis, *haemophilus influenzae* b, pneumococcal conjugate vaccine,[**] meningococcal C conjugate vaccine
6 months	Diphtheria, pertussis, tetanus, poliomyelitis,[†] *haemophilus influenzae* b, pneumococcal conjugate vaccine
12 months	Measles, mumps, rubella,[††] varicella,[‡] pneumococcal conjugate vaccine
18 months	Diphtheria, pertussis, tetanus, poliomyelitis, *haemophilus influenzae* b
4–6 years	Diphtheria, pertussis, tetanus, poliomyelitis
9–13 years	Hepatitis B[‡‡]
14–16 years	Diphtheria, tetanus, poliomyelitis, meningococcal C conjugate vaccine[§]

Notes:

[*] *Haemophilus influenzae* b requires a series of immunizations. The exact number and timing of each may vary with the brand of vaccine used.

[**] Recommended schedule, number of doses, and subsequent use of pneumococcal vaccine depends on the age of the child when vaccination is begun.

[†] If oral polio virus vaccine is used exclusively in a series of immunizations, this dose may be omitted.

[††] A second dose of MMR vaccine is recommended for children and youth. It may be administered any time after a minimum one-month waiting period; provincial schedules differ.

[‡] Children aged 12 months to 12 years should receive one dose of varicella vaccine. Individuals aged 13 years or older should receive two doses at least 28 days apart.

[‡‡] Hepatitis B requires a series of immunizations. In some jurisdictions, they may be administered at a younger age.

[§] Recommended schedule and number of doses of meningococcal vaccine depends on the age of the child.

Source: Adapted from *Canadian Immunization Guide,* 6th ed., Health Canada, 2002. Reproduced with the permission of the Minister of Public Works and Government Services Canada, 2007.

TABLE 12.4

Adult Immunization Schedule—Routinely for All

Vaccine	Dosing schedule (no record or unclear history of immunization)	Booster schedule (primary series completed)
Tetanus and diphtheria given as Td; and pertussis given as Tdap	Doses 1 and 2, 4–8 weeks apart and dose 3 at 6–12 months later; one of the doses should be given as Tdap for pertussis protection	Td every 10 years; 1 dose should be given as Tdap if not previously given in adulthood
Measles, mumps and rubella given as MMR	1 dose for adults born in or after 1970 without a history of measles or those individuals without evidence of immunity to rubella or mumps; second dose for selected groups	Not routinely required
Varicella	Doses 1 and 2, at least 4 weeks apart for susceptible adults (no history of natural disease or seronegativity)	Not currently recommended

Source: Health Canada, 2009©. Adapted and Reproduced with the permission of the Minister of Public Works and Government Services Canada, 2009.

TABLE 12.5
Adult Immunization Schedule—Specific Risk Situations

Vaccine or toxoid	Indication	Schedule
Influenza	Adults ≥ 65 years; Adults < 65 years at high risk of influenza-related complications, their household contacts, health-care workers, and all those wishing to be protected against influenza.	Every autumn, using current recommended vaccine formulation
Pneumococcal polysaccharide	Adults ≥ 65 years; Adults < 65 who have conditions putting them at increased risk of pneumococcal disease.	1 dose
Hepatitis A	Occupational risk, life-style, travel and living in areas lacking adequate sanitation. Outbreak control, post-exposure immunoprophylaxis. Patients with chronic liver disease.	2 doses 6–12 months apart
Hepatitis B	Occupational risk, life-style, post-exposure immunoprophylaxis. Patients with chronic liver disease.	3 doses at 0, 1, and 6 months
Bacille Calmette-Guérin (BCG)	Rarely used. Consider for high-risk exposure in selected cases.	1 dose
Cholera	High-risk exposure in travellers to endemic area(s).	1 oral dose of live attenuated vaccine; 2 doses at least 1 week apart but not greater than 6 weeks of oral inactivated vaccine
Japanese encephalitis	Travel to endemic area(s) or other exposure risk.	3 doses at days 0, 7, and 30
Poliomyelitis	Travel to endemic area(s) or other risk group.	Primary series doses 1 and 2, 4–8 weeks apart and dose 3 at 6–12 months later; 1 booster dose if > 10 years since primary series
Meningococcal conjugate	Young adults	1 dose
Meningococcal polysaccharide	High-risk exposure groups	1 dose
Rabies, pre-exposure use	Occupational or high-risk travellers	3 doses at days 0, 7, and 21
Typhoid	High-risk travellers to endemic area(s) or other high-risk exposure	Parenteral capsular polysaccharide 1 dose; live attenuated 3–4 oral doses depending on preparation
Yellow fever	Travel to endemic area(s) or if required for foreign travel	1 dose with booster every 10 years if required
Smallpox	Laboratory staff working with vaccinia or other orthopoxviruses	1 dose

Source: Health Canada, 2009©. Adapted and Reproduced with the permission of the Minister of Public Works and Government Services Canada, 2009.

itching or discharge. (See Figure 12.1 for signs that may indicate an STI.) Left untreated, however, some STIs have grave consequences, such as sterility, blindness, central nervous system destruction, disfigurement, and even death. Infants born to mothers with STIs are at risk of a variety of health problems.

Similar to other communicable diseases, much of the pain, suffering, and anguish associated with STIs could be eliminated or substantially reduced through education, responsible action, and prompt treatment when symptoms first occur. Overcoming the tendency to pass moral judgments on those who contract an STI would certainly lower the barriers to treatment. Similarly, being prepared to deal with the pressure to engage in sexual activity as well as the responsibility required when choosing to be sexually active can also be helpful.

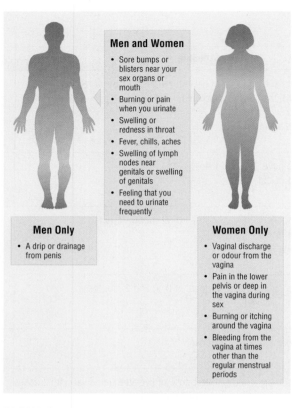

Men and Women
- Sore bumps or blisters near your sex organs or mouth
- Burning or pain when you urinate
- Swelling or redness in throat
- Fever, chills, aches
- Swelling of lymph nodes near genitals or swelling of genitals
- Feeling that you need to urinate frequently

Men Only
- A drip or drainage from penis

Women Only
- Vaginal discharge or odour from the vagina
- Pain in the lower pelvis or deep in the vagina during sex
- Burning or itching around the vagina
- Bleeding from the vagina at times other than the regular menstrual periods

FIGURE 12.1
Signs and Symptoms of STIs

Possible Causes: Why Me?

STIs affect men and women of all socioeconomic levels, ages, ethnicities, and regions of the world. Several reasons have been proposed to explain the present high rates of STIs. The first relates to the moral and social stigma associated with them. Shame and embarrassment often keep infected people from seeking treatment. Unfortunately, these people usually continue to be sexually active, thereby infecting others. People uncomfortable with discussing sexual issues may also be less likely to use, or to ask their partners to use, condoms as a means of protection against STIs.

Another reason proposed for the STI epidemic is the current casual attitude about sex. Bombarded by a media hype that glamorizes sex and the ease of being sexually active, many people engage in sexual activity without considering the consequences or being responsible for their actions. Others are pressured into sexual relationships they do not really want. Generally, the more sexual partners a person has, the greater the risk for contracting an STI. Evaluate your beliefs and attitudes about STIs by taking the Rate Yourself box self-assessment.

Ignorance about the infections themselves and an inability to recognize actual symptoms or to

acknowledge that a person may be asymptomatic yet still have an infection are also factors behind the current rise in STIs. A person infected but asymptomatic may unknowingly spread an STI to an unsuspecting partner, who may then ignore or misinterpret symptoms that appear. By the time either partner seeks medical help, they may have infected several others.

Modes of Transmission

STIs are generally spread through some form of sexual contact. Vaginal and anal intercourse, oral–genital contact, and hand–genital contact are (in decreasing order of likelihood) the most common modes of transmission. More rarely, pathogens for STIs are transmitted from mouth to mouth or, even more infrequently, through contact with fluids from body sores. While each STI is a different infection caused by a different pathogen, all STI pathogens prefer dark, moist places, especially the mucous membranes lining the reproductive organs. The majority of these organisms are susceptible to light, excess heat, cold, and dryness, and many die quickly on exposure to air. (The toilet seat is not a likely breeding ground for most bacterial or viral STIs.) Although most STIs are passed on by sexual contact, other kinds of close contact, such as sleeping on the sheets used by someone who has pubic lice or using their towel, may also result in transmission from one person to another. One method of preventing the spread of STIs is to use a condom during any sexual activity, including vaginal, anal, and oral sex as well as during hand-genital contact. To fully protect yourself, follow these basic rules:

- Decide ahead of time that you will only have sex using a condom. Make sure you have one with you.
- Never reuse a condom.
- Use only latex condoms.
- Store condoms in a cool, dry place—not in the glove compartment of your car or in your wallet.
- If a condom appears brittle or sticky, don't use it.
- Put the condom on (correctly) before any sexual activity, including oral sex and hand–genital contact.
- Apply a water-based lubricant containing spermicide to the condom for additional protection.
- If the condom breaks, tears, or becomes dislodged, wash the genitals thoroughly with soap and water, apply a spermicide, and put on another condom before additional contact. It takes only a fraction of a second to become infected with disease-laden body fluids or to infect someone else.
- Hold the condom in place during withdrawal to make sure it does not come off.

STI Attitude and Belief Scale

The following quiz will help you evaluate whether your beliefs and attitudes about STIs lead you to behaviours that may heighten your risk for contracting an STI.

DIRECTIONS

Read each statement. Circle T if you think the statement is true or F if you think the statement is false. Then consult the answer key that follows.

1. You can usually tell whether someone is infected with an STI, especially HIV.

   T   F

2. Chances are that if you have not caught an STI by now, you probably have a natural immunity and will not get infected in the future.

   T   F

3. A person successfully treated for an STI does not need to worry about getting it again.

   T   F

4. So long as you keep yourself fit and healthy, you do not need to worry about STIs.

   T   F

5. The best way for sexually active people to protect themselves from STIs is to practise safer sex.

   T   F

6. The only way to catch an STI is to have sex with someone who has one.

   T   F

7. Talking about STIs with a partner is so embarrassing that you are best off not to discuss them.

   T   F

8. STIs are a problem only for people who are promiscuous.

   T   F

9. You do not need to worry about contracting an STI so long as you wash yourself thoroughly with soap and hot water immediately after sex.

   T   F

10. You do not need to worry about AIDS if no one you know has ever had it.

   T   F

SCORING KEY

1. False. Several STIs, such as chlamydia, gonorrhea (especially in women), internal genital warts, and even HIV infection in its early stages, cause few if any obvious signs or symptoms.

2. False. If you practise unprotected sex and have not contracted an STI to this point, count your blessings.

3. False. Successful treatment does not render immunity against reinfection.

4. False. Even people in prime physical condition can be felled by the tiniest of microbes that cause STIs.

5. True. If you are sexually active, practising safer sex is the best protection against contracting an STI. Of course, abstinence is the only sure way to not contract an STI through sexual activity.

6. False. STIs can also be transmitted through nonsexual means, such as by sharing contaminated needles or, in some cases, through contact with disease-causing organisms on towels and bed sheets or even toilet seats.

7. False. Do not let embarrassment prevent you from taking steps to protect your and your partner's welfare.

8. False. STIs are a potential problem for anyone who is sexually active.

9. False. While washing your genitals immediately after sex may have limited protective value, it is no substitute for practising safer sex.

10. False. Symptoms of HIV infection may not appear for years after initial infection with the virus.

INTERPRETING YOUR SCORE

First, add up the number of items you got right. A score of eight or better indicates that your attitudes toward STIs should decrease your risk of contracting them. Yet even one wrong response on this test increases your risk of contracting an STI. Knowledge alone is not sufficient to protect yourself from STIs. You need to ask yourself how you are going to put knowledge into action by changing your behaviours to reduce your chances of contracting an STI.

Source: Adapted from Jeffrey S. Nevid with Fern Gotfried, *Choices: Sex in the Age of STDs*, 10–13. © 1995 by Allyn & Bacon. Reprinted by permission.

Like other communicable diseases, STIs have both pathogen-specific incubation periods and periods of time during which transmission is most likely, called periods of communicability.

Although there are more than 20 different types of STIs, we discuss only those most likely to pose a risk for the average adult.

Chlamydia

Genital **chlamydia** (*Chlamydia trachomatis*) first became nationally reportable in 1990 and emerged as the most prevalent bacterial STI in Canada. Preventable and treatable, genital chlamydia remains high in Canada—in 2007 the chlamydia rate (217.3 per 100 000; 149.8 in men and 283.0 in women)[15] was much greater than the national rate for gonorrhea (34.9 per 100 000; 41.3 in men and 28.6 in women).[16] Current chlamydia infection rates are higher than in past years and have been increasing since 1997. The increase is likely due to more screening being done with newer, non-invasive technologies (see Table 12.6).

The name of the infection is derived from the Greek verb *chlamys*, meaning "to cloak," because, unlike most bacteria, chlamydia can live and grow only inside other cells. Although many people classify chlamydia as either nonspecific or nongonococcal urethritis (NGU), a person may have NGU without having the organism for chlamydia. In more than half of the cases of NGU (infections of the urethra and surrounding tissues not caused by gonococcal bacteria), however, *Chlamydia trachomatis*, the bacterial organism that causes chlamydia, is present. For this reason, the two disease terms tend to be used interchangeably, even though NGU may be caused by other organisms.

In males, early symptoms include painful and difficult urination, frequent urination, and a watery, pus-like discharge from the penis. Symptoms in females may include a yellowish discharge, spotting between periods, and occasional spotting after intercourse. Unfortunately, many individuals with chlamydia have no symptoms and therefore do not seek help until the infection has done secondary damage. Females are especially likely to be asymptomatic, with more than 70 percent unaware they have the infection until secondary damage occurs.

The secondary damage resulting from chlamydia is serious for males and females. Males suffer damage to the prostate gland, seminal vesicles, and bulbourethral glands, as well as arthritis-like symptoms and damage to the blood vessels and heart. In females, secondary damage from chlamydia includes inflammation that damages the cervix or fallopian tubes, causing sterility and damage to the inner pelvic structure and leading to pelvic inflammatory disease (PID, see next section). If an infected woman becomes pregnant, she has a high risk for miscarriages and stillbirths. Chlamydia may also be responsible for one type of **conjunctivitis**, an eye infection that affects not only adults but also infants, who contract the disease from an infected mother during delivery. Untreated conjunctivitis can cause blindness.

Chlamydia can be controlled through responsible sexual behaviours and familiarity with the early symptoms of the disease. If detected early enough, chlamydia is easily treatable with antibiotics such as tetracycline, doxycycline, or erythromycin. In most cases, treatment is successfully completed in two to three weeks.

TABLE 12.6
Screening for STIs

Screening to detect asymptomatic STIs is divided into three categories:

Case Finding: A patient-based strategy in individuals with an increased likelihood of one or more STIs—for example, sexual contacts to gonorrhea

Focused Screening: A group-based strategy in subpopulations with high STI prevalence rates—for example, street youth, core groups, adolescents, and those with a history of STI

General Screening: A population-based strategy in certain members of the general public who are not considered to be at increased risk for STI but in whom serious consequences may occur if infected—for example, syphilis and HIV testing in pregnancy

	Case Finding	Focused Screening	General Screening
Procedures			
Sexual history	X	X	X
Physical examination			
External genital	X	X	X
Internal genital	Adults, adolescents	Adults, adolescents	—
Targeted extragenital	X	X	X
Laboratory tests			
Chlamydia trachomatis	X	X	—
Treponema pallidum	X	X	X
Pap smear	Adults, adolescents	Adults, adolescents	—
Hepatitis B (HBV)	Optional	Optional	X
HIV	X	X	X
Chlamydia trachomatis	X	X	—

Source: Health Canada, 2009©. Adapted and Reproduced with the permission of the Minister of Public Works and Government Services Canada, 2009.

what do you THINK?

Why do many post-secondary students, even though they have heard of the risks of STIs and HIV, fail to use condoms and in general act irresponsibly regarding their sexual health? What actions do you think could be taken to help you and your friends engage in sexually responsible behaviours?

Pelvic Inflammatory Disease (PID)

Pelvic inflammatory disease (PID) is actually not one disease but a term used to describe a number of infections of the uterus, fallopian tubes, and ovaries. Although PID is often the result of an untreated STI, especially chlamydia or gonorrhea, it is not actually an STI. Nonsexual causes of PID are also common, including excessive vaginal douching, cigarette smoking, and substance abuse. PID is not a notifiable disease in Canada; thus, estimating prevalence is difficult. A study undertaken by Health Canada's Laboratory Centre for Disease Control found that the rate of PID declined appreciably over 10 years. A study done in Manitoba came to a similar conclusion.[17]

Symptoms may include acute inflammation of the pelvic cavity, severe pain in the lower abdomen, menstrual irregularities, fever, nausea, painful intercourse, tubal pregnancies, and severe depression.[18] The major consequences of untreated PID are infertility, ectopic pregnancy, chronic pelvic pain, and recurrent upper genital infections. Risk factors include young age at first sexual intercourse, multiple sexual partners, high frequency of sexual intercourse, and change of sexual partners within the last 30 days.[19] Regular gynecological examinations and early treatment for STI symptoms reduce risk.

Gonorrhea

Gonorrhea still exists in Canada, though it has declined more than tenfold since 1980. The most recent data (2007) indicate a national incidence of 24.9 per 100 000.[20] This dramatic decline has been attributed to better control programs involving diagnostic services, contact tracing, and effective treatment.[21]

Currently, the majority of endemic gonococcal infections is thought to reside within core groups: a small subset of the population whose members frequently acquire new sexual partners. The highest rates of infection are found in the territories, particularly the Yukon (426.9 per 100 000), and the Northwest Territories (335.5 per 100 000) followed by Manitoba

(133.7 per 100 000) and Saskatchewan (96.6 per 100 000).[22] More research needs to be conducted to assess and describe core groups within a Canadian context; appropriate prevention and control strategies, aimed at reducing or ideally eliminating indigenous gonococcal infections, can then be implemented.[23]

Caused by the bacterial pathogen *Neisseria gonorrhoea*, this infection primarily infects the linings of the urethra, genital tract, pharynx, and rectum. It may be spread to the eyes or other body regions via the hands or body fluids.

In males, a typical symptom is a white milky discharge from the penis accompanied by painful, burning urination two to nine days after contact. This is usually enough to send most men to their physician for treatment. Only about 20 percent of all males with gonorrhea are asymptomatic.

In females, the situation is the opposite. Only about 20 percent of all females experience any form of discharge, and few develop a burning sensation upon urinating until much later in the infection (if ever). The organism can remain in the woman's vagina, cervix, uterus, or fallopian tubes for long periods with no apparent symptoms other than an occasional slight fever. Thus, a woman can be unaware that she has been infected and that she may be infecting her sexual partners.

Upon diagnosis, an antibiotic regimen using penicillin, tetracycline, spectiomycin, ceftriaxone, or other drugs is begun. A penicillin-resistant form of gonorrhea may require a particularly strong combination of antibiotics. Treatment is generally completely effective within a short period of time if the disease is detected early.

If the disease goes undetected in a woman, it can spread throughout the genital–urinary tract to the fallopian tubes and ovaries, causing sterility—or, at the very least, severe inflammation and pelvic inflammatory disease symptoms. If an infected woman becomes pregnant, the disease can cause conjunctivitis in her infant. In the past, to prevent this, physicians and midwives routinely administered silver nitrate or penicillin preparations to the eyes of newborn babies. Currently, an antibiotic ointment or drops are used, not only to prevent the spread of STIs but also to prevent other eye infections that might result because of bacteria.

Chlamydia: Bacterially caused STI of the urogenital tract.

Conjunctivitis: Serious inflammation of the eye caused by any number of pathogens or irritants; can be caused by STIs such as chlamydia.

Pelvic inflammatory disease (PID): Term used to describe various infections of the female reproductive tract.

Gonorrhea: Second most common STI in Canada; if untreated, may cause sterility.

Untreated gonorrhea in the male may spread to the prostate, testicles, urinary tract, kidney, and bladder. Blockage of the vasa deferentia due to scar tissue formation may cause sterility. In some cases, the penis develops a painful curvature during erection.

Syphilis

Syphilis, the other well-known STI, is also caused by a bacterial organism, the spirochete known as *Treponema pallidum*. Because it is extremely delicate and dies quickly on exposure to air, dryness, or cold, the organism is generally transferred only through direct sexual contact. Typically, this means contact between sexual organs during intercourse, but in rare instances the organism enters the body through a break in the skin, through deep kissing in which body fluids are exchanged, or through some other transmission of body fluids.

With the arrival of HIV in the 1980s, syphilis took on new importance. It increases sexual transmission of HIV by six- to sevenfold, and neurosyphilis in HIV-infected patients is particularly difficult to treat. Early detection and treatment of STIs can have a major impact on the sexual transmission of HIV2-9. Because of this synergy, syphilis control can have a significant impact on the HIV epidemic in Canada.[24]

Syphilis is called the "great imitator" because its symptoms resemble those of several other diseases. Only an astute physician who has reason to suspect the presence of the disease will order the appropriate tests for a diagnosis. Unlike most of the other STIs, syphilis generally progresses through several distinct stages.

Primary Syphilis

The first stage of syphilis, particularly for males, is often characterized by the development of a sore known as a **chancre** (pronounced "shank-er"), located most frequently at the site of the initial infection. This chancre is usually about the size of a dime and is painless, but it oozes bacteria, ready to spread to an unsuspecting partner. Usually the chancre appears between three and four weeks after contact.

In males, the site of the chancre tends to be the penis or scrotum because this is where the organism first made entry into the body. But, if the infection was contracted through oral sex, the sore can appear in the mouth, throat, or other "first contact" area. In females, the site of infection is often internal, on the vaginal wall or high on the cervix. Because the chancre is not readily apparent, the likelihood of detection is not great. In males and females, the chancre will completely disappear in three to six weeks.

A chancre on the site of the initial infection is a symptom of primary syphilis

Secondary Syphilis

From a month to a year after the chancre disappears, secondary symptoms may appear, including a rash or white patches on the skin or on the mucous membranes of the mouth, throat, or genitals. Hair loss may occur, lymph nodes may become enlarged, and the individual infected may run a slight fever or develop a headache. In rare cases, sores develop around the mouth or genitals. As during the active chancre phase, these sores contain infectious bacteria, and contact with them may spread the disease. In some people, symptoms follow a textbook pattern; in others, there are no symptoms at all. In a few cases, there may be arthritic pain in the joints. Because symptoms vary so much and because the symptoms that do appear are so far removed from previous sexual experience that the individual infected seldom connects the two, the infection often goes undetected even at this second stage. Symptoms may persist for a few weeks or months and then disappear, leaving the infected individual thinking that all is well.

Latent Syphilis

The syphilis spirochetes begin to invade body organs after the secondary stage. There may be periodic reappearance of previous symptoms, including the presence of infectious lesions, for between two and four years after the secondary period. After this period, the infection is rarely transmitted to others, except during pregnancy, when it can be passed on to the fetus. The child will then be born with congenital syphilis, which can cause death or severe birth defects such as blindness, deafness, or disfigurement. Because in most cases the fetus does not become infected until after the first trimester, treatment of the mother during this period will usually prevent infection of the fetus.

In some instances, a child born to an infected mother will show no apparent signs of the disease at birth but within several weeks will develop body rashes, a runny nose, and symptoms of paralysis. Congenital syphilis is usually detected before it progresses much further. But sometimes the child's immune system will ward off the invading organism, and further symptoms may not surface until the teenage years.

In addition to causing congenital syphilis, latent syphilis, if untreated, will continue to progress, infecting more and more organs until the infection reaches its final stage, late syphilis.

Late Syphilis

Most of the horror stories concerning syphilis involve the late stages of the infection. Years after syphilis has entered the body and progressed through the various organs, its net effects become clearly evident. Late-stage syphilis indications include heart damage, central nervous system damage, blindness, deafness, paralysis, premature senility, and, ultimately, insanity.

Treatment for Syphilis

Treatment for syphilis resembles that for gonorrhea. Because the organism is bacterial, it is treated with antibiotics, usually penicillin, penicillin G benzathine, or doxycycline. Blood tests are administered to determine the exact nature of the invading organism, and the doses of antibiotics are much stronger than those taken by the typical gonorrhea patient. The major obstacle to treatment is misdiagnosis of this "imitator" disease.

Pubic Lice

Often called "crabs," **pubic lice** are more annoying than dangerous. Pubic lice are small parasites usually transmitted during sexual contact. They prefer the dark, moist regions of the body and, during vaginal and anal sex, move easily from partner to partner. Although sexual contact is the most common mode of transmission, you can become infected with pubic lice from lying on sheets an infected person slept on or from using their towel. Sleeping in hotel and dormitory rooms in which blankets and sheets are not washed regularly, using someone else's towel at the gym, or sitting on toilet seats where the nits or larvae have been dropped and lie in wait for a new carrier may put you at risk.

Venereal Warts

Venereal warts (also known as genital warts or condylomas) are caused by a small group of viruses known as human papilloma viruses (HPVs). A person becomes infected when an HPV penetrates the skin and mucous membranes of the genitals or anus through sexual contact. The virus appears to be relatively easy to catch. The typical incubation period is from six to eight weeks. Many people have no apparent symptoms, particularly if the warts are located inside the reproductive tract. Others may develop a series of itchy bumps on the genitals, which range in size from a small pinhead to large cauliflower-like growths that can obstruct normal urinary or reproductive activity. On dry skin (such as on the shaft of the penis), the warts are commonly small, hard, and yellowish-grey, resembling warts that appear on other parts of the body. Venereal warts are of two different types: (1) full-blown genital warts noticeable as tiny bumps or growths, and (2) the much more prevalent flat warts not usually visible to the naked eye.

Risks of Venereal Warts

Many venereal warts will eventually disappear without treatment. Others will grow and generate unsightly flaps of irregular flesh on the external genitalia. The greatest threat from venereal warts may be in the apparent relationship between them and a tendency for dysplasia, or changes in cells that may lead to a precancerous condition, usually on the cervix. Exactly how HPV infection leads to cervical cancer is uncertain. What is known is that within five years of infection, 30 percent of all HPV cases progress to the precancerous stage. Of those cases that become precancerous and are left untreated, 70 percent will eventually result in cancer. As mentioned previously in Chapter 11, a vaccination is now available for young women to protect them from the HPV virus. In addition, venereal warts may pose a threat to a pregnant woman's unborn fetus if the fetus is exposed to the virus during birth. Caesarean deliveries may be considered in serious cases.

Treatment for Venereal Warts

Treatment for venereal warts may take several forms:

1. Warts are painted with a medication called podophyllin during a visit to the doctor's office.

Syphilis: An STI caused by a bacterial infection, cured with antibiotics, spread through direct sexual contact.

Chancre: Sore often found at the site of syphilis infection.

Pubic lice: Parasites that inhabit various body areas, especially the genitals; also called "crabs."

Venereal warts: Warts that appear in the genital area or the anus; caused by the human papilloma viruses (HPVs).

Genital warts are caused by the human papilloma virus and can be full blown or flat.

The podophyllin is washed off after about four hours, and a few days later the warts begin to dry up and fall off. Sometimes more than one application is necessary. This procedure is relatively painless.

2. Warts may be removed by cryosurgery, a procedure in which an instrument treated with liquid nitrogen is held to the affected area, "freezing" the tissue. Within a few days, the warts fall off.

3. Depending on size and location, some warts are removed by simple excision.

4. For larger warts, laser surgery is often used. This is a major procedure that normally requires general anesthesia. The frequency of laser use for wart removal is currently questioned by many health experts. (Precautions must also be taken during this procedure to shield medical staff from infection by viral spray.)

5. Creams containing 5-Fluoracil (an anticancer drug) are used to prevent further precancerous cell development.

6. For warts located externally, injections of interferon are sometimes given to keep the virus from spreading to healthy tissue. This treatment shows promise, but it is expensive and, when administered in large doses, may cause flu-like symptoms.

Prevention is clearly a better approach. What is true about protecting yourself from HIV infection is also true about protecting yourself from genital warts and other STIs (see the section on AIDS prevention later in this chapter).

Candidiasis (Moniliasis)

Unlike many of the other STIs caused by pathogens that come from outside the body, the yeast-like fungus caused by the *Candida albicans* organism normally inhabits the vaginal tract in most women. Only under certain conditions will these organisms multiply to abnormal quantities and begin to cause problems.

The likelihood of **candidiasis** (also known as moniliasis) is greatest if a woman has diabetes, if her immune system is overtaxed or malfunctioning, if she is taking birth control pills or other hormones, if she is pregnant, or if she is taking broad-spectrum antibiotics. All of the above factors decrease the acidity of the vagina, making conditions more favourable for the development of a yeast-like infection.

Symptoms of candidiasis include severe vaginal itching, a white, cheesy discharge, swelling of the vaginal tissue due to irritation, and a burning sensation. These symptoms are often collectively called **vaginitis**. When this microbe infects the mouth, whitish patches form and the condition is referred to as thrush. This monilial infection also occurs in males and is easily transmitted between sexual partners.

Antifungal drugs applied on the surface or by suppository usually cure the infection in a few days. For approximately 10 percent of women, however, nothing seems to work, and the organism returns again and again. In women with this chronically recurring infection, symptoms are often aggravated by contact of the vagina with soaps, douches, perfumed toilet paper, chlorinated water, and spermicides. Further, tight-fitting jeans and pantyhose can provide the combination of moisture and irritant the organism thrives on. Some women report that a "natural" treatment with probiotics (yoghurt or acidophilus capsules, either taken orally or used as a vaginal suppository) is effective for this problem.

Trichomoniasis

Unlike many of the other STIs, **trichomoniasis** is caused by a protozoan. Although many men and women have this organism, most remain free of symptoms until their bodily defences are weakened. Men and women may transmit the disease, but women are the more likely candidates for infection. The "trich" infection may cause a foamy, yellowish discharge with an unpleasant odour that may be accompanied by a burning sensation, itching, and painful urination. These symptoms are most likely to occur during or shortly after menstruation, but they can appear at any time or be absent altogether. Although usually transmitted by sexual contact, the "trich" organism is easily spread by toilet seats, wet towels, or other items that have discharged fluids on them. You can also contract trichomoniasis by sitting naked on the bench of the dressing room of your local health spa or locker room. Treatment includes oral metronidazole, usually given to both sexual partners to avoid the possible "ping-pong" effect of repeated cross-infection typical of STIs.

General Urinary Tract Infections

Although general urinary tract infections (UTIs) can be caused by various factors, some forms are sexually transmitted. Any time invading organisms enter the genital area, there is a risk that they may travel up the urethra and enter the bladder. Similarly, organisms normally living in the rectum, urethra, or bladder may travel to the sexual organs and eventually be transmitted to another person.

You can also get a UTI through autoinoculation (transmission to yourself by yourself). This frequently occurs during the simple task of wiping yourself after defecating. Wiping from the anus forward may transmit organisms found in feces to the vaginal opening or to the urethra. Contact between the hands and the urethra and between the urethra and other objects are also common means of autoinoculation of bacterial and viral pathogens. Women, with their shorter urethras, are more likely to contract UTIs. Treatment depends on the nature and type of pathogen.

Herpes

Herpes is a general term for a family of diseases characterized by sores or eruptions on the skin. Herpes infections range from mildly uncomfortable to extremely serious. One subcategory, herpes simplex, is caused by a virus. Herpes simplex virus type 1 (HSV-1) causes the cold sores and fever blisters that most of us have experienced at one time or another. The herpes simplex virus (HSV) is one of the most common infectious agents in Canada; in 1994, more than 14 000 cases were identified in laboratory tests, and many more undoubtedly went unreported.[25] HSV infection has overtaken bacterial STI infection as the most common cause of genital ulceration worldwide.[26] HSV-2 (genital herpes) is not a reportable STI in Canada; therefore, we have little baseline data available. The data we do have suggest that genital herpes is as great a concern in Canada as in the rest of the world.[27]

Genital herpes, caused by herpes simplex virus type 2 (HSV-2), is one of the most widespread STIs in the world. Typically, genital herpes is characterized by distinct phases. First, the herpes virus must gain entrance to the body, which it usually does through the mucous membranes of the genital area. Once these organisms invade, the infected individual will experience the prodromal (precursor) phase of the disease, characterized by a burning sensation and redness at the site of the infection. This phase is typically followed by the formation of a small blister filled with a clear fluid containing the virus. If you pick at this blister or otherwise spread this clear fluid by your hands, you can autoinoculate other body parts. Particularly dangerous is the possibility of spreading the infection to your eyes this way, because a herpes lesion on the eye may cause blindness.

Over a period of days, this unsightly blister will crust, dry, disappear, and the virus will travel to the base of an affected nerve supplying the area and become dormant. Only when the individual infected becomes overly stressed, when dietary intake is inadequate, when the immune system is overworked, or when there is excessive exposure to sunlight or other stressors will the virus reactivate (at the same site every time) and begin the blistering cycle all over again. This cyclical recurrence can be painful, unsightly, and, most important, highly contagious. Fluids from these blisters may readily be transmitted to sexual partners. Through oral sex, herpes simplex type 2 may be transmitted to the mouth. Symptoms are similar to those of herpes simplex type 1. Figure 12.2 summarizes the herpes cycle.

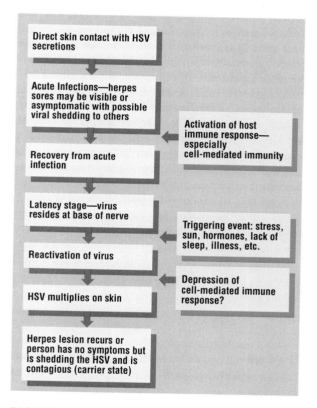

FIGURE 12.2

The Herpes Cycle

Candidiasis: Yeast-like fungal disease often transmitted sexually.

Vaginitis: Set of symptoms characterized by vaginal itching, swelling, and burning.

Trichomoniasis: Protozoan infection characterized by foamy, yellowish discharge and unpleasant odour.

Genital herpes: STI caused by herpes simplex virus type 2.

(a) Genital herpes is a highly contagious and incurable STI. (b) Oral herpes is caused by the same virus as genital herpes.

(a)   **(b)**

Genital herpes is especially serious in pregnant women because of the danger of infecting the baby as it passes through the vagina during birth. For that reason, women who have herpes should be prescribed anti-viral drugs before delivery; if they have active lesions at the time of labour, a Caesarean section will be recommended.[28] Additionally, women with a history of genital herpes also appear to have a greater risk of developing cervical cancer.

Although there is no cure for herpes at present, certain drugs have shown some success in reducing symptoms. Unfortunately, they seem to work only if the infection is confirmed during the first few hours after contact. As you may guess, this is rather rare. The effectiveness of other treatments, such as L-lysine, is largely unsubstantiated to date. Although lip balms and cold-sore medications may provide temporary anesthetic relief, it is useful to remember that rubbing anything on a herpes blister may spread herpes-laden fluids to other tissues or, via the hands, to other body parts.

Preventing Herpes

If you are worried about contracting herpes, these precautions should be followed:

- Avoid any form of kissing if you notice a sore or blister on your partner's mouth. Kiss no one, not even a peck on the cheek, if you know that you have a herpes lesion. Allow a bit of time after the sores go away before you start kissing again.

- Be extremely cautious if you have casual sex. Not every partner will feel obligated to tell you that he or she may have an STI. Protecting yourself against an infection is up to you.

- Wash your hands immediately with soap and water after any form of sexual contact.

- If you have herpes, reduce the risk of a herpes episode by avoiding excessive stress, sunlight, or whatever else appears to trigger a herpes outbreak in you.

- If you have questionable sores or lesions, seek medical help at once. Do not be afraid to name your sexual contacts.

- Since the herpes organism dies quickly upon exposure to air, toilet seats, soap, and similar sources are not likely means of transmission.

- If you have herpes, be responsible in your sexual contact with others. If you have herpes lesions that put your partner at risk, let that person know. Although it is not necessary to announce openly a herpes problem, use common sense in determining the appropriate time and place for a candid herpes discussion with your partner.

❋ ACQUIRED IMMUNE DEFICIENCY SYNDROME (AIDS)

Acquired immune deficiency syndrome (AIDS) is aptly named because it is a disease that is acquired. Since the virus suppresses the immune system, it is termed *immuno* and renders the body immune's system deficient, therefore *deficiency* is the third word. Finally, because the symptoms of AIDS all occur together, it is called a *syndrome*.[29]

Since 1981, when the first case of AIDS was diagnosed, the number of AIDS-diagnosed individuals and of persons infected with **human immunodeficiency virus (HIV)** skyrocketed, in North America and worldwide. Few regions of the world have been

State of the HIV/AIDS Epidemic

HIV/AIDS is a global threat that knows no boundaries. Epidemiological evidence shows that the developing world is bearing the brunt of the epidemic; more than 95 percent of new infections in 2000 were in developing countries. Sub-Saharan Africa accounts for a full 70 percent of the world's HIV-positive population, with the disease gaining strength in East Asia. Rates in Eastern Europe, the Middle East, Latin America, and the Caribbean are also on the rise. The Public Health Agency of Canada estimates that the epidemic is increasing in Canada as well—and at disproportionate rates for various subgroups.

An estimated 40 million people worldwide are living with HIV, more than 17.6 million of whom are women. In 2000, about 5 million people became infected, 800 000 of them children. In 2005, 4.3 million new people became infected. Since the epidemic began, AIDS has killed 24.8 million people, a significant majority of them in Sub-Saharan Africa. In 2005, it was estimated to have claimed almost 3 million lives. HIV/AIDS has also orphaned more than 13 million children under the age of 15.

Health Canada estimates show that at the end of 2005, 57 780 people had tested positive for the HIV virus in Canada. Further, the number of new HIV infections per year continues to increase by approximately 2300 to 4500. Not only have the number of positive HIV tests risen, the composition of these new infections has changed. This prevalence data clearly illustrates the changing face of the Canadian HIV epidemic, highlighting a potential resurgence of the epidemic among men who have sex with men and an increasingly urgent situation among women and Aboriginal and African Canadian populations. Although the estimates show a reduction among injection drug users, the number of new infections per year in this group is still unacceptably high.

Source: Health Canada, 2009©. Adapted and Reproduced with the permission of the Minister of Public Works and Government Services Canada, 2009.

spared. It has been estimated that more than 21 million people have died as a result of AIDS and that 57 million individuals had been infected with HIV.[30] The WHO reports that in 2006, 4.3 million people world-wide became infected with HIV and 2.9 million died of HIV/AIDS-related illnesses.[31] Individuals living in countries in southern and central Africa and South Asia account for three-quarters of these infections.[32]

The first case of AIDS in Canada was reported in 1982. Since HIV testing began in Canada in November 1985, there have been almost 60 000 positive HIV tests. The actual number of individuals in Canada living with HIV is expected to be higher than this number because not all individuals infected with HIV are actually tested for it.[33] It is estimated that between 2300 and 4500 new cases will be identified in 2005 (the most recent year for which estimates have been made).[34] Of the new cases testing positive each year, approximately 75 percent are men.[35] It should be pointed out, however, that there has been a disproportionate rise in the number of women testing positive for HIV since 1995, when fewer than 10 percent of new cases were found in women; now 27 percent of new cases are in women.[36] Even though ethnic status is not available on approximately one-third of all positive HIV reports, disproportionate increases in newly identified cases have been found among black Canadians (15.5 percent) and Aboriginal Canadians (14.8 percent).[37] The Focus on Canada box gives a detailed picture of the global face of AIDS.

what do you THINK?

Why do you think HIV infection is increasing among some groups and not others? What actions can we take to reduce the spread of HIV/AIDS? Why should the global HIV/AIDS epidemic be of concern to Canadians?

✳ How HIV Is Transmitted

HIV typically enters the body when another person's infected body fluids (semen, vaginal secretions, blood, etc.) gain entry through a breach in body defences. Mucous membranes of the genital organs and the anus

Acquired immune deficiency syndrome (AIDS): Extremely virulent STI that renders the immune system inoperative.

Human immunodeficiency virus (HIV): The slow-acting virus that causes AIDS.

provide the easiest route of entry. If there is a break in the mucous membranes (as can occur during sexual intercourse, particularly anal intercourse), the virus enters and begins to multiply. After initial infection, the HIV typically begins to multiply rapidly in the body, invading the bloodstream and cerebrospinal fluid. It progressively destroys helper T-lymphocytes, weakening the body's resistance to disease. The virus also changes the genetic structure of the cells it attacks. In response to this invasion, the body quickly begins to produce antibodies.

Despite some rather hysterical myths, HIV is not a highly contagious virus. Countless studies of people living in households with a person with HIV/AIDS have turned up no documented cases of HIV infection due to casual contact.[38] Other investigations provide overwhelming evidence that insect bites do not transmit the virus. In fact, the virus is actually quite selective in the way it transmits itself from person to person.

Engaging in High-Risk Behaviours

HIV is not a disease of certain groups. People are not predestined to get the disease because they belong to a group or associate with a group. Thus, HIV is not a gay disease, or a disease of minority groups, or Haitians, or any other class of people. It is a disease of high-risk behaviours. If you engage in these behaviours, you increase your risk for the disease. If you do not engage in these behaviours, your risk is minimal. Promiscuous sex—in males and females of all ages, ethnicities, sexual orientations, and socioeconomic conditions—is the greatest threat. Anyone who engages in unprotected sex at any time with a person who has engaged in high-risk behaviours is at risk. A celibate or monogamous gay man or a drug-injecting woman who never shares her needles is at very low risk for HIV. But a person who has had sex with someone who has, even once, had sex with an injecting drug user could be infected. You cannot tell by looking at someone; you cannot tell by questioning, unless the person has been tested recently and is HIV-negative. So, what should you do? The Building Communication Skills box offers some direct advice.

Of course, the best method of protection is abstinence. If you do not exchange body fluids, you will not get the disease. As a second line of defence, if you decide to be intimate, the best option is to use a condom. The following activities are high-risk behaviours.

Exchange of Body Fluids

The exchange of HIV-infected body fluids during sexual intercourse is the greatest risk factor. Substantial research indicates that blood, semen, and vaginal, cervical, and anal secretions are the major fluids of concern. Although the virus was found in one person's saliva (out of 71 people in a study population), most health officials state that saliva is not a high-risk body fluid.

Initially, public health officials also included breast milk in the list of high-risk fluids because a small number of infants apparently contracted HIV while breast-feeding. Subsequent research indicated that HIV transmission could have been caused by bleeding nipples rather than actual consumption of breast milk. Infection through contact with feces and urine is believed to be highly unlikely (though technically possible).

Receiving a Blood Transfusion Prior to 1986

A small group of people became infected with HIV as a result of a blood transfusion before 1986. Since then, the Canadian Red Cross has implemented a stringent testing program for all donated blood. And Canada's blood supply is now controlled by Canadian Blood Services, which screens donors for a number of potential risks, including, but not limited to, dental work in the previous three days; a cold, flu, or sore throat; ear piercing or body tattooing in the past three months; handling monkeys in or out of a laboratory setting; travelling to Africa in the past year; as well as a number of questions regarding illicit drug use with needles and questions regarding sexual activity in the past year.) Because of these massive

You cannot tell if someone has an STI, including HIV, just by looking at them. Being open and honest with your partners (and expecting the same from them) about sexual history and STI testing is an important part of prevention.

Communicating with Your Partner about STIs

The more people know about STIs and the more they internalize personal susceptibility, the greater the chance that they will adopt safer behaviours. Yet, despite large-scale public awareness and education programs, infection continues to rise. Many medical, education, and youth officials feel that the major obstacle to preventing STIs among young people is the discomfort most have about discussing personal needs and feelings regarding these infections and practising safer sex behaviours. For many young people, discussing STI status and safer sex practices, such as condom use, can be uncomfortable. Some fear that raising the issue suggests lack of trust in the partner; others worry that safer behaviours will hinder their sexual enjoyment; and still others fail to recognize their personal vulnerability. As a result, a great many put themselves at risk for infection rather than hurt the other person's feelings. Therefore, a major goal in the fight against STIs is to improve one-on-one communication between young people. The following tips can help open the lines of communication.

- Remember that you have a responsibility to your partner to disclose your status. You also have a responsibility to yourself to do what needs to be done to stay healthy and infection free. Do not be afraid to ask about your partner's STI status. If either person's status is unknown, suggest going through the testing together—before engaging in any sexual activity—as a means of sharing something important with each other.

- Be direct, honest, and determined in talking about sex before you become involved. Do not act silly or evasive. Get to the point, ask clear questions, and do not be put off receiving a response. Remember, a person who does not care enough to talk about sex probably does not care enough to take responsibility for his or her actions.

- Discuss the issues without sounding defensive or accusatory. Develop a personal comfort level with the subject prior to raising the issue with your partner. Be prepared with complete information and articulate your feelings clearly. Reassure your partner that your reasons for desiring abstinence or safer sex arise from respect rather than distrust. Sharing feelings is easier in a calm, suspicion-free environment in which both people feel comfortable.

- Encourage your partner to be honest and to share feelings. This will not happen overnight. If you have never had a serious conversation with this person before you get into an intimate situation, you can not expect honesty and openness when the lights go out.

- Analyze your beliefs and values ahead of time. The worst thing you can do is to get yourself into an awkward situation before you've had time to think about what is important to you and what you believe in. Know where you will draw the line, and be very clear with your partner about what you expect. If you believe that using a condom is necessary, make sure you communicate this to your partner.

- Decide what you will do if your partner does not agree with you. Anticipate your partner's potential objections or excuses and prepare your responses accordingly.

- Ask questions about past history. Although it may seem as though you are prying into another person's business, your current and future health depends upon knowing basic information about your partner's past. An idea of your partner's past sexual practices and use of injected drugs is valuable. Again, it is important to let your partner know why you are concerned and that you are not inquiring due to jealousy or other ulterior motives.

- Ask about the significance of monogamy in your partner's relationships. A basic question to ask before becoming involved in a sexual relationship is: "How important is a committed relationship to you?" You will need to decide early how important this relationship is to you and how much you are willing to work at arriving at an acceptable compromise on lifestyle.

screening efforts, the risk of receiving HIV-infected blood or any other blood-borne pathogen is almost nonexistent.

Injecting Drugs

Another source of infection is sharing or using HIV-contaminated needles. Injection drug use (IDU) has increasingly been a route of HIV transmission in Canada. In 2005, the percentage of new HIV infections in Canada estimated as a result of IDU was 17

percent.[39] This number has decreased significantly over the years due to increased attention focused on preventing HIV transmission in IDU.[40]

While illegal drug users are the people we usually think of in this category, it is important to remember that others may also share needles—for example, individuals with type 1 diabetes who inject insulin. People who share needles and engage in sexual activities with members of high-risk groups, such as those who exchange sex for drugs, increase their risks dramatically. Any needle prick with an HIV-contaminated needle provides a risk of infection. Thus, tattooing, body piercing, and any practice using unsterilized needles presents a potential risk. Similarly, dentists or physicians who work with HIV-positive individuals have increased risk of infection should there be any fluid transfer such as what might occur if their surgical gloves became torn and there were a cut or abrasion in the skin beneath.

Mother-to-Infant Transmission (Perinatal)

Infants may contract HIV from their infected mothers while in the womb or while passing through the vaginal tract during delivery.

Symptoms of the Disease

A person may go for months or years after acquiring HIV before any significant symptoms appear. The incubation time varies greatly from person to person. Children have shorter incubation periods than adults. Newborns and infants are particularly vulnerable to HIV infection because they are not fully immunocompetent (that is, their immune system is not fully developed) until they are 6 to 15 months old. New information suggests that some very young children show the "adult" progression of the disease. In adults, the average length of time it takes the virus to cause the slow, degenerative changes in the immune system that result in AIDS is 8 to 10 years. During this time, the person may experience a large number of opportunistic infections (infections that gain a foothold when the immune system is not functioning effectively). Colds, sore throats, fever, tiredness, nausea, night sweats, and other generally non-life-threatening conditions commonly appear.

Testing for HIV Antibodies

Once antibodies have begun to form in reaction to the presence of HIV, a blood test known as the **ELISA** test may detect their presence. If sufficient antibodies are present, this test will be positive. When a person who previously tested negative (no HIV antibodies present) has a subsequent test that is positive, "seroconversion" is said to have occurred. In such a situation, the person would typically take another ELISA test, followed by a more expensive, more precise test known as the **Western blot** to confirm the presence of HIV antibodies.

Although the ELISA is viewed as quite accurate, it is a conservative test in that it errs on the side of caution, meaning that it produces a large number of false positive results. It was deliberately designed to do this because it was intended as a test for screening the nation's blood supply. There have also been instances of false negative results. Some health professionals believe there are chronic carriers of HIV who, for unknown reasons, continually show false negative results on the ELISA and the Western blot test. False negative HIV tests raise serious concerns about risks for these people's sexual partners. It should be noted that these tests are not AIDS tests per se. Rather, they detect antibodies for the disease, indicating the presence of HIV in the person's system. Whether or not the person will develop AIDS depends to some extent on the strength of the immune system. However, the vast majority of infected people do develop some form of the disease.

Women carry not only the burden of their own health, but frequently that of a child infected before birth or at the time of delivery.

Numerous demonstrations have successfully called attention to the need for AIDS research and treatment programs.

As testing for HIV antibodies improves, scientists have explored ways of making it easier for individuals to be tested. Health officials distinguish between reported and actual cases of HIV infection because it is believed that many people who are HIV-positive avoid being tested. One reason is fear of knowing the truth. Another is the fear of negative consequences or judgmental attitudes from employers, insurance companies, and health professionals. However, early detection and reporting are important, because immediate treatment for someone in the early stages of HIV infection is critical and necessary to prevent further spread of the virus.

what do you THINK?

Should there be mandatory reporting of HIV and AIDS? Why or why not? Would you have an HIV test if you knew that your name and vital statistics would be "on file" if you tested positive? Why or why not?

Preventing HIV Infection

Although scientists have been searching for more than a decade for a vaccine to protect people from HIV infection, one has not been found. The only known effective prevention strategies relate to the means by which people contract HIV. HIV infection and AIDS are not uncontrollable conditions. You can reduce your risks by making responsible choices in your sexual and drug use behaviours. The Skills for Behaviour Change box suggests ways to reduce your risk for contracting HIV.

Because the status of your immune system is an important factor in whether you are susceptible to any of the STIs, it is important that you do everything possible to protect yourself. Engaging in physical activity regularly, eating a healthy dietary intake, getting enough sleep, managing your stress, ensuring that your vaccinations are up-to-date, and taking other preventive measures can do a great deal to ensure your long-term health.

NONINFECTIOUS DISEASES

Typically, when we think of the major ailments and diseases affecting people today, we think of "killer" diseases such as cancer and heart disease. Although these diseases capture much of the media attention, other forms of chronic disease cause substantial pain, suffering, and disability. The majority of these diseases can be prevented or their onset delayed.

To prevent the development of certain noninfectious and chronic diseases, we must identify the major common characteristics. They are not transmitted by any pathogen or by any form of personal contact. They usually develop over a long period of time, and they cause progressive damage to human tissues. Although these conditions normally do not result in death, they do lead to illness and suffering for many people. Lifestyle and personal health habits appear to be major contributing factors to the general increase

ELISA: Blood test that detects the presence of antibodies to HIV.

Western blot: More precise test than the ELISA to confirm presence of HIV antibodies.

Reducing Your Risks for HIV

Contracting HIV is not uncontrollable. HIV cannot, like cold or flu viruses, be caught casually. The transmission of HIV depends upon specific behaviours. Therefore, HIV infection can be prevented. The following list suggests ways to reduce your risk.

- Avoid casual sexual partners. Ideally, have sex only in a long-term, mutually monogamous relationship and with a partner whose HIV status is negative.

- Avoid unprotected sexual activity with people whose present or past behaviours put them (and thus you) at risk for infection. Do not be afraid to ask intimate questions about your partner's sexual history and past injection drug use. You expose yourself to your partner's history whenever you choose to have sexual relations. Postpone sexual involvement until you are assured that he or she is not infected.

- Sexually active adults not in a lifelong monogamous relationship should practise safer sex by using latex condoms. Remember, condoms do not provide 100-percent protection.

- Never share injecting needles with anyone for any reason.

- Never share any devices through which the exchange of blood could occur, including needles, razors, tattoo instruments, any body-piercing instruments, and any other sharp objects.

- Avoid injury to body tissue during sexual activity. HIV can enter the bloodstream through microscopic tears in anal or vaginal tissues.

- Avoid unprotected oral sex or any sexual activity in which semen, blood, or vaginal secretions could penetrate mucous membranes through breaks in the membrane. Always use a condom or a dental dam during all kinds of sex.

- Avoid using drugs that may dull your senses and affect your ability to make decisions about responsible precautions with potential sex partners.

- Wash your hands before and after sexual encounters. Urinate after sexual relations and, if possible, wash your genitals.

- Although total abstinence is the only absolute means of preventing the sexual transmission of HIV, abstinence can be a difficult choice to make. If you are in doubt about the potential risks of having sex, consider other means of intimacy, at least until you can ensure your safety. Enjoyable and safer alternatives include massage, dry kissing, hugging, holding and touching, and masturbation (alone or with a partner).

- When receiving care from medical professionals such as dentists or doctors, make sure they take appropriate precautions to prevent potential transmission, including washing their hands and wearing gloves and masks. Be sure that all equipment used for treatment is properly sterilized.

- If you are worried about your own HIV status, get tested!

- If you are a woman and HIV-positive, you should take the steps necessary to ensure that you do not become pregnant.

- If you suspect that you may be infected or if you test positive for HIV antibodies, do not donate blood, semen, or body organs.

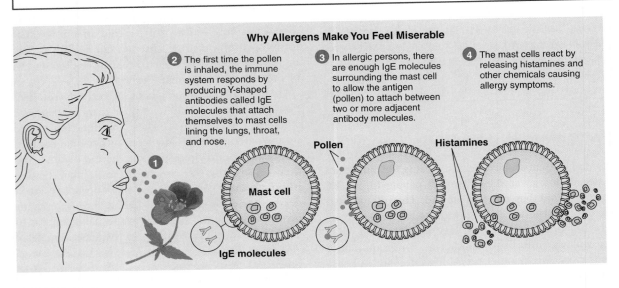

Why Allergens Make You Feel Miserable

2 The first time the pollen is inhaled, the immune system responds by producing Y-shaped antibodies called IgE molecules that attach themselves to mast cells lining the lungs, throat, and nose.

3 In allergic persons, there are enough IgE molecules surrounding the mast cell to allow the antigen (pollen) to attach between two or more adjacent antibody molecules.

4 The mast cells react by releasing histamines and other chemicals causing allergy symptoms.

Pollen

Histamines

Mast cell

IgE molecules

FIGURE 12.3

Steps of an Allergy Response

observed in the incidence of chronic diseases in Canada in recent years. Education, reasonable changes in lifestyle behaviours, and public health efforts aimed at prevention and control could minimize the effects of many of these diseases.

RESPIRATORY DISORDERS

Allergy-Induced Problems

An **allergy** occurs as a part of the body's attempt to defend itself against a specific antigen or allergen by producing antibodies in response to its presence. When foreign pathogens such as bacteria or viruses invade the body, the body responds by producing antibodies to destroy them. Under normal conditions, the production of antibodies is a positive element in the body's defence system. However, for unknown reasons, in some people the body overreacts by developing an overly elaborate protective mechanism against relatively harmless allergens or antigens. The resultant hypersensitivity reaction to specific allergens or antigens in the environment is fairly common, as anyone who has awakened with a runny nose or itchy eyes will testify. Most commonly, these hypersensitivity, or allergic, responses occur as a reaction to environmental antigens such as moulds, animal dander (hair and dead skin), pollen, ragweed, or dust. Once excessive antibodies to these antigens are produced, they trigger the release of **histamines**, chemical substances that dilate blood vessels, increase mucous secretions, cause tissues to swell, and produce other allergy-like symptoms (see Figure 12.3).

Although many people think of allergies as childhood diseases, in reality allergies tend to become progressively worse with time and with increased exposure to allergens. In these circumstances, allergic responses become chronic in nature, and treatment becomes difficult. Many people take allergy shots to reduce the severity of their symptoms. In most cases, once the offending antigen has disappeared, allergy-prone people suffer few symptoms. Although allergies cause numerous problems, the most significant is on the immune system.

Hay Fever

Perhaps the best example of a chronic respiratory disease is **hay fever**. Usually considered a seasonally related disease (most prevalent when ragweed and flowers are blooming), hay fever is common throughout the world. Hay fever attacks, characterized by sneezing and itchy, watery eyes and nose, cause a great deal of misery for many people.

Hay fever appears to have a genetic component, with research indicating that lifestyle is not as great a factor in its development as in other chronic diseases. Instead, an overzealous immune system and an exposure to environmental allergens including pet dander, dust, pollen from various plants, and other substances appear to be the critical factors that determine vulnerability. For some people, a change in setting may help; for others, medical assistance in the form of injections or antihistamines may provide the only possibility of relief.

✳ Asthma

Unfortunately for many hay fever sufferers, their condition is often complicated by the development of another chronic respiratory disease, **asthma**. Asthma is characterized by attacks of wheezing, difficulty breathing, shortness of breath, and coughing spasms. Although most asthma attacks are mild, they can trigger bronchospasms (contractions of the bronchial tubes in the lungs) of such a severe nature that, unless treatment is rapid, death may occur. Between attacks, most people have few symptoms.

Asthma attacks can be brought on by something as commonplace as physical activity. This does not mean that individuals with asthma should not participate in sports or other physical activities, but rather that they should create a plan that takes into account their limitations.

In the majority of cases, asthma first occurs in children under the age of ten, afflicting boys nearly twice as often as girls. Although many children outgrow the condition, a number of them continue to experience asthma as adults.

Although exposure to allergens such as dust, pollen, and animal dander may trigger many asthmatic episodes, emotional factors and excessive anxiety or stress can also trigger an attack. Exercise-induced asthma (EIA) is a type of asthma that has gained increasing attention. Relaxation techniques

---

Allergy: Hypersensitive reaction to a specific antigen or allergen in the environment in which the body produces excessive antibodies.

Histamines: Chemical substances that dilate blood vessels, increase mucous secretions, and produce other allergy-like symptoms.

Hay fever: A chronic respiratory disorder most prevalent when ragweed and flowers bloom.

Asthma: A chronic respiratory disease characterized by attacks of wheezing, shortness of breath, and coughing spasms.

Asthma attacks can be brought on by something as common place as physical activity. This does not mean that individuals with asthma shouldn't participate in sports or other physical activities, but rather that they should create a plan that takes into account their limitations.

appear to help some individuals who have asthma. Drugs may be necessary for serious cases. Doctors warn against using over-the-counter inhalers without medical advice: some over-the-counter products have serious side effects, depending on the type of asthma and other drugs used. Determining the specific allergen that provokes asthma attacks and taking steps to reduce your exposure, adjusting for triggers such as physical activity or stress, and finding the most effective medications are big steps in asthma control.

Emphysema

Emphysema involves the gradual destruction of the alveoli (tiny air sacs) of the lungs. As the **alveoli** are destroyed, the affected person finds it more and more difficult to exhale. The individual typically struggles to take in a fresh supply of air before the air held in the lungs has been expended. The chest cavity gradually begins to expand, producing the barrel-shaped chest characteristic of individuals with chronic emphysema.

The exact cause of emphysema is uncertain. There is, however, a strong relationship between the development of emphysema and long-term cigarette smoking and exposure to air pollution. Individuals with emphysema often suffer discomfort over a period of many years. What we all take for granted—the easy, rhythmic flow of air in and out of our lungs—becomes a continuous struggle for people with emphysema. Inadequate oxygen supply, combined with the stress of overexertion on the heart, eventually takes its toll on the cardiovascular system and leads to premature death.

Unfortunately, little can be done to reverse the effects of emphysema.

Chronic Bronchitis

Although often dismissed as "smoker's cough" or a bad case of the common cold, **chronic bronchitis** may be a serious, if not life-threatening, respiratory disorder. In this ailment, the bronchial tubes become so inflamed and swollen that normal respiratory function is impaired. Symptoms of chronic bronchitis include a productive cough and shortness of breath that persist for several weeks over the course of the year. Cigarette smoking is the major risk factor for this disease, although fumes, dust, and particulate matter in the air are contributing factors. Individuals with chronic bronchitis must often use respiratory devices similar to those used by individuals with emphysema. They must also avoid factors—such as cigarette smoking—that contributed to the development of bronchitis. Bronchitis coupled with a severe cold may be serious enough to warrant immediate medical attention.

NEUROLOGICAL DISORDERS

Headaches

Almost all of us have experienced at least one major headache in our lives, whether it is the mild, throbbing variety or the severe, pounding ache that makes us nauseated or dizzy. Not all headaches are equal, and more important, it is possible that not all headaches have the same cause. Some experts suggest that all serious headaches share the same basic causes and fall along a spectrum, with ordinary tension headaches at one end and full-blown migraines at the other.[41] Headaches may result from dilated blood vessels within the brain, underlying organic problems, or excessive stress and anxiety. The following are the most common forms of headaches and the most effective methods of treatment.

Tension Headaches

Tension headaches are generally caused by muscle contractions or tension in the neck or head. This tension may be caused by actual strain placed on the neck or head muscles due to overuse, static positions held for long periods of time, or tension triggered by stress. Research indicates that tension headaches may be a product of a more "generic mechanism" in which chemicals deep inside the brain cause the muscular tension, pain, and suffering often associated with an attack. Triggers for this chemical assault may be red wine, lack of sleep, fasting, menstruation, or other factors, and the same symptoms (sensitivity to light and sound, nausea, and/or throbbing pain)

Tension headaches are triggered by many factors, including lack of sleep, stress, and strain on head and neck muscles

may be characteristic of different types of headaches. Symptoms may vary in intensity and duration. Relaxation, hot water treatment, and massage have surfaced as the new "holistic treatments," while Aspirin, Tylenol, and Advil are the old standby forms of pain relief.

Migraine Headaches

If you have ever experienced pulsating pain on one side of the head in combination with dizzy spells, nausea, and intolerance for light and noise, you are probably one of those who suffer from **migraines**, a type of headache that has severe debilitating symptoms. Many migraine sufferers feel excruciatingly painful, recurring headaches that last for minutes, hours, or even days and may also experience some temporary visual impairment. Symptoms vary greatly by individual and attacks typically last anywhere from 4 to 72 hours, with distinct phases. In about 15 percent of cases, migraines are preceded by a sensory warning sign known as an aura, such as flashes of light, flickering vision, blind spots, or tingling in the arms or legs, or sensations of odour or taste. Symptoms of migraine include excruciating pain behind or around one eye and usually on the same side of the head. In some people, there is sinus pain, neck pain, or an aura without headache. Usually migraine incidence peaks in young adulthood (ages 20–45), the prime years for postsecondary students.[42]

Migraines may occur when blood vessels dilate in the membrane that surrounds the brain. Historically, treatments have centred on reversing or preventing this dilation. Critics of this theory question why only blood vessels of the head dilate in these circumstances. Other researchers believe that migraines are started by disturbances that keep the pain-regulating chemical serotonin from doing its job.

When true migraines occur, relaxation is only minimally effective as a treatment. Often, strong pain-relieving drugs prescribed by a physician are necessary.

Emphysema: A respiratory disease in which the alveoli become distended or ruptured and no longer functional.

Alveoli: Tiny air sacs of the lungs.

Chronic bronchitis: A serious respiratory disorder in which the bronchial tubes become so inflamed and swollen that respiratory function is impaired.

Migraine: A condition characterized by localized headaches that result from alternating dilation and constriction of blood vessels.

Secondary Headaches

Secondary headaches arise as a result of some other underlying condition. An example is a person with a severe sinus blockage that causes pressure in the sinus cavity. This pressure may induce a headache. Hypertension, allergies, low blood sugar, diseases of the spine, the common cold, poorly fitted dentures, problems with eyesight, and other types of pain or injury can trigger this condition. Relaxation and pain relievers are of little help in treating secondary headaches. Rather, medications or other therapies designed to relieve the underlying organic cause of the headache must be included in the treatment regimen.

Psychological Headaches

With this type of headache, the "it's all in your head" diagnosis may, in fact, be correct. Rather than having a physical cause, psychological headaches stem from anxiety, depression, and other emotional factors. Psychological headaches result from the stress of emotional disturbances, particularly depression. Unlike tension headaches, no muscles or blood vessels appear to be involved, thereby making relaxation and painkillers ineffective as treatment. Only therapy designed to treat the underlying depression or emotional problem appears to be effective in reducing this kind of headache.

Seizure Disorders

The word **epilepsy** is derived from the Greek *epilepsia*, meaning "seizure." Reports of epilepsy appeared in Greek medical records as early as 300 BCE. Ancient peoples interpreted seizures as invasions of the body by evil spirits or as punishments by the gods. Although much of the mystery surrounding epileptic seizures has been solved in recent years, the stigma and lack of understanding remain.

These disorders are generally caused by abnormal electrical activity in the brain and are characterized by loss of control of muscular activity and unconsciousness. Symptoms vary widely from person to person. There are several forms of seizure disorders. The most common are the following:

1. Grand mal, or major motor seizure: These seizures are often preceded by a shrill cry or a seizure aura (body sensations such as ringing in the ears or a specific smell or taste). Convulsions and loss of consciousness generally occur and may last from 30 seconds to several minutes or more. Keeping track of the length of time elapsed is one aspect of first aid.

2. Petit mal, or minor seizure: These seizures involve no convulsions. Rather, a minor loss of consciousness that may go unnoticed occurs. Minor twitching of muscles may take place, usually for a shorter time than grand mal convulsions.

3. Psychomotor seizure: These seizures involve mental processes and muscular activity. Symptoms may include mental confusion and a listless state characterized by activities such as lip smacking, chewing, and repetitive movements.

4. Jacksonian seizure: This is a progressive seizure that often begins in one part of the body, such as the fingers, and moves to other parts, such as the hand or arm. Usually only one side of the body is affected.

In the majority of cases, people with seizure disorders can lead normal, seizure-free lives under medical supervision. Epilepsy is seldom fatal. The greatest risk for individuals with epilepsy whose seizures are uncontrolled is motor vehicle or other accidents. Public ignorance about these disorders is one of the most serious obstacles confronting individuals with seizure disorders. Improvements in medication and surgical interventions to reduce some causes of seizures are among the most promising treatments today.

---

what do you THINK?

Do you suffer from recurrent headaches or other neurological problems? What do you do to relieve the symptoms? Have you addressed the underlying causes? If not, why not? What actions might you take to prevent headaches?

SEX-RELATED DISORDERS

Fibrocystic Breast Condition

Fibrocystic breast condition is a common, noncancerous problem among women in Canada. Symptoms range in severity from a small palpable lump to large masses of irregular tissue found in both breasts. The underlying causes of the condition are unknown. Although some experts believe it is related to hormonal changes during the normal menstrual cycle, many women report that their conditions neither worsen nor improve during their cycles. In fact, in most cases, the condition appears to run in families and to become progressively worse with age, regardless of pregnancy or other hormonal disruptions. Although the majority of these cyst formations consist of fibrous tissue, some are filled with fluid. Treatment often involves removal of fluid from the affected area or surgical removal of the cyst itself.

✳ Premenstrual Syndrome (PMS)

Premenstrual syndrome (PMS) refers to as many as 150 physical and emotional symptoms that occur prior to menstruation in some women and vary from woman to woman and from month to month. These symptoms usually begin a week to 10 days before the menstrual period and include depression, tension, irritability, headaches, tender breasts, bloated abdomen, backache, abdominal cramps, acne, fluid retention, diarrhea, and fatigue. It is believed that women with PMS develop a predictable pattern of symptoms during the menstrual cycle and that the severity of their symptoms is influenced by external factors, such as stress.

Women usually experience PMS for the first time after the age of 20, though younger women can experience it too, and it may remain a regular part of their reproductive life unless they seek treatment. For many women, the first day of their period brings immediate relief. For others, the depressive symptoms persist all month and are simply heightened before the menstrual period.

Most believe that the most plausible cause of PMS is a hormonal imbalance related to the rise in estrogen levels preceding the menstrual period. This theory is substantiated by the fact that women with PMS given prescriptions for progesterone often experience relief of symptoms. Critics of this theory argue that controlled research has not yet been conducted on the effects of progesterone on PMS.

Common treatments for PMS include hormonal therapy in addition to drugs and behaviours designed to relieve the symptoms. These include Aspirin for pain, diuretics for fluid retention, decreases in caffeine and salt intake, increases in complex carbohydrate intake, stress-reduction techniques, and physical activity. Some women claim they find relief through alternative treatments such as traditional Chinese medicine (acupuncture and herbs).

Endometriosis

Whether the incidence of **endometriosis** is on the rise or whether the disorder is simply attracting more attention is difficult to determine. Women who develop endometriosis tend to be between the ages of 20 and 40 years. Symptoms include severe cramping during and between menstrual cycles, irregular periods, unusually heavy or light menstrual flow, abdominal bloating, fatigue, painful bowel movements with periods, painful intercourse, constipation, diarrhea, menstrual pain, infertility, and low back pain. What is this disease? What causes it? What are the common methods of treatment?

Although much remains unknown about the causes of endometriosis, we do know that the disease is characterized by the abnormal growth and development of endometrial tissue (the tissue lining the uterus) in regions of the body other than the uterus. Among the most widely accepted theories concerning the causes of endometriosis are the transmission of endometrial tissue to other regions of the body during surgery or through the birthing process; the movement of menstrual fluid backward through the fallopian tubes during menstruation; and abnormal cell migration through body-fluid movement. Women with cycles shorter than 27 days and those with flows lasting over a week are at increased risk. The more aerobic physical activity a woman engages in and the earlier she starts, the less likely she is to develop endometriosis.

Treatment of endometriosis ranges from bed rest and reduction in stressful activities to **hysterectomy** (the removal of the uterus) or the removal of one or both ovaries and the fallopian tubes. In some areas, where the rate of hysterectomy is high, physicians have been criticized for overreliance on this procedure. More conservative treatments that involve dilation and curettage—surgically scraping endometrial tissue off the fallopian tubes and other reproductive organs—and combinations of hormone therapy are considered more acceptable. Hormonal treatments include gonadotropin-releasing hormone (GnRH) analogues, various synthetic progesterone-like drugs (Provera), and oral contraceptives.

what do you THINK?

Which of the preceding health problems do you think cause the most problems for women in Canada? Why is there stigma related to these "women's issues"? What actions should be taken to increase awareness and understanding of these conditions?

Epilepsy: A neurological disorder caused by abnormal electrical brain activity; can be accompanied by altered consciousness or convulsions.

Fibrocystic breast condition: A common, noncancerous condition in woman whose breasts contain fibrous or fluid-filled cysts.

Premenstrual syndrome (PMS): A series of physical and emotional symptoms that may occur in women prior to their menstrual periods.

Endometriosis: Abnormal development of endometrial tissue outside the uterus resulting in serious side effects.

Hysterectomy: Surgical removal of the uterus.

DIGESTION-RELATED DISORDERS

Diabetes

According to the Canadian Diabetes Association more than 2 million Canadians have **diabetes**; approximately 10 percent of all cases are type 1 diabetes and 90 percent are type 2.[43] Aboriginal people are three to five times more likely to develop type 2 diabetes than the general population. The number of Canadians with diabetes is expected to rise to 3 million by 2010.[44] An increase in prevalence is expected because (1) the population is aging, (2) obesity rates are rising, (3) Canadian lifestyles are increasingly sedentary, and (4) 80 percent of new Canadians come from high-risk groups for developing type 2 diabetes (that is, those of Hispanic, Asian, South Asian, or African descent).[45] Further, it should be pointed out that approximately one-third of persons with diabetes are undiagnosed.[46]

Contrary to popular belief, diabetes does not result from eating too much sugar, although it does relate to insulin and the body's ability or inability to use sugar. In healthy people, the pancreas, a powerful enzyme-producing organ, produces the hormone **insulin** in sufficient quantities to allow the body to use or store glucose (blood sugar). When this organ fails to produce enough insulin to regulate sugar metabolism, or when the body fails to use insulin effectively, diabetes occurs. Individuals with diabetes exhibit **hyperglycemia**, or elevated blood sugar levels, and high glucose levels in their urine. Other symptoms include excessive thirst, frequent urination, hunger, tendency to tire easily, wounds that heal slowly, numbness or tingling in the extremities, changes in vision, skin eruptions, and, in women, a tendency toward vaginal yeast infections.

Many individuals with diabetes remain unaware of their condition until they begin to show overt symptoms. Type 1 (insulin-dependent) diabetes or diabetes mellitus, usually begins early in life. Individuals with type 1 diabetes typically depend on insulin injections or oral medications for the rest of their lives, because insulin is not available in their bodies. Non–insulin dependent diabetes (formally termed "adult-onset"), or type 2 diabetes, in which insulin production is deficient, tends to develop in later life. Individuals with type 2 diabetes can often control the symptoms of their disease with minimal medical intervention through a healthy dietary intake, weight control, and regular physical activity (see Chapter 11 for more details). If they follow this regimen, they may be able to avoid oral medications or insulin indefinitely.

Diabetes tends to run in families, and a tendency to being overweight, coupled with inactivity, dramatically increases a person's risk. Older persons and mothers of babies weighing over 4 kilograms also run an increased risk. Approximately 80 percent of all individuals are overweight and sedentary at the time of diagnosis. Weight loss and regular physical activity are important factors in lowering blood sugar and improving the efficiency of cellular use of insulin. Both can help to prevent overwork of the pancreas and the development of diabetes. People who develop diabetes today have a much better prognosis than those who developed it 20 or 25 years ago.

Many physicians attempt to control diabetes with a variety of insulin-related drugs. Most of these drugs are taken orally, although self-administered hypodermic injections are prescribed when oral treatments are inadequate. Recent breakthroughs in individual monitoring and the implanting of insulin monitors and insulin infusion pumps that regulate insulin intake "on demand" have provided many individuals with diabetes the opportunity to lead normal lives. Other individuals with diabetes find they can control their diabetes by eating foods rich in complex carbohydrates, low in sodium, and high in fibre, by losing weight, and by getting regular physical activity.

Colitis and Irritable Bowel Syndrome (IBS)

Ulcerative colitis is a disease of the large intestine in which the mucous membranes of the intestinal walls become inflamed. Individuals with severe cases may have as many as 20 bouts of bloody diarrhea a day. Colitis can also produce severe stomach cramps, weight loss, nausea, sweating, and fever. What causes colitis? We are not sure. Although some experts believe that it occurs more frequently in people with high stress, this theory is controversial. Hypersensitivity reactions, particularly to milk and certain foods, have also been considered as possible causes. It is difficult to determine the cause of colitis because the disease goes into unexplained remission and then recurs without apparent reason. This pattern often continues for years and may be related to the later development of colorectal cancer. Because the cause of colitis remains unknown, treatment focuses exclusively on relieving the symptoms. Effective measures include increasing fibre intake and taking anti-inflammatory drugs, steroids, and other medications designed to reduce inflammation and soothe irritated intestinal walls.

Many people develop a condition related to colitis known as **irritable bowel syndrome (IBS)**, in which nausea, pain, gas, diarrhea, or cramps occur after eating certain foods or when a person is under unusual stress. IBS symptoms commonly begin in early adulthood. Symptoms vary from week to week and fade for long periods of time only to return. The cause of IBS is unknown, but researchers suspect that people with IBS have digestive systems overly sensitive to certain foods and beverages, stress, and certain hormonal changes. They may also be more sensitive to pain signals from the stomach. Stress management, relaxation techniques, regular physical activity, and a healthy dietary intake can bring IBS under control in the vast majority of cases.

Diverticulosis

Diverticulosis occurs when the walls of the intestine become weakened for undetermined reasons and small pea-sized bulges develop. These bulges often fill with feces and, over time, become irritated and infected, causing pain and discomfort. If this irritation persists, bleeding and chronic obstruction may occur, either of which can be life-threatening. If you have a persistent pain in the lower abdominal region, seek medical attention at once.

Peptic Ulcers

An ulcer is a lesion or wound that forms in body tissue as a result of some irritant. A **peptic ulcer** is a chronic ulcer that occurs in the lining of the stomach or the section of the small intestine known as the duodenum. It had long been thought to be caused by the erosive effect of digestive juices on these tissues. Now, research indicates that most peptic ulcers result from an infection from a common bacteria, *Helicobacter pylori*, and require powerful antibiotics to treat them. This is a dramatic departure from the treatment that was typical in the past, which used acid-reducing drugs known as H2 blockers, such as cimetidine (Tagamet) or ranitidine (Zantac). The new treatment recommends a two-week course of antibiotics. H2 blockers are still used in ulcer cases in which excess stomach acid or overuse of drugs such as Aspirin and ibuprofen have caused the irritation.

Ulcers appear to run in families and to be more prevalent in people who are highly stressed over long periods of time and who consume high-fat foods or excessive alcohol. People with ulcers should avoid high-fat foods, alcohol, and substances such as Aspirin that irritate organ linings or cause increased secretion of stomach acids and thereby exacerbate this condition. In some cases, surgery has been necessary to relieve persistent symptoms.

Gallbladder Disease

Gallbladder disease, also known as cholecystitis, occurs when the gallbladder has been repeatedly irritated by chemicals, infection, or overuse, thus reducing its ability to release bile for the digestion of fats. Usually, gallstones, consisting of calcium, cholesterol, and other minerals, form in the gallbladder itself. When the individual eats foods high in fats, the gallbladder contracts to release bile; these contractions cause pressure on the stone formations. One of the characteristic symptoms of gallbladder disease is acute pain in the upper right portion of the abdomen after eating fatty foods. This pain, which can last several hours, may feel like a heart attack or an ulcer attack and is often accompanied by nausea.

Not all gallstones cause acute pain. In fact, small stones that pass through one of the bile ducts and become lodged may be more painful than gallstones that are the size of golf balls. Many people find out that they have gallstones only after undergoing ultrasound and diagnostic X-rays to rule out other conditions. The absence of symptoms is significant because gallstones are considered a predisposing factor for gallbladder cancer.

Current treatment of gallbladder disease usually involves medication to reduce irritation, restriction of fat consumption, and surgery to remove the gallstones. New medications designed to dissolve small gallstones are currently used with some patients. In addition, some doctors use a technique known as lithotripsy, in which a series of noninvasive shock waves break up small stones. Lasers and laparoscopic surgery now reduce the risks associated with large surgical incisions.

MUSCULOSKELETAL DISEASES

Most of us will encounter some form of chronic musculoskeletal disease during our lifetime. Some form of arthritis will afflict half of us over the age of 65; low back pain hits most of us at some point in our life.

Diabetes: A disease in which the pancreas fails to produce enough insulin or the body fails to use insulin effectively.

Insulin: A hormone produced by the pancreas; required by the body for the metabolism of carbohydrates.

Hyperglycemia: Elevated blood sugar levels.

Ulcerative colitis: An inflammatory disorder that affects the mucous membranes of the large intestine, producing bloody diarrhea.

Irritable bowel syndrome (IBS): Nausea, pain, gas, or diarrhea caused by certain foods or stress.

Diverticulosis: A condition in which bulges form in the walls of the intestine; results in irritation and infection of the intestine.

Peptic ulcer: Damage to the stomach or intestinal lining, usually caused by digestive juices.

Arthritis

Arthritis is much more than occasional aches or pains; it is a serious and urgent problem in Canada. Currently, more than four million Canadians suffer from some form of arthritis, and more than 600 000 Canadians are disabled by it.[47] **Osteoarthritis** is a progressive deterioration of bones and joints associated with the "wear and tear" of aging. More recent research indicates that as joints are used, they release enzymes that digest cartilage while other cells in the cartilage try to repair the damage. When the enzymatic breakdown overpowers cellular repair, the pain and swelling characteristic of arthritis may occur. Weather extremes, excessive strain, and injury often lead to osteoarthritis flare-ups. But a specific precipitating event does not seem to be necessary. It is estimated that 85 percent of Canadians will be affected by osteoarthritis by age 70.[48] Although age and injury are undoubtedly factors in the development of osteoarthritis, heredity, abnormal use of the joint, dietary intake, abnormalities in joint structure, and impaired blood supply to the joint may also contribute. Osteoarthritis of the hands seems to have a particularly strong genetic component. Extreme disability as a result of osteoarthritis is rare. However, when joints become so distorted that they impair activity, surgical intervention is often necessary. Joint replacement and bone fusion are common surgical repair techniques. For most people, anti-inflammatory drugs, pain relievers, and cortisone-related agents ease discomfort. In some, applications of heat, mild physical activity, and massage may also relieve the pain.

Rheumatoid arthritis is similar to but far more serious than osteoarthritis. Rheumatoid arthritis is an inflammatory joint disease that can occur at any age, but most commonly appears between the ages of 20 and 45 years. It is three times more common among women than men during early adulthood but equally common among men and women in the over-70-years-of-age group. Symptoms may be gradually progressive or sporadic, with occasional unexplained remissions.

Rheumatoid arthritis typically attacks the synovial membrane, which produces the lubricating fluids for the joints. Advanced rheumatoid arthritis often involves destruction of the bony ends of joints. The remedy for this condition is typically bone fusion, which leaves the joint immobile. In some instances, joint replacement may be a viable alternative.

Although the exact cause of this form of arthritis is unknown, some experts theorize that it is an autoimmune disorder, in which the body responds as if its own cells were the enemy, eventually destroying the affected body parts. Other theorists believe that rheumatoid arthritis is caused by some form of invading microorganism that takes over the joint. Certain toxic chemicals and stress have also been mentioned as possible causes. Regardless of the cause, treatment of rheumatoid arthritis is similar to that for osteoarthritis. Emphasis is placed on pain relief and attempts to improve the functional mobility of the patient. In some instances, immunosuppressant drugs are also given to reduce the inflammatory response.

Fibromyalgia

Fibromyalgia is a chronic, painful rheumatological-like disorder. Symptoms include widespread pain; stiffness and numerous tender points; weakness; swelling; and neurovascular complaints including coldness, numbness, tingling, mottled skin, headaches, auditory sensitivity, irritable bowel syndrome, sleep disorders, depression, and dysmenorrhea. The cause of fibromyalgia remains a mystery, with many theories under investigation. Acute sleep disturbances, muscular irregularities, and forms of psychopathological disturbance have been considered as possible culprits. What is known is that the disease primarily affects women (particularly in their 30s and 40s), that the disease causes more chronic pain and debilitation than other musculoskeletal disorders, and that significant research must be conducted before an effective, long-term treatment will be available.

Systemic Lupus Erythematosus (SLE)

Lupus is a disease in which the immune system attacks the body, producing antibodies that destroy or injure organs such as the kidneys, brain, and heart. The symptoms vary from mild to severe and may disappear for periods of time. A butterfly-shaped rash covering the bridge of the nose and both cheeks is common. Nearly all individuals with SLE have aching joints and muscles, and 60 percent develop redness and swelling that moves from joint to joint. Extensive research has not yet found a cure for this sometimes fatal disease.

❋ Low Back Pain (LBP)

Most people (about 80 percent) will experience low back pain at some point during their life. Although some of these low back pain episodes may result from muscular damage and be short-lived and acute, others may involve dislocations, fractures, or other problems with spinal vertebrae or discs and be chronic or require surgery. LBP is epidemic throughout the world.

Risk Factors for Low Back Pain

Health experts believe that the following factors contribute to LBP:

- advancing age
- certain body types
- poor posture
- poor muscular strength and endurance
- psychological factors
- occupational risks

Preventing Back Pain and Injury

Almost 90 percent of all back problems occur in the lumbar spine region (lower back). Consciously protecting this region of the body from blows, excessive strain, or sharp twists when muscles are not warmed up is essential. You can reduce many problems by consciously attempting to maintain good posture when sitting, standing, and sleeping. In addition, physical activity, particularly activities that strengthen the abdominal muscles and the muscles that support the spine and stretch the back muscles, is important. It is also important to sleep on a supportive mattress, to work in an ergonomically friendly environment (supportive chair with feet flat on the floor, computer at eye level, keyboard appropriately placed, etc.), to lift heavy objects with your knees rather than your back, to avoid high-heeled and otherwise poorly fitting shoes, and to engage in regular physical activity. If you injure your back, be sure to consult with at least two different experts in rehabilitation and therapy to determine your best options. Consult an exercise physiologist, biomechanist, ergonomist, physical therapist, chiropractor, or physician specializing in bone and joint injuries for recommended physical activities.

OTHER MALADIES

During the last decade or so, numerous afflictions have surfaced that seem to be products of our times. Some of these health problems relate to specific groups of people, some are due to technological advances, and some are unexplainable. Still other diseases have been present for many years and continue to cause severe disability (see Table 12.7).

Among conditions that have received attention in recent years are chronic fatigue syndrome and disorders related to the use of video display terminals.

Chronic Fatigue Syndrome (CFS)

In the late 1980s, a characteristic set of symptoms was noted that included chronic fatigue, headaches, fever, sore throat, enlarged lymph nodes, depression, poor memory, general weakness, nausea, and symptoms remarkably similar to mononucleosis. Researchers initially believed that individuals were really talking about a series of symptoms caused by the Epstein-Barr virus, the same virus as mononucleosis. In some instances, the symptoms were so severe that individuals required hospitalization. Since those initial studies, researchers have all but ruled out the possibility of a mysterious form of the Epstein-Barr virus. Despite extensive testing, no viral cause has been found.

Today, in the absence of a known pathogen, many researchers believe that the illness, now commonly referred to as chronic fatigue syndrome (CFS), may have strong psychosocial roots.

The diagnosis of chronic fatigue syndrome depends on two major criteria and eight or more minor criteria. The major criteria are debilitating fatigue that persists for at least six months and the absence of diagnoses of other illnesses that could cause the symptoms. Minor criteria include headaches, fever, sore throat, painful lymph nodes, weakness, fatigue after physical activity, sleep problems, and rapid onset of these symptoms. Because an exact cause is not apparent, treatment of CFS focuses on improved dietary intake, rest, counselling for depression, judicious physical activity, and development of a strong support network.

Job-Related Disorders

During the last decade, a new potential health risk for computer users has been the topic of growing debate. Adverse health effects have been noted in people who work at computer video display terminals (VDTs) for several hours or more each day. Many post-secondary students are regular high-volume users of VDTs and are therefore at risk. Further adding to students' risk is their usage of cell phones.

Most of these problems relate to eyestrain and discomfort in the low back, neck, shoulders, and wrists. Questions about the danger posed by radiation from the electrical fields produced within the circuits of the VDT and about the potential effects on pregnant women and their fetuses remain unanswered.

Arthritis: Painful inflammatory disease of the joints.

Osteoarthritis: A progressive deterioration of bones and joints associated with the "wear and tear" of aging.

Rheumatoid arthritis: A serious inflammatory joint disease.

Lupus: A disease in which the immune system attacks the body.

Managing Your Disease Risks

Infectious diseases pose serious challenges throughout the world. In particular, STIs, including HIV, present an increasing health risk to young people. Infectious diseases can be prevented by practising safe and responsible behaviours. In addition, many noninfectious diseases can be prevented or their onset delayed by making positive personal health choices.

MAKING DECISIONS FOR YOU

Protecting yourself from infectious diseases is not always easy. Because most pathogens are microscopic, exposure to one can occur without your knowledge. Therefore, you need to be aware of your risks. What can you do to improve your awareness of your potential exposure to disease-causing pathogens?

What are some actions you can take to reduce your risk of contracting an STI? What steps could you take right now to ensure the sexual health of your partners? Finally, if you thought you had been exposed to HIV, where would you seek testing?

CHECKLIST FOR CHANGE: MAKING PERSONAL CHOICES

- Be aware of factors that threaten your health. Know your disease and immunization history.

- Take the precautions needed to protect yourself from exposure to infectious pathogens.

- Know the health status of your intimate partners.

- Communicate openly and honestly with your partners about your feelings regarding sexual intimacy.

- Wash your hands frequently and thoroughly with soap and water.

- Limit travel to places where outbreaks of infectious diseases have not been controlled. When travel to these places cannot be avoided, immunize yourself when possible for diseases that can be prevented.

- Maintain a healthy routine of adequate sleep, a healthy dietary intake following Eating Well with Canada's Food Guide, and regular physical activity.

- Cook foods at their appropriate temperatures. Keep hot foods hot, and cold foods cold.

- Recognize the symptoms that indicate a possible infection and seek treatment immediately.

- Recognize your responsibility for the health of others.

- Behave in sexually responsible ways.

- Limit your sexual partners.

- Limit alcohol or other drug use during intimate sexual encounters.

- Assess your level of risk for acquiring an STI, including HIV.

- Respect the rights and needs of individuals affected by an infectious disease.

- Adopt personal health habits that will reduce your risk of a chronic disease.

- Identify actions you can take today to reduce your risks for the diseases and disorders discussed in this chapter.

CHECKLIST FOR CHANGE: MAKING COMMUNITY CHOICES

- Does your student health service offer testing for all STIs, including HIV?

- Do you support government spending for HIV research and health promotion?

- Does your local school system offer a sex education curriculum including discussion about how to stop the spread of STIs, including HIV?

- If you worked for a government agency charged with helping people improve their personal health habits, what approaches would you take?

- Have you done anything to support campaigns raising money for research into chronic illnesses?

- What role should businesses play in improving employee health? Should the federal government provide tax credits to help businesses support employee health?

CRITICAL THINKING

You have been in a relationship for several months that has grown from a friendship to passionate sexual intimacy. During this time, a close and trusting bond has also developed. You have remained monogamous and believe that your partner has as well, although you have never discussed it. Nor has any discussion arisen about each other's sexual history or HIV status. You have been involved in sexual relationships in the past and have never been tested for HIV, and you are quite certain your partner is experienced as well. You trust your partner but recognize that, without complete information, you are both at risk for HIV infection. You want to take some precautionary steps but worry about insulting your partner's feelings.

Use the DECIDE model described in Chapter 1 to decide what you would do in this situation. Develop several different strategies and approaches for reaching the desired result.

TABLE 12.7
Other Modern Afflictions

Disease	Description	Treatment
Parkinson's disease	Disease affecting mostly people over the age of 55. Symptoms include tremors, rigidity, slowed movement, loss of autonomic movements, and difficulty walking.	Unknown cause makes prevention difficult. Tranquillizers are useful in controlling nerve responses.
Multiple sclerosis	Disease that affects women more than men. Precise cause uncertain. Symptoms include vision problems, tingling and numbness in extremities, chronic fatigue, and neurological impairments.	Medication to control symptoms and slow progression of the disease. Stress management may be helpful.
Cystic fibrosis	Inherited disease occurring in 1 out of every 1600 births. Characterized by pooling of large amounts of mucus in lungs, digestive disturbances, and excessive sodium excretion. Results in premature death.	Most treatments are geared toward relief of symptoms. Antibiotics are administered for infection. Recent strides in genetic research suggest better treatments and potential cure in the near future.
Sickle cell disease	Inherited disease affecting mostly blacks. Disease affects hemoglobin, forming sickle shaped red blood cells that interfere with oxygenation. Results in severe pain, anemia, and premature death.	Reduce stress and attend to minor infections immediately. Seek genetic counselling.
Cerebral palsy	Disorder characterized by the loss of voluntary control over motor functioning. Believed to be caused by a lack of oxygen to the brain at birth, brain disorders or an accident before or after birth, poisoning, or brain infections.	Follow preventive actions to reduce accident risks; improved neonatal and birthing techniques.
Graves' disease	Thyroid disorder characterized by swelling of the eyes, staring gaze, and retraction of the eyelid. Can result in loss of sight. The cause is unknown and it can occur at any age.	Medication may help control symptoms. Radioactive iodine supplements also may be administered.

Carpal tunnel syndrome is a common occupational injury in which the median nerve in the wrist becomes irritated, causing numbness, tingling, and pain in the fingers and hands. This condition is worsened by the repetitive typing motions made by computer users and is often classified as a common repetitive motion injury. For those who must work on a computer for hours at a time, day after day, ergonomists recommend regular breaks. Remove your hands from the keyboard to move them about every 20 minutes; stretch other body parts such as the neck and shoulders periodically. Physically remove yourself from your computer at least once every hour for several minutes, perhaps walking around the room or doing some simple stretches. Paying attention to the design, height, and support of your chair, and placing your keyboard at a comfortable angle and height, can save countless hours of suffering—though these precautions do not remove the need to get up and move every so often.

Working in front of a computer for several hours a day can put you at risk for eyestrain and back, neck, shoulder, and wrist pain.

Carpal tunnel syndrome: A common occupational injury in which the median nerve in the wrist becomes irritated, causing numbness, tingling, and pain in the fingers and hands.

Go to MyHealthLab at **www.pearsoned.ca/myhealthlab**. Here you will find self-assessments, case studies, links to health on the net, and much more.

DISCUSSION QUESTIONS

1. What is a pathogen? What are the similarities and differences between pathogens and antigens?

2. What is the difference between natural and acquired immunity?

3. Identify five STIs and their symptoms in men and women. How do they develop? How are they treated? What are their potential long-term risks?

4. Why might it be inappropriate to identify groups as at high risk for HIV infection? Why might HIV infection be better referred to as a sexually transmissible infection than as a sexually transmitted infection?

5. What are some of the major noninfectious chronic diseases affecting Canadians today? What are the common risk factors? How are they treated?

6. List the common respiratory diseases affecting Canadians. Which of these has a genetic basis? An environmental basis? An individual basis?

7. Compare and contrast the different types of headaches, including their symptoms and treatments. What can be done to prevent them? Treat them?

8. Do you believe that PMS is a disorder or disease or simply a catchall name for many naturally occurring events in the menstrual cycle? Why?

9. What are the medical risks of fibrocystic breast condition and endometriosis? How can they be treated? Prevented?

10. Describe the symptoms and treatment of diabetes. What is the difference between type 1 and type 2 diabetes?

11. How can you tell whether your stomach is reacting to final exams or telling you that you have a serious medical condition?

APPLICATION EXERCISE

Reread the "Consider This . . ." scenario at the beginning of this chapter and answer the following questions.

1. What was your initial reaction to this scenario? Why?

2. What are some legal issues that could arise or that already exist regarding all infectious diseases, including STIs? Why do the rights of all the individuals involved in relationships need to be considered?

3. What services exist on your campus for people living with HIV infection or AIDS? What services focus on informing people about STIs?

MYSEARCHLAB EXERCISE

1. Log on to www.MySearchLab.com.

2. Retrieve article AN 36006045, "Chlamydia in Female Reproductive Tract," by Deeksha Pandey, Jyoti Shetty, Muralidhar V. Pai, and Pratapkumar.

3. Read the article.

4. Summarize the key findings in a PowerPoint presentation or a one-page handout that could be shared with students on campus.

CHAPTER 13

ENVIRONMENTAL HEALTH

Thinking Globally,
Acting Locally

CONSIDER THIS . . .

Leo decided to live off campus this year, so for the first time he is in charge of all aspects of his day-to-day living, including the cleaning of his apartment. Though environmentally friendly in his previous lifestyle habits (that is, he recycled as much as possible), he is not sure what to look for when buying cleaning products, nor does he know where to look for help.

What suggestions would you give to Leo to find more information and specific products he could purchase to clean effectively without causing too much damage to the environment?

CHAPTER OBJECTIVES

* Explain the impact of global population growth on the environment.

* Identify the major causes of air pollution, including photochemical smog and acid rain, and make suggestions for reducing it.

* Identify major sources of water pollution and make suggestions for reducing it.

* Describe the consequences of noise pollution and what you can do to protect yourself.

* Identify the major causes of land pollution and what can be done to reduce it.

Human health, well-being, and survival are ultimately dependent on the integrity of the planet. Today, the natural world is under attack from the pressure of the number of people who live in it and the wide range of their activities. Effective management of the environment is critical to avoiding at least 25 percent of all preventable diseases worldwide.[1] In fact, as many as 13 million deaths could be prevented each year if we made our environment healthier. Worldwide, one-third of all diseases and about 4 million deaths in children under the age of five years are due to unsafe water and air pollution.[2] In fact, improved management of the environment could prevent as many as 40 percent of deaths from malaria, 41 percent from lower respiratory infections, and 94 percent from diarrhoeal disease—three of the world's biggest childhood killers. In the least developed countries, one-third of death and disease can be attributed to environmental causes. Though some environmental issues are managed better in developed countries, targeted interventions such as promoting safe household water storage, better hygiene measures, and the use of cleaner and safer fuels would reduce the incidence of cancers, cardiovascular diseases, asthma, lower respiratory infections, musculoskeletal diseases, road traffic injuries, poisoning, and drowning.[3]

Other interventions such as increasing the safety of buildings; promoting safe, careful use and management of toxic substances at home and in the workplace; and better water resource management would also result in improvements in population health and wellness.[4]

Canadians' concern about the environment has intensified since the initial outpouring on the first Earth Day in April 1970. The federal, provincial/territorial, and municipal governments share responsibility for the environment. Public health agencies are becoming more responsive to public concerns regarding the environment. While Canadians get most of their environmental information from the media, the majority look to public health professionals for answers to their concerns.

Health agencies are involved in defining the problems and seeking solutions in many of the approaches taken to address environmental health issues.[5] And this is supported by thousands of individual Canadians changing their habits and working to improve the environment. People are exposed to contaminants in water, air, food, and soil in various ways:[6]

- Ingesting food, water, soil, objects, or liquids containing contaminants. The mouth, throat, stomach, and intestines can absorb ingested materials rapidly and at different rates, depending on the contaminant.

- Inhalation of a contaminated gas or vapour, or of airborne particles. This includes small amounts of soil and dust inhaled into the lungs. The lungs often absorb gasses and vapours quickly and efficiently.

- Dermal (skin) contact with contaminants in water, soil, or air. Some contaminants are absorbed through the skin, while in other cases the skin acts as an efficient barrier.

- In the case of radioactivity, exposure can occur through penetration of the skin by radioactivity in the atmosphere or released from radionuclides in the air or on the ground. The radionuclide does not actually need to be in contact with the skin.

See Figure 13.1 for a diagram of major exposure pathways.

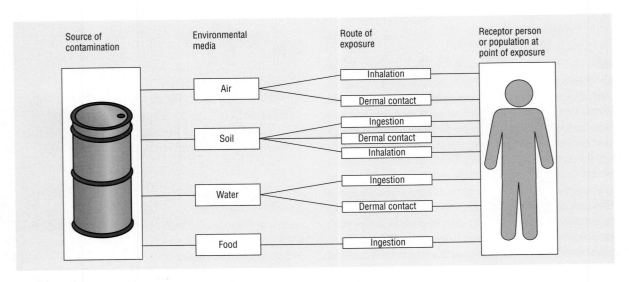

FIGURE 13.1

Major Pathways of Human Exposure to Environmental Contaminants

✓ OVERPOPULATION

Our most challenging environmental problem is population growth. The anthropologist Margaret Mead wrote, "Every human society is faced with two population issues: how to beget and rear enough children and how not to beget and rear too many."[7]

The United Nations' "World Populations Prospects: The 2006 Revision" estimates that the world's population will be 6.9 billion people in 2010.[8] Compared to the estimate made for 2005, an increase of 392 million people is expected, equivalent to a gain of approximately 78 million people per year. Despite the decreases in fertility projected for 2005 to 2050, the world population is expected to reach 9.2 billion people by 2050 and will be increasing by 59 million persons per year.

The majority (that is, 95 percent) of the population growth occurs in the developing world.[9] In fact, between 2005 and 2050, the population of the more developed countries is expected to remain about the same. At the same time, the less developed regions' population is estimated to increase from 5.3 to 7.9 billion, adding 58 million people annually. The population of the least developed countries is expected to more than double from 2005 to 2050, with an annual increase of 22 million people. The population is expected to triple between 2005 and 2050 in Afghanistan, Burkina Faso, Burundi, Chad, Congo, the Democratic Republic of Congo, the Democratic Republic of Timor-Leste, Guinea-Bissau, Liberia, Mali, Niger, and Uganda. On the other hand, the population of 51 countries or areas, including Germany, Italy, Japan, the Baltic States, and most of the successor states of the former Soviet Union, are expected to be lower in 2050 than in 2005. Given these findings, nine countries are expected to account for half of the world's projected population increase. In order of population growth, these countries are India, Pakistan, Nigeria, the Democratic Republic of China, Bangladesh, Uganda, the United States, Ethiopia, and China.

Estimates for population growth are highly dependent upon predicted fertility rates.[10] In the projections presented previously, worldwide average fertility was expected to slowly decrease from 2.55 in 2005–2010 to 2.02 children per woman in 2050. A fertility path half a child above or below the estimates would result in a world population in 2050 of 10.6 billion or 7.6 billion, respectively. Global fertility has decreased from 5.02 children per woman in 1950 to 2.65 children per woman in 2000–2005. In more developed regions fertility is currently 1.60 children per woman and is expected to increase to 1.79 children per woman by 2045–2050. In the least developed countries, fertility is currently 4.63 children per woman and is expected to drop to 2.50 by 2045–2050. In the rest of the developing world (that is, less developed regions), fertility is currently 2.75 and is expected to decrease to 2.05 children per woman by 2045–2050.

Another factor to consider with regard to world population is life expectancy. Current world life expectancy at birth is 67.2 years (63.9 years for men; 68.3 years for women).[11] World life expectancy for 2045–2050 is predicted to be 75.4 years (73.1 years for men; 77.8 years for women). Individuals living in more developed regions have a much longer life expectancy at birth in 2005–2010, at 76.5 years (72.9 years for men; 79.3 years for women), and a predicted life expectancy in 2045–2050 of 82.4 years (79.4 years for men; 85.4 years for women). As mentioned in Chapter 1, life expectancy at birth in 2003 (the most recent data available) is 79.9 years (77.4 years for men; 82.4 years for women). In the least developed countries, an individual's current life expectancy at birth is 54.6 years (53.4 years for men; 55.8 years for women). In other less developed regions, current life expectancy at birth is 65.4 years (63.7 years for men; 67.2 years for women). In 2045–2050, individuals in the least developed countries are expected to live 67.2 years (65.4 years for men; 69.1 years for women), while those living in less developed regions are predicted to live 74.3 years (72.1 years for men; 76.5 years for women). As a result of increases in life expectancy, the world population is expected to age. Currently, in more developed regions 20.1 percent of the population is over the age of 60 years; this is expected to increase to 32.6 percent. In the least developed countries, only 5.1 percent of the current population is over the age of 60 years, with a projected increase to 10.3 percent by 2050. In the less developed regions, current estimates are that 8.1 percent of the population is over the age of 60 years; this is expected to increase to 20.1 percent by 2050.

As the global population expands, so does the competition for the earth's resources. Environmental

As world population increases, the world's resources cannot keep up. In fact, in many parts of the world, governments struggle to meet the needs of its increasing number of citizens.

degradation caused by loss of topsoil, pesticides, toxic residues, deforestation, global warming, air pollution, and acid rain seriously threatens the food supply and undermines world health. However, population growth doesn't tell the whole story. North Americans consume more energy and raw materials per person than people from other regions of the world. Many of these resources come from other countries, and our consumption is depleting the resource balances of those countries. Therefore, we must start by living environmentally conscious lives.

what do you THINK?

What do you think we, as a world community, ought to do about population growth? How would you react to a government-imposed restriction on family size? What about mandatory limitations in developing nations?

✳ AIR POLLUTION

As our population has grown, so have the number and volume of the environmental pollutants produced. It is estimated that air pollution causes approximately 2 million deaths worldwide per year.[12] Concern about air quality prompted Parliament to pass the Clean Air Act in 1970. This was consolidated in 1985 into the Canadian Environmental Protection Act (CEPA). CEPA was further updated and revised in 1999 and came into effect March 31, 2000.[13] The Canadian Environmental Assessment Act (CEAA) provides a legal basis for federal environmental assessment and came into force on January 19, 2005.[14] Various agreements (that is, high-level commitments entered into by two or more parties that identify the actions, roles, and commitments of the parties involved in dealing with environmental pollution) have also been established. The Canada-Wide Accord on Environmental Harmonization, Pollution Prevention Policy Agreement, Comprehensive Air Quality Management Framework for Canada, and the Canada–United States Air Quality Agreement are examples of current agreements in place within the Canadian government and between the Canadian and U.S. governments.[15] These acts and agreements cover pollution prevention, management of toxic substances, clean air and water, control of pollution and waste, information gathering, and the setting of guidelines and enforcement of environmental laws and regulations.

Sources of Air Pollution

Sulphur Dioxide

Sulphur dioxide is a yellowish-brown gas that is a by-product of burning fossil fuels. Electricity generating stations, smelters, refineries, and industrial boilers are the main source points. In humans, sulphur dioxide aggravates symptoms of heart and lung disease, obstructs breathing, and increases the incidence of respiratory diseases such as colds, asthma, bronchitis, and emphysema. It is toxic to plants, destroys some paint pigments, corrodes metals, impairs visibility, and is a precursor to acid rain.

Particulates

Particulates are tiny solid particles or liquid droplets suspended in the air. Cigarette smoke releases particulates. They are also by-products of some industrial processes and the internal combustion engine. Particulates irritate the lungs and carry heavy metals and cancer-causing agents deep into the lungs. When combined with sulphur dioxide, particulates exacerbate respiratory diseases. Particulates also corrode metals and obscure visibility.

Carbon Monoxide

Carbon monoxide is an odourless, colourless gas that originates primarily from motor vehicle emissions. Carbon monoxide interferes with the blood's ability to absorb and carry oxygen and impairs thinking, slows reflexes, and causes drowsiness, unconsciousness, and death. When inhaled by a pregnant woman, it threatens the physical and mental growth and development of the fetus. Long-term exposure increases the severity of circulatory and respiratory diseases.

Nitrogen Dioxide

Nitrogen dioxide is an amber-coloured gas emitted by coal-powered electrical utility boilers and by motor vehicles. High concentrations of nitrogen dioxide can be fatal. Lower concentrations increase susceptibility to colds and flu, bronchitis, and pneumonia. Nitrogen dioxide is also toxic to plant life and causes a brown discolouration of the atmosphere. It is a precursor of ozone and, along with sulphur dioxide, of acid rain.

Ozone

Ozone is a form of oxygen produced when nitrogen dioxide reacts with hydrogen chloride. These gases release oxygen, which is altered by sunlight to produce ozone. In the lower atmosphere, ozone irritates the mucous membranes of the respiratory system, causing coughing and choking. It impairs lung functioning, reduces resistance to colds and pneumonia, and aggravates heart disease, asthma, bronchitis, and pneumonia. This ozone corrodes rubber and paint and injures or kills vegetation. It is also one of the irritants found in smog. A Canadian study concluded that there is no safe level of human exposure to ground-level ozone.[16]

The natural ozone found in the upper atmosphere serves as a protective layer against heat and radiation from the sun. This atmospheric layer, called the ozone layer, is discussed later in the chapter.

Lead

Lead is a metal pollutant found in the exhaust of motor vehicles powered by fuel containing lead and in the emissions from lead smelters and processing plants. Lead often contaminates drinking water systems in homes with plumbing installed before 1930. Lead negatively affects the circulatory, reproductive, and nervous systems, the blood and kidneys, and accumulates in bone and other tissues. Lead is particularly detrimental to children and fetuses, resulting in birth defects, behavioural abnormalities, and decreased learning ability.

Hydrocarbons

Hydrocarbons encompass a wide variety of chemical pollutants in the air. Sometimes known as volatile organic compounds, **hydrocarbons** are chemical compounds containing various combinations of carbon and hydrogen. The principal source of polluting hydrocarbons is the internal combustion engine. Most automobile engines emit hundreds of different types of hydrocarbon compounds. By themselves, hydrocarbons cause few problems, but when combined with sunlight and other pollutants they form such poisons as formaldehyde, various ketones, and peroxyacetylnitrate (PAN), all of which are respiratory irritants. Hydrocarbon combinations such as benzene and benzopyrene are carcinogenic (that is, cancer-causing). In addition, hydrocarbons play a major part in the formation of smog.

Photochemical Smog

Photochemical smog is a brown, hazy mix of particulates and gases that forms when oxygen-containing compounds of nitrogen and hydrocarbons react in the presence of sunlight. Photochemical smog is sometimes called ozone pollution because ozone is created when vehicle exhaust reacts with sunlight. Such smog is most likely to develop on days with little wind and high traffic congestion. In most cases, it forms in areas that experience a **temperature inversion**, a weather condition in which a cool layer of air is trapped under a layer of warmer air, preventing air circulation. When gases such as hydrocarbons and nitrogen oxides are released into the cool air layer they cannot escape, and thus remain suspended until wind conditions move the warmer air layer. Sunlight filtering through the air causes chemical changes in the hydrocarbons and nitrogen oxides, which results in smog. Smog is more likely to be produced in valley regions blocked by hills or mountains.

The most noticeable adverse effects of exposure to smog are difficulty in breathing, burning eyes, headaches, and nausea. Long-term exposure to smog poses serious health risks, particularly for children, the elderly, pregnant women, and people with chronic respiratory disorders such as asthma and emphysema. According to the Canadian Lung Association, repeated exposure to smog accelerates the aging of the lungs and increases susceptibility to infections by hindering immune system functioning.[17]

Acid Rain

Acid rain is precipitation that falls through acidic air pollutants, particularly those containing sulphur dioxides and nitrogen dioxides. This precipitation, in the form of rain, snow, or fog, has a more acidic composition than unpolluted precipitation. In lakes and ponds, acid rain gradually acidifies the water. At a certain level, acid rain creates conditions in lakes and ponds where plants and animals cannot survive. Ironically, acidified lakes and ponds become a crystal-clear deep blue, creating an illusion of beauty and health.

Ozone: A gas formed when nitrogen dioxide interacts with hydrogen chloride.

Hydrocarbons: Chemical compounds that contain carbon and hydrogen.

Photochemical smog: The brownish-yellow haze resulting from the combination of hydrocarbons and nitrogen oxides.

Temperature inversion: A weather condition occurring when a layer of cool air is trapped under a layer of warmer air.

Acid rain: Precipitation contaminated with acidic pollutants.

It's Not Easy Being Green

Circle the number of each item that describes what you have done or are doing for the environment.

1. When walking, cycling, camping, or spending time at beaches, I never leave anything behind.

2. I ride my bike, walk, carpool, or use public transportation whenever possible.

3. I write my municipal, provincial/territorial, and federal representatives about environmental issues.

4. I avoid turning on the air conditioner or increasing the heat whenever possible.

5. I take short showers and my shower has a low-flow shower head.

6. I do not run the water while brushing my teeth, shaving, or hand-washing clothes.

7. I take short showers instead of baths.

8. My sink taps have aerators installed in them.

9. I have a water displacement device in my toilet(s).

10. I snip or rip plastic six-pack rings before I throw them out.

11. I choose recycled and recyclable products as often as possible.

12. I avoid noise pollutants. (I sit away from speakers at concerts, select an apartment away from busy streets or airports, and so on.)

13. I make sure my car is tuned with functional emission control equipment.

14. I try to avoid known carcinogens such as vinyl chloride, asbestos, benzene, mercury, X-rays, and so on.

15. When shopping, I choose products with the least amount of packaging and I use cloth shopping bags.

16. I dispose of hazardous materials (used batteries, paint, oil, and antifreeze) at appropriate sites.

17. If or when I have children, I will use cloth rather than disposable diapers.

18. I store food in reusable containers rather than using plastic wrap.

19. I use as few paper products as possible.

20. I take my own bag along when I go shopping.

21. I avoid products packaged in plastic and unrecycled aluminum.

22. I recycle newspapers, glass, cans, and all other recyclables.

23. I run the clothes dryer only as long as it takes my clothes to dry. I dry as many clothes as possible outdoors or indoors on a laundry line or clothes drying rack.

24. I turn off lights and appliances when not in use.

25. I compost organic wastes.

SCORING AND INTERPRETATION

Count how many items you have circled. Ideally, you should be doing all these things, but if you are trying to do at least some, you can score yourself as follows:

20–25: Good contributions to maintaining the environment.

14–19: Moderate contributions to maintaining the environment.

Below 13: Need to consider the recommendations made in this chapter to help the environment.

Sources of Acid Rain

More than 95 percent of acid rain originates from human actions, chiefly the burning of fossil fuels. When industries burn fuels, the sulphur and nitrogen in the emissions combine with the oxygen and sunlight in the air to become sulphur dioxide and nitrogen oxides (precursors of sulphuric acid and nitric acids, respectively). Small acid particles are then carried by the wind and combine with moisture to produce acidic rain, snow, or fog. Because of higher concentrations of sunlight in the summer months, rain is more strongly acidic in the summertime. Additionally, the rain or snow that first falls is more acidic than that which falls later. Southern Ontario experiences some of the highest concentrations of acid aerosols in North America.[18]

Effects of Acid Rain

The damage caused to lake and pond habitats is not the worst of the problems created by acid rain. Each year, acid rain is responsible for the destruction of millions of trees in forests in Europe and North America. Scientists concluded that 75 percent of Europe's forests are now experiencing damaging levels of sulphur deposition by acid rain. Forests in every country on the continent are affected.[19]

Doctors believe that acid rain aggravates and may even cause bronchitis, asthma, and other respiratory problems. In Southern Ontario, several air pollution epidemiological studies demonstrated that increases in acid aerosols and ground-level ozone positively correlate with increased hospital admissions due to respiratory problems.[20] In other words, the greater the acid aerosols and ground-level ozone, the greater the hospital admissions related to respiratory issues. People with emphysema or a history of heart disease as well as unborn children may also suffer from exposure to acid rain.

Acidic precipitation can cause metals such as aluminum, cadmium, lead, and mercury to **leach** (dissolve and filter) out of the soil. If these metals make their way into water or food supplies (particularly fish), they can cause cancer in humans who consume them.

Acid rain is also responsible for crop damage, which, in turn, contributes to world hunger. Laboratory experiments showed that acid rain reduced seed yield by up to 23 percent. Actual crop losses are reported with increasing frequency. In May 1989, China's Hunan Province lost an estimated $260 million worth of crops and seedlings to acid rain. Similar losses have been reported in Chile, Brazil, and Mexico.[21] Another consequence of acid rain is the destruction of public monuments and structures, with billions of dollars in damage each year.[22]

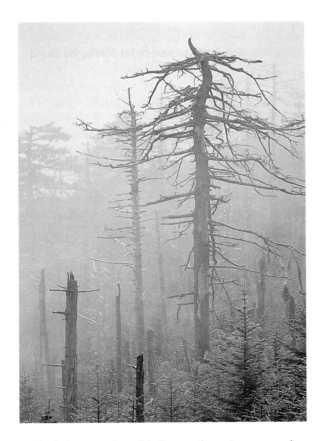

Acid rain has many harmful effects on the environment and poses numerous health hazards, including the risk of cancer from heavy metals that can make their way into the food chain.

Indoor Air Pollution

A growing body of research indicates that the air within our homes and other buildings can be 10 to 40 times more hazardous than outdoor air even in the most industrialized cities. This is a concern for the most vulnerable people in our population, particularly the young, the elderly, and the chronically ill, who spend more than 90 percent of their time indoors.[23]

There are 20 to 100 potentially dangerous compounds in the average home. Most indoor pollution comes from sources that release gases or particles into the air. Inadequate ventilation, particularly in heavily insulated buildings with airtight windows, may increase pollution by not allowing outside air in. Some sources, such as building materials, furnishings, and household products such as air fresheners, release pollutants continuously. Others release pollutants intermittently. Several factors affect risk, including age, pre-existing medical conditions, individual sensitivity, room temperature and humidity, and liver, immune, and respiratory system functions.[24]

Prevention should focus on three main areas: source control (eliminating or reducing individual contaminants), ventilation improvements (increasing the amount of outdoor air coming indoors), and air cleaners (removing particulates from the air).[25] Indoor air pollution comes primarily from woodstoves, furnaces, asbestos, passive smoke, formaldehyde, radon, and household chemicals and cleaners. In certain parts of Canada, mould may also be a significant source.

Wood Stove Smoke

Wood stoves emit significant levels of particulates and carbon monoxide in addition to other pollutants, such as sulphur dioxide. If you rely on wood for heat, make sure your stove is properly installed, vented, and maintained. Proper adjustments and emission controls taken to recombust potential pollutants can help to reduce pollution levels from wood stoves. Burning seasoned wood also reduces the amount of particulates released into the air.

Furnaces

People who rely on oil- or gas-fired furnaces also need to make sure that these appliances are properly installed, ventilated, and maintained. Inadequate cleaning and maintenance can lead to a buildup of carbon monoxide in the home, which can be deadly.

Leach: A process by which chemicals dissolve and filter through soil.

Asbestos

Asbestos is another indoor air pollutant that poses serious threats to human health. **Asbestos** is a mineral commonly used in insulating materials in buildings constructed before 1970. When bonded to other materials, asbestos is relatively harmless, but if its tiny fibres become loosened and airborne, they can embed themselves in the lungs and cannot be expelled. Their presence leads to cancer of the lungs, stomach, and chest lining, and is the cause of a fatal lung disease called mesothelioma.

Passive Smoke

Typically, **passive smoke** (or environmental tobacco smoke) is encountered as secondhand or sidestream smoke from cigarettes. Similar to active smoking, lengthy exposure to passive smoke can cause serious negative health effects. Nonsmokers who live with smokers are at a higher risk for heart disease and some cancers. Passive smoke is a major cause of respiratory problems, especially in infants and children. Though widespread bans are now in place—limiting smokers from lighting up in restaurants, the workplace, shopping malls, schools, and in some cases while in a vehicle—many people, including children and youth, remain susceptible to passive smoke at home. Avoiding regular exposure to secondhand tobacco smoke will reduce your risks of heart and lung disease.

Formaldehyde

Formaldehyde is a colourless, strong-smelling gas present in some carpets, draperies, furniture, particle board, plywood, wood panelling, countertops, and many adhesives. It is released into the air in a process called outgassing. Outgassing is greatest in new products, but the process can continue for many years. Exposure to formaldehyde can cause respiratory problems, dizziness, fatigue, nausea, and rashes. Long-term exposure can lead to central nervous system disorders and cancer. If you experience symptoms of formaldehyde exposure, your home should be tested by a municipal, regional, or provincial/territorial health agency.

Radon

Radon, an odourless, colourless gas, is the natural by-product of uranium or radium decay in the soil. Radon may penetrate homes through cracks, pipes, sump pits, and other openings in the foundation. At toxic levels, it can cause lung cancer. However, Health Canada does not consider radon pollution a widespread problem in Canadian homes. In fact, studies indicate that less than one-tenth of 1 percent of all homes in Canada—fewer than 8000 out of a total of 8 million—could have levels of radon sufficiently high to warrant efforts aimed at lowering the level. Population studies based on a survey of 14 000 homes in 19 Canadian cities did not show a correlation between radon levels in homes and lung cancer.[26]

Household Chemicals

Cleansers and other cleaning products should be used only in well-ventilated rooms. Further, regular cleaning will reduce the need to use potentially harmful cleaning products. Cut down on dry cleaning, as the chemicals used by many cleaners can cause cancer. If your newly cleaned clothes smell of dry cleaning chemicals, either return them to the cleaner or hang them in the open air until the smell is gone. Avoid the use of household air freshener products containing the cancer-causing agent dichlorobenzene. It is recommended that you clean with non-toxic, phosphate-free, and environmentally friendly products.

Ozone Layer Depletion

We earlier defined ozone as a chemical produced when oxygen interacts with sunlight. In people, ozone can lead to respiratory distress. Farther away from the earth, it forms a protective membrane-like layer in the earth's stratosphere—the highest level of the earth's atmosphere, located from 20 to 50 kilometres above the earth's surface. The ozone layer in the stratosphere protects the planet and its inhabitants from ultraviolet B (UV-B) radiation, a primary cause of skin cancer. Ultraviolet B radiation may also damage DNA and be linked to weakened immune system functioning in humans and animals.

> ## what do you THINK?
> When you clean, what products do you use? Do you read the labels of these products? Why or why not? What influences your choice of cleaning products?

In the early 1970s, scientists began to warn of a depletion of the earth's stratospheric ozone layer. Special instruments developed to test atmospheric contents indicated that specific chemicals used on the earth contributed to the rapid depletion of this vital protective layer. These chemicals are called

A Breath of Fresh Air: Made-in-Canada Solutions to Meet Canada's Environmental Challenges

Although the Government of Canada is viewed as a leader on environmental sustainability issues and a strong promoter of sustainable development opportunities, there remains a large number and variety of issues for Canada to deal with. Current efforts aimed at protecting the health and well-being of Canadians and their communities from air pollution have not matched our reputation. Since ratifying the Kyoto Protocol, Canada's greenhouse gas emissions are up 24 percent—a far cry from the target of 6 percent below 1990 levels. Further, Canada ranked 28th overall out of 30 countries on 29 environmental indicators in the "Maple Leaf in the OECD: Comparing Progress Toward Sustainability" report. More specifically, Canada ranked 26th in greenhouse gas emissions, 29th in water consumption, 27th in pollution from sulphur oxides, and 26th on species at risk.

As result, we need to take action; we need to clean the air we breathe. It is critical that we act. It is critical that we act now. In a report from a 2004 British Columbia Provincial Officer of Health, it was estimated that air pollution would cause between 140 and 400 premature deaths, 700 to 2100 hospital stays, and between 900 and 2700 emergency room visits per year.

Further, the direct and indirect costs of air pollution are staggering. In Ontario (in 2005 dollars) these costs were estimated at $374 million for lost productivity and work time, $507 million for indirect healthcare costs, $537 million in pain and suffering, and $6.4 billion in social welfare due to premature death.

In the summer of 2005, there were 53 smog advisory days in Ontario, 24 in Quebec, and three in the Atlantic Provinces. Ten winter smog advisory days were also issued in Quebec, and five more in Ontario.

Given these findings, the solutions proposed must address greenhouse gases and air pollution—not separately, as has been done in the past. Thus, the federal government will develop—in conjunction with the provinces and territories, municipalities, and aboriginal communities—a new Canadian Clean Air Act. Canadians will be encouraged "to get out of their cars and get onto public transit by providing a federal tax credit to offset part of the costs of monthly transit passes. Increasing the use of public transit will help reduce traffic congestion in Canadian cities, reduce greenhouse gases and fight pollution." Those who cannot get out of their cars will be encouraged to use cleaner fuel.

It is expected that offering these cleaner choices and inviting Canadians to work with the government in making solutions will result in a cleaner Canada and a cleaner world.

Source: Adapted from "A Breath of Fresh Air: Made in Canada Solutions to Meet Canada's Environmental Challenges," speaking notes for an address by the Honourable Rona Ambrose, Minister of the Environment of Canada, Vancouver BC, March 31, 2006. Retrieved on May 19, 2006, from www.ec.gc.ca/minister/speeches/2006/060331_s_e.htm.

chlorofluorocarbons (CFCs) (see Figure 13.2). In 1979, a satellite measurement showing a large hole in the ozone layer over Antarctica shocked scientists. Since then, satellite measurements of the ozone layer have regularly shown increases in the size of the hole. As a result, Canada banned the production of CFCs in 1993 and their importation in 1996. Methyl chloroform was also banned in 1996.

In 2001, the Government of Canada published its Interim Plan 2001 on Particulate Matter and Ozone to share its plans to achieve Canada-wide standards for Particulate Matter and Ozone. Five years later, a progress report indicated that major advances had been made in reducing smog-producing pollutants in the transportation sector, transboundary sources of air pollution, and establishing strong air quality monitoring networks across the country.[27] It was also noted that further work is still needed to achieve the Canada-wide standards by 2010.

Global Warming

More than 100 years ago, scientists theorized that carbon dioxide emissions from fossil-fuel burning would create a buildup of "greenhouse" gases in the earth's atmosphere and that this accumulation would have a warming effect on the earth's surface. The century-old predictions are now coming true, with alarming effects. Average global temperatures are higher today

Asbestos: A substance that separates into stringy fibres and lodges in lungs, where it cannot be expelled.

Passive smoke: Secondhand or sidestream cigarette smoke.

Formaldehyde: A colourless, strong-smelling gas released from products through outgassing.

Radon: A naturally occurring radioactive gas resulting from the decay of certain radioactive elements.

Chlorofluorocarbons (CFCs): Chemicals that contribute to the depletion of the ozone layer.

4. A free oxygen molecule breaks up the chlorine monoxide. The chlorine is free to repeat the process.

Ozone molecules

Free chlorine

Chlorine monoxide

Sun

Oxygen molecule

Ultraviolet light

3. The chlorine atom attacks an ozone molecule, breaking it apart. An oxygen molecule and a molecule of chlorine monoxide are formed.

2. In the upper atmosphere, ultraviolet light breaks off a chlorine atom from a chlorofluorocarbon molecule.

1. Chlorofluorocarbon molecule released from air conditioners, refrigerators, etc.

FIGURE 13.2

This diagram shows the depletion of the stratospheric ozone layer.

Climate change

Stratospheric ozone depletion

Diverse pathways

Desertification and land degradation

Agroecosystem productivity

UV exposure

Human health

Population displacement

Decline in several ecosystem services

Water quantity and safety

Altered precipitation

Biodiversity loss and ecosystem function

Freshwater decline

FIGURE 13.3

Large-scale and global environmental hazards to human health include climate change, stratospheric ozone depletion, loss of biodiversity, changes in hydrological systems and the supplies of fresh water, land degradation, and stresses on food-producing systems.

Source: World Health Organization, www.who.int/globalchange/en/.

than at any time since global temperatures were first recorded, and the change in atmospheric temperature may be taking a heavy toll on humans and crops. Climate researchers predicted in 1975 that the buildup of greenhouse gases would produce life-threatening natural phenomena, including drought, severe forest fires, flooding, extended heat waves over large areas of the earth, and killer hurricanes. Figure 13.3 illustrates the complex interactions and the influence of climate change on human health.

Greenhouse gases include carbon dioxide, CFCs, ground-level ozone, nitrous oxide, and methane. These chemicals become part of a gaseous layer that encircles the earth, allowing solar heat to pass through and then trapping it close to the earth's surface (as if in a greenhouse). The most predominant of these chemicals is carbon dioxide, which accounts for 49 percent of all greenhouse gases. Eastern Europe and North America are responsible for approximately half of all carbon dioxide emissions. Since the late 19th century,

carbon dioxide concentrations in the atmosphere increased 25 percent, with half of this increase occurring since the 1950s. Not surprisingly, these greater concentrations coincide with world industrial growth.

Rapid deforestation of the tropical rainforests of Central and South America, Africa, and Southeast Asia is also contributing to the rapid rise of greenhouse gases. Trees take in carbon dioxide, transform it, store the carbon for food, and then release oxygen into the air. Thus, as we lose forests we lose the capacity to dissipate carbon dioxide.

The potential consequences of global warming are dire. The rising atmospheric concentration of greenhouse gases may be the most economically disruptive and costly change of our modern industrial society. Ozone causes damage to leaf tissue, inhibiting photosynthesis, the process by which plants use light energy for growth. Some forest species at risk include northern red oak, eastern white pine, black oak, and sugar maple. Ground-level ozone has been linked to the forest decline observed in Germany and other European countries.[28]

Reducing Air Pollution

Canada's air pollution problems are rooted in our energy, transportation, and industrial practices. Comprehensive national strategies are required to reduce air pollution and clean the air for future generations. We must support policies that encourage the use of renewable resources such as solar, wind, and water power as the providers of most of the world's energy.[29] The atmosphere has no borders.

Most experts agree that shifting away from gas-powered automobiles as the primary source of transportation is the only way to reduce air pollution significantly, which would reduce the greenhouse effect and, consequently, global warming. Some cities have taken steps in this direction by setting high parking fees, imposing bans on city driving, and establishing high road-usage tolls. Further, community governments should be encouraged to provide convenient, inexpensive, and, most importantly, easily accessible public transportation.

Auto makers must be encouraged to manufacture automobiles that provide excellent fuel economy and low rates of toxic emissions. Incentives given to manufacturers to produce such vehicles, tax breaks for purchasers who buy them, and "gas-guzzler" taxes on inefficient vehicles are three promising suggestions that may effectively help to reduce air pollution.

Similarly, primary suppliers of gasoline have been encouraged and regulated to reduce the proportion of benzene in their products. The Benzene in Gasoline Regulations came into effect on July 1, 1999. These regulations state that concentration of benzene in gasoline may only be 1 percent by volume and that the aromatics (or equivalent tailpipe emissions) must be frozen at 1994 levels.[30]

✳ WATER POLLUTION

Seventy-five percent of the earth is covered with water in the form of oceans, seas, lakes, rivers, streams, and wetlands. Still, a lack of water affects 40 percent of the worlds' population.[31] Beneath the landmass are reservoirs of groundwater. We draw our drinking water either from this underground source or from surface freshwater sources. The status of our water supply reflects the pollution level of our communities and, ultimately, the whole earth.

The federal government passed the Canada Water Act in 1970 and created the Department of the Environment in 1971, entrusting the Inland Waters Directorate with providing national leadership for freshwater management. Under the Constitution Act (1867), the provinces are "owners" of the water resources within their boundaries and have wide responsibilities in their day-to-day management. The federal government has certain specific responsibilities relating to water, such as fisheries and navigation, as well as exercising certain overall responsibilities such as the conduct of external affairs.[32]

Water Contamination

Any substance that gets into the soil has the potential to get into the water supply. Contaminants from industrial air pollution and acid rain eventually work their way into the soil and then into the groundwater. Pesticides sprayed on crops wash through the soil into the groundwater. Oil spills and other hazardous wastes flow into local rivers and streams. Underground storage tanks for gasoline may develop leaks. The list continues.

Pollutants can enter waterways through a number of routes. These routes may be divided into two general categories: point-source and non-point-source. Pollutants that enter a waterway at a specific point, through a pipe, ditch, culvert, or other such conduit, are referred to as **point-source pollutants**. The two major sources of this type of pollution are sewage treatment plants and industrial facilities.

Non-point-source pollutants—commonly called runoff and sedimentation—seep into waterways from broad areas of land rather than through a discrete pipe or conduit. It is currently estimated that 99 percent of the sediment in our waterways, 98 percent of the bacterial contaminants, 84 percent of the phosphorus, and 82 percent of the nitrogen come from non-point sources.[33] Non-point-source pollution results from a variety of human land-use practices

Greenhouse gases: Gases that contribute to global warming by trapping heat near the earth's surface.

Point-source pollutants: Pollutants that enter waterways at a specific point.

Non-point-source pollutants: Pollutants that seep into waterways from broad areas of land.

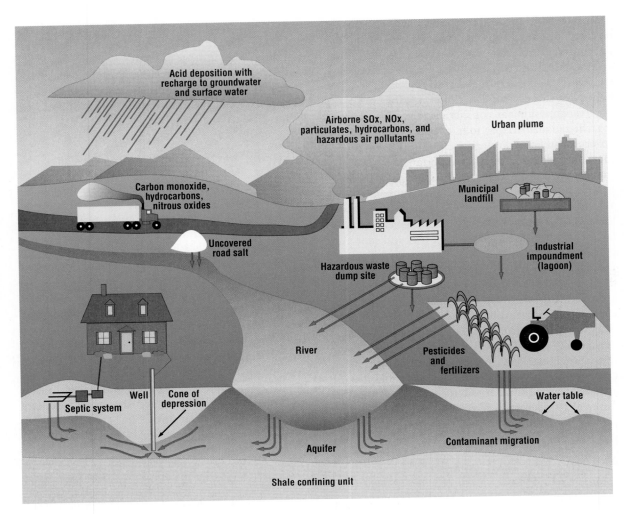

FIGURE 13.4

Sources of Groundwater Contamination

including soil erosion and sedimentation, construction wastes, pesticide and fertilizer runoff, urban street runoff, wastes from engineering projects, acid mine drainage, leakage from septic tanks, and sewage sludge.[34] (See Figure 13.4.)

Septic Systems

Bacteria from human waste can leach into the water supply from improperly installed septic systems. Toxic chemicals disposed of directly into septic systems also get into the groundwater supply.

Landfills

Landfills and dumps generate a liquid called leachate, a mixture of soluble chemicals that come from household garbage, office, biologic, and industrial waste. If a landfill has not been properly lined, leachate trickles through the layers of garbage and eventually into the water supply.

Gasoline and Petroleum Products

Underground storage tanks for gasoline and petroleum products are common; most are located at gasoline filling stations. A number of these underground tanks are thought to be leaking.[35] These tanks are slowly being replaced over time, since many were installed 30 to 35 years ago and were made of fabricated steel that was unprotected from corrosion. As a result, over time pinpoint holes developed in the steel and the petroleum products stored in the tanks leaked into the groundwater. The most common way to detect the presence of petroleum products in the water supply is to test for benzene, a component of oil and gasoline. Benzene is highly toxic and associated with cancer development.

Dioxins

Dioxins are chlorinated hydrocarbons contained in herbicides (chemicals used to kill vegetation) and produced during certain industrial processes. Dioxins have the ability to bioaccumulate and are much more toxic than PCBs (see below).

Chemical Contaminants

Most chemicals designed to dissolve grease and oil are called organic solvents. These extremely toxic substances, such as carbon tetrachloride, tetrachloroethylene, and trichloroethylene (TCE), are used to clean clothing, painting equipment, plastics, and metal parts. Many household products, such as stain and spot removers, degreasers, drain cleaners, septic system cleaners, and paint removers, also contain these toxic chemicals.

Organic solvents work their way into the water supply in different ways. Consumers often dump leftover products into the toilet. One example of this is pharmaceuticals; many consumers dispose of unused medications by flushing them—whereas they should be returned to pharmacies. Another example is paint thinner; some consumers will flush this as well. Industries pour leftovers into large barrels, which are then buried. After a while, the chemicals eat their way out of the barrels and leach into the groundwater.

A related group of toxic substances contains chlorinated hydrocarbons. The most notorious of these substances are the polychlorinated biphenyls (PCBs), their cousins the polybromated biphenyls (PBBs), and the dioxins.

PCBs

Polychlorinated biphenyls (PCBs) are fire-resistant and stable at high temperatures and therefore used for many years as insulating materials in high-voltage electrical equipment such as transformers. PCBs bioaccumulate, which means the body does not excrete them but instead stores them in fatty tissues and the liver. PCBs are associated with birth defects and known to cause cancer. PCBs have not been manufactured in North America since the late 1970s, but millions of kilograms of PCBs have been dumped into landfills and waterways, where they continue to pose an environmental threat.[36]

The long-term effects of bioaccumulation of these toxic substances include possible damage to the immune system, increased risk of infection, and elevated risk of cancer. Exposure to high concentrations of PCBs or dioxins for a short period of time can also have severe consequences, including nausea, vomiting, diarrhea, painful rashes and sores, and chloracne, an ailment in which the skin develops hard, black, painful pimples that may never go away.

Pesticides

Pesticides are chemicals designed to kill insects, rodents, plants, and fungi. Canadians use millions of kilograms of pesticides each year, with only 10 percent actually reaching the targeted organisms. The remaining pesticides settle on the land and in the water. Pesticide residues also cling to many fresh fruits and vegetables and are ingested when people eat them. Most pesticides accumulate in the body. Potential hazards associated with long-term exposure to pesticides include birth defects, cancer, liver and kidney damage, and nervous system disorders.

Trihalomethanes

Most Canadians drink water treated with chlorine to kill harmful bacteria. Trihalomethanes (THMs) are synthetic organic chemicals formed at water treatment plants when the added chlorine reacts with natural organic compounds in the water. Any chlorinated drinking water supply is likely to contain THMs, which include such substances as chloroform, bromoform, and dichlorobromomethane. Chloroform in high doses is known to cause liver and kidney disorders, central nervous system problems, birth defects, and cancer. Recent research indicates that THM concentrations can be substantially reduced by adjusting the chlorine dose, improving filtration practices to remove organic material, or adding chlorine after filtration rather than before.[37]

Lead

Lead might be ingested in household water if coming from lead pipes. Water, particularly acidic water, will leach some of the lead from the pipes. One way to reduce the possibility of ingesting lead if it does exist in your home's water system is to run tap water for several minutes to flush out water that has been standing overnight. Although leaded paints and ceramic glazes also pose health risks, particularly for small children who put toys in their mouths, the use of leads in such products has been effectively reduced in recent years in Canada and the United States.

Dioxins: Highly toxic chlorinated hydrocarbons contained in herbicides and produced during certain industrial processes.

Polychlorinated biphenyls (PCBs): Toxic chemicals once used as insulating materials in high-voltage electrical equipment.

Pesticides: Chemicals designed to kill insects and other pests that interfere with growth of a particular product (for instance, grass).

Chronic low-level exposure to lead may result in serious health consequences: anemia, malaise, and damage to the nervous system.[38] As mentioned, children are particularly vulnerable as even low-level exposure can reduce their IQ and result in learning disabilities, poor school performance, and violent behaviour.[39]

what do you THINK?

What can you do to ensure clean water in your home? In your community? What actions can you take to conserve water in your home? Elsewhere?

❋ NOISE POLLUTION

Loud noise has become commonplace. We are often painfully aware of construction crews working on our streets, jet airplanes roaring overhead, stereos blaring next door, and trucks rumbling down nearby freeways. We also use various devices to listen to music privately with earphones directly in our ears. Your body has a physiologic response to loud sounds, and when they are perceived as noise, they can become a source of physical and mental distress.

Prolonged exposure to some noises results in hearing loss. Short-term exposure reduces productivity, concentration levels, and attention spans, and may affect mental and emotional health. Symptoms of noise-related distress include disturbed sleep patterns, headaches, and tension. Physically, our bodies respond to noises in a variety of ways. Blood pressure increases, blood vessels in the brain dilate, and vessels in other parts of the body constrict. The pupils of the eyes dilate. Cholesterol levels in the blood rise and some endocrine glands secrete additional stimulating hormones, such as adrenaline, into the bloodstream.

At this point, it is necessary to distinguish between sound and noise. Sound is anything that can be heard. Noise is sound that can damage the hearing or cause mental or emotional distress. When sound becomes distracting or annoying, it becomes noise.

Despite increased awareness that noise pollution is more than a nuisance, government representatives continue to give noise-control programs low priority. In order to prevent hearing loss, it is important that you avoid exposure to excessive noise. Playing stereos in your vehicle, home, and in your ear at reasonable levels, wearing earplugs when you use power equipment, and establishing barriers (closed windows, etc.) between you and noise will help prevent hearing loss.

what do you THINK?

In your current lifestyle, what places your hearing at risk? What changes can you make to reduce these risks?

LAND POLLUTION

Many communities in Canada face serious problems in safely and effectively managing their garbage.

Solid Waste

Municipal solid waste is outstripping available landfill sites, and the opening of new landfill sites is usually controversial as people become more aware of the hazards they pose to nearby land and water. Toronto, for instance, has had to scramble to find communities in other parts of Ontario that would take its overflow garbage.

Part of the answer to this worsening problem is increased personal commitment to reducing, reusing, and recycling. Experts believe that as much as 90 percent of our garbage is ultimately reusable or recyclable.

◄◉ Hazardous Waste

Hazardous wastes are defined as wastes with properties that make them capable of harming human health or the environment.

The Canadian Environmental Protection Agency (CEPA) established an overall program to deal with hazardous wastes. The CEPA divides hazardous materials into two groups for elimination or reduction. Persistent, bioaccumulative, toxic hazardous wastes that are primarily the result of human activity will be targeted for virtual elimination from the environment; substances that do not meet these criteria are candidates for full life-cycle management to prevent or minimize their release into the environment.[40]

Industry education and cooperation are important for achieving a safer environment with less hazardous wastes. In cooperation with provincial/territorial and municipal authorities, the following procedures are in place:

- Many wastes are banned from land disposal or treated in such a way that their toxicity is reduced before they are dumped.

- Hazardous-waste handlers must clean up contamination resulting from past waste management practices in addition to current activities.

- CEPA is exploring ways to create economic incentives to encourage ingenuity in hazardous waste minimization practices and recycling.

A Brief History of the Kyoto Protocol

The Kyoto Protocol represents a crucial first step in the world's fight to stop climate change. The Kyoto Protocol is signed by 128 nations, and commits participating industrialized countries to cut deadly greenhouse gas emissions by 5 percent between 2008 and 2012. These are the highlights leading up to the Kyoto Protocol.

1972–First Earth Summit, in Stockholm, Sweden

World leaders announced their intention to hold a gathering every 10 years to determine the health of the planet.

1988–The International Panel on Climate Change (IPCC), First Report

Created by the UN to find scientific answers to climate change, it released its first report in 1990, stating that it believed the planet was warming and that human activity was causing this warming, but that it needed to do more research to be certain.

1988–Toronto Conference on the Changing Atmosphere

Former Canadian prime minister Brian Mulroney and former Norwegian prime minister Gro Harlem Bruntland hosted one of the world's first major scientific conferences on climate change. It called for a 20 percent cut to 1988 greenhouse gas emissions by 2005 and called the effect of climate change, "second only to global nuclear war."

1992–Second Earth Summit, Rio de Janeiro, Brazil

The largest gathering of world leaders ever, the Earth Summit created the United Nations Framework Convention on Climate Change, also known as the Rio Convention. This convention called on the world to stabilize 1990 greenhouse gas emissions by 2000.

Canada and the United States signed and ratified this convention. Former US president George Bush Sr. negotiated an agreement to allow developing nations to increase emissions–which is the reason they are not included in the Kyoto Protocol. The treaty is legally binding on countries that ratified it.

1995–COP I in Berlin, Germany

Each year, the countries that ratified the Rio Convention held a Conference of Parties (COP). The first of these happened in 1995 and reviewed the adequacy of the Rio Convention's goal of stabilizing greenhouse gas emissions.

1995–The IPCC's Second Report

The IPCC released its second report saying "the balance of evidence" pointed to a "discernable human influence on the global climate system."

1997–COP III in Kyoto, Japan

After reviewing the original targets of the Rio Convention and finding them too weak, the countries came up with new targets. Now, 1990 greenhouse gas emissions would be cut by 5 percent between 2008 and 2012. Though 5 percent is a global target, different countries have different targets. The European Union's target is an 8 percent cut (Germany committed to a 25 percent cut and the UK to 15 percent). The United States had a target of 7 percent and Canada a target of 6 percent.

1998–COP IV in Buenos Aires, Argentina

Here, the Buenos Aires Plan of Action was developed to decide how the Kyoto mechanism (emissions trading, carbon sinks, clean development in the developing world, etc.) would be implemented. The countries agreed that the mechanism through which targets would be achieved would be finalized by COP VI, or by 2000.

2001–COP V½ in Bonn, Germany

Just before dawn on July 29, 2001, 180 countries (that is, the whole world except for the United States and Australia) agreed to the rules for implementing the Kyoto Protocol. Now each country must officially ratify the accord.

2002–Update

Canadian Parliament ratified Canada's participation in the agreement. Currently, Canada produces less than 2 percent of total greenhouse-gas emissions. The United States, the largest producer of greenhouse-gas emissions in the world, decided not to ratify the accord.

Source: Adapted from Greenpeace Canada, "A Brief History of the Kyoto Protocol." Retrieved May 18, 2006, from www.greenpeace.org/canada//e/campaign/climate_energy/depth/kyoto/history.php. Reprinted with permission.

✳ what do you THINK?

Do you consciously "reduce"? Why or why not? Do you recycle? Why or why not? Do you reuse? Why or why not? What barriers exist that make your efforts at the three Rs more difficult? What can be done to reduce these barriers?

Municipal solid waste: Includes durable goods, nondurable goods, containers and packaging, food wastes, yard wastes, and miscellaneous wastes from residential, commercial, institutional, and industrial sources.

Hazardous waste: Solid waste that poses a hazard to humans or to the environment.

RADIATION

A substance is considered radioactive when it emits high-energy particles from the nuclei of its atoms. There are three types of radiation: alpha particles, beta particles, and gamma rays. Alpha particles are relatively massive particles not capable of penetrating human skin. They pose health hazards only when inhaled or ingested. Beta particles are capable of slight penetration of the skin and are harmful when ingested or inhaled. Gamma rays are the most dangerous radioactive particles because they pass right through the skin, causing serious damage to organs and other vital structures.

Ionizing Radiation

Exposure to ionizing radiation is an inescapable part of life. **Ionizing radiation** is caused by the release of particles and electromagnetic rays from atomic nuclei during the normal process of disintegration. Some naturally occurring elements, such as uranium, emit radiation. Other radiation-producing elements, such as deuterium, develop as part of the decay process of uranium or are created by scientists in laboratories. Radiation, whether naturally occurring or human-made, can damage genetic material in the reproductive cells of living organisms. It can also cause mutations, miscarriages, physical and mental deformities, cancer, eye cataracts, gastrointestinal illnesses, and shortened life expectancies.

Scientists cannot agree on a safe level of radiation. Reactions to radiation differ from person to person. Exposure is measured in radiation absorbed doses, or "rads" (also called roentgens). Recommended maximum "safe" dosages range from 0.5 to 5 rads per year. Approximately 50 percent of the radiation we are exposed to comes from natural sources, such as building materials. Another 45 percent comes from medical and dental X-rays. The remaining 5 percent comes from computer screens, microwave ovens, television sets, luminous watch dials, and radar screens and waves. Most of us are exposed to far less radiation than the "safe" maximum dosage per year.

Radiation can cause damage at dosages as low as 100 to 200 rads. At this level, signs of radiation sickness include nausea, diarrhea, fatigue, anemia, sore throat, and hair loss. Death is unlikely at this dosage. At 350 to 500 rads, the previously mentioned symptoms increase in severity, and death may result because bone marrow production of the white blood cells that we need to protect us from disease is hindered. Dosages above 600 to 700 rads are invariably fatal. The effects of long-term exposure to relatively low levels of radiation are unknown. Some scientists believe that such

While we may feel that many of the environmental problems facing the world today are beyond individual control, we can play a significant role in keeping our own little part of it clean, green, and beautiful.

exposure can cause lung cancer, leukemia, skin cancer, bone cancer, and skeletal deformities.

Nonionizing Radiation

The lower-energy portions of the electromagnetic spectrum, ranging from lower-energy ultraviolet radiation down through infrared, radar, radio, and the electric and magnetic fields associated with many household appliances and electric power lines, are **nonionizing radiation**. Although the biologic effects of ionizing radiation have been recognized for some time, we still do not know very much about the effects of certain types of nonionizing radiation—in particular, the photons associated with electric and magnetic fields. Techniques for assessing radiation from many such sources continue to evolve.[41]

Nuclear Power Plants

Nuclear power plants account for less than 1 percent of the total radiation we are exposed to. Other producers of radioactive wastes include medical facilities that use radioactive materials for treatment and diagnostic procedures (for instance, MRI, CT scans, etc.) and nuclear weapons production facilities.

Proponents of nuclear energy believe it is a safe and efficient way to generate electricity. Initial costs of building nuclear power plants are high, but actual power generation is relatively inexpensive. A 1000-megawatt reactor produces enough energy for 600 000 homes and saves 1590 million litres of fossil fuels each year. In some areas where nuclear power plants were decommissioned, electricity bills tripled when power companies turned to hydroelectric or fossil fuel sources.

Nuclear reactors also discharge fewer carbon oxides into the air than fossil fuel–powered generators. Advocates believe that conversion to nuclear power could slow the global warming trend.[42]

All of these advantages of nuclear energy must be weighed against the disadvantages. First, disposal of nuclear wastes is extremely problematic for the entire world. Additionally, the chances of a reactor core meltdown pose serious threats to the immediate environment of nuclear plants—and to the world in general.

A nuclear **meltdown** occurs when the temperature of the core of the reactor increases to a point that it melts the nuclear fuel and its containment vessel. Most modern facilities seal their reactors and containment vessels in concrete buildings with pools of cold water on the bottom. Then, if a meltdown occurs, the building and the pool should prevent the radioactive release.

Human error and mechanical failure were the reported causes of the 1986 reactor core fire and explosion at the Chernobyl nuclear power plant in Russia. In just four and a half seconds, the temperature in the reactor rose to 120 times normal, causing an explosion. Eighteen people were killed immediately, 30 died later from radiation sickness, and 200 others were hospitalized for severe radiation sickness. Officials evacuated people living nearby the plant. Some medical workers estimate that the eventual death toll from radiation-induced cancers exceeded 100 000. Direct costs of the disaster were more than $13 billion, including lost agricultural output and the cost of replacing the power plant.

Opponents of nuclear energy believe that there is no safe place to dispose of, contain, or store the escalating supply of nuclear waste.

FOOD QUALITY

For most Canadians, food accounts for 80 to 95 percent of their daily intake of the most persistent toxic contaminants, while air contributes 10 to 15 percent and drinking water contributes very little. Compared with other countries, the food available in Canada is some of the safest. Still, contamination remains a concern. Aside from microbial contamination, as discussed in Chapter 5, environmental contamination can occur in several fashions. Chemical contaminants enter the food supply through uptake from water or soil, and by air deposition on leaves and fruit. Some contaminants can bioaccumulate to become more toxic when at the top of the food chain, as with mercury concentration in game fish in a number of Canadian water systems. Also, chemicals used in food production and handling can leave residues on food products—for example, the hormones and antibiotics used to increase meat and dairy production, or the substances used to preserve freshness or enhance flavour.[43] Refer back to "Food Safety Concerns" in Chapter 5 for steps you can take to reduce your risk.

Ionizing radiation: Radiation produced by photons with enough energy to ionize atoms.

Nonionizing radiation: Radiation produced by photons associated with lower-energy portions.

Meltdown: An accident that results when the temperature in the core of a nuclear reactor increases sufficiently to melt the nuclear fuel and its containment vessel.

Managing Environmental Pollution

Environmental health begins at home. We must overcome our inertia and make efforts and/or sacrifices that contribute to the good of the planet. By understanding how political and economic issues affect the environment, we can pressure corporations and elected representatives to change policies harmful to the environment. For example, environmentalists pressured the World Bank to stop issuing development loans leading to the destruction of rainforests. Discussing issues with lawmakers and making decisions at the polls are two ways you can influence environmental policy.

MAKING DECISIONS FOR YOU

One of the most significant decisions we make as consumers is whether to pay more for environmentally safe products. As a student on a tight budget, are you willing to pay more for products such as environmentally friendly soap and laundry detergent? If so, how much more? If not, are you willing to buy a *less* environmentally unfriendly product? While it's not likely that you can increase your budget enough to buy all environmentally safe products, you can start now. Think about the products you buy: Which could you substitute with more environmentally friendly brands? Could you use less of the environmentally damaging products?

CHECKLIST FOR CHANGE: MAKING PERSONAL CHOICES

- Do you vote? Do you know the difference between rhetoric and reality when it comes to environmental issues?
- Do you conserve water? Do you fix leaky taps quickly? Do you wash only full loads? Do you overwater lawns or gardens?
- Do you think before you buy? Do you buy products in recyclable packaging? Do you reuse containers rather than buy new ones?
- Do you think before you throw household chemicals away? Finish them, give them away, or save them for a household hazardous waste collection. Consider nonhazardous substitutes.
- Do you recycle used oil? Oil dumped down storm drains or on the ground can pollute streams, killing insects, fish, birds, and wildlife.
- Do you recycle tin cans, glass, newspaper, paper, plastic, and cardboard?
- Have you considered reporting people who litter?
- Have you considered walking, riding the bus, using your bike, or carpooling whenever possible?
- Have you thought about the amount of fertilizers and pesticides you use? Rain can wash them off lawns and carry them into lakes and streams. Use low-phosphorus fertilizers.

- Do you ask yourself if you really need a product before you buy it?
- Do you consider whether a product is practical and durable, well made, and of timeless design?
- Do you buy used and rebuilt products whenever possible? Do you sell unused/lightly used items at yard or garage sales or donate them to charities?
- Do you compost leaves, grass clippings, and kitchen scraps?

CHECKLIST FOR CHANGE: MAKING COMMUNITY CHOICES

- Do you work in your community to create and enforce laws that protect drinking water and prohibit the manufacture, use, storage, transport, or disposal of hazardous substances in your water supply area?
- Do you volunteer to take part in cleanup activities in your community?
- Does your community have a hazardous materials ordinance?

CRITICAL THINKING

Your health teacher is leading a protest next week to the corporate headquarters of "one of the country's worst polluters." You are told that this company has a terrible record of point- and non-point-source pollutants and that the "corporate bigwigs refuse to do anything about it." After hearing the brief appeal to join the protest, you decide it's your duty as a citizen to go. As your teacher hands out maps to the protest site, you realize that the company in question is your employer! Now you are really confused: your company claims to have spent billions of dollars to reduce pollution and considers itself an innovator in cleaning up sites it polluted in the past. You are upset because only one side of the story is being told. Should you speak up in class? What else could you do?

Using the DECIDE model in Chapter 1, decide what you would do. First, decide why you are upset. Then decide what you would like to accomplish by speaking up. In addition, consider the best setting to communicate your message to your teacher (in class, during office hours, by email, etc.).

Go to MyHealthLab at **www.pearsoned.ca/myhealthlab**. Here you will find self-assessments, case studies, links to health on the net, and much more.

❋ DISCUSSION QUESTIONS

1. Describe the issues surrounding global population and how they differ among the developed, developing, and least developed regions.

2. How does an increasing global population affect the environment locally, provincially, nationally, and globally?

3. List the primary sources of air pollution, acid rain, and indoor air pollution in Canada. What can be done individually and collectively to reduce each type of pollution?

4. What are the environmental consequences of global warming? What can Canadian citizens do to slow the deforestation of tropical rainforests? How might the Kyoto Protocol help in the fight to stop/reduce climate change?

5. Explain point- and non-point sources of water pollution. Discuss how water pollution can be reduced or prevented altogether in Canada. What actions can you as a student take?

6. Given all the open land in Canada, do you think solid waste disposal is a problem? Why or why not?

7. Are the advantages of nuclear power worth the risks involved with storage? Put another way, if you lived near a nuclear power plant, would you be willing to pay two or three times as much for electricity in order to have the nuclear power plant closed? Why or why not?

APPLICATION EXERCISE

Reread the "Consider This ..." scenario at the beginning of the chapter and answer the following questions.

1. What resources are available on your campus to help students become environmentally friendly in their day-to-day living? In your community?

2. How much time and effort are students willing to put into conserving the environment? Is it seen as a real issue? Why or why not?

MYSEARCHLAB EXERCISE

1. Log on to www.MySearchLab.com.

2. Find an article to share with the class related to more effectively managing the environment to improve individual, community, or global health. This article can relate to world population levels (and/or life expectancy and/or birth rate), global warming, climate change, air pollution, land pollution, noise pollution, or water pollution.

3. Summarize the article, creating a five-slide/five-minute presentation. Be sure to include the purpose of the article, the main findings, limitations, and suggestions to improve current environmental management (either from a personal or community perspective).

CHAPTER 14

PERSONAL SAFETY

Reducing Violence, Abuse, and Injury

CONSIDER THIS . . .

Kyle is wakened by the sound of loud voices. His parents are fighting again. His father is calling his mother awful names. She is shouting back. Kyle creeps to the top of the stairs. They are just below him. He hears a sickening "whack" as his father hits his mother. Then his father kicks her. There is a knock at the door. The police have been called by the neighbours. They take his father away and talk to his mother. Kyle goes back to his room, where he lies awake wondering what has happened, why it happened, and what he could have done differently.

What factors in Canadian society have contributed to our increased awareness of violence in the family? What attitudes and beliefs do you have regarding family violence? Do you think violence in the home is increasing? What is the effect of family violence—on the perpetrator? the victim? the other family members?

CHAPTER OBJECTIVES

- Define violence and the extent of it in Canada. Include homicide, suicide, youth violence, and hate and bias crimes.

- Identify domestic violence (abuse against women, children, men, and the elderly committed by their family members) and its causes.

- Describe sexual victimization, including sexual assault, and the culture surrounding it.

- Describe the steps you can take to prevent personal assaults at home, on the street, or in your car.

- Identify methods by which Canadians can reduce the incidence of injury to themselves and others.

Chances are that if you turn on the TV, watch a movie, or play a video game, you will see graphic images of violent acts and their outcomes. Some of these will be real and others created for our entertainment. We live in a world caught in an epidemic of violence. The World Health Organization defines **violence** as "the intentional use of physical force or power, threatened or actual, against oneself, another person or against a community, that either results in or has a high likelihood of resulting in injury, death, psychological harm, maldevelopment or deprivation."[1] The focus of this chapter is the kinds of violence that may have particular relevance to you.

✔· VIOLENCE IN CANADA

Violence is a worldwide problem. Each year, more than 1.6 million people across the world lose their lives to violence.[2] Worldwide, violence is among the leading causes of death for individuals between the ages of 15 and 44, accounting for 14 percent of male and 7 percent of female deaths. Further, for every person who dies as a result of violence, many more are injured, resulting in a myriad of physical, sexual, social, spiritual, and mental health problems. Although violent incidents may not be as common in Canada as other countries, we have had riots after sporting events and political confrontations: the 2000 melee at the Ontario provincial legislature and the 1995 standoff at Gustafson Lake in British Columbia are notable examples. We have also had police strikes with no change in the crime rate, and most cities are relatively safe to work, play, and live in. Canadians are less likely to take precautions against crime when going out than are people in other industrialized countries.[3] Yet violence exists here, in overt forms such as assault or homicide and in more subtle but nonetheless intimidating forms such as stalking. Violence can flare up between groups—as it did at Oka in 1990, between First Nations peoples and the town of Oka over disputed land—or in families, as in child, spousal, and elder abuse. In fact, the most violent setting in Canadian society today is the family.

The 1987 General Social Survey estimated that only 31 percent of violent crimes were reported to police. Why do victims not report violence? Stated reasons were that the victims felt the incident was minor, believed the police could do nothing about it, were fearful, or had dealt with it informally.[4] Although there was little change between 1988 and 1996 in the percentage of people who reported being a victim of crime, 75 percent of Canadians in 1997 reported that they thought crime had increased.[5]

In a 1995 report, the Department of Justice noted that Canada has a long history of violence toward ethnic minorities. In Vancouver in 1907, a mob of whites attacked the Chinese and Japanese communities, resulting in several fatalities and damage to stores.[6] The internment of Japanese Canadians during World War II and the confiscation of their property is another example.[7] The federal government gave compensation and an apology to the Japanese-Canadian community many years later.

Vulnerable groups such as women, children, and the elderly witnessing or experiencing violence in families is of concern. The issue of violence by men toward women and children and by adult children toward their parents is now recognized as a major social problem in Canadian society. The opening of sexual assault centres and battered women's shelters in the 1970s made this type of violence more visible to the public and indicates some of the efforts made to treat the effects of it. Still not enough is done for prevention and there remains a need to raise awareness of the various types of violence that continue to be pervasive in our society today.

Acts of violence result in injuries and deaths as well as the subtler forms of damage caused by actual or threatened violence, such as stress, poor mental health, conduct disorders, and lack of social and emotional responsiveness. In addition to these social and emotional costs, the economic costs of violence are very high.[8]

Although the underlying causes of violence and abuse are as varied as the individual crimes and people involved, several social, cultural, and individual factors increase the likelihood of violence occurring. Poverty, unemployment, hopelessness, lack of education, inadequate housing, poor parental role models, cultural beliefs that objectify women and allow men to act as aggressors, lack of social support systems, discrimination, ignorance about people who are different, religious self-righteousness, breakdowns in the criminal justice system, stress, economic uncertainty, and a host of other factors may precipitate violent acts.

By learning more about the root causes of homicide, suicide, and other violent acts, you will reduce your risk of becoming a victim or perpetrator and protect your health. Further, by taking steps to prevent violence against others, you will safeguard the health of society.

Violence: Refers to intentional behaviours that produce injuries, as well as the outcomes of these behaviours (the injuries themselves).

Homicide

There were 594 **homicides** in Canada in 2007 (12 less than in 2006), a rate of 1.80 per 100 000 people.[9] Nunavut (22.50 per 100 000 people) has the highest rate, followed by the Yukon Territory (6.45 per 100 000 people), Manitoba (5.22 per 100 000 people) and the Northwest Territories (4.69 per 100 000 people). The lowest rate was in Prince Edward Island, with 0.00 homicides per 100 000 people; Newfoundland and Labrador (0.39 per 100 000 people); New Brunswick (1.07 per 100 000 people) and Quebec (1.17 per 100 000 people). Stabbing continues to occur the most frequently across Canada (190), followed closely by shooting (188), beating (116), strangulation (50), fire (4), and other/not known methods (44).[10] Most victims were males (432 versus 162), with the greatest number (119) being between the ages of 18 and 24.[11] Similarly, a higher number of males were accused of homicide (474 versus 53), with the highest number between the ages of 18 and 24 (177), followed by 30 to 39 (78). Seventy-four youths (aged 12–17), 66 male and 8 female, were accused of homicide in 2007.[12] Despite popular fears of the violent stranger, a homicide is most likely to be committed by someone known to the victim (47 percent by an acquaintance, 36 percent by a spouse).

In the United States, 48 percent of households owned at least one firearm. In Canada, individuals owning firearms must register them. Currently, there are about 1.86 million valid firearms licences issued to individuals under the Firearms Act; 889 526 are possession only licenses (allows the holder to possess, but not acquire firearms, and to possess and acquire ammunition), 962 887 are possession and acquisition licenses (holder is allowed to possess and acquire firearms and ammunition), and 7088 are minor's licenses (for individuals under the age of 18).[13] More than 7.3 million firearms are currently registered, with 6.65 million registered as non-restricted firearms, 450 635 as restricted firearms, and 210 407 as prohibited firearms.

Suicide

When anger, rage, and hopelessness turn inward rather than outward, violence against the self results. Suicide is the most extreme form of this violence. As discussed in Chapter 2, suicide attempts occur for a number of reasons. They can be "a cry for help" and/or a signal of extreme distress and emotional pain. The physical pain of self-injury distracts the person from what is perceived as never-ending emotional pain. A suicide attempt may be an explosive outburst of rage at the self; such attempts are usually fatal. Or, the suicide may be motivated by a balance of sadness, resignation, and a desire for dignity, in the case of a terminally ill person. Why some people choose suicide is unclear. Studies indicate that a combination of neurobiological,[14] psychological,[15] and social[16] factors combine to enable suicide.

According to the World Health Organization, an estimated 815 000 people killed themselves in 2000—a rate equivalent to 16.0 per 100 000 people, or roughly one suicide every 40 seconds.[17] The most recent Statistics Canada data indicate that there were 3613 suicides in Canada in 2004, equivalent to 11.3 per 100 000 people.[18] Men, on average, are more likely than women to commit suicide.[19] Men between the ages of 45 and 49 and 50 and 54 have the highest rates (25.5 and 25.7 per 100 000), while men aged 10 to 14 and 15 to 19 (1.6 and 14.7 per 100 000) have the lowest rates. Similarly, women between the ages of 45 and 49 and 50 and 54 have the highest rates, at 9.4 and 9.7 per 100 000, while women between the ages of 10 and 14 and age 90 and older have the lowest rates (1.1 and 2.5 per 100 000).

Suicides accounted for 80 percent of all firearm deaths in Canada, with the proportion of suicides involving firearms declining over the last two decades. Fewer than a quarter of the suicides in 1995 involved a firearm, usually a rifle or shotgun. While suicides are more frequent in urban areas, the percentage involving a firearm is higher in rural areas.[20]

Those who attempt suicide are a very mixed group and may differ markedly from those who complete suicide. Most people who attempt suicide do not ultimately die from their attempt(s), though they may try frequently, and many people who die from suicide have not attempted previously.[21] There is a need to understand suicide more completely so we can respond more appropriately.

The suicide rate among Aboriginal youth is at least two to seven times greater than that of the population as a whole.[22] The Canadian Institute of Child Health[23] interprets these statistics as a warning that these youth need more support, recognition, respect, and hope for the future, and that society as a whole must rethink the way we work with and serve Aboriginal youth.

Youth Violence

As previously mentioned, violence is among the leading causes of death for people aged 15 to 44

Violence in the form of fatal stabbings, beatings, and spousal, child and elder abuse is a major cause of death and physical and emotional disability in Canada.

worldwide, accounting for 14 percent of all male deaths and 7 percent of all female deaths.[24] Also as noted previously, the greatest number of male homicides in Canada occurred in those between the ages of 18 and 24. Similarly, the greatest number of males accused of homicide are males between the ages of 18 and 24. In 2007, 23 homicides occurred in males between the ages of 12 and 17. In females, 21 of the 162 homicides were committed by women between the ages of 18 and 24, and another 8 by women between the ages of 12 and 17.[25] Of the 474 males accused of homicide, 177 were between the ages of 18 and 24 and 66 between the ages of 12 and 17. In females, 12 of the 53 accused of homicide were between 18 and 24 and 8 were between the ages of 12 and 17.[26]

In 1991, 22 percent of federal statute charges were against youths. A higher proportion of youths than adults were criminally charged. In 1997–98, one in five cases (20 percent) involved violent crimes; about half were common assaults. The rate of property crime cases has dropped by 25 percent since 1992, whereas the rate of violent crime has risen by 4 percent. The rate of youth court cases has increased for females (by 5 percent) and decreased for males (by 12 percent) over this period.[27] Total charges in 1991 against youths were double the number charged in 1986. Does this statistic truly represent an increase in youth crime? Or does it reflect an increased sensitivity toward youth violence with more pressure to apply societal justice?

The youth involved in violent crime are generally in their late teens (16- and 17-year-olds account for 51 percent of offenders), and the victims are generally youths between the ages of 12 and 17 (36 percent of minor assaults), usually male (76 percent of aggravated assaults). Assaults most commonly occur in a public place (35 percent in 1997 occurred in a parking lot or on public transportation), dwellings (26 percent), or schools (22 percent).[28]

Although some attention is given to alternative methods in Canada, a high proportion of young offenders continue to be jailed. Unlike in the adult justice system, there is no parole for youth. Aboriginal youth, youth from certain ethnic and cultural groups, and young people from lower-income families are overrepresented in our justice system. Yet it should be remembered that more than 95 percent of Canada's young people are never in trouble with the law.[29]

✳ The Violence of Hate

Canada has always welcomed people from other cultures—while marginalizing Aboriginal people. The degree of acceptance, however, decreases with the immigrants' physical and cultural differences from Northern European peoples. Much as we may wish otherwise, prejudice and racism have always been and continue to be a part of Canadian society.

Historically, established leaders in Canadian society (individual and institutional) have made key contributions to interracial violence—for example, to the anti-Chinese riot of 1887 and the anti-Chinese and Japanese riot of 1907 in Vancouver. In both cases, the local newspapers, respectable individuals (businessmen, clergymen, politicians), and organizations played a very prominent role in at least preparing the groundwork and instigating the violence, which claimed "scores" of Chinese lives. The timing of the riots seems to have been related to white workers' alleged fears of economic competition, especially at a time of recession.[30]

Homicide: Death as a result of another's intent to injure or kill.

Preventing Hate and Bias Crimes

Canadian data relating to hate-motivated conduct are not collected and reported systematically by police forces on a national scale. In contrast, countries such as England, France, and the United States put in place reporting mechanisms that provide a more comprehensive national picture of the scale of hate-motivated behaviours in their respective countries.

Although the causes of intolerance remain in question, it is believed that much of it stems from a fear of change and a desire to blame others when forces such as the economy and crime seem to be out of control. Think about yourself, your family, your friends, and your community and your interactions with them. How do you—and they—talk about and treat others? What can you do to reduce the violence of hate in your home, on campus, and in your community?

- Support educational programs designed to foster understanding and appreciation for differences in people. Many colleges and universities require diversity classes as part of their academic curriculum.
- Examine your attitudes and behaviours. Are you intolerant of others? Do you have beliefs about a particular group? Do you engage in behaviours that demean any group or individuals?
- Discourage racist, sexist, and homophobic jokes and other forms of social or ethnic bigotry. Do not participate in such behaviours and express your dissatisfaction with others who do. Silence condones others' behaviours.
- Vote for community leaders who respect the rights of others, value diversity, and do not have racially or ethnically motivated hidden agendas.
- Educate yourself. Read, interact with, and try to understand people who appear to be different from you. Respecting people's right to be different is part of being a healthy, integrated individual.
- Examine your values in determining the relative worth of your friends and the others in your life. Are you judgmental? Are you somewhat intolerant of others' differences? How do you resolve your tendencies to be judgmental and bigoted? Do you judge people on appearances? Do you take time to get to know who they are as individuals? Do you respect them as individuals?

what do you THINK?

What bias or hate crimes are you aware of? Who were the victims? Who were the perpetrators? What do you think motivates people to initiate such crimes against others? What should be done locally, provincially, and nationally to prevent these kinds of behaviours? How can you be involved?

Violence against Women

Canadians were shocked out of denying the existence of violence toward women by the Montreal Massacre at École Polytechnique in Montreal in 1989, when a young man shot and killed 14 women at the school because, as his writings amply explained, he hated women.

The first major empirical study on violence toward women noted that one in ten women living with a man would be abused each year.[31] This figure, which was initially ridiculed, is now accepted as an underestimate: more recent figures indicate that more than one woman in four (29 percent) experiences some form of domestic violence from her partner.[32] Assaults are eight times more likely in a relationship of less than two years than in partnerships lasting more than 20 years.[33] Almost half (45 percent) of assault cases result in physical injury to the woman. The most frequent types of injuries are bruises (90 percent); cuts, scratches, and burns (33 percent); and broken bones and fractures (33 percent).[34]

The shelter movement (begun in England in 1972 and in Canada in 1974) lobbied for zero tolerance of abuse and mandatory charging of abusers. This policy was adopted in virtually all jurisdictions in Canada in 1982, when Canada's attorney general urged police chiefs to lay charges in all cases of suspected wife abuse. The Royal Canadian Mounted Police introduced a formal policy in 1984 specifically instructing its members to lay charges in all cases where there were "reasonable and probable grounds" to believe that assault occurred. The abusive partner may be charged under the assault sections of the Criminal Code of Canada. A police charge not only highlights the criminal nature of the act but also relieves the victim of the burden of laying charges.[35]

Discrimination and violence toward women is a global issue. At the urging of Canada, among other nations, the United Nations Convention on the Elimination of All Forms of Discrimination Against Women adopted a resolution in 1992 accepting that states are responsible for acts of domestic violence between individuals. In December 1993, the UN passed a Declaration Against Violence Against Women.

How many times have you heard of a woman being repeatedly beaten by her partner or spouse and wondered, "Why doesn't she just leave him?" There are many reasons some women find it difficult, if not impossible, to leave their abusers. Many women, particularly those with small children, are financially dependent on the abuser. Others fear retaliation against themselves or their children. There are women who hope that the situation will change with time (it rarely does); those who feel that the good times are so very good, they think they can put up with the bad times; and others who stay because their cultural or religious beliefs forbid divorce. Finally, there are women who still love their partner, despite the abuse and are concerned about what will happen to him if they leave.[36]

✱ Cycle of Violence Theory

Psychologist Lenore Walker developed a theory known as the "cycle of violence" to explain how women (and men) can get caught in a downward spiral without knowing what is happening to them.[37] The cycle has three phases:

- Phase One: Tension Building. In this phase, minor battering occurs, and the victim may become more nurturant, more pleasing, and more intent on anticipating the abuser's needs in order to forestall another violent scene. The victim assumes guilt for doing something to provoke the abuser and tries hard to avoid doing it again.

- Phase Two: Acute Battering. At this stage, pleasing the abuser does not help and the victim can no longer control or predict the abuse. Usually, the abuser claims to be trying to "teach a lesson," and will not stop until enough pain has been inflicted. When the acute attack is over, the abuser may respond with shock and denial about his or her behaviours. Usually, both the abuser and the victim soft-pedal or deny the seriousness of the attacks and the resulting physical and mental damage.

- Phase Three: Remorse/Reconciliation. During this "honeymoon" period, the abuser may be kind, loving, and apologetic, swearing to never act violently again. The abuser may "behave" for several weeks or months, and the victim may question whether she (or in some cases he) overrated the seriousness of past abuse. Then the kind of tension that precipitated abusive incidents in the past resurfaces, the abuser loses control again, and once more beats his or her partner. Unless some form of intervention breaks this downward cycle of abuse, contrition, further abuse, denial, and contrition, it will repeat again and again, ending perhaps only when the abuser kills the victim or, less often, when the victim kills the abuser.

It is very hard for most women who get caught in this cycle of violence (which may include forced sexual relations and psychological and economic abuse as well as physical beatings) to find the courage and resolution to extricate themselves. Most need effective outside intervention.

Despite obvious physiological and psychological injury, it can be difficult for a woman to leave her abusive partner.

✱ Domestic Violence

The extent of spousal violence has only recently been well documented. Statistics Canada conducted its first Violence Against Women survey in 1993. It found that 29 percent of Canadian women experienced violence at the hands of a current or past marital partner. Between 1974 and 1992, 1435 women were killed by their husbands and 451 men were killed by their wives.[38] In late 2008, the most recent report—the eleventh annual Family Violence in Canada report produced by the Canadian Centre for Justice Statistics under the Federal Family Violence Initiative—was released. This report includes statistics on spousal violence, family violence against children and youth, family violence against older adults, and family homicides.[39] Although there has been a steady decrease in police-reported incidents of spousal violence from 1998 to 2006, more than 38 000 incidents—or 15 percent of all police-reported violent incidents—were reported to police across Canada.[40] Spousal violence reported to the police was most prevalent in Nunavut and Quebec (20 percent) and least reported in British Columbia (8 percent), Nova Scotia (8 percent), and New Brunswick (8 percent).

Females (83 percent of all victims) continue to be the most likely victims of police-reported spousal violence, and incidents are most common between current (69 percent) versus former (31 percent) partners. Common assault (61 percent) is the most

A Week without Violence

Violence can and does happen anywhere—at home, at school, at work, and at play—and it takes many forms. When we think of violence, we often think of physical violence and underestimate the effect of psychological violence such as verbal putdowns and degrading gestures. Many people endure emotional, psychological, economic, social, physical, and sexual violence in silence. Women, Aboriginal peoples, visible minorities, and gays and lesbians confront systemic forms of violence almost every day of their lives. This is the harsh reality of the violence that permeates our society.

Speaking about violence can help us to identify feelings of loss and anger, and to heal from them. Organized by the YWCA, the Week without Violence is a nationwide effort that encourages people to identify realistic and sustainable alternatives to violence; this event occurs during the third week of October. It is believed that with active support from schools,

politicians, law enforcement agencies, faith groups, and national and local community agencies safer places to live, work, and play will be created.

In 2004, more than 45 000 people and 600 schools, workplaces, and community organizations participated. For example, in Kamloops a native drumming circle of friendship was created; in Brockville a youth day focused on sports rather than violence; in Lethbridge discussions on racism and eliminating discrimination were held; and in Vancouver a mask-making workshop to empower women was hosted. For more ideas and to read more about this initiative, see www .weekwithoutviolence.ca.

Source: Adapted from YWCA of Canada. Retrieved May 5, 2006, from www.weekwithoutviolence.ca.

prevalent reported violent offence, followed by major assault (14 percent), uttering threats (11 percent), and criminal harassment (8 percent). The rate of spousal violence is twice the average in those couples who are gay or lesbian (15 versus 7 percent), and Aboriginal peoples are 3 times more likely to be victims of domestic violence (21 versus 7 percent).

Only 27 percent of those who experience spousal abuse report the incident(s) to the police, with a greater proportion of females making the reports (37 versus 27 percent). Approximately one-third (32 percent) of those who report their abuse to the police obtain restraining orders or protective orders against their abusers. Thirty-four percent of those who experience spousal violence seek help from a formal agency because of the violence, with

more females than males seeking this help (47 versus 20 percent).[41]

Causes of Domestic Violence

There is no single explanation for why people tend to be abusive in relationships. Although alcohol abuse is often associated with **domestic violence**, marital dissatisfaction seems to predict physical abuse more effectively than any other variable.[42] Numerous studies also point to differences in the communication patterns between abusive relationships and non-abusive relationships.[43] While some argue that the hormone testosterone is the cause of male aggression, studies have failed to show a strong association between physical abuse in relationships and this hormone.[44] Many experts believe that men who engage in severe violence are more likely than other men to suffer from personality disorders.[45]

The dynamics that people bring to a relationship can result in violence and allow it to continue. Obtaining help from community support and counselling services may help to determine the underlying basis of the problem and help the victim and the abuser come to a better understanding of the actions necessary to stop the cycle of abuse. The Rate Yourself box may help you to determine if you are a victim (or perpetrator) of abuse.

Violence against Children

Child abuse is found in all societies and is almost always a highly guarded secret wherever it takes place.

what do you THINK?

Do you know a woman who you think might be a victim of domestic violence? Can you think of a man whom you consider a likely victimizer? What about him has contributed to his current situation? Similarly, can you think of a man who you think might be a victim of domestic violence? Can you think of a woman whom you consider a likely victimizer? What about her has contributed to her current situation? In either of these situations, how could you intervene such that the anticipated violence does not occur?

In countries with reliable mortality reporting, the World Health Organization (WHO) estimates that as many as 1 in 5000 to 1 in 10 000 children under the age of five die each year from physical violence. In the same countries, every year from 1 in 1000 to 1 in 180 children are either taken to a health-care facility or are reported to child welfare services as a consequence of abuse.

A second nation-wide study of reported child maltreatment in Canada estimated that, of the estimated 217 319 investigations, 47 percent were substantiated—equivalent to an incidence rate of 21.71 per 1000 cases of maltreatment in children.[46] It was pointed out in this report that only cases investigated by child welfare services were included, and those that were screened out or only investigated by the police were not reported. Further, it was noted that there was a change in reporting that may relate to the increase in rates of investigated and substantiated cases of maltreatment between 1998 and 2003. Of the confirmed cases of maltreatment, 15 percent involved emotional maltreatment, 28 percent of the children were exposed to domestic violence (that is, witnessing violence against another family member), 3 percent were sexually abused, 24 percent were physically abused, and 30 percent were neglected.

Physical violence often originates when the parents lack parenting skills. Typically, abusive parents are unable to respond to a young child's needs and have unrealistic expectations for the stage of a child's development. Another factor is the cultural acceptance of corporal punishment and violence within a society.

Sympathetic and sensitive therapy can help abused children cope with the mental and physical pain inflicted on them.

Other stresses contributing to child maltreatment may include an unwanted child, an unsupported single-parent household, the absence of social support, financial pressures, and unemployment. Child maltreatment can be aggravated by substance abuse on the part of the parent or guardian. Families in which there is substance abuse are also likely to experience physical violence, sexual abuse, and domestic violence. Further, these violent acts are most often directed at family members, particularly women and young children.

The perpetrators of violence against or sexual abuse of children are often trusted individuals in a position of authority, usually males, and often family members.[47] In fact, for every 100 000 young persons (under age 18) living in Canada, 334 have been victims of physical or sexual violence, with 187 (or 56 percent) experiencing the violence by a family members and 101 (or 30 percent) at the hand of a stranger.[48] More specifically, 107 (or 32 percent) of the victims were physically of sexually assaulted by a parent. Physical violence and sexual abuse in the home is a factor contributing to the phenomenon of street children in developed and developing countries. Further abuse on the street is an everyday reality.[49]

Child victims of violence or sexual abuse have a high risk of becoming perpetrators of similar forms of abuse toward younger children. In later years, they may be physically violent toward children in their care or toward their own children. The normal reactions to harm are the expression of anger and pain. The child who is abused is usually forbidden to express anger and cannot bear to endure the pain alone. To survive, the child must repress the feelings and even the memory. The repressed emotions will gain expression in destructive acts—against others, as in criminal behaviours and even mass murder, or self-directed, as with drug and alcohol abuse.[50] Suppressed memories of child abuse can also surface later in adult years, with post-traumatic stress experienced as a result (see Chapter 2).

The use of threat and power by an adult against a child breaks the trust the child has in the adult. That the adult would turn against the child is unthinkable, and so the child divorces awareness of the abuse from everyday thoughts and manages to forget the trauma. But the fear influences the child's

Domestic violence: The use of force to control and maintain power over another person in the home environment; it includes actual physical harm or psychological harm and the threat of harm.

Child abuse: The systematic harming of a child by a caregiver, generally a parent.

Dealing with Family Violence in Canada

What Factors Contribute to Family Violence?

There is no single cause of family violence, and many people–regardless of status–are vulnerable to it. Most experts believe that family violence is linked to inequalities and power imbalances in our society. Most abusers are in a position of power over their victims.

A person's vulnerability to abuse may be increased by factors such as dislocation, racism, sexism, homophobia, disability, poverty, isolation, and by lack of access to community services and support and the child welfare and criminal justice systems. For example, in the past, many children from marginalized groups in our society who were sent to institutions (such as residential schools or orphanages) experienced abuse.

What Are the Consequences of Family Violence?

Individuals who experience–or are exposed to–family violence, can experience psychological, physiological, behavioural, academic, sexual, interpersonal, self-perceptual, or spiritual consequences, which are fatal in some cases.

Consequences for Abusers

In some cases, abusers may have been abused–or exposed to abuse–themselves and learned that abuse is a way of exerting power and control over others. They may continue to harm others even if it destroys their relationships or has other negative consequences for their lives.

Societal Consequences

Family violence has enormous economic costs for Canadian society. The first research study to estimate the costs of various forms of violence against women, including abuse in intimate relationships, found it costs Canadian society an estimated $4.2 billion per year in social services, education, criminal justice, labour, employment, health, and medical costs.

Preventing and Responding to Family Violence

Victims and abusers are involved in intimate or dependent relationships, and often have strong emotional ties. Community services and supports for victims, such as shelters, are essential. All levels of government are working together to ensure that the criminal justice system responds more effectively to protect victims and hold abusers accountable via legal reform, public and professional education, research, and support for programs and services.

DISCUSSION QUESTION

Besides reforming the law and enhancing its implementation, what other strategies are you aware of to prevent and respond to family violence in Canada? What interventions or programs are offered in your community? What impact do these programs have on the incidence or impact of family violence for the victims and Canadian society at large?

Source: *Family Violence: Department of Justice Canada Overview Paper,* http://canada.justice.gc.ca/eng/pi/fv-vf/facts-info/fv-vf/index.html, Department of Justice Canada, 2009. Reproduced with the permission of the Minister of Public Works and Government Services Canada, 2010.

attitudes, behaviours, and interactions with others, often in destructive ways. Later in life, when it is safer, the memory may resurface and the person can begin to heal.

Not all child violence is physical. A child's health can be severely affected by psychological violence—assaults on personality, character, competence, independence, or general dignity as a human being. The negative consequences of this kind of victimization in close relationships can be harder to discern and therefore harder to combat. They include depression, lowered self-esteem, sub-optimal growth[51] and a pervasive fear of doing something that will offend the abuser.

what do you THINK?

What factors in society lead to child maltreatment? What are common characteristics of children's abusers? Why are family members often the perpetrators of child abuse including sexual abuse? What actions can be taken to prevent such behaviours? How can the cycle of the abused becoming the abuser be stopped?

TABLE 14.1

Elder Abuse: The Victims and the Abusers

Number and proportion of older adult victims of violent crime by sex of victims and relationship to accused, 2000[*]

Relationship of accused to victim	Total		Female		Male	
	No.	%	No.	%	No.	%
Total[**]	3627	100	1792	100	1835	100
Unknown	214	6	91	5	123	7
Non-family	2407	66	1052	59	1355	74
Family	1006	28	649	36	357	19
Total family[***]	1006	100	649	100	357	100
Spouse[†]	312	31	236	36	76	21
Parent	53	5	28	4	25	7
Adult child[††]	398	40	243	37	155	43
Sibling[‡]	110	11	60	9	50	14
Extended family[§]	133	13	82	13	51	14

Percentages may not total 100 percent due to rounding.

[*]Data are not nationally representative. Based on data from 166 police departments representing 53 percent of the national volume of crime in 2000.

[**]Excludes one case where relationship between victim and accused was unknown.

[***]Excludes cases where relationship between victim and accused was unknown.

[†]Includes current and former spouses, either by legal marriage or common-law relationship.

[††]Includes a small number of cases where age or the relationship between the accused and the victim may have been miscoded.

[‡]Sibling includes natural, step, half, foster, or adopted brother or sister.

[§]Extended family includes others related to the victim either by blood or by marriage, for example, aunts, uncles, cousins, and in-laws.

Source: "Number and Proportion of Older Adult Victims of Violent Crime by Sex of Victims and Relationship to Accused, 2000," adapted from Statistics Canada, *Revised Uniform Crime Reporting Survey* (UCR2), 2000.

Violence against Men

While women are most often the targets of violence by men, men can also be the target. In 1999, males committed 85.5 percent of violent crimes. Thirty-nine percent of violent crimes in 1999 involved males attacking other males. Men under the age of 34 are more likely to be perpetrators in major assaults (65 percent). In only 6 percent of reported cases did a woman commit a violent act on a man.[52] Thus, the task of overcoming violence in our society is largely a male issue. The principal reason seems to be that boys are taught—overtly or subtly—that competitiveness, power, and control are valued male attributes. Violence can be seen as an expression of frustration and stress.

Violence against Older Adults

Violence toward older adults (elder abuse) has more recently been getting attention. The first national survey of abuse toward the elderly was done in 1989 at Ryerson University; the researchers found that 4 percent of Canadians over 65 living in private dwellings (or 98 000 seniors) reported experiencing at least one type of abuse in the last 12 months. The most prevalent types of abuse reported (listed in order of prevalence) were material abuse (such as forcing older adults to hand over money or valuable goods), chronic verbal aggression, physical abuse, and neglect.[53] The victim was more often female (67 percent), and the abuser was most frequently a spouse or a child of the victim. (See Table 14.1.) Recent data from Statistics Canada indicates that 56 percent of violence against seniors was by someone they knew.[54] The vulnerability of this group is reflected in the lack of formal charges laid against the perpetrators, with only 13 percent of older adults who were abused laying charges.

Statistics Canada reports that older women are more likely than their male counterparts to be victims of family violence, with almost 40 percent of older

Are You a Victim of Abuse?

Ask yourself if you are being abused. Start with the following questions, responding yes or no. Be honest.

1. Does your partner continually criticize what you wear, what you say, how you act, and how you look? _____

2. Does your partner often call you insulting or degrading names? _____

3. Do you feel like you need to ask permission to go out and see your friends and family? _____

4. Do you feel that no matter what you do, everything is your fault? _____

5. Do you feel like you're walking on eggshells trying to avoid an argument? _____

6. When you are late getting home, does your partner harass you about where you were and whom you were with? _____

7. Is your partner so jealous that you are always being accused of having affairs? _____

8. Has your partner threatened to hurt you or the children if you leave? _____

9. Does your partner force you to have sex? _____

10. Has your partner threatened to hit you? _____

11. Has your partner ever pushed, shoved, or slapped you? _____

12. Has your partner ever purposely broken anything of value to you? _____

If you answered yes to one or more of these questions, you may be suffering abuse.

WHERE TO GO FOR SUPPORT SERVICES

- Transition house or shelter
- Police department/RCMP unit
- Distress centre
- Sexual assault centre/women's resource centre
- Social service agency
- Health centre/doctor's office

Telephone numbers can be found at the front of your phone book.

DO YOU WANT TO LEARN MORE?

The National Clearinghouse on Family Violence can provide you with a list of publications that can be ordered free of charge. The Clearinghouse can also tell you about films and videos on abuse that can be borrowed through the National Film Board's regional offices.

Source: Deborah Prieur and Mary Rowles, *Taking Action: A Union Guide to Ending Violence Against Women* (BC Federation of Labour and the Women's Research Centre, 1992) 14. Reprinted by permission of the BC Federation of Labour.

female victims assaulted by a family member compared to 20 percent of older male victims.[55] Most (55 percent) older adult victims of family-related violence experience common assaults, while another 19 percent experience verbal aggression. The perpetrators of these assaults are most often males.

SEXUAL VICTIMIZATION

In 1997, sexual offences reported to police represented 10 percent (30 735 sexual offences) of violent crimes. The offenders are mostly male (98 percent in 1997) and somewhat older (average age 32) than the norm for all violent offenders (average age 29). The 1997 rate was 25 percent lower than the peak in 1993.[56]

✱ Sexual Assault

Sexual assault can be understood in terms of a power imbalance in society "in which violence is implicit" as the base upon which sexual exploitation is built.[57] In Canada, sexual assault is defined as incidents of unwanted sexual activity, including sexual attacks and sexual touching.[58] The prevalence of sexual assault is difficult to quantify in Canada because an overwhelming majority of such assaults (91 percent) are not reported to the police.[59] The most recent published data, in 2004, indicated a rate of 1977 per 100 000 persons.[60] A survey of more than 6000 post-secondary students found that 84 percent of women who had been sexually assaulted knew their attacker and that 57 percent of the rapes happened on a date.[61] Of male offenders, 19 percent were between the ages of 18 and 24, 32 percent were between 25 and 34, and 23 percent were between 35 and 44. Many universities coordinate "safe walk" programs, during which a person can be accompanied at night on campus from building to building or to and from the parking lots. Self-defence courses can provide some protection against attackers as well as improve self-confidence. The Skills for Behaviour Change box discusses preventing sexual assault when dating.

Why Some Males Sexually Assault Women

Over the years, psychologists and others have proposed many theories to explain why so many males sexually victimize women. One study found that almost two-thirds of the male respondents had engaged in sexual activity that was unwanted by the woman, primarily because of male peer pressure.[62]

Peer pressure is certainly a strong factor in such behaviours, but a growing body of research suggests that sexual assault is encouraged by the normal socialization processes that males experience daily.[63] One Canadian study investigated the characteristics of stalkers.[64] A physically violent stalker is more likely to have had a strong previous attachment with the victim, be highly fixated on the victim, have a higher degree of perceived negative affect toward the victim, engage in significant verbal threats to the victim, and have a history of battering or abusing the victim. Overall, the author describes the physically violent stalker as someone with significant anger, vengeance, emotional arousal, humiliation, projection of blame, and insecure attachment. Another Canadian study examined male erotomania, a particularly dangerous form of sexual harassment. These men have a severely paranoid thought disorder which combines jealously, projection, and interpretation. The typical behaviour of these men is characterized by escalating violence in their contact with women who they believe love them.[65]

Social Assumptions

According to many experts, certain common assumptions in our society prevent the recognition by the perpetrator and the wider public of the true nature of sexual assault.[66] The most important of these assumptions are[67]

- Minimization: It is assumed that sexual assault of women is rare because official crime statistics show relatively few offences; however, sexual assault is the most underreported of all serious crimes—with 91 percent not reported in Canada!

- Trivialization: Incredibly, sexual assault of women is often not viewed as a major issue; in fact, it is often treated in a jocular matter by many men.

- Blaming the victim: Many discussions of sexual violence against women display a sometimes unconscious assumption that the woman did

Emergency call boxes are becoming a common sight on college campuses as school administrators beef up their safety and emergency alert systems.

something to provoke the attack—that she dressed too revealingly or flirted too much or she put herself in a compromising position.

- "Boys will be boys": This is the assumption that men can not control themselves once they become aroused. The myth that men cannot stop once they start is millennia old and typically suggests that males are slaves to their sexual organs or that physical harm can happen to the unfortunate male denied ejaculation. These notions can be countered by pointing out the following: (a) If a woman's parents walked into the room where sex was occurring, it's a sure bet that the man could stop; and (b) there has never been a documented case where a male died due to coitus interruptus.

✳ PREVENTING PERSONAL ASSAULTS

After a violent act is committed against someone we know, we acknowledge the horror of the event, express sympathy for the victim, and then go on with our lives. But the brutalized person often takes a longer time to recover—and sometimes complete recovery from the assault is not possible (see Table 14.2 for a summary of

Sexual assault: Any act in which one person is sexually intimate with another person without consent.

Preventing Date Rape

Men and women need to proactively protect themselves from date rape in their potential roles as perpetrators and victims. The following suggestions—created specifically and separately for women and men—help to reduce the risk of date rape.

WOMEN

- Decide ahead of time how far you are willing to go. Remember that it is your game, your rules, and no one should pressure or force you to go beyond your limits.

- Think ahead and try to avoid "compromising" situations. If you have not implicitly decided to have sex, stay out of your date's bedroom, the back seat of the car, or other quiet spots away from the rest of the crowd where intimacy can result.

- Communicate directly. Do not be wishy-washy. If things start to go farther than you want them to, say "no" loudly and with conviction. Do not worry about hurting feelings, disappointing your partner, or seeming aggressive. Be firm and stick to your words.

- Be aware that some men, in some situations, will interpret a low-cut, sexy dress or other clothing as a come-on. Although this is obviously wrong on their part, it is important that you do not naively assume that everyone is enlightened. Be direct and firm with anyone who seems to be assuming too much from your attire or interactions.

- Limit your consumption of alcohol and other drugs that reduce your ability to think clearly. Do not accept a drink from anyone. Do not leave your drink unattended.

- Pay attention to the nonverbal and verbal cues that your date is giving you. If he is indicating that he is interested in more, let him know that you are not.

- Be concerned about any of the following behaviours or expressions exhibited by your date:

  - Continued suggestive or dirty language indicating disrespect for you and others.

  - Failure to listen to or to value your opinions about where to go, whom to spend time with, etc.

  - Unusual displays of jealousy or rage concerning your interactions with others.

  - Unusual roughness and forceful pushing or shoving to get you to comply with his wishes.

  - Wild anger and violent acts toward others.

  - Inability to control drinking and to display appropriate behaviours.

  - Lack of concern for your feelings; laughter or derisive comments when you say no.

MEN

- Take stock of your past behaviours in sexual situations and in potentially sexual situations. How have you behaved, what have been the outcomes of the encounters, etc.? Have you felt uncomfortable about pushing too hard to have sex with your dates in the past? Have you felt pushed yourself?

- Know and express your sexual limits. If you feel that you are beginning to lose control in an intimate situation, communicate your feelings and indicate why it is time to stop.

- Understand that NO means NO—and that it is not a sign of rejection. Respect your partner's right to say no, regardless of how far you have gone or what you thought she might have wanted. Stop NOW and do not try "another line." Think about how you would want your sister or close female friend to be treated by another guy in a similar situation.

- Just because you may have been intimate with the woman before does not mean it is okay now. When you hear the word NO, or if the woman struggles in any way, STOP.

- Limit alcohol and other drugs that cause you to think less clearly. Do not accept a drink from anyone or leave your drink unattended. Do not purchase a drink for someone unless they ask for it.

- Avoid situations likely to get you into trouble. Until you are sure of your intentions and your date's intentions, stay out of bedrooms, the back seats of cars, or any other places away from people where there is the potential to be intimate.

- If you encounter a particularly aggressive woman, it is not unmanly to tell her you do not want to have sex and are not interested in being intimate in any way. Say NO and avoid situations that may cause you to be caught in a compromising position. Forget about what she may say or what your friends will say. Remember, it is up to you whether or not you have sex.

TABLE 14.2

Common Consequences of Victimization

Psychological	Medical
Recurrent and intrusive recollections, dreams, or flashbacks involving traumatic incidents	Death
Generalized anxiety, mistrust, and/or social isolation	Sexual/reproductive symptoms/consequences: chronic pelvic pain, HIV infection, urinary act infections, premenstrual pain, fertility problems, trauma-specific pain, orgasmic difficulty
Difficulty in forming or maintaining non-exploitive intimate relationships	Battering-related symptoms: bruises, black eyes, fractured ribs, broken teeth, subdural hematomas, detached retinas, other head injuries
Chronic depression	Stress-mediated symptoms: headaches, backaches, TMJ symptoms, high blood pressure, hyperalertness, sleep disorders, gastrointestinal disorders
Dissociative reactions: phobic avoidance, often generalized to apparently unrelated situations; feelings of "badness," stigma, and guilt; impulsive or self-defeating behaviour	Eating disorders
	Self-mutilation

Source: From Marjorie Whitaker Leidig, "The Continuum of Violence against Women: Psychological and Physical Consequences," *Journal of American College Health*, 40 (1992): 151.

the most common consequences of victimization). In this section, we discuss prevention of violence and abuse rather extensively because it is far better to stop a violent act than to have to recover from it.

Self-Defence against Sexual Assault

To reduce your risk of sexual assault, there are some common-sense self-defence tactics that you can learn. Self-defence is a process that includes increased awareness, learning self-defence techniques, taking reasonable precautions, and developing the self-confidence and judgment needed to determine appropriate responses to different situations.[68]

> ## what do you THINK?
> Why do you think women are reluctant to report sexual assault? How can we help women in this regard? Why do you think men are not aware of their sexually harassing behaviours? What can be done to increase their awareness? And that of society in general?

Taking Control

Most sexual assaults by assailants unknown to the victim are planned in advance. They are frequently preceded by a casual, friendly conversation. Although many victimized women said that they started to feel uneasy during such a conversation, they denied the possibility of an attack on themselves until it was too late. Listen to your feelings and trust your intuition. Be assertive and direct to someone who is getting out of line or threatening—this may convince the would-be assailant to back off. Stifle your tendency to be "nice," and don't be afraid of making a scene. Let him know that you mean what you say and are prepared to defend yourself:[69]

- Speak in a strong voice and use statements like "Leave me alone" rather than questions like "Will you please leave me alone?" Avoid apologies and excuses.

- Maintain eye contact with the would-be attacker.

- Mean what you say. Speak assertively.

- Stand up straight, be confident, and remain alert. Walk as if you own the sidewalk.

Many assailants use certain ploys to initiate their attacks. Among the most common are:

- Request for help. This allows him to get close—to enter your house to use the phone, for instance.

- Offer of help. This can also help him gain entrance to your home: "Let me help you carry that package."

Managing Campus Safety

University and college campuses today may be healthy places for student interactions, or they may be settings for violent and aggressive interactions between students. Most campuses have initiated programs, services, and policies designed to protect students from possible violations of their personal health and safety. Respond to the following to determine yours and your college administrators' degree of interest in and commitment to proactive violence protection and to a violence-free setting.

MAKING DECISIONS FOR YOU

Setting limits on where you go, at what time, and with whom seems to be a running theme of this chapter. What types of limits do you set for yourself? Think for a moment about your next night out with friends or with your lover. What limits will you set for yourself? Will you decide ahead of time to limit your drinking? What time do you want to be home? How far will you go sexually? Will you use condoms? Decide how you will achieve your goals

CHOICES FOR CHANGE: MAKING PERSONAL CHOICES

- Do you decide before a date to limit your sexual behaviours?
- Do you travel in groups whenever possible?
- Do you avoid being out alone at night?
- Do you avoid high-crime areas?

CHOICES FOR CHANGE: MAKING COMMUNITY CHOICES

- Does your campus have a student health centre with a trained staff?
- Does your health centre offer workshops on prevention of sexual assault?
- Does your campus offer courses focusing on understanding human diversity?
- Does your campus offer workshops or seminars for men to help them understand their sexuality and refrain from all forms of sexual assault against women?
- Does your campus offer workshops and information for students to help them avoid situations that put them at risk for violent sexual or other interactions?
- Does your campus offer confidential counselling or assistance to victims of sexual assault?
- Does your campus offer workshops or educational sessions dealing with suicide?
- Does your campus offer information, workshops, or services dealing with domestic violence?
- Does your campus offer information, workshops, or services dealing with child abuse and/or sexual abuse?
- Does your campus offer workshops or seminars that help males learn how to confront peers who express attitudes supportive of "overcoming" women sexually?
- Does your campus have strict substance-use policies designed to reduce the likelihood of sexual assaults?
- Are sessions designed to negate myths and to increase understanding between the sexes offered in "safe" environments where discussions are open and positive role models encourage positive actions?
- Are services such as rides and escort services available to students after hours to prevent assaults? Do security guards patrol the campus?
- Is your campus well-lit and open in the evenings?
- Are campus health educators, counsellors, and other professionals trained to spot victimization in clients and recommend appropriate services?
- Does your campus have a code of conduct that mandates swift and prudent punishment for alcohol and other drug abuse and acts of campus violence?

CRITICAL THINKING

Your best friend and roommate was accused of date rape; if the charge is substantiated, he could be dismissed. The way your friend tells it, they had a few drinks, started making out, and eventually had sex. He claims that she did not try to stop him. Your friend asks you to talk to the girl; after all, she is a friend of yours from high school and you introduced them. He wants you to "find holes in her story" and see if you can get her to "forget about the whole thing." It is hard to believe your best friend is a rapist. But then you have not talked to the accuser yet.

Using the DECIDE model described in Chapter 1, decide what you will do. Reconsider the information about date rape in the chapter. Would it make a difference if she came to you to talk?

- Guilt trip. "Gee, no one is friendly nowadays . . . I cannot believe you will not talk with me for just a little while."
- Authority. Some victimized women have been fooled by the "police officer at the door" ruse. If anyone comes to your door dressed in the uniform of a police officer, firefighter, repair person, or any other individual, ask him to show you his ID before you unlock the door. You can also call the employer to get a confirmation on his ID.

If you are attacked, act immediately:

- Do not worry about causing a scene. Draw attention to yourself and your assailant. Scream for help.
- Report the attack to the appropriate authorities immediately.

To prevent an attack from occurring:

- Always be vigilant. Even the safest cities and towns have sexual assaults. Do not be fooled by a sleepy, little-town atmosphere.
- Use campus escort services whenever possible.
- Be assertive in demanding a well-lit campus and safe-walk programs.
- Do not use the same routes all the time. Think about your movement patterns and vary them accordingly.
- Do not leave a bar alone with a friendly stranger. Stay with your friends, and let the friendly stranger come along. Do not give your address or phone number to anyone you do not know.

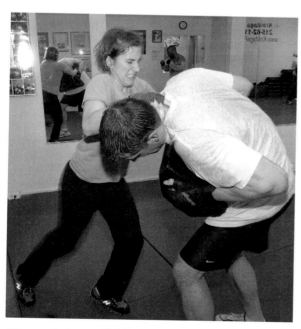

Women who learn self-defence techniques and remember to take reasonable safety precautions lower their risk for assault.

- Never accept a drink from another person and never leave your drink unattended. Rohypnol (often called the date rape drug) is odourless and colourless and you cannot tell if it has been put in your drink.
- Let friends or family know where you are going, what route you plan to take, and when to expect your return.
- Stay close to others. Avoid shortcuts through dark or unlit paths. Do not be the last one to leave the lab or library late at night.
- Keep your windows and doors locked. Do not answer the door to strangers.

What to Do When a Sexual Assault Occurs

If you are a victim of sexual assault, it should be you who reports the attack. This gives you a sense of control. Call 911 immediately. Do not bathe, shower, douche, clean up, or touch anything the attacker may have touched. Do not throw away or launder the clothes you were wearing. They will be needed as evidence. Bring a clean change of clothes to the clinic or hospital. Contact the Rape Crisis Centre in your area and ask for advice on therapists or counselling for additional support.

If you want to help a victim of sexual assault, the best thing you can do is to believe her. Do not ask questions that appear to implicate her in the assault. Your hindsight may find some questionable judgment on her behalf, but that does not mean she's to blame. Sexual assault is a violent act against someone; the victim was certainly not looking or asking for it. Encourage her to talk, and when she does, listen. Hold back on advice.

Encourage her to see a doctor immediately, as she may have medical needs but be too embarrassed to seek help on her own. Be supportive of her reporting the crime. Continue to be her friend. It may take six months to a year for emotional recovery, and you should be empathetic during this time. Encourage her to seek counselling if problems persist.

Preventing Assaults at Home

When at home, there are several precautions you can take to avoid being assaulted:[70]

- Get deadbolts and peepholes and make sure the entryway to your house is well lit and free of shrubs.
- Put a lock, solid-core door, and extension phone with a lighted dial in your bedroom.
- Get to know your neighbours and organize a neighbourhood watch.

- Do not hide your keys under a fake rock or other device. These are dead giveaways to experienced criminals.
- Do not open your door to anyone you do not know.
- Ask for identification from repair people, police officers, firefighters, and any others who come to your door offering services. Call to verify that this person was sent.
- Keep lights on in at least one room other than the one you are in to make it look as if you are not home alone.
- Do not put your full name on your mailbox or in the phone book; use your initials instead.
- Use a "Beware of Dog" sign to deter assailants. Be careful of "doggy doors." Many assailants have entered a house through a pet door.

Preventing Assaults on the Street

There are several suggestions to prevent an assault when you walk or jog:[71]

- Walk or jog at a steady pace. Be confident and alert to your surroundings.
- Walk or jog with others. There is safety in numbers.
- Vary your running or walking routes.
- At night, avoid dark parking lots, wooded areas, and all other good hiding places for assailants.
- Listen for footsteps and voices. Change the pace of your walk if you think you are being followed to see if the person behind you does likewise. If he or she does, walk down the middle of the street, staying near the streetlights. Run and yell if you feel threatened.
- Be aware of cars that keep driving around in your area.

<hr>

what do you THINK?
How safe are you in your own home? How about on campus? What can you do to reduce your risk?

<hr>

Preventing Assaults in Your Car

Carjackings and murders of individuals driving expensive cars, rental cars, and other vehicles point out the necessity for personal actions to prevent assaults when you are in your car:[72]

- Keep your doors locked and your windows rolled up.

- Do not stop for vehicles in distress. Drive on and call for help.
- If your car breaks down, lock the doors and wait for help from the police. Do not accept assistance from strangers, particularly from individuals on isolated roads.
- If you think someone is following you, do something to attract attention. Stay in your car with locked windows and doors and drive to a fire station, police station, all-night grocery, restaurant, or other place where there are people. If you are forced to stop on a deserted road, leave your engine running and in gear. Wait until your pursuer gets out of his car, then drive away as fast as you safely can.
- Stick to well-travelled routes. Avoid dark, isolated shortcuts.
- Fill your car with gas and keep it in good running order.
- Do not put your name and address on your key ring.
- Before getting into your car, walk around it and check the back seat, floor, and undercarriage.
- On long trips, do not make it obvious that you are travelling alone. Never take a map into a restaurant.
- Do not sleep in your car along the highway. This is no longer safe in many areas.
- When you stop at a traffic light, leave a car's length ahead of you so that if you are approached you will have room to pull out. If someone does approach, blow your horn and attract attention.
- If someone bumps into you, never get out of the car until a police officer arrives. Murders and carjackings have involved assailants ramming victims' cars from behind and then shooting or attacking those who investigate.

VIOLENCE AND HEALTH

If the health sector is to adequately understand and respond to violence, greater emphasis is needed on the Population Health Model adopted by the various levels of government, which views health as embracing not only medical services and personal health practices, but also the physical, social, and economic environment (see Chapter 1). Prevention of violence must be based on the creation of life conditions that reduce the occurrence of violence and lessen its effects.

Clearly, a violence-free environment is a prerequisite for health. Violence is a barrier to health and a consequence of an unhealthy environment. The

Ottawa Charter for Health Promotion (an international statement on health promotion) states:

> The fundamental conditions and resources for health are peace, shelter, education, food, income, a stable ecosystem, sustainable resources, social justice and equity. Improvement in health requires a secure foundation in these basic prerequisites.[73]

Injury Prevention

Intentional acts of violence and abuse receive more media coverage and public awareness than unintentional injuries, which kill and disable Canadians every day. Unintentional injuries—the result of falls, motor vehicle crashes, railway and pedestrian injuries, drowning and suffocation, poisoning, and fires—are the leading cause of death among Canadians up to the age of 44, and they kill more young people between the ages of 1 and 20 than all other causes of death combined. Why, then, do we not view injury as a serious population health problem? It is likely because we tend to call unintentional injuries "accidents." This suggests that the injury was due to some unavoidable circumstance over which the individual had no control. However, most injuries are predictable and preventable. Not wearing seatbelts or bicycle helmets drastically increases the risk of injury. Falls account for about 40 percent of the total injuries to Canadians, while motor vehicle crashes account for about 20 percent.

Who Are the Victims of Unintentional Injury?

The injury rate resulting in death or hospitalization is higher for seniors than for any other age group in Canada, and is expected to grow as the population ages. The most common cause of injury among seniors is falls. More than $980 million is spent each year to cover the cost of direct medical care to treat these falls. Canadians of all ages face hazards in their everyday environment that might cause falls—ice-coated sidewalks and stairs, loose banisters, and unsafe play or work equipment.

Falls are by far the most common reason that Canadians are admitted to hospital for injury. The Canadian Institute for Health Information reports that falls account for more than 50 percent of all people admitted to hospital, 67 percent of all days spent in hospital due to trauma, and 75 percent of all people who die in hospital due to trauma.

Preventable injuries account for almost 70 percent of injury-related deaths among children and youth. Of the 3000 people per year who die in motor vehicle crashes in Canada, 40 percent (1200 deaths) are attributed to alcohol. Up to $25 billion is spent annually for emergency care, rehabilitation, and other costs resulting from traffic collisions.

What Can Be Done?

SmartRisk suggests that each individual has the power to control the level of risk in his or her life. Smart risk-taking means that you have identified all risks beforehand and that you fully understand the consequences of your actions. Preparing for the risky activity will reduce the amount of risk you take and enable you to make good decisions when a risky scenario presents itself. You must be prepared to choose behaviours that will reduce the likelihood of injury. Buckle up. Drive sober. Wear a bicycle helmet. Get trained. Wear the safety gear. Look first. (For more on practising smart risk, check out www.smartrisk.ca.)

All-Terrain Vehicles: Handle with Care

All-terrain vehicles (ATVs) were introduced to Canada sometime in the early 1970s. Since then, Canada has become the biggest market per capita in the world, with approximately 2.5 million Canadians riding ATVs and approximately 850 000 owning one or more.

Along with increased use has come an increase in the number of ATV-related injuries and hospitalization. In fact, according to the Canadian Institute for Health Information, from 1996 to 2001 ATV-related hospitalizations increased by 50 percent. Children and adolescents between the ages of 5 and 19 account for more than one-third of these injuries. Currently, ATV-related injuries are the third most common serious injury in the sports and recreational category, after cycling and snowmobiling.

Helmets must be worn when riding an ATV, though not all riders abide by this mandatory regulation. Each province legislates the minimum age restriction for ATV use, from no restrictions in British Columbia, to age 12 and over on public property in Ontario, 14 and older in Newfoundland and Labrador, and 16 and older in the Yukon Territory and Nova Scotia. In addition to not wearing helmets, young riders are also likely to ride double and on public roads.

To reduce risk of injury, the Canadian Health Network recommends that riders

- Buckle up. Although ATVs do not have seatbelts, you should securely fasten the straps on your helmet and gloves.
- Look first. Become familiar with the terrain you are going to be driving on and know where you are going. If you plan a day-long or overnight trip, ensure that a responsible adult is aware of your plans. Take a cellphone.
- Wear the gear. In addition to wearing a helmet, wear wrist and eye protection. During the winter, dress for the weather.
- Get trained. Riders of all ages should take certification of training from a club or manufacturer. The Canada Safety council offers ATV riders' courses, including one geared for those under the age of 14.
- Drive sober. Do not drive an ATV under the influence of alcohol or any other drug that affects your ability to think clearly.

Further, the Canadian Paediatric Society recommends the following:

- Children under 16 should *not* operate ATVs.
- Children should never ride as passengers.
- ATVs should not be used at night.

Source: Adapted from Canadian Health Network, "All-Terrain Vehicles: Handle with Care." Retrieved on May 18, 2006, from www.canadian-health-network.ca/servelet/ContentServer?cid=1146231807156&pagename=CHN-RCS/CHNResiource/CHNResourcePagePrint.

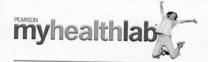 Go to MyHealthLab at **www.pearsoned.ca/myhealthlab.** Here you will find self-assessments, case studies, links to health on the net, and much more.

DISCUSSION QUESTIONS

1. Identify the types of violence in Canada as well as the prevalence of each.
2. What are the health issues of violence on your campus? And in society?
3. What leads to domestic violence? Compare spousal abuse against men and women: What are the differences? What are the similarities?
4. What puts a child at risk for abuse? What can be done to prevent or to decrease the amount of child abuse?
5. Detail the actions you can take to protect yourself from personal assault in your home, on the streets, or in your car.
6. If your friend called to tell you she or he was just sexually assaulted, what would you do? What would you suggest that she or he do?
7. Think about a time when you did something risky. Was it a smart or foolish risk? What steps did you take to manage or limit the risk? If you had the same opportunity, what, if anything, would you do differently?

APPLICATION EXERCISE

Reread the "Consider This . . . " scenario at the beginning of the chapter and answer the following questions.

1. From what you have read in this chapter, do you think what Kyle has witnessed is common in Canadian society?
2. How do you think Kyle might react to the police taking his father away?
3. How might Kyle react to his mother?
4. How can Kyle break the cycle of violence and not become an abuser himself?
5. Where can Kyle go for help for himself?

MYSEARCHLAB EXERCISE

1. Log on to www.MySearchLab.com.
2. Retrieve article AN 23652084, "Active versus Passive Commuting to School: What Children Say," by S. M. Lee and C. Tudor-Locke.
3. Read the article, then provide a response to the following:
   a. What are the risks of using active transportation (that is, walking, cycling, scootering, in-line skating) for getting to school for children in Grade 6? Do the risks differ for boys and girls?
   b. What are your risks for travelling actively to and from school? Between classes? In the evening or later at night?
   c. What measures have been taken on your campus to ensure student safety?

CHAPTER 15

CONSUMERISM

*Using Health-Care
Products and Services*

CONSIDER THIS . . .

Petra is 25 years old with a history of chronically painful menstrual periods and excessive bleeding. She seeks care from a gynecologist, who immediately tells her that she must have a hysterectomy. Because she has not yet had children and does not want to risk early menopause, Petra seeks a second opinion from the gynecologist's colleague. Without giving her much of an exam, the second doctor agrees with the first, so Petra seeks yet another opinion—but this time from a gynecologist outside the original group's practice. This third doctor adamantly disagrees and suggests a more conservative treatment not involving surgery.

Which doctor's advice should Petra follow? Is it appropriate to seek more than one opinion? Is it appropriate to seek more than two opinions? How much say should the individual have in his or her course of treatment?

CHAPTER OBJECTIVES

- Outline a method for making informed health-care choices, including evaluating online medical resources.

- Explain when self-diagnosis and self-care are appropriate, when to seek medical care, and how to assess health professionals.

- Compare and contrast allopathic and non-allopathic medicine, including the types of treatments that fall into each category.

- Discuss Canada's health-care system, including the current problems associated with it.

There are many reasons for you to be an informed health-care consumer. Most important, you have only one body, and it is up to you to maintain it. Doing everything you can to be healthy and to recover rapidly when not healthy enhances every other part of your life. Canada's history has brought about a commitment to share the liability of illness and injury among the entire population because our health-care system is based on shared values of equity, fairness, compassion, and respect for the dignity of all.[1] This is not the case in all other countries.

In the 1990s, the federal government cut its health-care transfer payments to the provinces in stages from a 50–50 share to a 15–85 share as part of its deficit reduction strategy. This shift had a profound impact on the provinces and territories, which are responsible for providing health care. In 2002, the Commission on the Future of Healthcare in Canada made recommendations aimed at sustaining our publicly funded health system by balancing investments in prevention and health maintenance with those directed to care and treatment.[2] As head of the Commission, Roy Romanow recommended comprehensive changes to ensure that our health-care system would be sustained for years to come.

As we continue to scrutinize the evolution of our health-care system, trends continue to emerge—including a shift from centralized governing bodies to regional health authorities, a shift in emphasis from institutionally focused care to community-based care, decision making based on need and the best available evidence, and funding of health services at sustainable levels.[3] Despite these changes, health care remains very important to Canadians, with 63 percent of those polled in a 2005 study indicating that health care should receive the greatest attention from the country's leaders.[4] At the same time, approximately 20 percent and fewer than 10 percent thought education and the economy, respectively, should be the main issue for Canada's leaders.

Even though our society tends to treat health as a social good to which everyone is entitled, you must still be knowledgeable about what resources are available and when to be assertive to obtain services in your best interests. Almost all Canadians use some type of health services each year. When asked in a Statistics Canada survey in 2007 if they had a regular medical doctor, 85 percent of Canadians said yes.[5] Six percent of Canadians said they could not find a doctor. Further, Canadians made approximately 14 million visits to a hospital emergency department in the past year.[6]

As you may already know, medical and health-care services are much harder to evaluate than are, say, clothing or fruit and vegetables. That said, 85 percent of Canadians were very or somewhat satisfied with the care they received in the past 12 months,.[7] Further, most Canadians rated the quality of care as excellent or very good. Although men and women across the country report similar levels of satisfaction overall regarding their health care, women were significantly more satisfied. In response to questions about access to health care, most Canadians (84 percent) did not have difficulty in accessing care.[8] The most common challenges to accessing health care were waiting too long to get an appointment, waiting too long in doctors' offices, and problems in contacting a physician. Another issue highlighted in the 2006 Statistics Canada survey included access time for elective or non-emergency surgeries, with almost 20 percent waiting more than three months.[9]

The federal and provincial governments have responded to the need to adapt the system to meet Canadians' needs, notably by[10]

- adopting a "determinant of health" framework that recognizes that while health care is obviously an important contributor to health, its role must be placed in context as only one component of a much broader set of determinants of health
- shifting the emphasis of the health-care system away from institutionally based delivery models (that is, physicians and hospital-based care) to integrated community-based models that place increased emphasis on prevention and health promotion
- developing strategies for the coordinated management of the health-care workforce, including the remuneration, geographical distribution, and appropriate use of various health-care providers
- reducing wait times for cancer care, cardiac care, hip and knee replacements, cataract surgery, and diagnostic imaging

This chapter will help you to become proactive in making decisions that affect your health and health care. Canada's health-care system is a shared responsibility of the federal, provincial, and territorial governments. It includes hospitals, home-care agencies, long-term care facilities, and people (physicians, nurses, social workers, midwives, and other health care providers).[11] In 2007, public- and private-sector health expenditure was $160 billion for a broad range of services—millions of physician visits, immunizations, prescriptions, lab tests, and hospital stays.[12]

✳ MAKING INFORMED HEALTH-CARE CHOICES

Perhaps the single greatest difficulty that we face as consumers is the sheer magnitude of options available. Many different companies aggressively market health

Are You a Good Health-Care Consumer?

Select the response that best describes your typical health behaviours. After completing this survey, total your points and assess your competence regarding health-care products and services.

1. I never act this way

2. I sometimes act this way

3. I act this way most of the time

4. I always act this way

1. When moving to a new location, I seek recommendations from friends and ask for referrals from physicians who treated me in the past, before I get ill.   1 2 3 4

2. I schedule an interview with health-care professionals prior to treatment to determine if I am comfortable with them.   1 2 3 4

3. I ask about costs of health-care procedures. 1 2 3 4

4. I carefully assess my symptoms and go to the doctor only when necessary.   1 2 3 4

5. I get second opinions when I am unsure of what my physician tells me.   1 2 3 4

6. I ask my physician why a test is given and what my options are before I allow that test to be performed.   1 2 3 4

7. I follow recommended guidelines for health exams, inoculations, and self-care.   1 2 3 4

8. Whenever I receive a prescription drug, I follow the directions exactly, including finishing the medication in the prescribed time period.   1 2 3 4

9. I am aware of differences in prices at various pharmacies and comparison-shop whenever possible.   1 2 3 4

10. When my peers make obviously incorrect statements about "health alternatives," I tactfully point out their errors.   1 2 3 4

11. I am aware of my body and seek medical care quickly when unusual changes occur.   1 2 3 4

12. I try to get my health information from reputable sources.   1 2 3 4

13. I carefully scrutinize health-related advertisements and news items.   1 2 3 4

14. I read the labels of health products and follow instructions carefully.   1 2 3 4

INTERPRETING YOUR SCORE

14–19 Health consumer skills dangerously weak

20–29 Health consumer skills below average

30–44 Health consumer skills about average, not adequate for many situations

45–56 Very good health consumer skills.

BEYOND INTERPRETATION

- Given your results above, where do you need the most improvement?

- What can you do to improve in these areas?

products and services to the public. Even medical professionals sometimes feel overwhelmed, confused, and frustrated by the many options. Informed consumers are aware that there is always more to learn. Wise consumers use every means at their disposal to ensure that they are acting responsibly in their own health-care choices. Check out your own knowledge in the Rate Yourself box.

Evaluating Online Medical Resources

The internet has increasingly become a source of health information for many Canadians. How can we be sure that the information we read on websites is credible? The National Centre for Complementary and Alternative Medicine suggests that we ask ourselves the following questions:[13]

- Who runs the site? Any good site will make it easy for you to find out who is responsible for the information presented on it.

- Who pays for the site? The source for the website's funding should be clearly stated. You should know how a website pays for its existence. Does it sell advertising? Is it sponsored by a pharmaceutical company? The source of funding may influence how information is presented.

- What is the purpose of the site? This is related to who runs and pays for the site. The site's purpose should be clearly stated and help you in evaluating the trustworthiness of the information included.

- Where does the information come from? If the information does not come from the website creator, the original source(s) should be identified.

- What is the basis of the information? In addition to providing a complete citation list, the site should describe what the materials presented are based upon. Facts and figures presented should have credible references. Opinions should be set apart from evidence-based information.

- How is the information selected? Was the presented material peer-reviewed? That is, did other appropriate health professionals review the material prior to posting?

- How current is the information? Good health websites are reviewed and updated on a regular basis to ensure that the information presented is current. The date when the website was most recently updated should be clearly stated.

- How does the site choose links to other sites? Credible websites have policies regarding what links they will establish.

- What information about you does the site collect, and why? Websites routinely track the paths visitors take to determine usage rates. Some websites may ask you to subscribe or become a member. This may be to collect a user fee or to assist in collecting information relevant to your concerns. Any credible website will tell you why it is requesting information.

- How does the site manage interaction with visitors? A credible site will provide a way for you to contact the site owner if you have any problems, questions, or feedback.

Financing Health Care

Canada has a predominantly publicly funded, privately delivered health-care system that rests on an interlocking set of 10 provincial and 3 territorial health insurance plans. Known to Canadians as medicare, the system provides access to universal, comprehensive coverage for medically necessary hospital, inpatient, and outpatient physician services. This structure results from the constitutional assignment of jurisdiction over most aspects of health care to provincial governments. The system is referred to as a "national" health insurance system because all provincial or territorial hospital and medical insurance plans are linked through adherence to national principles set at the federal level. The provinces and territories plan, finance, and evaluate the provision of hospital, physician, and allied health care, some aspects of prescription care, and public health.[14] Figure 15.1 details how health care in Canada is funded.

Accepting Responsibility for Your Health Care

While income is generally not a barrier to universally insured medical services, disparities in access to

uninsured health services remain. Most agree that dental care, vision care, and counselling services are not "frills." For many people, access to these services is essential to basic health, yet many have restricted or no access to these services because of lack of private or publicly assisted insurance.[15]

Even though most health care you need is publicly funded, you still need to learn how, when, and where to enter the system and how to obtain the care you need without incurring unnecessary risk or wasting resources. Acting responsibly in times of illness can be difficult, but the person best able to act on your behalf is you. Being knowledgeable about self-care and its limits is critical for responsible consumerism.

Why Some False Claims May Seem True

Many marketing strategies revolve around trendy news items. A good example of this is the concern about trans fat. Whereas food advertisements and product labels previously focused on "low calories," "low cholesterol," "low fat," or "low in saturated fat" they now emphasize "0 trans fat." Many of these products, despite having 0 grams of trans fat, have high levels of saturated fats—this puts an individual at risk for heart disease. When it comes to gathering health information, it is your responsibility to approach advertisers' claims with a "buyer beware" mindset firmly in place.

The same skepticism should be used when evaluating advertising for medical cures. Because of Canadian restrictions and limitations on pharmaceutical advertising, we have not experienced as much of this as Americans have, whose laws in this regard are not as stringent. People often fall victim to false health-care claims because they mistakenly believe that a product or provider has helped them. This belief often arises from two conditions: spontaneous remission and the placebo effect.

Spontaneous Remission

It is commonly said that if you treat a cold, it will disappear in a week, but if you leave it alone, it will last seven days. A **spontaneous remission** from an ailment refers to the disappearance of symptoms without any apparent cause or treatment. Many illnesses, like the common cold and even back strain, are self-limiting and will improve in time, with or without treatment. Other illnesses, such as multiple sclerosis and

Spontaneous remission: The disappearance of symptoms without any apparent cause or treatment.

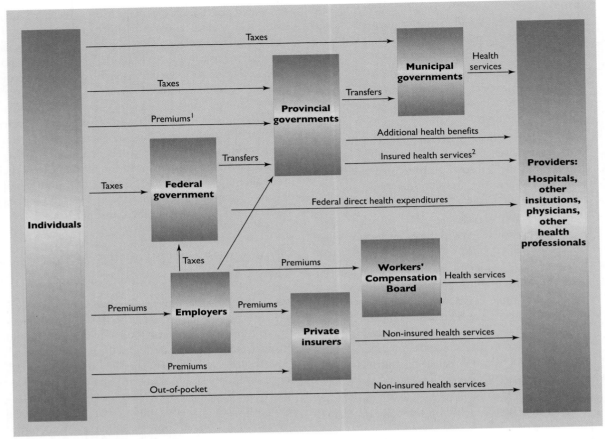

Taxes

Municipal governments

Health services

Taxes

Provincial governments

Transfers

Premiums[1]

Additional health benefits

Transfers

Insured health services[2]

Taxes

Federal government

Providers:

Hospitals, other insitutions, physicians, other health professionals

Individuals

Federal direct health expenditures

Taxes

Premiums

Workers' Compensation Board

Health services

Premiums

Employers

Premiums

Premiums

Private insurers

Non-insured health services

Premiums

Out-of-pocket

Non-insured health services

1. Some provinces levy health premiums.
2. Medically necessary hospital and physician services.

FIGURE 15.1

The Funding Structure of the Health System in Canada

Source: Health Canada, 1998. © Minister of Public Works and Government Services Canada, 2006.

some cancers, are characterized by alternating periods of severe symptoms and sudden remissions. Because of this phenomenon, people seeking profit may exploit consumers by claiming that their particular treatment, procedure, or drug cured the condition. People experiencing spontaneous remissions can easily attribute their "cure" to a treatment, drug, or provider that had no real effect on the disease or condition.

Placebo Effect

The **placebo effect** is an apparent cure or improved state of health brought about by a substance, product, or procedure that has no therapeutic value. It is not uncommon for individuals to report improvements based on what they expect, desire, or were told would happen after taking simple sugar pills believed to be powerful drugs. About 10 percent of the population is believed to be exceptionally susceptible to the power of suggestion; the remainder may be influenced to varying

degrees. Those most susceptible to the placebo effect may be victimized by aggressive marketing of products and services. Although the placebo effect is often harmless, it does account for the expenditure of millions of dollars on worthless health products and services every year. Further, people who mistakenly use placebos when medical treatment is needed are not likely to get better.

SELF-HELP OR SELF-CARE

Self-care is a composite of individual identity and specific attitudes and behaviours associated with looking after the "self."[16] As medical technologies become more sophisticated and as health-care consumers become better informed, we can perform many health-care tasks that were formerly the exclusive responsibility of formal caregivers in institutional

For parents, knowing when to seek help for a sick child is often a challenge since young children are unable to assess their own symptoms and may not be able to describe them adequately.

settings.[17] We can also interpret basic changes in our physical and emotional health and treat minor afflictions without professional help. Self-care consists of knowing your body, recognizing its signals, and taking appropriate action to stop the progression of illness or injury or to improve your overall health.

> ## try it NOW!
> Be prepared for an unexpected medical emergency. Even though you take measures to be safe and healthy, you do not know when you will be in an emergency medical situation, such as a car accident. Make sure your health card is in your wallet, as well as information on who to contact (parents, friends, other family members, etc.) in the event of an emergency.

When to Seek Help

Effective self-care requires the knowledge of when to seek professional medical attention rather than treat a condition on your own. Generally, consult a physician if you experience any of the following:

- a serious accident or injury
- sudden or severe chest pains resulting in difficulty breathing

- trauma to the head or spine accompanied by a headache, blurred vision, loss of consciousness, vomiting, convulsions, or paralysis
- sudden high fever or recurring high temperature (over 38.5°C for adults and 39.5°C for children) or sweats
- tingling sensation in the arm accompanied by slurred speech or impaired thought processes
- adverse reactions to a drug or insect bite (shortness of breath, throat constriction, severe swelling, itchiness, or dizziness)
- unexplained bleeding or loss of bodily fluid from any body opening
- unexplained and sudden weight loss
- persistent or recurrent diarrhea or vomiting
- blue-coloured lips, eyelids, or nail beds
- any lump, swelling, thickness, or sore that does not subside or that grows for over a month
- any marked change in or pain accompanying bowel or bladder habits
- yellowing of the skin or the whites of the eyes
- any unusual symptom that recurs over time
- signs that suggest possible pregnancy

With the vast array of home diagnostic devices currently available, it appears to be relatively easy for most people to take care of themselves. A strong word of caution is in order: although many of these devices are valuable for making an initial diagnosis, home health tests should not be a substitute for regular, complete examinations by a trained practitioner. The Skills for Behaviour Change box offers valuable information about taking an active part in your health care.

✓• Assessing Health Professionals

Suppose you decide that you do need medical attention. You must then identify what type you need and where to obtain it. Initially, selecting a doctor may seem a simple matter, yet many people have no idea how to assess the qualifications of a medical practitioner. Knowledge of traditional medical specialties and alternative medicine is critical to making intelligent selections. You also need to be aware of criteria for evaluating a health professional. Studies indicate that many people's greatest concerns when choosing a doctor have less to do with medical qualifications than with availability and personality. While a warm and caring personality is certainly a valuable attribute, doctors who lack in bedside manner may, in fact, be

Placebo effect: An apparent cure or improved state of health brought about by a substance or product with no medicinal value.

Being Proactive in Your Health Care

Personal involvement in your wellness is critical. Taking a proactive approach to practising preventive behaviours goes a long way toward ensuring a long and healthy life. Sometimes, regardless of the steps taken to care for yourself, you still get sick. At such a time, it is important that you continue to be involved in your care. The more you know about your body and the factors that affect your health, the better you are able to communicate with your doctor. It also helps you to make informed decisions and to recognize when a certain treatment may not be right for you. The following points may be helpful.

- Know your and your family's medical history.
- Be knowledgeable about your condition—causes, physiological effects, possible treatments, prognosis. Do not rely only on the doctor for this information. Do some research of your own.
- Bring a friend or relative along for medical appointments to help you review what the doctor says and possibly write down the doctor's answers to your questions.
- Ask the practitioner to explain the problem and appropriate treatments, tests, and drugs in a way that you understand.
- If the doctor prescribes medications, ask for their generic names so that you can pay less for them.
- Ask for a written summary of the results of your visit and any lab tests.
- If you have any doubt about the doctor's recommended treatment, seek a second opinion.

Afterward:

- Write down an account of what happened and what was said. Be sure to include the names of the doctor and all other people involved in your care, the date, and the place.
- Shop around at various drugstores for the best prices in the same way that you would when shopping for clothes.
- When filling prescriptions, ask to see the pharmacist's package inserts that list medical considerations concerning the prescribed drug and any possible interactions.
- Have clear instructions written on the label to avoid risk to others who may take the drug in error.

Doctors are human; their decisions are based on the best information available to them and may be influenced by a number of factors including—but not limited to—workload, limited information, personal views. Therefore, in addition to the practical steps listed above, being proactively involved in your health care also means that you should be aware of your rights as a patient. The following are the basic rights of all individuals seeking care from a health-care professional. You have the right to

1. Informed consent. Before receiving any care, you have the right to be fully informed of what is planned, the risks and potential benefits, and possible alternative forms of treatment, including the option of no treatment. Your consent must be voluntary and without any form of coercion. It is critical that you read consent forms carefully and amend them as necessary before signing.
2. Know whether the treatment you receive is standard or experimental. In experimental conditions, you have the legal and ethical right to know if the study is one in which some people receive treatment while others do not and if a drug is used in the research project for a purpose not approved by the Health Protection Branch of Health Canada.
3. Privacy, which includes protecting your right to make personal decisions concerning all reproductive matters.
4. Refuse or stop treatment at any time.
5. Receive care.
6. Access your medical records.
7. Confidentiality of your records.
8. Seek the opinions of other health-care professionals regarding your condition.

better trained and qualified than more cordial practitioners. That being said, it is critical to find a physician who is willing and able to listen to your concerns. Carefully consider the following factors about prospective health-care providers:

- What professional education/training do they have? What licence or board certification do they hold?
- Are they affiliated with an accredited medical facility or institution? Accreditation Canada requires these institutions to verify all education, licensing, and training claims of their affiliated practitioners.
- Do they indicate clearly how long a given treatment may last, or do they have you returning week after week with no apparent end in sight?
- Do their diagnoses, treatments, and general statements appear to be consistent with established scientific theory and practice?
- Do they listen to you, appear to respect you as an individual, and give you time to ask questions?

Finding a Personal Physician

Consider the following situation. Mary wakes one morning with a chest cold. In a few days, the cold worsens and she thinks she developed bronchitis. Mary knows she should see a doctor but she does not have a primary care physician, so she decides to let the cold take its course, without medical attention. Unfortunately for Mary, this approach does not work, as her cold worsens, resulting in pneumonia and a much longer recovery time.

Unfortunately, a great many people hesitate about seeking early care because they do not have a physician. In these cases, emergency room care or drop-in clinics are used. As a result, no long-term relationship can be established between the health-care practitioner and patient. If Mary (and others) had a primary care physician, she could have called him or her as soon as her symptoms worsened.

One of the most important decisions a person or family makes is choosing a primary care physician. Your physician plays a critical role in the prevention and treatment of illnesses. When you are ill or develop symptoms that need attention, having someone to contact in whom you have confidence can relieve a great deal of anxiety. Yet, despite the importance of identifying and regularly visiting a primary care physician, a great many people wait until they are ill to seek a doctor. Depending on the severity of the illness, waiting this long can limit a person's options. Selecting a doctor long before an illness develops allows you to identify and interview several doctors to find the one to best fit your needs and with whom you feel the most comfortable. In Canada, you may have easier access to a primary care physician (general or family practitioner) if another family member visits that practitioner or if you are new to the area. It may be difficult to change doctors when remaining in the same location. This difficulty makes it all the more important to properly assess a doctor at the outset. (Another issue to keep in mind is that there is a physician shortage in many areas in Canada, with some physicians not taking new patients.)

The following procedure can help you with this process.

1. First, consider the following questions:
   - Would you feel more comfortable with a male or female health professional? Why?
   - Is age an important factor to you? Why?
   - Do you have a pre-existing condition for which specialization may be helpful?
   - Do you prefer to see primarily one physician or are you comfortable visiting a service with a team of doctors (like what you would find in a health clinic)?

2. Next, assemble a list of names of doctors in your area. Names of potential physicians can be identified by
   - Asking friends and colleagues for recommendations. These are often your best sources of information about a doctor's availability and promptness as well as overall general concern.
   - Calling the local medical association, local health advocacy groups (many communities provide references as a service), or the local hospital for names of doctors accepting new patients.

- Researching medical directories at your local library. The Canadian Medical Directory, for example, includes information about every physician who belongs to the CMA (Canadian Medical Association).

3. Call the offices of the physicians on your list and explain that you are seeking a primary care physician. Ask the receptionist about the doctor's hospital affiliation, office hours, and the kind of coverage the physician has for emergency situations outside normal office hours. Take into consideration the receptionist's tone and how your questions are answered. Find out how much time is allotted for appointments (30 to 45 minutes for a routine physical is average).

4. Narrow the list to two or three physicians and make appointments for brief consultations.

5. While visiting with each doctor, you should find answers to the following questions:
   - Is the doctor's educational and experiential background appropriate?
   - While visiting, do you feel that he or she cares about you as a person?
   - Do you feel relaxed in his or her presence?
   - Are you encouraged to ask questions? Are answers explained clearly?
   - Does the physician use a lot of medical jargon? If so, how does that make you feel?
   - Does the doctor use a condescending tone?
   - Does the physician attend to you personally or does he or she serve primarily as a "gatekeeper" to specialists?

6. Develop some direct questions about treatment that identify the physician's philosophy on care. For example, you could ask how the physician would treat a terminally ill patient or about his or her willingness to accommodate your religious feelings.

7. Once you choose a physician, get the most from your visits by creating and maintaining an open line of communication. You can do this by
   - Being prepared for appointments. Know your medical and family history and be specific and detailed about the symptoms you experience.
   - Not bringing up irrelevant questions regarding your partner's, children's, or parent's health when the appointment is about you. If these individuals need an appointment, book one.
   - Being an educated patient. Expect and insist on a diagnosis explained in a way that you fully understand. Never leave your doctor's office with questions unanswered.

- Taking a proactive role in your health care. Treatment will work only if you follow it. Listen to and follow instructions, find out when you can call with follow-up questions, and be sure that the doctor reports any test results to you promptly. "No news is good news" is not an appropriate adage to follow.
- Communicating your needs to the doctor. If you have concerns about communication or treatment, speak up.

Asking the right questions at the right time may save you personal suffering. Many individuals find that writing their questions down ahead of time helps them to get all their inquiries answered. You should not accept a defensive or hostile response; asking questions is your right as a patient. The Building Communication Skills box discusses finding a personal physician in more detail.

what do you THINK?

If you had the choice of seeing a practitioner of your own sex and ethnicity, would you? Why or why not? Have you ever had difficulty finding a practitioner with whom you were comfortable?

CHOICES OF MEDICAL CARE

Familiarizing yourself with the various health professions and health subspecialties will help you choose the right provider for your needs. There are more than 62 000 physicians and 252 000 registered nurses in Canada.[18] Those you are most familiar with probably subscribe to allopathic medical procedures. Most people believe that **allopathic medicine**, or traditional, Western medical practice is based on scientifically validated methods, but you should consider that only about 20 percent of all allopathic treatments have been found to be clinically effective in research trials. Medical practitioners who adhere to allopathic principles are bound by a professional code of ethics.

Traditional (Allopathic) Medicine

Selecting a **primary care practitioner**—a medical practitioner whom you can go to for routine ailments, preventive care, general medical advice, and appropriate referrals—is not an easy task, particularly given the shortage of general practitioners in various parts of Canada. The primary care practitioner for most people is a family practitioner. Others use nontraditional providers as their primary source of care. The common denominator is continuity in services over a period of time. Having a "usual source of care" is important to the quality of care you receive.

Some of what is done in medicine either does not improve health outcomes or creates iatrogenic disease (illness caused by the medical treatment itself). An essential part of medical care is informed consent. This refers to your right to have explained to you—in language you can understand—possible side effects, benefits, and consequences of a specific procedure and treatment regimen as well as available alternatives. It also means that you have the right to refuse a specific treatment or to seek a second or even third opinion from unbiased, noninvolved health-care providers.[19]

Informed consent gives you the right to ask questions such as

- What will happen if I choose not to have a particular test or treatment?
- Can other tests be performed instead? What are their risks? Why should I choose this test instead of an alternative?
- How often has the doctor performed this test, surgery, or procedure, and with what success?
- Are the risks from the treatment greater than the risks from the condition?
- What are the side effects of the diagnostic tests? Can these side effects be prevented, treated, or reduced?
- Does this procedure require an overnight stay at a hospital or can it be performed in a doctor's office?
- Why has this test been ordered? What is the doctor trying to find or exclude?
- Are these medications necessary? What are their possible side effects? What will happen if I decide not to take them? What alternatives are available? Is there a generic version that costs less? Will they interact with the other drugs I currently consume (other prescription or OTC drug, caffeine, alcohol, or any other drug that I may be taking)?
- Why do I have this problem? What can I do to prevent if from happening again?

what do you THINK?

Have you ever taken a list of questions to your practitioner's office? If you have, were your questions answered fully? Did you feel intimidated or rushed? Do you think people have the right to question their practitioners' recommendations? Why or why not?

Allied Professionals

Canada lags behind other countries in its creative use of allied health professionals. For example, the official recognition of midwifery occurred recently and in only a few provinces. The use of nurse practitioners is relatively rare except in isolated northern communities, and the Dentacare Program in Saskatchewan, which relied mostly on dental therapists, folded.[20]

Nurses are highly trained and strictly regulated health practitioners who provide a wide range of services for patients and their families, including patient education, counselling, community health and disease prevention information, and administration of medications. They have the designation RN (registered nurse). Although nurses may work in health service organizations (HSOs), clinics, doctors' offices, student health centres, nursing homes, public health departments, schools, businesses, and other health-care settings, many are employed in the hospital setting. There has, however, been an increasing trend away from hospital-based employment as the demand for nurses in other settings has increased.

Nurse practitioners are professional nurses with advanced training obtained through either a master's degree program or a specialized nurse practitioner program. Nurse practitioners have the training and authority to conduct diagnostic tests and prescribe medications. They work in a variety of settings, particularly in hospitals, clinics, and client homes. They have become an increasingly popular source of health care in recent years. Nurses may also earn a bachelor of science and nursing degree (BScN), a master of science and nursing (MScN), or a research-based PhD in nursing.

✳ Non-allopathic Medicine

While people in other parts of the world consider **non-allopathic medicine** the "traditional" form of treatment, in North America we tend to think of non-allopathic medicine as "alternative medicine." As the government, private payers, and consumers evaluate the costs, effectiveness, and quality of traditional health care, many have found it wanting. The two core services under the Canada Health Act, hospital and physician services, count for 43 percent of the total health spending of $130 billion in 2004.[21] Although these two core services account for a smaller part of the total health-care spending than in the past, they have increased more than 51 percent since 1994. However, it should be pointed out that the increase in spending on public health and administration (6 percent of the total) outpaced increases for hospital and physician services. Further, the cost of prescription

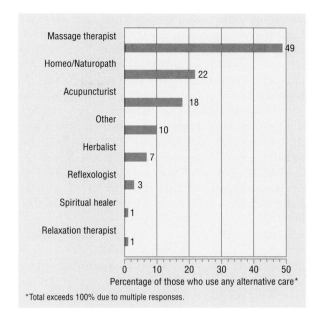

FIGURE 15.2

Percentage of Canadians Aged 12+ Who Use Alternative Health-Care Practitioners, by Type, Canada, 1996–97.

Source: Adapted from the Statistics Canada publication *National Population Health Survey Overview,* catalogue no. 82-567, released July 29, 1998.

and OTC drugs has been the fastest-growing component of the total bill. As a result of dissatisfaction with traditional methods of care and the financing of the health-care system, each year more and more people seek non-allopathic or alternative medical care from providers other than licensed medical doctors. One survey found that 7 percent of Canadians aged 12 and over used alternative health services. If this category is expanded to include complementary and alternative treatments such as herbal remedies, the figure rises to 42 percent.[22] See Figure 15.2 for the types of practitioners used.

Numerous non-allopathic alternatives are available. Many people turn to non-allopathic medicine only after more traditional (allopathic) methods have failed

Allopathic medicine: Traditional, Western medical practice; based on scientifically validated methods and procedures.

Primary care practitioner: A medical practitioner who treats routine ailments, advises on preventive care, gives general medical advice, and makes appropriate referrals when necessary.

Nurse: Health practitioner who provides many services and may work in a variety of settings.

Non-allopathic medicine: Medical alternatives to traditional, allopathic medicine.

to improve their conditions. Because they are often "providers of last resort," these unconventional treatments may appear to produce more negative outcomes overall than traditional medicine. This has given them a bad reputation even though it was the failure of traditional medicine that sent many to non-allopathic practitioners in the first place. Although some alternative therapies are controversial and may be dangerous, many offer significant benefits at reasonable costs. It is the consumer's job to ascertain the credentials of non-allopathic practitioners, because not all are licensed or regulated; this job of verifying credentials may, therefore, be even more difficult than in traditional medicine.

Similar to self-care and accessing allopathic practitioners, you must be assertive in asking providers of non-allopathic medicine about their training, licensing (if relevant), and affiliations. You should also ask how many patients with your specific complaint they have treated and what their success rate is. A potential danger in seeking the assistance of an alternative medical practitioner is that it may keep you from obtaining effective conventional treatment (if any is available).

Chiropractic Treatment

Chiropractic medicine has been practised for many years. At one point, allopathic and chiropractic medicine were in direct competition.[23] Although there have always been medical doctors who collaborate with chiropractic doctors, their numbers have recently increased. Some chiropractic treatments are covered by provincial health insurance, and many private insurance companies pay for treatment if a medical doctor recommends it.

Chiropractic medicine is based on the premise that a life-giving energy flows through the spine via the nervous system. Ill health occurs then if the spine is subluxated (partly misaligned or dislocated) because that force is disrupted. Chiropractors, in their treatment, use a variety of techniques to manipulate the spine back into alignment so the life-giving energy can flow unimpeded through the nervous system. It has been established that their treatment is effective for chronic low back pain, neck pain, and headaches.

The average chiropractic training program requires four years of intensive courses in biochemistry, anatomy, physiology, diagnostics, pathology, nutrition, and related topics, combined with hands-on clinical training. Currently, the only school in Canada where you can learn to become a chiropractor is Canadian Memorial Chiropractic College, located in Toronto. Many chiropractors continue their training to obtain specialized certification—for example, in women's health, gerontology, or pediatrics.

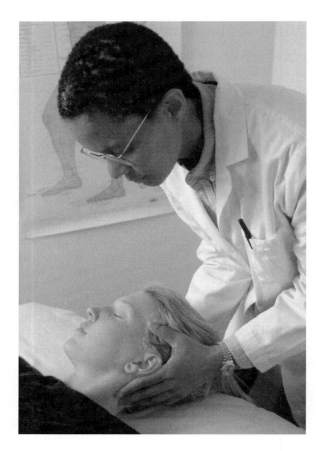

A chiropractor uses a variety of techniques to manipulate the spine into alignment.

You should investigate and question a chiropractor as carefully as you would a medical doctor. As with many health-care professionals, you may note vast differences in technique among specialists. It is recommended that you choose a chiropractor who follows standard chiropractic regimens for treating musculoskeletal conditions.

Massage Therapy

Massage therapy refers to the assessment and treatment of the body's soft tissues.[24] More specifically, massage therapy is used to treat soft-tissue injuries and dysfunctions (whiplash, sprains, strains, muscle spasms), diseases and disorders (osteoarthritis, rheumatoid arthritis, bronchitis), painful conditions such as low back or neck pain, and conditions with psychological implications such as stress, anxiety, or depression. The Canadian Massage Therapy Alliance recommends a two-year intensive program, equivalent to approximately 2200 hours of training. All provinces and territories have different requirements to become a registered massage therapist. Check out the Canadian Massage Therapist Alliance website at www.cmta.ca for the specific requirements related to where you live.

Many have found acupuncture an effective treatment for a variety of complaints.

Acupuncture and Acupressure

Acupuncture is the ancient (more than 2000 years old) Chinese art of inserting fine needles at points on the skin that fall along 14 major meridians, or pathways of energy (called *qi*), that flow through the body. These points and meridians are thought to be associated with particular internal organs and bodily functions. Proponents of acupuncture believe that the vital forces of life—the yin and the yang—are restored to equilibrium when these points are stimulated. Acupuncture has been effective for treating chronic pain and for blocking acute pain briefly.[25] Acupuncturists treat complaints as diverse as back and neck pain, menstrual cramps, morning sickness, addiction, asthma, infections, and arthritis. They also help women in labour and people who want to quit smoking.

The Acupuncture Foundation of Canada Institute teaches licensed health practitioners about acupuncture. Some licensed MDs and chiropractors have also trained in acupuncture. If you decide to have acupuncture, it is very important to ensure that the needles the acupuncturist uses are disposable or properly sterilized using an autoclave, because needles reused without sterilization can transmit hepatitis and HIV.

Acupressure is similar to acupuncture, but does not use needles. Instead, the practitioner applies pressure to points critical to balancing yin and yang. Practitioners must have the same basic understanding of energy pathways as acupuncturists. Acupressure should not be applied by an untrained person to pregnant women or anyone with a chronic condition.

Herbalists and Homeopaths

Herbalists practise herbal medicine, which is based on the medicinal qualities of plants or herbs. Homeopaths use herbal medicine (as well as minerals and chemicals), and at the root of their practice is the theory that administering extremely diluted doses of potent natural agents that produce disease symptoms in healthy persons will cure the disease in the sick. Herbal and homeopathic medicines are common in Europe and Asia, but not nearly as accepted in Canada.

try it NOW!

Find out from your college or university's health clinic what type of alternative therapies (non-allopathic treatments) are offered. Further, find out which alternative therapies you have coverage for and in what circumstances.

Although plants have been used for medicinal purposes for centuries and form the basis of many modern "wonder drugs," herbal medicine should not be taken lightly. Because something is natural—or grows on its own—does not necessarily mean that it is safe. Many plants are poisonous, and others can be toxic if consumed in high doses. One of the greatest dangers with this kind of therapy is that practitioners who mix their own tonics do not use standardized measures. It is therefore imperative that you carefully investigate the chemical properties of herbs yourself before you ingest them.

Naturopathy

Naturopaths believe that illness results from violations of natural principles of life in modern societies. They view diseases as the body's effort to ward off impurities and harmful substances from the environment. Naturopathic treatment uses substances and forces found in nature: water, magnets, gravity, heat, crystals and minerals, herbs, and even the sun. Practitioners argue that returning to a natural, purified state will restore health.

Thorough training to become a Naturopath is only provided at three naturopathic medical schools in the United States and Canada. Those who receive a naturopathic doctor (ND) degree from one of these schools have been through a four-year graduate program that emphasizes humanistically oriented family medicine. If you decide to be treated by a naturopath, you should carefully check his or her credentials.

Chiropractic medicine: A form of medical treatment that emphasizes the manipulation of the spinal column.

Health Care in Canada 2005: Executive Summary

Consistently identified as a top issue for Canadians, access to care is a priority from coast to coast. What matters most differs between regions of the country and over time—sometimes the focus is on wait times for hip replacements, sometimes finding a family doctor is a priority—but the underlying challenge is shared. Reflecting this reality, Canada's first ministers put timely access to quality care for all at the top of their agenda in the recent Ten-Year Plan to Strengthen Health Care.

The goal of *Health Care in Canada 2005* was to provide a window into the $130 billion health system by highlighting what we do and do not know about access to care and other emerging issues. This report focused on the relationship between surgical volumes and patient outcomes.

WHAT THE RESEARCH SAYS

Many studies across a variety of procedures, diseases, and health-care settings indicate that patients treated in centres with higher numbers of cases are less likely to die after surgery. A systematic review commissioned for this report—the largest ever conducted—found 161 journal articles on this topic published worldwide between 1979 and the spring of 2004. In more than two-thirds (68 percent) of the analyses, the greater the volume of procedures performed by a hospital or a physician, the better the outcomes. In a further 31 percent, the relationship between volumes and outcomes was either not statistically significant or undetermined. Only a few analyses (one percent) showed a significant association between higher volumes and poorer patient outcomes.

There are two theories often used to explain why higher volumes associate with better outcomes. The first is that "practice makes perfect." That is, high volume centres may have more experienced teams and a broader range of resources. The second is that these hospitals and care providers have better outcomes because physicians tend to refer more patients to centres of excellence. This theory is known as "selective referral." Regardless of which theory is correct (or if both have some merit), much remains to be learned about the nature of the link between volumes and outcomes and the potential effects of consolidating care in centres of excellence.

NEW FINDINGS FOR CANADA

The bulk of existing volume-outcome research (about 80 percent) comes from the United States. To further explore the relationship in Canada, we studied the risk of dying in hospital within 30 days of admission for nine different types of surgery. Our analyses covered more than 180 000 surgeries performed between 1998–1999 and 2003–2004 (excluding procedures in Quebec and parts of Manitoba). Adjusted mortality rates ranged from 0.2 percent to 5.9 percent.

The results confirm that hospitals that perform higher numbers of selected procedures tend to have better outcomes, but the nature and strength of the relationship varies. In three of the nine selected procedures, we found a steady drop in the risk of death with higher volumes, after taking patient characteristics and the year the procedure was performed into account. For example, for every 10 additional procedures

performed in a hospital, the risk of mortality was 44 percent lower for esophagectomies (complete or partial surgical removal of the esophagus) and 46 percent lower for pancreatic cancer surgery. A smaller, but still statistically significant, effect was also seen for angioplasty (one percent reduction). For the six other procedures, either no statistically significant relationship was observed, or a difference was seen only between hospitals performing the highest and lowest volumes of surgery.

CONSOLIDATING CARE: TRADE-OFFS TO BE MADE?

Across the country, decisions are made to concentrate care in centres of excellence—or not to—on a regular basis. For both relatively rare operations and more common procedures, there are large variations in the number of hospitals performing different types of surgery. Many hospitals conduct a very small number of procedures. A much smaller number of centres perform higher volumes of surgery. Cardiac surgery is among the most highly concentrated, reflecting decisions in many parts of the country to consolidate care within high-volume centres.

The issues involved in deciding how and when to consolidate care are clearly complex. The "right" balance likely varies from procedure to procedure and place to place. The potential travel burden for patients and families is just one of many factors that may weigh in the balance. A new survey of adults aged 20 and older across the country found that many respondents would prefer to have surgery at a hospital close to their home. But if forced to choose, quality was more important than closeness. Only 9 percent of those surveyed were primarily concerned with how close to home they received their care. More valued having a surgeon recommended by their family doctor (42 percent) or the number of similar procedures the surgeon had performed in the past (41 percent). However, less than half (38 percent) of those who actually had a procedure in the past two years said that they had been aware of the number of procedures that their surgeon had performed recently.

MONITORING KEY TRENDS

Almost all Canadians receive some type of health services each year. Visiting a doctor and taking medication are the most common types of care. In 2003, 80 percent of teens and adults said that they had consulted a physician in the past year. About the same number (84 percent) reported having taken prescription or non-prescription medication.

In addition to the detailed analyses of this year's focus topic, *Health Care in Canada 2005* highlights broad trends related to these and other health services.

Two chapters profiled health expenditures:

- Canada spent an estimated $130 billion on health care in 2004. That's approximately $4078 per Canadian. The amount spent represents about 10 percent of Canada's gross domestic product, placing fifth among OECD countries in 2002.

- Both public and private health expenditures are higher than in the past, but recent public-sector spending growth has outpaced that of the private sector.

- Hospitals, drugs, and physician services are the three largest categories of expenditures. In 2004, hospitals accounted for an estimated $39 billion—about 30 percent of all health-care expenditures. Hospital spending has grown an average of 7 percent per year since 1975. Retail spending on prescribed drugs, over-the-counter medications, and personal health supplies has doubled since 1996. It reached an estimated $21.8 bilon in 2004, about 17 percent of total health expenditures.

There were about 59 000 physicians practising in Canada. Spending on physician services rose 4.8 percent between 2003 and 2004, reaching an estimated $16.8 billion or 13 percent of total health spending.

The report also looked at Canadians' views on health care. For example:

- Most Canadians give high marks to their care. A 2003 Statistics Canada survey found that 85 percent of Canadians were very or somewhat satisfied with the care they had received in the last year, about the same number as in 2000–2001.

- As in other countries, Canadians tended to give higher ratings to the care that they or their families received than to the health-care system in general. In 2004, only 1 to 3 percent of adults in Canada, Australia, New Zealand, the United Kingdom, and the US said that their medical care in the past year was poor.

More (13 percent to 33 percent) said that their health system needed to be completely rebuilt. About one in seven Canadians (14 percent) felt this way. This is down from 23 percent in 1998, but higher than the 1988 level of 5 percent.

In addition, Health Indicators 2005 highlights how health, health care, and patient outcomes vary across the country. It offers comparative data on a range of health and health system indicators for health regions with a population of 75 000 or more and for provinces and territories, representing 95 percent of the Canadian population.

The thousands of Canadians wheeled into operating rooms every year all hope for good outcomes from surgery. Their age, state of health, and even where they live can make a difference. Other factors may also contribute to outcomes, including how early a diagnosis is made, the skills and experience of the health-care team, and the setting in which the surgery takes place. In recent years, researchers in several countries have explored the relationship between surgical volume and patient outcomes. Many studies—across a variety of procedures, diseases, and health-care settings—show improved clinical outcomes when patients are cared for by physicians or in hospitals performing a higher volume of procedures. The bulk of this research comes from the United States, but a few studies are from other countries. *Health Care in Canada 2005* provides new information on the relationship between volumes and outcomes of care in Canada.

Understanding this relationship, and what might be influencing it, is more than an academic question. There are practical implications for health policy and patient care that flow from this research and how results are interpreted. For example, policy-makers may consider the results as they weigh decisions about where different types of care should be provided. Individual Canadians also indicate that they want information that will inform their own choices. This report is a first step in responding to both sets of information needs.

To download a copy of the full report, go to: http://secure.cihi.ca/cihiweb/dispPage.jsp?cw_page=PG_376_E&cw_topic=376&cw_rel=AR_43_E

Canada produces a *Health Care in Canada* report each year, to download the most recent report, go to http://secure.cihi.ca/cihiweb/dispPage.jsp?cw_page=AR_43_E

Source: Canadian Institute for Health Information, *Health Care in Canada 2005*. Retrieved on May 19, 2006, from www.cihi.ca. The last two paragraphs of this box are extracted from the Introduction of *Health Care in Canada;* the rest is extracted from the Executive Summary.

✱ Other Alternative Therapies

Many other therapies exist, including reflexology (zone therapy), iridology (light therapy), aromatherapy, and auramassage. Some of these may work, but they have yet to be substantiated scientifically. Others may be harmful to your health or may delay you from seeking more efficacious forms of care. Until you can sort through the proliferation of new therapies, it's a good idea to follow the maxim "buyer beware."

what do you THINK?

Should people be allowed to choose any type of practitioner they want—regardless of whether the treatment has been scientifically proven to be safe or effective? How much should the government spend to investigate and/or regulate new and/or alternative therapies?

TYPES OF MEDICAL PRACTICES

Many health-care providers combine resources into a **group practice**, which can be single- or multi-specialty. Physicians share their offices, equipment, utility bills, and staff costs. Proponents of group practice maintain that it reduces unnecessary duplication of equipment and improves the quality of health care through peer review. **Solo practitioners** are medical providers who practise independently.

Hospitals and Clinics

Hospitals and clinics provide a range of health-care services. These include emergency treatment, diagnostic tests, and inpatient and outpatient (ambulatory) care.

There are several ways to classify hospitals: by profit status (non-profit or for-profit), by ownership (private, public), by specialty (children's, chronic care, psychiatric, general, acute), by teaching status (teaching-affiliated or not), and by size. **Non-profit (voluntary) hospitals** have traditionally been administered by religious or other humanitarian groups. Before universal health care, such hospitals cared for patients whether they could pay or not. Today, some hospitals retain religious ties and orientations; others are administered by independent hospital boards. There are few **for-profit (proprietary) hospitals** in Canada, though they are increasing in number as our health-care system continues to struggle to balance needs and services in a timely manner. For-profit hospitals do not receive tax breaks and tend to focus on particular specialties.

More treatments or services, including surgery, are delivered on an **outpatient (ambulatory) care** basis (care which does not involve an overnight stay) by hospitals, traditional clinics, student health clinics, and nontraditional clinical centres. One type of ambulatory facility is the surgicentre—a place where minor, low-risk procedures such as vasectomies, tubal ligations, tissue biopsies, cosmetic surgery, abortions, and minor eye operations are performed.

Hospitals have made efforts to improve the quality of care and patient outcomes. Many hospitals are now designated as trauma centres. They have helicopters available to transport patients to the hospital quickly, specialty physicians in-house (not just on call) around the clock, and specialized diagnostic equipment. This combination of rapid transport and readily available specialty equipment and staff has dramatically reduced mortality rates for trauma patients. One drawback, however, is that trauma centres are exceptionally expensive to run.

PROMISES AND PROBLEMS OF CANADA'S HEALTH-CARE SYSTEM

Since the beginning, Canada's health-care system has been a work in progress.[26] Over the past 40 to 50 years, reforms have been made and will continue to be made in response to changes within medicine and demands from society. Regardless, the underlying concepts of Canada's health-care system, known to Canadians as "medicare," remain the same: universal coverage for medically necessary health-care services provided on the basis of need, rather than the ability to pay.

Even though we have one of the best health-care systems in the world, there are problems with the system. First, several levels of government are involved in delivering the services. The federal government funds health care, provided the provinces meet the guidelines. The federal government also funds and administers health programs for special groups such as First Nations peoples, war veterans, and prisoners. Using federal dollars, the provinces allot monies to health care. As governments struggle to reduce deficits and/or manage the recession, there is less money available even though health-care costs continue to rise. Reduced or limited health-care spending, often results in downsizing and restructuring. These organizational divisions and increased fiscal pressures add tension between the federal and provincial governments over power, dollars, and responsibilities.

Physicians and provincial governments have also been in conflict. The provinces are responsible for medical programs and the allocation of dollars, while physicians control access to programs and institutions. Some provinces provide bonuses for physicians working in remote areas or reduce payments to physicians working in over-serviced areas. As well, other stakeholders such as midwives, nurses, and dietitians vie for financial resources and recognition for their contributions to the health status of Canadians.

Another source of pressure for funding is the many voluntary organizations that help Canadians, some long-established. For example, the Canadian National Institute for the Blind has been in operation since before Confederation. These organizations (for instance, Heart and Stroke Foundation, Canadian Cancer Society, etc.) also solicit funds from the general population.

Health research is also supported by federal monies. Direct-care health services (hospitals and physicians, for example) compete for dollars with research and prevention. Prevention runs a weak third, accounting for only about 5 percent of total health spending in 1996. Figure 15.3 shows Canada's place on a spectrum of public versus private health systems.

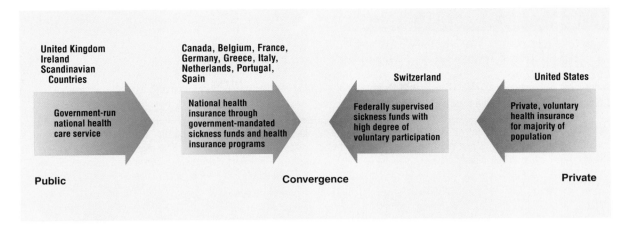

FIGURE 15.3

The Convergence of Public/Private Health-Care Systems

Source: Reprinted with permission from Gunter Becher, "European Health Issues," *Employee Benefits Journal* 38 (March 1993), published by the International Foundation of Employee Benefit Plans, Brookfield, WI.

Access

Your access to health care is determined by numerous factors, including the supply of providers and facilities and your health status. Doctors are generally not well distributed by specialty and geographic area. Some rural areas face constant shortages of physicians.

Quality Assurance

The Canadian health-care system employs several mechanisms for ensuring quality services overall: education, licensure, certification or registration, accreditation, peer review, and, as a last resort, the legal system of malpractice litigation. Some of these mechanisms are mandatory before a professional organization may provide care, while others are purely voluntary. Consumers should note that licensure, although provincially mandated for some practitioners and facilities, is only a minimum guarantee of quality.

Detecting Fraud and Abuse in the System

Becoming knowledgeable and acting responsibly when selecting health-care providers and payers reduces the likelihood of financial or physical abuse. Nevertheless, with the number of options in health products and services available, even the most careful consumer can be victimized. Individual provinces

maintain boards for quality assurance in the medical system. If you find yourself in a situation you cannot deal with, remember that the Health Protection Branch of Health Canada, the provincial ministries of health, and the colleges/universities of various professions are responsible for protecting you and other health consumers. Do not hesitate to contact them if you have suspicions about a provider, service, or product.

what do you THINK?

What do you think about Canada's health-care system? Do you think it is in crisis? Why or why not? Do you think the system will be able to continue to handle the needs of the population? Why or why not?

Group practice: A group of physicians who combine resources, including offices, equipment, and staff, to render care to patients.

Solo practitioner: Physician who renders care to patients independently of others.

Non-profit (voluntary) hospitals: Hospitals funded by the people through taxes.

For-profit (proprietary) hospitals: Hospitals that provide a return on earnings to the investors; not funded by the government.

Outpatient (ambulatory) care: Treatment that does not involve an overnight stay in a hospital.

Canadians Open to Health User Fees, Poll Finds

Most Canadians are open to major changes to Medicare, including digging into their own pockets for services, as long as a single-tier, universally accessible system is preserved, a recent survey suggests.

The Environics Research poll of 2000 health professionals and 3300 other adults finds that most Canadians believe the health-care system is in a state of crisis.

The greatest concern relates to the amount of time people have to wait for medical services. However, most people oppose ratcheting up government spending to solve the problems.

"People are saying, 'If the system is overloaded and it can't sustain itself, then I'm willing to pay a small user fee,'" said Diana MacDonald, a senior associate with Environics Research.

The poll found that eight in 10 respondents want significant reforms to Medicare, but only one in 10 would approve of a system in which those who can afford to pay for medical services get better or faster care.

"People really do believe in universality," said MacDonald. "They don't want to see a private and a public system."

A minority of Canadians said they would be willing to pay higher taxes, but a majority said they favoured a variety of reforms, including measures that would reduce the need for large infusions of cash.

Overall, two-thirds of respondents said they were open to a range of strategies that included user fees—as long as low-income Canadians were exempt—and more intensive use was made of nurses and other health practitioners instead of doctors.

However, 45 percent of those asked said they favoured market-oriented changes such as private delivery of health-care services, provided those services also remained publicly funded.

"We're always told that (people) are not open to a lot of reform, they want things as they are," said MacDonald. "But they are open to reform and we think that's startling."

Half of those surveyed said they favoured a greater emphasis on prevention and health promotion.

Environics billed the survey as the most comprehensive ever done in Canada of the attitudes and behaviours of the public and health professionals toward health-care issues.

However, the company cited client confidentiality in refusing to release a breakdown of the actual questions posed or even a detailed breakdown of the results.

Source: The Canadian Press

HEALTH SERVICE ORGANIZATIONS: A NEW MODEL OF HEALTH CARE

The dominant model of medicine in Canada is fee-for-service. A practitioner, most often a physician, performs a service and bills the provincial health plan. Planners have been searching for other models that would contain costs while providing improved services and encouraging prevention and shared responsibility. One model already in place is the health service organization (HSO). The patient registers with the organization, which is funded a set amount per patient per year (capitation), and is responsible for the patient's overall care. The originators of this model believed it would encourage practitioners and patients alike to emphasize prevention.

There are currently 87 HSOs in Ontario alone, serving more than half a million patients. Many are run by community-based boards. In Ontario, the community health branch of the provincial Ministry of Health is responsible for the HSOs, and defines the program's objectives as follows:

- to create an atmosphere that supports physicians and other health-care personnel, and that allows flexibility in responding to health-care needs
- to develop a coordinated system of health-care delivery that makes the most appropriate use of health-care resources and is accessible, efficient, and economical
- to provide special attention to health maintenance and illness prevention
- to decrease institutional health care by giving emphasis to outpatient care, self-care, and home care

HSOs may offer a more comprehensive range of services than the conventional system. For example, counselling is available through HSOs as part of the service. If you live in Ontario, your physician may be a member of an HSO, so additional services may be available at no cost to you.

TAKING CHARGE

Managing Your Health-Care Needs

Throughout this text, we have emphasized behaviours important to keeping you healthy. Now we focus your attention on your attitudes and behaviours about when and how to seek medical attention. Most people wait until a problem arises to seek medical care and take the first available physician or medical facility. But by looking ahead to future needs, you can take charge of your choices and make positive moves toward getting more effective and efficient health care.

MAKING DECISIONS FOR YOU

As you have seen in this chapter, many health-care decisions are dictated by physicians and government agencies. Still, many decisions rest with you.

CHECKLIST FOR CHANGE: MAKING PERSONAL CHOICES

Considering the following questions may help you in obtaining excellent health care from your medical practitioner.

- How long did you have to wait before getting an appointment?
- How long did you have to wait in the waiting room before being seen?
- Do the clerical staff convey their concern for you when delays occur?
- Are there educational materials available in the waiting areas?
- Are the medical practitioner's credentials clearly displayed?
- Does the medical practitioner treat you as if he or she is concerned about you?
- Do you feel comfortable discussing your problems with the medical practitioner?
- Are you confident that your medical practitioner knows what he or she is talking about?
- Is the medical practitioner willing to talk about issues such as credentials, hospital affiliations, and qualifications of referrals for special needs?

- Are you able to understand answers to your questions? Does the medical practitioner seem interested in whether you understand? Seem willing to answer questions? Encourage you to ask questions?
- Does the medical practitioner tell you why one test is being given rather than another? About risks of the test? About preparation for the tests? About what to expect concerning certain results?
- Does the medical practitioner support you in obtaining a second opinion, or does he or she seem irritated with such a request?
- If you became seriously ill and had to see a lot of this medical practitioner, would you feel comfortable with him or her, or would you rather have someone else?

CHECKLIST FOR CHANGE: MAKING COMMUNITY CHOICES

The following questions may help you in determining the level of health-care service available in your community.

- What health-care services are located in your community?
- How long has your doctor been practising in your community?
- How many hospitals are within a 30-minute drive of your home? Are any of them teaching hospitals?

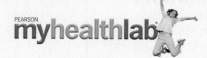

PEARSON
myhealthlab

Go to MyHealthLab at **www.pearsoned.ca/myhealthlab**. Here you will find self-assessments, case studies, links to health on the net, and much more.

DISCUSSION QUESTIONS

1. Describe one dubious claim made by a health-care product (such as fat-reducing creams, hair-growth tonics, muscle-building milkshakes, etc.). Why do marketers use such claims when advertising their products? Why do consumers buy such products?

2. List some conditions (resulting from illness or accident) for which you do not need to seek medical help. If the symptoms increase in severity, at what point would you seek medical attention? How do you decide to whom and where to go for treatment?

3. What are the differences in education between allopathic and non-allopathic practitioners? Under what circumstances would you seek treatment from a non-allopathic practitioner? Which types of non-allopathic medicine appeal to you? Why? Which types of non-allopathic medicine do not appeal to you? Why not?

4. What are the benefits and risks of group practices?

5. Discuss the problems of the Canadian health-care system. If you were Minister of Health, what would you propose as a solution—provincially and/or nationally? Which groups might oppose your plan? Which groups might support it?

6. Should governments dictate costs for various medical tests and procedures in an attempt to manage the finances of the health-care system?

APPLICATION EXERCISE

Reread the "Consider This ..." scenario at the beginning of the chapter and answer the following questions.

1. When you have a medical problem like Petra's, where do you go for medical attention? How do you know if you are getting good advice?

2. Make up a list of questions for Petra to ask each physician so that she has a better understanding of her diagnosis and the recommended treatment plan.

MYSEARCHLAB EXERCISE

1. Log on to www.MySearchLab.com.

2. Retrieve article AN 20612601, "The Health Care Philosophy That Nearly Destroyed Medicare in Canada in a Single Decade," by I. T. Beck and M. Thomson.

3. Read the article and respond to the following:

   a. What health-care philosophy almost destroyed medicare?
   b. What happened as a result?
   c. What was put in its place?
   d. Has the health-care system rebounded (that is, is adequate care provided)? Has it rebounded effectively? Why or why not?
   e. What currently challenges Canada's health-care system? How are these challenges similar to and different from previous challenges?

CHAPTER 16

LIFE'S TRANSITIONS

The Aging Process

CONSIDER THIS . . .

Choi, aged 82, is a springboard diver. She walks 10 blocks every morning to the city pool, where she practises her diving and swims for about an hour. Susan, aged 79, is an internationally recognized expert in family dysfunction. She travels extensively, giving several lectures a week, volunteering her services to community groups and maintaining an active social life. Andre, aged 83, is a professional writer and recently learned how to run the latest versions of software programs on his computer. He keeps in touch with his children and grandchildren using various modes of electronic communication.

What do all these people have in common? Are these people atypical? Why or why not? What factors do you think contributed to their healthy aging? Do you know any elderly people like them? How do these people compare to your grandparents?

CHAPTER OBJECTIVES

- Define aging, and explain the related concepts of biologic, psychological, social, legal, and functional age.

- Discuss the biological and psychosocial theories of aging along with the major physiological and psychological changes that occur as a result of the aging process.

- Define death and explain why people deny it.

- Describe the grief process, grief work, and strategies for coping more effectively.

- Identify the ethical concerns that arise from the concepts of the right to die and rational suicide.

Growing old does not have to entail declining physical and mental health. Health promotion, disease prevention and wellness-oriented activities prolong vigour and productivity, even among those who may not have always led a model lifestyle or made healthy choices a priority. Getting older can mean getting better in many ways—particularly socially, psychologically, spiritually, and intellectually.

The manner in which you view aging (either as a natural part of living or as an inevitable move toward disease and death) is an important factor in how successfully you will adapt to life's transitions. If you view these transitions as opportunities for growth—as changes that lead to improved mental, emotional, spiritual, and physical phases in your development as a human being—your journey will be smooth. Explore your own knowledge of aging in the Rate Yourself box.

Aging has traditionally been described as the patterns of life changes that occur in members of all species as they grow older. Some believe that it begins at the moment of conception. Others contend that it starts at birth. Still others believe that true aging does not begin until we reach our 40s. Typically, chronologic age (that is, age based on birthdate) is used to assign a person to a particular life-cycle stage. However, people of different chronologic ages view age very differently. To the 4-year-old, a university or college student seems quite old. To the 20-year-old, parents in their 40s are over the hill. Have you ever heard your 65-year-old grandparents talking about "those old people down the street"? Views of aging are also coloured by occupation. For example, a professional linebacker may find himself too old to play football in his mid-30s. Airline pilots and police officers often retire in their 50s, while professors, senators, and prime ministers may work well into their 70s.

❋ REDEFINING AGING

Discrimination against people based on age is known as **ageism**. When directed against the elderly, this type of discrimination carries with it social ostracism and negative portrayals of older people. A developmental task approach to life-span changes tends to reduce the potential for ageist or negatively biased perceptions about what occurs as a person ages chronologically. The study of individual and collective aging processes, called **gerontology**, explores the reasons for aging and the ways in which people cope with and adapt to this process. Gerontologists have identified several types of age-related characteristics that should be used to determine where a person is in terms of biologic,

psychological, social, legal, and functional life-stage development:[1]

- *Biologic age* refers to the relative age or condition of the person's organs and body systems. Arthritis and other chronic conditions often accelerate biologic age.

- *Psychological age* refers to a person's adaptive capacities, such as coping abilities and intelligence, and to the person's awareness of his or her individual capabilities, self-efficacy, and general ability to adapt to a given situation.

- *Social age* refers to a person's habits and roles relative to society's expectations. People in a particular life stage often share similar tastes in music, television shows, and decor.

- *Legal or chronologic age* is probably the most common definition of age in Canada. Legal age is based on chronological years and is used to determine such things as voting rights, driving privileges, drinking age, eligibility for Old Age Security and Canada Pension Plan benefits, and a host of other rights and obligations.

- *Functional age* refers to the ways in which people compare to others of a similar age. It is difficult to separate functional aging from other types of aging, particularly chronologic and biologic aging.

WHAT IS NORMAL AGING?

Contemporary gerontologists analyze the vast majority of people who continue to live full and productive lives throughout their later years. In the past, our youth-oriented society viewed the onset of the physiological changes of aging as something to be dreaded. The aging process was seen primarily from a pathological (disease) perspective, and therefore as a time of decline; the focus was not on the gains and positive aspects of normal adult development throughout the life span. Many of these positive developments occur in the areas of emotional and social life as older adults learn to cope with and adapt to the many changes and crises that life has in store for them.

Aging: The patterns of life changes that occur in a species as they grow older.

Ageism: Discrimination based on age.

Gerontology: The study of individual and collective aging processes.

Aging Quiz

Test your knowledge of healthy aging by taking the following test. Answer true or false to each statement. The answers are listed below.

1. Men usually outlive women.
2. If your parents had Alzheimer's disease, you will also get it.
3. Dietary intake and physical activity can reduce the risk of developing osteoporosis.
4. Heart disease affects women as much as men.
5. The older you get, the less sleep you need.
6. People should reduce their caloric intake as they age.
7. People take more medications as they age.
8. As your body changes with age, so does your personality.
9. Intelligence declines with age.
10. Most older people live alone.
11. Most people become "senile" if they live long enough.
12. Physical strength tends to decline with age.
13. Most older adults limit their travel to be closer to home.
14. Older adults have the lowest income of all adult groups.
15. Most older adults have no interest in, or capacity for, sexual activity.
16. People tend to become more religious with age.
17. People tend to change their driving habits as they age.
18. Older people are more likely to commit suicide than younger people.
19. Many older people are preoccupied with death.
20. Most older people new to Canada speak neither English nor French.

ANSWERS

1. False. Women have an average life expectancy greater than men. In 2003, a boy born is expected to live to 77.4 years, while a girl born in the same year is expected to live to 82.4 years or 5 years longer.
2. False. Between 90 and 95 percent of people with Alzheimer's disease have a form of the disease not necessarily linked to family history. Only 5 percent of Alzheimer's cases are a result of a genetic link.
3. True. Bone loss can be reduced by eating foods rich in calcium (for example, milk and other dairy products; dark green, leafy vegetables; canned salmon; sardines; and tofu) and engaging in regular, weight-bearing physical activity, such as walking and resistance training.
4. True. Heart disease is one of the leading causes of death for men and women.
5. False. Although quality of sleep declines when we age, required sleep time does not. Further, sleep tends to get more fragmented as we get older.
6. True. Older people need fewer calories because of decreases in metabolic function and physical activity. If an involuntary

weight gain or loss of 5 kilograms or more occurs in six months, a physician should be consulted.
7. True. Most Canadian older adults take some form of prescription or over-the-counter medication. Further, older adults (85+) are more likely than younger older adults (65–74) to take more than one medication (65 versus 52 percent).
8. False. Other than personality changes associated with Alzheimer's disease and other forms of dementia, personality does not change appreciably as you age.
9. False. Although studies show that the elderly have a slower reaction time and take longer to learn something new, their intellect is maintained and can be improved as they get older.
10. False. The majority of Canadian older adults (69 percent) live with their family or extended family.
11. False. Dementia ("senility" is not the correct term) is not a normal part of aging. One in 50 older adults between the ages of 65 and 74, one in nine older adults between the ages of 75 and 84, and one in three older adults over the age of 85 will develop dementia.
12. True. Physical strength does decrease with age—as does the quality of the muscles. Decreases in strength can be reduced by regular participation in physical activity, including resistance training.
13. False. In fact, some older adults are more likely to travel abroad than younger adults.
14. True. In 1997, 19 percent of all older adults (65+) had an income below the low-income cut-off. Women (24 percent) are more likely than men (11.7 percent) to have a low income.
15. False. Aging does not equate to a loss of interest in or capacity for sex.
16. False. Despite a perception that people tend to become more religious with age, this is not true. This perception may reflect a difference between generations rather than a characteristic of aging.
17. True. To accommodate the changes associated with aging many older adults modify their driving behaviour by planning their trips, driving less, limiting highway travel, and avoiding driving in poor weather or at night.
18. False. Overall, older adults in Canada are less likely to commit suicide than are younger adults.
19. False. Older adults' attitudes toward death are variable, though some trends can be noted. Specifically, older adults are less anxious and more matter-of-fact about death. Most young adults avoid thinking about or discussing death.
20. True. The majority (61 percent) of older immigrants to Ontario from 1996 to 1999 spoke neither English nor French.

Source: Adapted from the Ontario Gerontology Association, "Aging Quiz." Retrieved on May 16, 2006, from http://ontgerontology.on.ca.

Gerontologists have devised several categories for specific age-related characteristics. For example, people who reach the age of 65 are considered to fit the general category of "old age." They receive special consideration in the form of government assistance programs such as the old age pension. People aged 65 to 74 are viewed as the **young-old**; those aged 75 to 84 are the **middle-old** group; those 85 and over are classified as the **old-old**.

You should note that chronological age is not the only component considered when objectively defining aging. The question is not how many years a person has lived, but how much life a person has packed into those years. This quality-of-life index, combined with the inevitable chronological process, appears to be the best indicator of the "aging gracefully" phenomenon. The eternal question then becomes, "How can I age gracefully?" Most experts agree that the best way to experience a productive, full, and satisfying old age is to take appropriate action to lead a productive, full, and satisfying life *prior* to old age. Essentially, older people are the product of their lifelong experiences, moulded over years of happiness, heartbreak, and day-to-day existence.

WHO ARE THE ELDERLY?

Contrary to popular belief, the elderly are not and never will be the "forgotten minority." The 65-and-over age group will unquestionably continue to be a major force in the social, political, and economic plans of the nation because of their sheer numbers (see Table 16.1) and buying power. Canadian seniors are living longer lives in better health than in the past. By the year 2010, a whole generation of 1960s "flower children," who once proclaimed that no one over 30 could be trusted, will become 65 years old. Whereas people aged 65 and older made up less than 10 percent of the population in 1981, they are projected to make up more than 20 percent by 2031. In 2006, it was estimated that 13.7 percent of the Canadian population were 65 years of age or older (see Table 16.2).[2]

> ## what do you THINK?
> How do you define aging? What do you think of becoming old? How much interaction do you have with people over the age of 65?

> ## ✳ try it NOW!
> Estimate your life expectancy. How long you live involves more than good genes. Health behaviours that you can control have a direct impact on whether or not you will live to see 100. Visit this life expectancy calculator to see how long you are likely to live, given your history and current habits: www.livingto100.com.

For a more detailed profile of today's elderly, download "Canada's Aging Population," a report prepared by Health Canada in collaboration with the Interdepartmental Committee on Aging and Seniors Issues, at www.globalaging.org/elderrights/world/canada.pdf.

THEORIES ON AGING

Biologic Theories

Explanations about the biologic causes of aging include:

- The wear-and-tear theory, which states that, like everything else in the universe, the human body wears out. Inherent in this theory is the idea that

TABLE 16.1
Canada's Elderly

Age	Total	Men	Women
65–69	1 193 500	574 400	619 100
70–74	1 042 600	488 600	554 000
75–79	864 300	377 700	486 500
80–84	625 300	241 700	383 600
85–89	322 500	107 100	215 400
90 and over	169 500	44 600	125 000

Source: Statistics Canada, "Population by Sex and Age Group." Retrieved on May 16, 2006, from www40.statcan.ca/101/cst01/demo10a.htm.

TABLE 16.2

Age Structure of Population, Medium-Growth Scenario (in millions)

Number

Age	2000	2006	2016	2026	2036	2051
0 to 14	5869	5527	5241	5382	5203	5053
15 to 64	21 018	22 400	23 477	23 056	22 765	22 440
65 and over	3863	4302	5702	7753	9067	9366
Total	30 750	32 229	34 420	36 191	37 035	36 860

Percentage

Age	2000	2006	2016	2026	2036	2051
0 to 14	19.1	17.1	15.2	14.9	14.0	13.7
15 to 64	68.3	69.5	68.2	63.7	61.5	60.9
65 and over	12.6	13.3	16.6	21.4	24.5	25.4

Source: Statistics Canada, "2006 Census: Portrait of the Canadian Population in 2006, by Age and Sex: Highlights." Retrieved on March 30, 2009, from www12.statcan.ca/census-recensement/2006/as-sa/97-551/p1-eng.cfm.

the more you abuse your body and/or the more you do not treat it as well as you can, the faster it will wear out.

- The cellular theory, which states that at birth we have only a certain number of usable cells, and these cells are genetically programmed to divide or reproduce only a limited number of times. Once these cells reach the end of their reproductive cycle, they begin to die and the organs they make up begin to show signs of deterioration. The rate of deterioration varies from person to person, and the impact of the deterioration depends on the system involved.

- The autoimmune theory, which attributes aging to the decline of the body's immunological system. Studies indicate that as we age, our immune systems become less effective in fighting disease. Lifestyle can contribute negatively to this process in bodies subjected to too much stress, lack of sleep, a poor dietary intake, inactivity, and so on. Although autoimmune diseases occur in all age groups, some gerontologists believe that they increase in frequency and severity with age.

- The genetic mutation theory, which proposes that the number of cells exhibiting unusual or different characteristics increases with age. In this theory, it is believed that aging relates to the amount of

For many, the secret to aging well is to remain physically active, eat well, and enjoy the company of good friends.

mutational damage within the genes. The greater the mutation, the greater the chance that cells will not function properly, leading to eventual dysfunction of body organs and systems.

Young-old: People aged 65 to 74 years.

Middle-old: People aged 75 to 84 years.

Old-old: People 85 years and over.

Psychosocial Theories

Numerous psychological and sociological factors also have a strong influence on the manner in which people age. Psychologists have formulated theories of personality development that encompass the human life span. These theories emphasize adaptation and adjustment. In the developmental model, it is noted that people must progress through eight critical stages during their lifetime. If a person does not receive adequate stimulation or develop effective methods of coping with life's stresses from infancy onward, problems are likely to develop later in life. According to this theory, attitudes, behaviours, and beliefs related to maladjustments in old age are often a result of problems encountered in earlier stages of a person's life. Specifically, the developmental theory focuses on the crucial issues of middle and old age because it is believed that during these periods people face a series of increasingly stressful tasks. Those who are poorly adjusted psychologically or who have not developed appropriate coping skills are likely to undergo a painful aging process.

A key element in these theories is the incorporation of age-related factors into lifelong behaviour patterns. Both models (biological and psychosocial) emphasize that successful aging involves maintaining emotional as well as physical well-being. Most probably, a combination of psychosocial and biologic factors as well as environmental "trigger mechanisms" cause each of us to age in a unique manner.

CHANGES IN THE BODY AND MIND

Answers to the question of what is "typical" or "normal" when applied to aging are highly speculative. In order to assess the typical aging process, we should ask ourselves what we can reasonably expect to happen to our bodies as we grow older. Keep in mind that despite physical changes that occur, 76 percent of seniors 65 to 74 years old and 68 percent of seniors over 75 years of age reported their health to be "good," "very good," or "excellent."[3]

Physical Changes

Although the physiological consequences of aging differ in their severity and timing from person to person, there are standard changes that occur.

The Skin

As we age, the skin becomes thinner and loses elasticity, particularly in the outer surfaces. Fat deposits, which add to the soft lines and shape of the skin, begin to diminish. Starting at about age 30, lines develop on the forehead as a result of smiling, squinting, and other facial expressions. These lines become more pronounced, with added "crow's-feet" around the eyes, during the 40s. During a person's 50s and 60s, the skin begins to sag and lose colour, leading to pallor in the 70s. Body fat in underlying layers of skin continues to be redistributed away from the limbs and extremities into the trunk region of the body. Age spots become more numerous because of excessive pigment accumulation under the skin. The sun tends to increase pigment production, leading to more age spots.

Bones and Joints

Bones are the most metabolically active tissue in our bodies, in a continual state of modelling or remodelling.[4] Bone mineral accrual exceeds bone mineral loss during our growing years. Then, once we are fully grown, our bone mineral accrual and loss are at about the same rate, with our bones maintaining their integrity and strength. Then, in mid-to-late adult life, generally during menopause in women, and a little later in men, bone mineral loss exceeds bone mineral accumulation, resulting in a deterioration of bone tissue in which bones become fragile and brittle and at an increased risk of fracture. This loss of bone mineral content occurs in men and women, although it tends to occur at a faster rate in women, especially after menopause. Loss of bone mineral content contributes to **osteoporosis**, a condition characterized by weakened, porous, and fractured bones.

Although many people consider osteoporosis a disease of the elderly, it is actually a progressive disorder with roots firmly established in childhood and adolescence. In fact, osteoporosis prevention begins in childhood by developing the strongest bones possible with the greatest reservoir of bone mineral content. When you hear of osteoporosis, you likely envision a slumped-over individual with a characteristic "dowager's hump" in the upper back, but this is the rare extreme. Bone loss occurs over many years and without symptoms until fractures occur. The spine, hips, and wrists are the most common sites of fractures, though other bones of the body may be involved.[5]

Osteoporotic fractures of the hip, vertebrae, proximal humerus, pelvis, and wrist increase in incidence with age and are more common among women. It is estimated that one in four women aged 60 years and over will have an osteoporotic fracture.[6] Further, about one-third of all women aged 65 and over have vertebral osteoporosis. About 70 percent of all fractures among individuals over the age of 45 result from osteoporosis. Several risk factors for developing osteoporosis have been identified:[7]

- Sex: Women's risk is four times greater than men's. Their peak bone mass is lower than men's, and they experience an accelerated rate of bone loss after menopause.

- Age: After the third and fourth decade of life, most individuals begin to lose bone mass and are more susceptible—particularly if sedentary.

- Low bone mass: Low bone mass is one of the strongest predictors of osteoporosis. Measurement of bone density is an important aspect of risk assessment. Low bone mass is often a result of inadequate bone-growth stimulation (inactivity), poor dietary intake (lack of total calories and insufficient calcium intake), estrogen suppression (delayed onset of menarche, amenorrhea), and smoking.

- Early menopause: The early occurrence of menopause, whether natural or caused by surgery, means that the positive effects of estrogen occur for a shorter period of time. (Decreases in sex hormones—estrogen in females and testosterone in males—increase risk for osteoporosis.) Menstrual disturbances, such as those caused by anorexia nervosa or bulimia nervosa or excessive exercise without an adequate dietary intake, may similarly result in an early loss of bone minerals.

- Thin, small-framed body: Petite, thin women usually have a relatively low bone mass and are therefore at greater risk for osteoporosis.

- Ethnicity: Caucasians and Asians are at higher risk of developing osteoporosis than individuals of African descent. Individuals of African descent have greater bone density, on average, than individuals of Caucasian or Asian descent. And women of African descent have about half the incidence of hip fractures of women of Caucasian descent.

- Lack of calcium and vitamin D: A lifetime of low calcium and vitamin D intake may result in a lower than expected peak bone mineral content and above-average loss of bone mineral content throughout adulthood.

- Lack of physical activity: Immobilized, bedridden, and inactive people have less muscle and bone mass.

- Cigarette smoking: Since cigarette smoking suppresses estrogen, bone mineral accrual is negatively affected.

- Heredity: Hereditary factors may play a role in the development of osteoporosis; these factors relate to body size as well as the body's efficiency at using calcium and other minerals to build bone.

The goal of treatment and prevention of osteoporosis is to decrease the likelihood and severity of bone fractures. Currently accepted treatments of established osteoporosis include enhancing calcium and vitamin D intake, engaging in daily weight-bearing physical activity, fall-prevention measures, and potentially hormonal supplementation (in individuals not at high risk for certain forms of cancer).[8] One study indicated that increasing calcium intake to 1380 mg per day—an amount that exceeds the current DRI for calcium—reduces bone loss and increases bone mineralization in women aged 58 to 77.[9] Other therapies for osteoporosis, such as sodium fluoride, various metabolites of vitamin D, and bisphosphonates, are under investigation.[10]

The most effective method of preventing osteoporosis is to develop strong, dense bones during growth. Critical to developing strong bones is sufficient calcium intake during childhood and young adulthood[11] as well as weight-bearing or weight resistance (that is, bone-growth-stimulating) physical activity. For adolescent males and females (ages 15 to 18 years), an adequate intake of calcium is 1300 mg per day.[12] Children and adolescents should also do 30 minutes of vigorous-intensity and 60 minutes of moderate-intensity physical activities almost every day of the week.[13] Once strong bones are developed, the next critical step is to maintain them and delay the onset of bone mineral loss. This can most effectively be done by maintaining a healthy dietary intake and remaining physically active. Regular physical activity of weight-bearing joints, maintenance of muscular strength and flexibility, and an adequate intake of calcium are probably your best routes of osteoporosis prevention during early, middle, and late adulthood.

Another bone condition that affects a large number of people is osteoarthritis, a progressive breakdown of joint cartilage. Osteoarthritis becomes more common with age and is a leading cause of disability.

The Head

With age, features of the head enlarge and become more noticeable. Increased cartilage and fatty tissue cause the nose to grow 1.25 cm wider and another 1.25 cm longer. Earlobes get thicker and grow longer, while overall head circumference increases 0.6 cm per decade, even though the brain itself shrinks.

The Urinary Tract

One problem often associated with aging is **urinary incontinence**, which ranges from passing a few drops

---

Osteoporosis: A degenerative bone disease characterized by loss of bone mineral density resulting in an increased fracture risk.

Urinary incontinence: The inability to control urination.

of urine while laughing or sneezing to having little or no control when and where urination takes place. This condition affects 22 percent of older men and 35 percent of older women.[14] Incontinence poses major social, physical, and emotional problems for the elderly. Embarrassment and fear of wetting oneself may cause an older person to become isolated and avoid social functions. Caregivers may become frustrated. Prolonged wetness and the inability to properly care for oneself can lead to irritation, infections, and other problems. However, incontinence is not an inevitable part of the aging process. Most cases are caused by highly treatable underlying neurological problems that affect the central nervous system, medications, infections of the pelvic muscles, weakness in the pelvic walls, or other problems. When the problem is treated, incontinence usually vanishes.[15]

The Heart and Lungs

Assuming physical fitness levels do not fluctuate dramatically, resting heart rate remains about the same during an adult's life. Stroke volume (the amount of blood the muscle pumps per beat), however, diminishes as heart muscles deteriorate. Vital capacity, or the amount of air that moves when you inhale and exhale at maximum effort, also declines with age. Aerobic physical activity is effective at reducing and slowing the age-related deterioration expected in heart and lung function.

✳ Eyesight

By the age of 30, the lens of the eye begins to harden, causing specific problems by the early 40s. The lens begins to yellow and loses transparency, while the pupil of the eye begins to shrink, allowing less light to penetrate. Activities such as reading become more difficult, particularly in dim light. By age 60, depth perception declines and farsightedness often develops. A need for glasses usually develops in the 40s that evolves into a need for bifocals in the 50s and trifocals in the 60s. **Cataracts** (clouding of the lens) and **glaucoma** (elevation of pressure within the eyeball) become more likely. There may eventually be a tendency toward colour-blindness, especially for shades of blue and green. **Macular degeneration** is the breakdown of the light-sensitive part of the retina responsible for the sharp, direct vision needed to read or drive. Its effects can be devastating to independent older adults.

✳ Hearing

Our ability to hear high-frequency consonants (for example, s, t, and z) diminishes with age. Much of the actual hearing loss experienced as we age relates to our inability to distinguish extreme ranges of sound from normal conversational tones—which can make it harder for older individuals to hear what someone is saying if the surrounding environment is noisy, compared to younger people in the same situation.

Taste

Our sense of taste declines as we age. At age 30, each tiny elevation on the tongue (called papilla) has 245 taste buds. By the age of 70, we have only 88 left. The mouth gets drier as salivary glands secrete less fluid. The ability to distinguish sweet, sour, bitter, and salty diminishes. Thus, many older people compensate for their diminished sense of taste by adding salt, sugar, and other flavour enhancers to their food.

Smell and Touch

Our sense of smell also diminishes with age. As a result of this loss, coupled with the loss in taste, food is often less appealing when we get older. This lack of appeal may be one factor that contributes to the tendency for our older population to be malnourished. Pain receptors also become less effective and our tactile senses decline.

Mobility

Nearly half of older Canadians report some disability, usually related to mobility and agility; one-third require help with housework and shopping. The incidence and severity of disability increase with age.[16]

Sexual Changes

As people age, they experience noticeable changes in sexual function. The degree and rate of change varies from person to person. As men age, the following changes generally occur:

- The ability to get and maintain an erection diminishes.
- The length of the refractory period between orgasms increases.
- The orgasm itself becomes shorter.

Women experience the following changes with age:

- Menopause usually occurs between the ages of 45 and 55. At this time, women may experience hot flashes, mood swings, weight gain, development of facial hair, and other hormone-related problems.
- The walls of the vagina become less elastic, and the epithelium thins, making sexual activity less comfortable.

- Vaginal secretions diminish, particularly during sexual activity (though this problem can be reduced with the use of a lubricant).
- The breasts decrease in firmness. Loss of fat in various areas leads to fewer curves, with a decrease in the soft lines of the body.

While these physiologic changes may sound discouraging, the fact is that many older people enjoy satisfying sexual activity throughout their lives.[17] Indeed, one study refuted long-held beliefs that sexual desire decreases as we age. The results showed that nearly half the population over 60 years of age engaged in sexual activity at least once a month, and 40 percent would like to have sex more frequently.[18]

Body Comfort

Because of the loss of body fat, thinning of the epithelium, and diminished glandular activity, elderly people generally have greater difficulty regulating body temperature. This change means that their ability to withstand extreme cold or heat may be limited, thus increasing their risks of hypothermia, heat stroke, and heat exhaustion.

Many of these changes related to body comfort are exacerbated by poor nutrition. For a variety of reasons, getting adequate nutrition is a problem for many seniors. Using assessments based on risk factors associated with malnutrition, researchers have determined that 40 to 50 percent of community-dwelling seniors have a moderate to high risk of becoming malnourished, especially among those who live alone. The limited data on frailer seniors suggest that the picture is much worse. Poor nutrition worsens the impact of chronic disease, reduces resistance to infections, slows healing, and increases use of the health-care system. Identifying seniors at risk for malnutrition is important to enable them to maintain an optimal quality of life and age successfully.[19]

<hr>

what do you THINK?
Of the health conditions listed in this section, which ones are preventable? Which ones can be delayed?

<hr>

Mental Changes

Intelligence

Stereotypes concerning inevitable intellectual decline among the elderly have been largely refuted. Research demonstrated that much of our previous knowledge about elderly intelligence was based on inappropriate testing procedures. Given an appropriate length of time, elderly people may learn and develop skills in a similar manner to younger people. Researchers have also determined that what many elderly people lack in speed of learning they make up for in practical knowledge—that is, the "wisdom of experience."

Memory

Have you ever wondered why your grandfather seems unable to remember what he did last weekend even though he can graphically depict the details of a social event that occurred 40 years ago? This phenomenon is not unusual among the elderly. Research indicates that although short-term memory may fluctuate on a daily basis, the ability to remember events from past decades remains largely unchanged.

Adaptability

Although it is widely believed that people become more like one another as they age, nothing could be further from the truth. Having lived through a multitude of experiences and faced diverse joys, sorrows, and obstacles, the typical older person has developed unique methods of coping. These unique adaptive variations make for interesting differences in how the elderly confront the many changes brought on by the aging process. Thus as a group, older Canadian are heterogeneous.

Depression

Most adults continue to lead healthy, fulfilling lives as they grow older. Some research indicates, however, that depression may be the most common psychological problem as we age. Still, those aged 25 to 44 years have greater depression rates (approximately 10 percent) than those older than 65 (5 percent).[20]

Dementia

Over the years, older people have often been the victims of ageist attitudes. People chronologically old were often labelled "senile" whenever they displayed memory failure, errors in judgment, disorientation, or erratic behaviours. (The term *senile* is seldom used

<hr>

Cataracts: Clouding of the lens that interrupts the focusing of light on the retina, resulting in blurred vision or eventual blindness.

Glaucoma: Elevation of pressure within the eyeball, leading to hardening of the eyeball, impaired vision, and possible blindness.

Macular degeneration: Disease that breaks down the macula, the light-sensitive part of the retina responsible for sharp, direct vision.

Georgia O'Keeffe retained her intellectual and artistic abilities into old age.

today except to describe a very small group of organic disorders.) Today, scientists recognize that these same symptoms can occur at any age and for various reasons, including disease or the use of OTC or prescription drugs. When the underlying problems are corrected, memory loss and disorientation also improve.

Alzheimer's Disease

Dementias are progressive brain impairments that interfere with memory and normal intellectual functioning. Although there are many types of **dementia**, one of the most common forms is **Alzheimer's disease**. Alzheimer's affects an estimated one in 20 people between the ages of 65 and 75 and one in five people over the age of 80. The total number of people with Alzheimer's disease is expected to increase. Estimates are that the incidence of dementia could triple by 2031.[21] This possibility presents a real economic burden for the future. While the disease is associated in most people's minds strictly with the elderly, it has been diagnosed in people as young as their late 40s. In fact, about 5 percent of all cases occur before age 65.

Alzheimer's refers to a degenerative disease of the brain in which nerve cells stop communicating with one another. Ordinarily, brain cells communicate by releasing chemicals that allow the cells to receive and transmit messages for various behaviours. In Alzheimer's patients, the brain does not produce enough of these chemicals, cells cannot communicate, and eventually the cells die. This degeneration happens in the sections of the brain that affect memory, speech, and personality, leaving the parts that control other bodily functions, such as heartbeat and breathing, working fine. Thus, the mind's ability to function decreases while the body continues to work more or less fine. Alzheimer's happens slowly and progressively, and it may be as long as 20 years before symptoms are noticed. It is generally detected first by family members, who note memory lapses and personality changes. Medical tests rule out other underlying causes and neurological tests confirm the diagnosis.

What are the symptoms of Alzheimer's? Alzheimer's disease is characteristically diagnosed in three stages. During the first stage, symptoms include forgetfulness, memory loss, impaired judgment, increasing inability to handle routine tasks, disorientation, lack of interest in one's surroundings, and depression. These symptoms accelerate in the second stage, which also includes agitation and restlessness (especially at night), loss of sensory perceptions, muscle twitching, and repetitive actions. Many patients become depressed at this stage and there is a tendency to be combative and aggressive. In the final stage, disorientation is often complete. The person becomes completely dependent on others for eating, dressing, and other activities. Identity loss and speech problems are common symptoms. Eventually, control of bodily functions may be lost.

Once Alzheimer's disease strikes, the patient's remaining life expectancy is cut in half. Treatment includes several prescription drugs. Some physicians prescribe vitamin E because it may help protect brain cells from free radical damage. Researchers are also examining anti-inflammatory drugs, theorizing that Alzheimer's may develop in response to an inflammatory ailment. Others are focusing on stimulating the brains of those prone to Alzheimer's, believing that as people learn, more connections between brain cells are formed that may offset those that are lost.

✓• HEALTH CHALLENGES OF OLDER CANADIANS

The elderly are disproportionately victimized by a number of societally induced problems. Other problems result when older people do not develop the

Canada's Aging Population Runs Greater Dementia Risk

by Steven Wharry, Canadian Medical Association Journal

The Alzheimer Society of Canada is warning that the number of Canadians battling dementia is set to explode as the population ages.

Steve Rudin, executive director of the Alzheimer Society told *CMAJ* that a study published in *Neurology* predicts that about 109 000 Canadians will develop dementia in the next year alone, while the total number of those suffering from the syndrome will reach 364 000.

"These numbers are very alarming and with this huge number of new cases the implications for our health care system are profound," said Rudin. "The financial and social costs risk being overwhelming."

The estimates are based on data from the Canadian Study of Health and Aging (CSHA) report, which dementia experts warn contain some dire predictions: in 2011, new cases of dementia are expected to reach 145 300 a year; the total number of cases will be 475 000; by 2031 there will be an estimated 778 000 Canadians with Alzheimer's disease and related dementias.

Rudin states that long-term care facilities and services to help these individuals and initiatives such as a national home care program need to be examined to help families cope with caring for stricken family members.

"The population in the 85-plus age group is the fastest growing segment of the population," states Joan Lindsay, co-investigator of the CSHA study and chief of the Aging Related Diseases Division of Health Canada. "The increase in the numbers of people with dementia is a direct result of the growth in the 'oldest of the old' segment of our population."

Dementia is a syndrome that includes loss of memory, judgment, reasoning, and ability to function. Alzheimer's disease is a degenerative brain disorder that destroys vital brain cells. The cause is unknown and the Alzheimer Society and other organizations continue to fund research aimed at finding a cure.

"Given the vast numbers of people predicted to get this disease, it's even more urgent for us to find a cause and a cure," said Rudin. "We must also develop better methods for diagnosis, caregiving and providing needed services."

ability to cope with life's various hurdles. Still other problems come from a perceived loss of control in older people over the circumstances of their lives—when they watch loved ones die, are forced to retire, face problems with personal health, and confront an uncertain economy on a fixed income. Developing adequate coping and decision-making skills in your earlier years, as well as strong social supports, may significantly reduce your risk for problems in old age.

Alcohol Use and Abuse

A person prone to alcoholism during their younger and middle years is more likely to continue drinking during his or her later years. The older individual addicted to alcohol is no more common than the younger person, despite the stereotype of the old, lost soul hiding his or her sorrows in a bottle. Alcohol abuse is five times more likely in older men than in older women. Almost half of all older men and even more older women do not drink at all. Those who do drink consume less than younger persons, at only five to six drinks per week.

Prescription Drug Use: Unique Problems for Older Canadians

It is extremely rare for older people to use illicit drugs, but some do overuse, misuse, and grow dependent upon prescription and OTC drugs. Beset with numerous aches, pains, and inexplicable as well as diagnosable maladies, some older Canadians take between four and six prescription drugs a day in addition to vitamin and/or mineral supplements and regular use of OTCs such as Aspirin. Anyone who combines drugs runs the risk of dangerous and/or uncomfortable drug interactions. The risks of adverse effects are greater for people with circulation impairments and declining kidney and liver functions. Older people displaying symptoms of these drug-induced effects, including bizarre behaviour patterns or an appearance of being out of touch, are often misdiagnosed as experiencing dementia.

Dementia: Refers to mental deterioration, loss of memory, and judgment and orientation problems.

Alzheimer's disease: A chronic condition involving changes in nerve fibres of the brain; results in mental deterioration.

Baby Boomers Sport Waistline Woes

In Andrew Wister's new book (*Baby Boomer Health Dynamics: How Are We Aging?* UTP, 2005), he calls obesity "the new tobacco." Despite today's baby boomers' making many healthier lifestyle choices such as not smoking, reducing alcohol consumption, and engaging in physical activity or exercise, they are not aging any better than their forefathers 25 years ago. One thing boomers experience at a much higher rate than their forefathers and -mothers is obesity. In fact, the number of people classified as obese has doubled in the past 15 years. Clearly the lifestyle improvements have not been sufficient to counteract the quantity and quality of our food consumption.

To examine the exercise–obesity paradox, Wister, Chair of the Department of Gerontology at Simon Fraser University, analyzed data from six Canadian health surveys. From these analyses, it was noted that 25 percent of the energy we take in (that is, calories) comes from the "other" food group of Canada's Food Guide to Healthy Eating (updated and now called Eating Well with Canada's Food Guide). Twenty percent of all meals were eaten outside the home, many at fast food restaurants which continue to serve exceedingly large portions. Further, it was noted that as many as 27 percent of people eat at least one meal per week in their car.

These changes have a direct impact on individual and national levels of obesity. Given the sheer number of boomers, combined with an increase in the number classified as obese, our health-care system is likely to become overburdened in the coming years as the boomers age.

Source: Adapted from Centre on Aging, "Research through the Life Course," *The Bulletin* 14.1 (January 2006): 12. Retrieved on May 16, 2006, from www.coag.uvic.ca.

Over-the-Counter Remedies

Although older Canadians today appear to be more receptive to medical treatment than previous generations, a substantial segment of the over-60 population avoid orthodox medical treatment, viewing it as only a last resort. As might be expected, ASA and laxatives head the list of commonly used OTC medications for relief of arthritic pain and the irregular bowel activity sometimes experienced by older Canadians.

Physical Activity

An inevitable physical change the body undergoes as it ages is **sarcopenia**, age-related declines in muscle mass. The less muscle you have, the less energy you require, even when physically active. The lower your metabolic rate, the more likely you will gain weight—particularly when your caloric intake remains the same. Regular moderate-intensity physical activity that gets your heart beating faster will help to reduce the expected age-related declines in quality and quantity of muscle (See also Chapter 4). Further, regular resistance training will increase (or maintain) muscle mass, boost metabolism, strengthen your bones, prevent osteoporosis, and in general help older Canadians to feel better and function more effectively and efficiently.

Canada's Physical Activity Guide to Healthy Active Living for Older Adults (available at www.phac-aspc. gc.ca/pau-uap/paguide/older/index.html) recommends that older adults choose a variety of endurance, flexibility, and strength and balance activities such that they accumulate 30 to 60 minutes of moderate-intensity physical activity most days of the week.[22] It is further noted that these activities can be accumulated in 10-minute blocks of time.

Dietary Concerns

As with many bodily processes, the digestion of food slows with age. Nevertheless, the body still requires nutrients consumed in moderate quantities and in the right combination. Certain nutrients are especially important to healthy aging:

- Calcium: Many elderly people do not consume adequate calcium, or they may take it as an individual supplement without vitamin D, which is necessary for calcium absorption in the body. Adequate calcium intake should be part of a lifelong regimen of preventive health care to reduce loss of bone mineral content. For individuals over the age of 50, a calcium intake of 1200 mg per day is recommended.[23]

- Vitamin D: As noted above, vitamin D is essential to enable adequate calcium absorption. As people age, particularly in and beyond their 50s and 60s, they do not absorb vitamin D as readily from foods. More recently, vitamin D has been

Learning to cope with challenges and make effective decisions early in life develops attitudes and skills that contribute to a full and satisfying old age.

identified as protective from a number of chronic diseases. Further, it is clear, particularly during the winter months in Canada, that most Canadians cannot obtain sufficient vitamin D from the sun. Supplementation may therefore be warranted.

- Protein: As older adults become concerned about cholesterol and fatty foods, and as their budgets shrink, one nutrient often cut back on is protein. Meat costs more, takes longer to cook, and has a "fat" stigma associated with it. Many older people cut back on protein to a point below the DRIs. Because protein is necessary to maintain muscle mass, deficiencies can spell trouble.

✱ Gender Issues: Caring for Older Canadians

According to the most recent census data, older women fill a disproportionate place in Canadian society. In 2005, for example, 56.5 percent of Canadians over the age of 65 years were women.[24] This difference in the number of older women increases with age. In the same year, women made up 58.4 percent of people aged 75 to 84, and 69.2 percent of Canadians aged 85 or older. This is also a relatively new phenomenon—as recently as 1950, there were more older men than women.[25] Because women live longer then men on average, older women are more likely than older men to be living alone, and thus to lack the support in the home that helps keep them independent. Women over the age of 75 were the largest consumers of home-care services, with 20 percent reporting using these services.[26]

The rate of institutionalization is twice as high among older people without a spouse as for married older people; one reason is that a married person has a built-in potential caretaker. Further, women are more likely than men to experience poverty and multiple chronic health problems, a situation referred to as **comorbidity**. Consequently, more older women than men are likely to need assistance from children, other relatives, friends, and neighbours.

✱ UNDERSTANDING DEATH AND DYING

Death eventually comes to everyone. Although this can be a depressing thought, we must accept the inevitable. The acceptance of death helps shape our attitudes about the importance of life. Throughout history, humans have attempted to determine the nature and meaning of death. This questioning continues today. Although we will touch on moral, spiritual, and philosophical questions about death, we will not explore such issues in depth in this chapter. Rather, our primary focus is to present dying and death as a normal part of life and to discuss how we can cope with it.

Confrontations with death elicit different feelings depending on many factors, including age, religious beliefs, family orientation, health, personal experience, and the circumstances of the death itself. To cope effectively with dying and death, we must address the individual needs of those involved. Why is it that we wish to deny, or even postpone, death?

Defining Death

Dying is the process of decline in body functions resulting in the death of an organism. **Death** can be

Sarcopenia: Age-related declines in the quality and quantity of muscle tissue.

Comorbidity: The presence of a number of diseases at the same time.

Dying: The process of decline in body functions resulting in the death of an organism.

Death: The "final cessation of the vital functions" and the state in which these functions are "incapable of being restored."

defined as the "final cessation of the vital functions" and refers to a state in which these functions are "incapable of being restored."[27] This definition has become more significant as medical and scientific advances have made it increasingly possible to postpone death. Although irreversible cessation of circulatory and respiratory functions acceptably defines death, irreversible cessation of brain function is also equivalent to death even though the heart continues to beat while the individual is on a respirator.

In 1968, following the publication of the Harvard criteria for the diagnosis of brain death, the Canadian Medical Association (CMA) provided guidelines, revised in 1974 and 1975. In 1976, guidelines were established in the United Kingdom, and in 1981, revised guidelines were published in the *Journal of the American Medical Association*. Brain death must be determined clinically by an experienced physician in accordance with accepted medical standards.[28] The following definitions facilitate classification of various phases of biologic death:

- Cell death: The gradual death of a cell after all metabolic activity has ceased. The rate of cellular death varies according to the tissue involved. For example, higher-functioning brain cells die five to eight minutes after respiration ceases; striated muscle cells die two to four hours later; kidney cells die after about seven hours; and epithelial cells (hair and nails) die several days later. Rigor mortis, the temporary stiffening of muscles, is associated with cell death.

- Local death: The death of a body part or portion of an organ without the death of the entire organism. For example, a kidney may fail, part of the heart muscle may die, or a limb or section of intestine may die as a result of loss of circulation.

- Somatic death: The death of the entire organism, as opposed to death of a part of an organ or an extremity.

- Apparent death: The cessation of vital physiologic functions, particularly spontaneous cardiac and respiratory activities, which produces a state simulating actual death but from which recovery is possible through resuscitative efforts.

- Functional death: Extensive and irreversible damage to the central nervous system, with respiration and circulatory function maintained by artificial means.

- Brain death: The cessation of brain function, as evidenced by loss of all reflexes and electrical activity of the brain or by irreversible coma. Brain death is confirmed by an electroencephalogram reading of electrical activity of brain cells.

The Canadian Medical Association established the following criteria for the clinical diagnosis of brain death:[29]

1. An etiology has been established capable of causing brain death, and potentially reversible conditions have been excluded (drug intoxication, treatable metabolic disorders, core temperature less than 32.2°C, shock, and peripheral nerve or muscle dysfunction due to disease or neuromuscular-blocking drugs).

2. The patient is in deep coma and shows no response within the cranial nerve distribution to stimulation of any part of the body. In particular, there should be no motor response within the cranial nerve distribution to stimuli applied to any body regions. There should be no spontaneous or elicited movements arising from the brain. However, various spinal reflexes may persist in brain death.

3. Brain-stem reflexes are absent. Pupillary light and corneal, vestibulo-ocular, and pharyngeal reflexes must be absent. The pupils should be midsize or larger and must be unresponsive to light. Care should be taken that atropine or related drugs that could block the pupillary response to light have not been given to the patient.

4. The patient does not breathe when taken off the respirator for an appropriate time.

5. The conditions listed above persist when the patient is reassessed after a suitable interval to ensure that the non-functioning state of the brain is persistent and to reduce the possibility of observer error.

The CMA also suggests that a physician consult with another experienced physician before determining death.

what do you THINK?

How long do you think you will live? Do you have concerns about the quality of your life up until you die? How can you obtain not only a long life, but also a healthy quality of life?

Denying Death

We can look at our attitudes toward death as falling on a continuum. At one end of the continuum, death is viewed as the enemy of humankind. Medical science promotes this idea of death. At the other end of the continuum, death is accepted and welcomed.[30] For people whose attitudes fall at this end, often those with

In some cultures, death is not feared but viewed as a passage to a better state of being that is to be celebrated.

a deep religious faith or spiritual belief, death is a passage to a better state of being. Most of us perceive ourselves somewhere in the middle of this continuum. From this perspective, death is a bewildering mystery that elicits fear and apprehension, as well as profoundly influencing our attitudes, beliefs, and actions throughout our lives.

In Canada, a high level of discomfort is associated with dying and death. As a result, we often avoid speaking about the subject. You may be denying death if you:

- avoid people who are grieving after the death of a loved one so you do not have to talk about it
- fail to validate a dying person's situation by talking to the person as if nothing were wrong
- substitute euphemisms for the word *death* (a few examples are "passed away," "kicked the bucket," "no longer with us," "gone to heaven," or "gone to a better place")
- give false reassurances to dying people by saying things like "everything is going to be okay"
- shut off conversation about death by silencing people trying to talk about it
- avoid touching a dying person

Although some experts indicate that the denial of death has always been a predominant characteristic of our society, we must keep in mind that societal norms contribute to this denial. The miraculous feats of science and medicine during the first half of the century created an attitude closer to death-defying than to death-denying. However, the pendulum appears to be swinging back. Today, a growing number of people are rejecting "high-tech" death—death postponed through the use of life-support technology—in favour of more personal, and perhaps more humane, alternatives. The concept of death as an enemy may be giving way to acceptance of dying as a natural part of life.

THE PROCESS OF DYING

Dying is a complex process that includes physical, intellectual, social, spiritual, and emotional dimensions. Accordingly, we must consider the process of dying from several perspectives. The preceding section primarily examined the physical indicators of death. It is also essential to consider the emotional aspects of dying and "social death" in establishing an appreciation for the multifaceted nature of life and death.

Coping Emotionally with Death

Science and medicine enable us to understand changes associated with growth, development, aging, and social roles throughout the life span, but they have not revealed the nature of death. This may partially explain why the transition from life to death evokes mystery and emotion. Although emotional reactions to dying vary, there seem to be many similarities in this process.

Much of our knowledge about reactions to dying stems from the work of Elisabeth Kübler-Ross, a major figure in modern **thanatology**, the study of death and dying. In 1969, Kübler-Ross published *On Death and Dying*, a sensitive analysis of the reactions of terminally ill patients.[31] This pioneering work encouraged the development of death education as a discipline and prompted efforts to improve the care of patients who were dying. In her book, Kübler-Ross identified five psychological stages that terminally ill patients often experience as they approach death: denial, anger, bargaining, depression, and acceptance. Health professions immediately embraced this "stage theory" and hastily applied it in clinical settings.[32] However, research evidence supporting the concept of stages of grief is neither extensive nor convincing. Although it is normal to grieve when a severe loss has been sustained, some people never go through this process and instead remain emotionally calm. Others pass back and forth between the stages.

Thanatology: The study of death and dying.

A summation of Kübler-Ross's five stages follows: [33]

- Denial: ("Not me, there must be a mistake.") This is usually the first stage, experienced as a sensation of shock and disbelief. A person intellectually accepts his or her impending death but rejects it emotionally. The individual is too confused and stunned to comprehend "not being" and thus rejects the idea. When this anxiety level diminishes, the individual is able to sort through the powerful web of emotions surrounding his or her impending death.

- Anger: ("Why me?") Anger is another common reaction to the realization of imminent death. The person becomes angry at the prospect of dying when others, including loved ones, are healthy and not threatened. The person dying perceives the situation as "unfair" or "senseless" and may be hostile to friends, family, physicians, and/or the world in general.

- Bargaining: ("If I am allowed to live, I promise . . .") This stage generally occurs at about the middle of the progression toward acceptance of death. During this stage, the dying person may resolve to be a better person in return for an extension of life or may secretly pray for a short reprieve from death in order to experience a special event, such as a family wedding or birth.

- Depression: ("It is really going to happen to me and I cannot do anything about it.") Depression eventually sets in as vitality diminishes and the person begins to experience distressing symptoms with increasing frequency. The individual's deteriorating condition becomes impossible for him or her to deny, and feelings of doom and tremendous loss may become unbearably pervasive. Feelings of worthlessness and guilt are also common in this depressed state because the person dying may feel responsible for the emotional suffering of loved ones and the arduous but seemingly futile efforts of caregivers.

- Acceptance: ("I am ready.") This is often the final stage. The individual stops battling with emotions and becomes tired and weak. The need to sleep increases, and wakeful periods become shorter and less frequent. With acceptance, the person does not "give up" and become sullen or resentfully resigned to death, but rather becomes passive. According to one dying person, the acceptance stage is "almost void of feelings . . . as if the pain had gone, the struggle is over, and there comes a time for the final rest before the long journey."[34] As he or she lets go, the dying person may no longer welcome visitors and may not wish to engage in conversation. Death usually occurs quietly and painlessly while the individual is unconscious.

Subsequent research indicated that each individual has a distinct mix and process of grieving. A person may move from denial to depression, to anger, to denial again, and so on. Even if it is not accurate in all its particulars, Kübler-Ross's theory offers valuable insights for those seeking to understand or cope with the process of dying.

Social Death

The need for recognition and appreciation within a social group is nearly universal. Although the size and nature of the social group may vary widely, the need to belong exists in all of us. Loss of value or of appreciation by others can lead to **social death**, an often irreversible situation in which a person is not treated like an active member of society. Dramatic examples of social death include the exile of nonconformists from their native countries or the excommunication of dissident members of religious orders. More often, however, social death is inflicted by avoidance of social interaction. Numerous studies indicate that people are treated differently when they are dying. The isolation that accompanies social death in terminally ill patients may be promoted by the following:[35]

- The dying person is referred to as if he or she were already dead.
- The dying person may be inadvertently excluded from conversations.
- Dying patients are often moved to terminal wards and given minimal care.
- Bereaved family members are avoided, often for extended periods, because friends and neighbours are afraid of feeling uncomfortable in the presence of grief.
- Medical personnel may make degrading comments about patients in their presence.

A decrease in meaningful social interaction often strips dying and bereaved people of recognition as valued members of society at a time when belonging is critical. Some dying people choose not to speak of their inevitable fate in an attempt to make others feel more comfortable and thus preserve vital relationships.

Near-Death Experiences

We cannot speak of the process of dying without mentioning near-death experiences. Thousands of similar reports have been given by people who almost died or were actually pronounced dead and subsequently recovered. The descriptions of feelings, perceptions, and visions associated with being near death have many common features. Three phases have been identified: resistance, life review, and transcendence. During the initial phase, resistance, the dying person is aware of extreme danger and struggles desperately to escape from the unseen threat. Many people report a sensation of expanding fear. The second phase, life review, has been described as a feeling of being outside one's body and beyond danger. During this period, the dying person feels a sensation of security while observing his or her physical body from an emotionally detached perspective. The dying person's life experiences may also seem to pass by in rapid review. The last phase, transcendence, is characterized by a reported feeling of euphoria, contentment, and even ecstasy. Some people recall a sensation of being unified with nature and of having an awareness of infinity. In February 2000, Pam Barrett, long-time leader of the Alberta New Democratic Party, abruptly resigned from politics after a near-death experience due to an allergic reaction. She termed the experience "a spiritual awakening," and said that it had forced her to re-evaluate all aspects of her life.

✴ Coping with Loss

The death of a loved one may be extremely difficult to cope with. The dying person, as well as close family and friends, frequently suffers emotionally and physically from the impending loss of critical relationships and roles. Words used to describe feelings and behaviours related to losses resulting from death include bereavement, grief, grief work, and mourning. These terms are related but not identical. A discussion of them may help you to understand the emotional processes associated with loss and the cultural constraints that often inhibit normal coping behaviours (see Figure 16.1).

Bereavement is generally defined as the loss or deprivation experienced by a survivor when a loved one dies. Because relationships vary in type and intensity, reactions vary. The death of a parent, spouse, sibling, child, friend, or pet will result in different kinds of feelings. The death of loved ones will leave "holes" in the lives of the bereaved or of close survivors. We can think of bereavement as the awareness of these holes. Time and courage are necessary to fill these spaces.

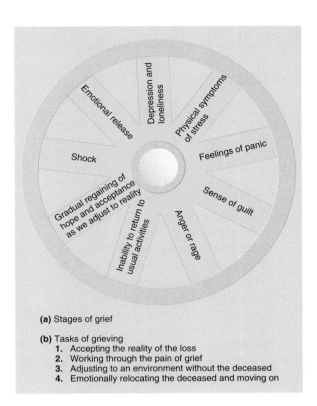

(a) Stages of grief

(b) Tasks of grieving
1. Accepting the reality of the loss
2. Working through the pain of grief
3. Adjusting to an environment without the deceased
4. Emotionally relocating the deceased and moving on

FIGURE 16.1
The Stages and Tasks of Grief

(a) People react differently to loss, and most eventually adjust. Generally, the stronger the social support system, the smoother the progression through the stages of grief.
(b) Worden's developmental tasks associated with grief are another way to understand the grieving process.

When a person experiences a loss that cannot be openly acknowledged, publicly mourned, or socially supported, coping may be much more difficult. This type of grief is referred to as **disenfranchised grief**.[36] Some examples of a death that may lead to disenfranchised grief include

- Death of a divorced spouse: Unresolved anger and hurt along with fond memories are conflicting feelings that may prevent the resolution of feelings surrounding the ex-spouse's death.

- Death of a secret lover: When a lover dies and no one but the partner knew of the relationship, grief

what do you THINK?
Have you, or someone close to you, experienced the stages of grief? What would you add to or take away from the description given?

Social death: An irreversible situation in which a person is not treated as an active member of society.

Bereavement: The loss or deprivation experienced when a loved one dies.

Disenfranchised grief: Grief concerning a loss that cannot be openly acknowledged, publicly mourned, or socially supported.

Bereavement and Grief

Each of us uses various methods to relieve sorrow and bereavement. Similar to other types of stress (see Chapter 3), the stress caused by grief affects people mentally and physically. If an individual is having an especially difficult time dealing with grief, he or she may become depressed or physically ill. There are a number of feelings that people experience while coming to terms with a loss, including:

- shock, numbness, bewilderment, a sense of disbelief, and possibly denial
- feelings of emptiness and intense suffering
- dreams or hallucinations that their loved one is still alive
- feelings of despair as one comes to terms with the loss
- feelings of sadness and the inability to feel pleasure
- tense, restless anxiety alternated with lethargy and fatigue
- avoiding reminders of the deceased alternated with reclaiming memories
- sadness mixed with anger
- self-blame for treating the deceased badly

Physical symptoms of grief include weakness, sleep disturbances, loss of appetite, headaches, back pain, indigestion, shortness of breath, heart palpitations, and occasional dizziness and nausea.

WHY WE GRIEVE

All cultures have various rituals to mourn the death of a loved one. Mourning customs help to confirm social bonds, reorder personal relationships, and establish a new identity for the bereaved. Within our society, people often die in hospitals or away from their families. These changes to the social fabric have made it difficult for some to see death as a natural part of life, and to come to terms with the death of a loved one. Friends and social groups are especially important for helping the bereaved adjust to their loss and move on with his or her life.

WHAT YOU CAN DO TO HELP THE BEREAVED

People who have experienced a death need sympathetic company, reassurance, and willingness among or by others to listen. What the bereaved say they want most are offers of specific practical support, expressions of concern, and the presence of people close to them. Statements such as "time heals" and vague offers of help that do not materialize are more annoying than helpful. People should not discourage expressions of grief or shut off discussions about the person who died, since that is part of the healing process. Understanding that this is a highly emotional time for the bereaved and assuring them that their anger, guilt, and other feelings are normal and part of the grieving process is the most supportive thing you can do.

is often hidden. Examples would include a partner in an extramarital relationship or a lover of a gay person who is not openly gay.

- Death of a gay lover: Gays and lesbians—even those who are "out"—may find it difficult to mourn the deaths of their lovers when they themselves are not accepted by their own families or the families of their lovers. The situation can be even more difficult if the lover died of AIDS, because of the unjust stigma and discrimination associated with this disease.

A special case of bereavement occurs in old age. Death is an intrinsic part of growing old. The longer we live, the more deaths we are likely to experience. These deaths include physical, social, spiritual, and emotional losses as our bodies deteriorate and more and more of our loved ones die. The theory of bereavement overload has been proposed to explain the effects of multiple deaths and the accumulation of sorrow in the lives of some elderly people. This theory suggests that the gloomy outlook, disturbing behaviour patterns, and apparent apathy that characterize these people may be related more to bereavement overload than to intrinsic physiological degeneration in old age.[37]

Grief is a mental state of distress that occurs in reaction to significant loss, including one's own impending death, the death of a loved one, or a quasi-death experience. Grief reactions include any adjustments needed for one to "make it through the day" and may include changes in patterns of eating, physical activity, sleeping, working, and even thinking.

The term **mourning** is often incorrectly equated with the term *grief.* As we have noted, grief refers to a wide variety of feelings and actions that occur in response to bereavement. *Mourning*, in contrast, refers to culturally prescribed and accepted time periods and behaviour patterns for the expression of grief. In Judaism, for example, "sitting shivah" is a designated mourning period of seven days that involves prescribed rituals and prayers. Depending on a person's relationship with the deceased, various other rituals may continue for up to a year.

By accepting dying as a part of the continuum of life, many people are able to make necessary readjustments after the death of a loved one. This holistic concept, which accepts dying as a part of the total life experience, is shared by believers and non-believers.

What Is "Normal" Grief?

Grief responses vary widely from person to person. Despite these differences, a classic acute grief syndrome often occurs when a person acknowledges a death. This common grief reaction can include the following:

- periodic waves of physical distress lasting from 20 minutes to an hour
- a feeling of tightness in the throat
- choking and shortness of breath
- a frequent need to sigh
- a feeling of emptiness
- a feeling of muscular weakness
- an intense feeling of anxiety described as actually painful

Other common symptoms of grief include insomnia, memory lapse, loss of appetite, difficulty in concentrating, a tendency to engage in repetitive or purposeless behaviours, an "observer" sensation or feeling of unreality, difficulty in making decisions, lack of organization, excessive speech, social withdrawal or hostility, guilt feelings, and preoccupation with the image of the deceased. Susceptibility to disease increases with grief and may even be life-threatening in severe and enduring cases.

Coping with Grief

A bereaved person may suffer emotional pain and exhibit a variety of grief responses for many months after the death of a loved one. The rate of healing depends on the amount and quality of "grief work" that a person does. **Grief work** is the process of integrating the reality of the death with everyday life and learning to feel better. Often, the bereaved person must deliberately and systematically work at reducing denial and coping with the pain that results from memories of the deceased. This process takes time and requires emotional effort.

Worden's Model of Grieving Tasks

William Worden, a researcher of the death process, developed an active grieving model suggesting four developmental tasks to complete in the grief work process (refer to Figure 16.1):[38]

1. Accept the reality of the loss. This task requires acknowledging and realizing that the person is dead. Traditional rituals, such as the funeral, help many bereaved people move toward this acceptance.

2. Work through the pain of grief. It is necessary to acknowledge and work through the pain associated with loss or it will manifest itself in other symptoms or behaviours.

3. Adjust to an environment in which the deceased is missing. The bereaved may feel lonely and uncertain about their identity without the person who has died. This loss brings the challenge of adjusting to their own sense of self.

4. Emotionally relocate the deceased and move on with life. Individuals never lose memories of a significant relationship. They may need help in letting go of the emotional energy that used to be invested in the person who has died, finding an appropriate place for the deceased in their emotional lives.

Models of the grief process can be viewed as "generalized maps"—each theory is an attempt by an investigator to understand and guide grieving people through their pain. However, each individual will travel through grief at his or her own speed using an appropriate route.

When an Infant or a Child Dies

The death of a child is terribly painful for the whole family. For several reasons, siblings of the deceased child have a particularly hard time with grief work. Bereaved children usually have limited experience with death and therefore have not learned how to deal with it. Children may feel uncomfortable talking about death, may have difficulty understanding it, and may also receive less social support and sympathy than their parents. Because so much attention and energy are devoted to the deceased child, the surviving children may also feel emotionally abandoned.

Grief: The mental state of distress that occurs in reaction to significant loss.

Mourning: The culturally prescribed behaviour patterns for the expression of grief.

Grief work: The process of accepting the reality of a person's death and coping with memories of the deceased.

Teenage suicide affects many people, but siblings and friends—who generally have little experience with death—are especially challenged in coping with their grief.

Quasi-Death Experiences

Social and emotional support for the bereaved in the aftermath of death is supported by many cultures. Typically, however, there is little support for many other significant losses in life. Losses that in many ways resemble death and carry with them a heavy burden of grief include a child running away from home, an abduction or kidnapping, a divorce, a move to a distant place, a move to a long-term care facility, the loss of a romance or an intimate friendship, retirement, job termination, finishing a "terminal" academic degree, or ending an athletic career.

These **quasi-death experiences**[39] resemble death in that they involve separation, termination, loss, and a change in identity or self-perception. If grief results from these losses, the pattern of the grief response will probably follow the same course as responses to death. Factors that complicate the grieving process associated with quasi-death experiences include uncomfortable contact with the object of loss (for example, an ex-spouse or ex-partner) and a lack of adequate social and institutional support.

✳ LIFE-AND-DEATH DECISION MAKING

Life-and-death decisions are serious, complex, and often expensive. We will not attempt to present the "answers" to death-related moral and philosophical questions. Instead, we offer topics for your consideration. We hope that discussion of the needs of the dying person and the bereaved will help you to make difficult decisions in the future. Problematic or controversial issues include questions concerning the right to die and euthanasia. Increasingly, Canadians living with terminal or life-threatening diagnoses are demanding to make decisions about their own lives. Options include pain and symptom management, extended palliative care, active and passive forms of euthanasia, and suicide.

The need to consider right-to-die issues accompanies the development of new reproductive technologies, increases in terminal AIDS cases, and a visible increase in public media coverage of actual cases in Canada and the United States. The right to self-determination is situated within the context of society, health and illness, and human rights and freedoms. Considerations of the economic, social, spiritual, and moral impact of the individual's choice are often

Many terminally ill people spend their last days in a hospice where maximum involvement of loved ones is emphasized.

Palliative Care

The needs of terminally ill patients are different from those of other patients. They require another approach and different services defined by different criteria. Palliative care is a compassionate form of health care for patients approaching the end of their life. Pain and symptom management and social, psychological, and spiritual support are components of palliative care. We need to understand more fully the meaning that death and dying have to seniors, and how to provide effective pain management for seniors experiencing the symptoms of several health conditions simultaneously.

Different models of care have been explored all over the world: St. Christopher's in London, the Maison Michel Sarrazin in Quebec, and the Elizabeth Bruyère Centre in Ottawa, for example, are highly specialized in pain control and offer supportive care and attention to dying patients. Friends and family are welcome at all times and special training is given to volunteers who can then assist the patients, their families, and the caregivers on staff.

In-home palliative care services are provided in collaboration with a care facility. If treatment is balanced, this type of service can ensure the full continuum of care and nurturing needed to allow terminally ill individuals to remain in their familiar surroundings for as long as possible. The family also needs to be supported and kept informed by being given clear explanations and directives. For individuals to derive maximum benefits from this situation, the home atmosphere needs to be calm and serene, and services must be of the same quality as those offered in hospital. If you are terminally ill, you can make your wishes regarding your care known in several ways:

- If you are facing a life-threatening illness, you should talk over your wishes with your family and let them know what you want.

- You can also put your wishes in writing so that, in the event you are unable to say what you want, your family and healthcare providers will know. Such documents are called advance directives or living wills (see the Taking Charge box). You should seek advice within your community about advance directives, as the laws concerning them vary from province to province.

- Your public library may have material on palliative care. You can also call help lines, such as the Canadian Hospice Palliative Care Association at 1-800-668-2785 or 613-241-3663, or the Cancer Information Service at 1-888-939-3333 or 905-387-1153.

Sources: The Legal Information Society of Nova Scotia (LISNS), Living Wills, www.legalinfo.org.

involved in decision making. A living will, discussed in the Taking Charge box, is one way in which people may express their wishes about life-and-death choices.

Dyathanasia is a form of "mercy killing" in which life-prolonging treatments are withheld or life-sustaining medical support is withdrawn, thereby allowing the person to die. It is believed that withholding food and water from terminally ill individuals may actually ease their suffering. **Euthanasia** is the active form of "mercy killing." An example of euthanasia is direct administration of a lethal drug overdose with the objective of hastening the death of a suffering person. Euthanasia is illegal and considered murder in Canada. After years of legal run-ins, the well-known American euthanasia proponent Dr. Jack Kevorkian was convicted of murder for assisting in euthanasia ("assisted suicide") in the late 1990s. Nevertheless, euthanasia continues to occur. In fact, it is believed that some doctors induce euthanasia upon the request of the patient. This type of euthanasia is accomplished by administering large doses of painkillers that depress the central nervous system to the extent that basic life-sustaining regulatory centres cease to function. The heart stops beating, breathing ceases, and total brain death follows shortly.

what do you THINK?

Have you ever thought about being in a situation where you might rather die than be kept alive? Have you ever talked with your parents, siblings, partner, or anyone else close to you about the "right to die"? Why or why not?

Quasi-death experiences: Losses or experiences that resemble death in that they involve separation, termination, significant loss, a change of personal identity, and grief.

Dyathanasia: The passive form of "mercy killing" in which life-prolonging treatments or interventions are withheld, thereby allowing a terminally ill person to die naturally.

Euthanasia: The active form of "mercy killing" in which a person or organization knowingly acts to hasten the death of a terminally ill person.

The Living Will

A living will is a written document in which you clearly identify your wishes for health care in the event that, some time in the future, you are unable to consent to treatment. Living wills deal with health care. They do not deal with property or assets. Living wills are needed if you are unable to consent when have a terminal illness or are seriously injured and unlikely to recover. In such cases medical staff will need to know what measures you would wish them to take to care for you.

There are no guarantees that every term of the living will be followed. Family members or your proxy in consultation with medical staff will have to make the decision taking into account the existing circumstances, including your expressed wishes. (A proxy is someone you have appointed to make decisions about your health care should you become unable to consent.) A living will may ease the emotional burden from family members or your proxy if they have to make decisions about your health. Many families consider a living will morally binding, especially if you have discussed it with them beforehand.

A living will is not a request to take positive steps to end your life. Euthanasia, or mercy killing, as it is sometimes called, is the term used when someone takes steps to end your life in order to relieve suffering. Assisted suicide is a term used when someone, at your request, takes steps to end your life, because your illness or condition prevents you from commit-ting suicide. Euthanasia and assisted suicide are illegal under Canadian criminal law.

The living will must have your name and address and the date. It should clearly identify what kind of life-sustaining treatments you would want in certain circumstances should you be incapable of consenting at the time. You must sign the living will and date it. Your signature should be witnessed by two adults. They should give their addresses. If you do not already have a proxy, you may also want to include the appointment of someone to consent to treatment on your behalf should you become unable to do so. You should choose someone whom you trust to carry out your wishes. The person must be at least 19 years of age but does not have to be your next of kin.

Source: The Legal Information Society of Nova Scotia (LISNS), Living Wills, www.legalinfo.org.

Go to MyHealthLab at **www.pearsoned.ca/myhealthlab.** Here you will find self-assessments, case studies, links to health on the net, and much more.

DISCUSSION QUESTIONS

1. Discuss the various definitions of aging. At what age would you place your parents or grandparents in each category?

2. As the population of older people grows, what implications are there for you? Would you be willing to pay higher taxes to support social programs for older Canadians?

3. List the major physiological changes that occur with aging. Which of these, if any, can you change? Which can you slow down? Specifically address dietary intake and physical activity in your response.

4. Identify the major physical and mental health challenges that older Canadians face.

5. List the varied definitions of death. How do they relate to one another?

6. Discuss why we deny death. How could death become a more socially accepted topic to discuss?

7. What are the stages that terminally ill patients theoretically experience? Do you agree with the five-stage theory? Explain why or why not.

8. Debate whether assisted suicide should be legalized for the terminally ill. What restrictions would you include in a law?

APPLICATION EXERCISE

Reread the "Consider This . . ." scenario at the beginning of the chapter and answer the following questions.

1. Do you think the individuals in the scenario are normal for their age? What is normal for a particular age? How is "normal" defined?

2. What changes have made it easier for older people to lead healthy lives? What changes have made it more difficult?

MYSEARCHLAB EXERCISE

1. Log on to www.MySearchLab.com.

2. Find an article on aging, death, dying, or the grief process.

3. Respond to the following questions:
   a. Why did you choose this article?
   b. Summarize the article in a way that you can share it with others in class (this might be as a poem, video, pamphlet/handout, short story, slide presentation, piece of artwork—you decide).
   c. Was this a difficult assignment for you? Why or why not?

Note: All red numbers indicate Canadian references.

CHAPTER 1

1. Statistics Canada, *Canada Year Book 1997* (Ottawa: Minister of Industry, Cat. No. 402-XPE, 1996) 116.

2. Statistics Canada, "Deaths," *The Daily,* Wednesday, December 21, 2005. Retrieved on May 31, 2006 from www.statcan.ca/Daily/English/051221/d051221b.htm.

3. C. F. Beckington, "The World Health Organization," in *World Health* (New York: Longman, 1975) 149.

4. World Health Organization, "Constitution of the World Health Organization," *Chronicles of the World Health Organization* (Switzerland: Geneva, 1947).

5. Rene Dubos, *So Human an Animal* (New York: Scribners, 1968) 15.

6. Wikipedia, "Biophilia Hypothesis." Retrieved on December 5, 2008 from en.wikipedia.org/wiki/Biophyilia.

7. Thompson Rivers University, "Spiritual Health." Retrieved on October 9, 2008 from www.tru.ca/wellness/spiritual.html.

8. The Secretariat for the Intersectoral Healthy Living Network in partnership with the F/P/T Healthy Living Task Group and the F/P/T Advisory Committee on Population Health and Health Security (ACPHHS), "The Integrated Pan-Canadian Healthy Living Strategy 2005." Retrieved on May 31, 2006 from www.phac-aspc.gc.ca/hl-vs-strat/pdf/hls_e.pdf.

9. Public Health Agency of Canada, "Healthy Living: Frequently Asked Questions (FAQ)." Retrieved on May 31, 2006 from www.phac-aspc.gc.ca/hl-vs-strat/faq_e.html.

10. Ibid.

11. Ibid.

12. Secretariat for the Intersectoral Healthy Living Network, "Pan-Canadian Healthy Living Strategy."

13. Lisa Miller, "Medical Schools Put Women in Curricula," *Wall Street Journal,* May 24, 1994: B1, B7.

14. M. Eichler, A. L. Reisman, and E. M. Borins, "Gender Bias in Medical Research," *Women and Therapy* 12 (1992): 61–70.

15. Ibid.

16. National Cancer Institute Statistics, "Breast Cancer Risk," *Health,* May/June 1994, 14.

17. Statistics Canada, "Selected Leading Causes of Death, by Sex." Retrieved on June 1, 2006 from ww40.statcan.ca/101/cst01/health36.htm.

18. M. DiMatteo, *The Psychology of Health, Illness, and Medical Care: An Individual Perspective* (Pacific Grove, CA: Brooks/Cole, 1994) 101–103.

19. Edward P. Sarafino, *Health Psychology* (New York: John Wiley & Sons, 1990) 189–191.

20. George D. Bishop, *Health Psychology* (Needham Heights, MA: Allyn & Bacon, 1994) 84–86.

21. I. Ajzen. "The Theory of Planned Behavior," *Organizational Behavior and Human Decision Processes* 50 (1991): 179–211.

22. A. Ellis and M. Bernard, *Clinical Application of Rational-Emotive Therapy* (New York: Plenum, 1985).

23. P. Watson and R. Tharp, *Self-Directed Behavior: Self-Modification for Personal Adjustment* (Pacific Grove, CA: Brooks/Cole, 1993) 13.

24. The Stanford DECIDE Drug Education Curriculum, Garfield Company, CA.

25. S. K. Powers, S. L. Dodd, A. M. Thompson, and C. C. Condon, *Total Fitness and Wellness,* Cdn. ed. (Toronto: Pearson, 2006).

CHAPTER 2

1. National Mental Health Association, *Mental Health* (Alexandria, VA: National Mental Health Association, 1988) 3–4; W. Menninger, "Emotional Maturity," in *A Psychiatrist for a Troubled World: Selected Papers of William Menninger,* ed. Bernard H. Hall (New York: Viking, 1967), 789–807; Gerald Caplan, *Principles of Preventive Psychiatry* (New York: Basic Books, 1964).

2. R. Pausch and J. Zaslow, *The Last Lecture* (New York: Hyperion, 2008), 180.

3. Wikipedia "Biophilia Hypothesis." Retrieved on December 5, 2008 from en.wikipedia.org/wiki/Biophyilia.

4. Canadian Mental Health Association, "Benefits of Good Mental Health." Retrieved on January 24, 2009 from www.cmha.ca/bins/print_page.asp?cid=2-267-1320&lang=1.

5. Canadian Mental Health Association, "Men and Mental Illness." Retrieved on January 24, 2009 from www.cmha.ca/bins/print_page.asp?cid=3-726&lang=1.

6. Richard Lazarus, *Emotion and Adaptation* (New York: Oxford Press, 1991).

7. Christine Ritter, "Social Supports, Social Networks, and Health Behaviors," in *Health Behavior: Emerging Research Perspectives,* ed. David Gochman (New York: Plenum, 1988).

8. Lester Lefton, *Psychology,* 5th ed. (Boston: Allyn & Bacon, 1994) 626.

9. B. Pesut "A Conversation on Diverse Perspectives of Spirituality in Nursing Literature," *Nursing Philosophy* 9.2 (April 2008): 98–109.

10. Thompson Rivers University, "Spiritual Health." Retrieved on October 9, 2008 from www.tru.ca/wellness/spiritual.html.

11. A. O'Connell and V. O'Connell, *Choice and Change: Psychology of Holistic Growth, Adjustment, and Creativity* (Englewood Cliffs, NJ: Prentice Hall, 1992).

12. J. A. Astin et al., "Mind–Body Medicine: State of the Science, Implications for Practice," *Journal of the American Board of Family Practice* 16 (2003): 131–147; J. Bishop et al., "Mindfulness: A Proposed Operational Definition," *Clinical Psychology* 11 (2004): 230–241.

13. Bishop et al., "Mindfulness."

14. Ibid.

15. Ibid.

16. K. Karen et al., *Mind/Body Health: The Effects of Attitudes, Emotions, and Relationships,* 3rd ed. (San Francisco: Benjamin Cummings, 2006).

17. A. Astin et al., "Spirituality in Higher Education: A National Study of College Students' Search for Meaning and Purpose," Higher Education Research Institute, Graduate School of Education & Information Studies, UCLA, 2004, www.spirituality.ucla.edu.

18. Z. Segal et al., *Mindfulness-Based Cognitive Therapy for Depression: A New Approach to Preventing Relapse* (New York: Guilford Publications, 2001); M. Weiss, J. W. Nordlie, and E. P. Siegel, "Mindfulness-Based Stress Reduction as an Adjunct to Outpatient

Psychotherapy," *Psychotherapy and Psychosomatics* 74.2 (2005): 108–112; J. Cohen-Katz et al., "The Effects of Mindfulness-Based Stress Reduction on Nurse Stress and Burnout, Part II: A Quantitative and Qualitative Study," *Holistic Nurse Practice* 1 (2005): 26–35; A. Tacon et al., "Mindfulness Meditation, Anxiety Reduction, and Heart Disease: A Pilot Study," *Family and Community Health* 26.1 (2003): 25–33.

19. D. Elkins, *Beyond Religion—A Personal Program for Building a Spiritual Life Outside the Walls of Traditional Religion* (Wheaton, IL: Quest Books, 1998).

20. Martin Seligman, *Learned Optimism* (New York: Knopf, 1990).

21. Ibid.

22. P. Zimbardo, A. Weber, and R. Johnson, *Psychology* (Boston: Allyn and Bacon, 2000) 403.

23. M.W. Kilpatrick, "Exercise, Mood, and Psychological Well-Being: A Practitioner's Guide to Theory, Research and Application," *ACSM's Health & Fitness Journal* 12.5 (2008): 14–20.

24. National Sleep Foundation, "NSF's 2007 Sleep in America Poll: Stressed-Out American Women Have No Time for Sleep," March 6, 2007, www.sleepfoundation.org.

25. K. Wright et al., "Effects of Sleep Inertia on Cognition," *Journal of the American Medical Association* 295.2 (2006): 163–165.

26. Karen et al., *Mind/Body Health.*

27. M. Lemonick, "The Biology of Joy," *Time* 165.3 (2005): A12–A14.

28. J. Kluger, "The Funny Thing about Laughter," *Time* 165.3 (2005): A25–A29.

29. Ibid.

30. R. Davidson et al., "The Privileged Status of Emotion in the Brain," *Proceedings of the National Academy of Sciences of the United States of America* 101.33 (2004).

31. E. Diener and M. E. P. Seligman, "Beyond Money: Toward an Economy of Well-Being," *Psychological Science in the Public Interest* 5 (2004): 1–31; C. Peterson and M. Seligman, *Character Strengths and Virtues* (London: Oxford University Press, 2004).

32. B. Fredrickson, "Cultivating Positive Emotions to Optimize Health and Well-Being," *Prevention and Treatment* 3 (March 7, 2000), article 0001a.

33. D. Grady, "Think Right, Stay Well," *American Health* 11 (1992): 50–54.

34. J. M. Gottman and N. Silver, *The Seven Principles of Making Marriage Work* (New York: Crown Publishers Inc., 1999).

35. Grady, "Think Right."

36. Health Canada, "Message from the Minister of Health: National Mental Health Week: May 1–7, 2006." Retrieved on May 8, 2006 from www.hc-sc.gc.ca/ahc-asc/minist/health-sante/messages/2006_05_01_e.html.

37. Statistics Canada, "Risk of Depression, by Age Group and Sex, Household Population Aged 12 and Over, Canada, 2000/01." Retrieved on May 30, 2006 from dissemination.stat.ca/English/freepubl/82-221-XIE/2005002/tables/html/1295.htm.

38. Adapted by permission of the author from Kathryn Rose Gertz, "Mood Probe: Pinpointing the Crucial Differences between Emotional Lows and the Gridlock of Depression," *Self* (November 1990): 165–168, 204.

39. The Canadian Mental Health Association, Ontario Division, Information Sheet: "Understanding," 1999.

40. Anthony J. Levitt and Michael H. Boyle, "The Impact of Latitude on the Prevalence of Seasonal Depression," *Canadian Journal of Psychiatry* 47 (2002): 361–367.

41. Levitan, "An Overview of Seasonal Affective Disorder," Psychiatry Rounds, Department of Psychiatry, University of Toronto Centre for Addiction and Mental Health, October 2, No. 7 (1998).

42. Canadian Mental Health Association, "Anxiety Disorders." Retrieved on January 24, 2009 from www.cmha.ca/bins/print_page.asp?cid=3-94&lang=1.

43. Ibid.

44. Canadian Mental Health Association, "Obsessive Compulsive Disorder." Retrieved on January 24, 2009 from www.cmha.ca/bins/print_page.asp?cid=3-94-95&lang=1.

45. Ibid.

46. Canadian Mental Health Association, "Phobias and Panic Disorders." Retrieved on January 24, 2009 from www.cmha.ca/bins/print_page.asp?cid=3-94-96&lang=1.

47. Canadian Mental Health Association, "Post Traumatic Stress Disorder." Retrieved on January 24, 2009 from www.cmha.ca/bins/print_page.asp?cid=3-94-97&lang=1.

48. Statistics Canada, "Risk of Depression."

49. Statistics Canada, "Suicides and Suicide Rate."

50. World Health Organization, "Self-Directed Violence."

51. Royal Commission of Aboriginal Peoples, *Special Report on Suicide.*

52. Canadian Mental Health Association, "Preventing Suicide."

53. Canadian Mental Health Association, "Youth and Suicide." Retrieved on January 24, 2009 from www.cmha.ca/bins/print_page.asp?cid=3-101-104&lang=1.

54. Canadian Mental Health Association, "Youth and Suicide."

55. Canadian Mental Health Association, "Preventing Suicide."

CHAPTER 3

1. Canadian Mental Health Association, "Coping with Stress." Retrieved on January 24, 2009 from www.cmha.ca/bins/print_page.asp?cid=2-28-30&lang=1.

2. Hans Selye, *Stress without Distress* (New York: Lippincott, 1974) 28–29.

3. Canadian Mental Health Association, "Coping."

4. Charles Morris, *Understanding Psychology* (Englewood Cliffs, NJ: Prentice Hall, 1993) 471–473.

5. W. B. Kannel and E. D. Eaker, "Psychosocial and Other Features of Coronary Heart Disease: Insights from the Framingham Study," *American Heart Journal* 112.5 (1986): 1066–1073.

6. R. Ader and S. Cohen, "Psychoneuroimmunology: Conditioning and Stress," *Annual Review of Psychology* 44 (1993): 53–85.

7. N. Cohen, D. Tyrrell, and A. Smith, "Negative Life Events, Perceived Stress, Negative Affect, and Susceptibility to the Common Cold," *Journal of Personality and Social Psychology* 64 (1993): 131–140.

8. Ader and Cohen, "Psychoneuroimmunology."

9. Ibid.

10. Selye, *Stress without Distress.*

11. Thomas Holmes and Richard Rahe, "The Social Readjustment Rating Scale," *Journal of Psychosocial Research* (1967): 213–217.

12. Ibid.

13. Richard Lazarus, "The Trivialization of Distress," in *Preventing Health Risk Behaviors and Promoting Coping with Illness,* ed. J. Rosen and L. Solomon (Hanover, NH: University Press of New England, 1985) 279–298.

14. Lester Lefton, *Psychology* (Boston: Allyn & Bacon, 1994) 471.

15. Ibid.

16. R. C. Kessler, K. S. Kendler, A. C. Heath, M. C. Neale, and L. J. Eaves, "Social Support, Depressed Mood, and Adjustment to Stress: A Genetic Epidemiological Investigation," *Journal of Personality and Social Psychology* 62 (1992): 257–272.

17. Morris, *Understanding Psychology,* 447–448.

18. Meyer Friedman and Ray H. Rosenman, *Type A Behavior and Your Heart* (New York: Knopf, 1974).

19. R. Ragland and R. Brand, "Distrust, Rage May Be Toxic: Cores That Put Type A Person at Risk," *Journal of the American Medical Association* 261 (1989): 813, 814.

20. Philip L. Rice, *Stress and Health* (Monterey, CA: Brooks/Cole, 1992) 471.

21. Ibid.

22. Robert Eliot, *Is It Worth Dying For?* (New York: Bantam, 1984), 225.

23. Canadian Mental Health Association, "Coping."

CHAPTER 4

1. World Health Organization, "Health and Development through Physical Activity and Sport." WHO/NHM/NPH/PAH/O3.2. (Geneva: WHO Document Production Services, 2003).

2. C. Bouchard, R. J. Shephard, T. Stephens, J. R. Sutton, and B. D. McPherson, "Exercise, Fitness, and Health: The Consensus Statement," in *Exercise, Fitness, and Health: A Consensus of Current Knowledge,* eds. C. Bouchard, R. J. Shephard, T. Stephens, J. R. Sutton, and B. D. McPherson (Champaign, IL: Human Kinetics, 1988) 4–27.

3. Bouchard et al., "Exercise, Fitness, and Health"; College of Family Physicians of Canada, "Exercise: A Healthy Habit to Start and Keep." Last modified October 31, 2002. Retrieved on February 9, 2003 from www.cfpc.ca/programs/education/pated/Exercise.asp.8.

4. D. E. R. Warburton, C. Whitney Nicol, and S. S. D. Bredin. "Prescribing Exercise as Preventive Therapy," *Canadian Medical Association Journal,* 174.7 (2006): 961–974. Erratum, 178.6 (2008): 731–732.

5. Statistics Canada, "Physical Activity, by Age Group and Sex, Household Population Aged 12 and Older." Retrieved on February 20, 2006 from www40.statcan.ca/l01/cst01/health46.htm?sdi=physical activity.

6. Canadian Fitness and Lifestyle Research Institute, "Survey Statistics Summaries—2004 Physical Activity Monitor." Retrieved on June 5, 2006 from www.cflri.ca/eng/statistics/index.php.

7. A. M. Thompson, P. D. Campagna, L. A. Rehman, R. J. L. Murphy, R. L. Rasmussen, and G. W. Ness, "Physical Activity and Body Mass Index in Grade 3, 7, and 11 Nova Scotia Students," *Medicine & Science in Sports & Exercise* 37.11 (2005): 1902–1908.

8. A. M. Thompson, M. L. Humbert, and R. L. Mirwald, "A Longitudinal Study of the Impact of Childhood and Adolescent Physical Activity Experiences on Adult Physical Activity Perceptions and Behaviours." *Qualitative Health Research* 13.3 (2003): 358–377.

9. Statistics Canada, "Physical Activity Level, Changes Between 1994/1995 and 2004/2005, by Age Group." Retrieved on August 20, 2008 from www40.statcan.ca/cbin/fl/cstprintflag.gci.

10. Health Canada: Physical Activity Unit, "Helpful Definitions." Retrieved on August 23, 2004 from www.hc-sc.gc.ca/hppb/fitness/definitions.html.

11. D. E. R. Warburton, C. Whitney Nicol, and S. S. D. Bredin, "Health Benefits of Physical Activity: The Evidence," *Canadian Medical Association Journal* 174.6 (2006) 801–809.

12. L. Bernstein et al., "Adolescent Exercise Reduces Risk of Breast Cancer in Younger Women," *Journal of the National Cancer Institute* (September 1994).

13. D. E. R. Warburton, P. T. Katzmarzyk, R. E. Rhodes, R. J. Shephard, "Evidence-Informed Physical Activity Guidelines for Canadian Adults," *Canadian Journal of Public Health* 98 (Suppl. 2007): S16–S68.

14. J. C. Spence, R. C. Plotnikoff, and W. K. Mummery, "The Awareness and Use of Canada's Physical Activity Guide to Healthy Living," *Canadian Journal of Public Health,* 93.5 (2002): 394–396.

15. Health Canada: Physical Activity Unit, "Helpful Definitions."

16. Ibid.

17. Public Health Agency of Canada, "Canada's Physical Activity Guide for Healthy Active Living." Ottawa.

18. W. L. Haskell, A. S. Leon, C. J. Caspersen, et al., "Cardiovascular Benefits and Assessment of Physical Activity and Physical Fitness in Adults," *Medicine and Science in Sports and Exercise* 24.6 (Suppl. 1992): S201–S220.

19. Ibid.

20. "Third Report of the National Cholesterol Education Program Expert Panel on Detection, Evaluation, and Treatment of High Blood Cholesterol in Adults," *Journal of the American Medical Association* 285.19 (2001): 1–19.

21. G. R. Herzberg, "Aerobic Exercise, Lipoproteins, and Cardiovascular Disease: Benefits and Possible Risks," *Canadian Journal of Applied Physiology* 29.6 (2004): 800–807.

22. W. H. Ettinger Jr, and R. F. Afable, "Physical Disability from Knee Osteoarthritis: The Role of Exercise as an Intervention," *Medicine and Science in Sports and Exercise* 26 (1994): 1435–1440.

23. P. A. Kovar, J. P. Allegrante, C. R. MacKenzie, et al., "Supervised Fitness Walking in Patients with Osteoarthritis of the Knee: A Randomized, Controlled Trial," *Annals of Internal Medicine* 116 (1992): 529–534; D. T. Felson, Y. Zhang, J. M. Anthony, et al., "Weight Loss Reduces the Risk of Symptomatic Knee Osteoarthritis in Women: The Framingham Study," *Annals of Internal Medicine* 116 (1992): 535–539.

24. H. M. Frost, "Skeletal Structural Adaptations to Mechanical Usage (SATMU): 1. Redefining Wolff's Law: The Bone Remodeling Problem," *The Anatomical Record* 226 (1990): 403–413.

25. B. L. Drinkwater, "Does Physical Activity Play a Role in Preventing Osteoporosis?" *Research Quarterly for Exercise and Sport* 65 (1994): 197–206.

26. C. E. Tudor-Locke, R. C. Bell, and A. M. Meyers, "Revisiting the Role of Physical Activity and Exercise in the Treatment of Type II Diabetes," *Canadian Journal of Applied Physiology* 25.6 (2000): 466–492.

27. S. P. Helmrich, D. R. Ragland, and R. S. Paffenbarger Jr, "Prevention of Non-Insulin-Dependent Diabetes Mellitus with Physical Activity," *Medicine and Science in Sports and Exercise* 26 (1994): 824–830.

28. R. Paffenbarger, R. Hyde, A. Wing, and C. Hsieh, "Physical Activity, All Cause Mortality, Longevity of College Alumni," *New England Journal of Medicine* 314 (1986): 605–613.

29. S. N. Blair, H. W. Kohl III, R. S. Paffenbarger, et al., "Physical Fitness and All-Cause Mortality: A Prospective Study of Healthy Men and Women," *Journal of the American Medical Association* 262.17 (1989): 2395–2401.

30. E. R. Eichner, "Infection, Immunity, and Exercise: What to Tell Patients?" *Physician and Sportsmedicine* (January 1993): 125–135.

31. D. C. Nieman, "Exercise, Immunity and Respiratory Infections," *Sports Science Exchange* (August 1992).

32. D. C. Nieman, L. M. Johanssen, J. W. Lee, et al., "Infectious Episodes in Runners before and after the Los Angeles Marathon," *Journal of Sports Medicine and Physical Fitness* 30 (1990): 316–328.

33. Eichner, "Infection, Immunity, and Exercise."

34. Canadian Society for Exercise Physiology, *The Canadian Physical Activity, Fitness & Lifestyle Approach (CPAFLA): CSEP Health & Fitness Program's Health-Related Appraisal and Counselling Strategy,* 3rd ed. (Ottawa: Canadian Society for Exercise Physiology, 2003).

35. E. Fox, R. Bowers, and M. Foss. *The Physiological Basis for Exercise and Sport* (Dubuque, IA: Brown and Benchmark, 1989).

36. B. Stamford, "Tracking Your Heart Rate for Fitness," *Physician and Sportsmedicine* (March 1993).

37. Public Health Agency of Canada, "Canada's Physical Activity Guide."

38. P. D. Wood, "Physical Activity, Diet, and Health: Independent and Interactive Effects," *Medicine and Science in Sports and Exercise* 26 (1994): 838–843.

39. R. T. Kell, G. Bell, A. Quinney, "Musculoskeletal Fitness, Health Outcomes, and Quality of Life," *Sports Medicine* 31.12 (2001): 863–873.

40. S. K. Powers, S. L. Dodd, A. M. Thompson, and C. C. Condon, *Total Fitness and Wellness,* Cdn. ed. (Toronto: Pearson, 2006).

41. P. A. Sienna, *One Rep Max: A Guide to Beginning Weight Training* (Indianapolis: Benchmark, 1989).

42. H. G. Knuttgen and W. J. Kraemer, "Terminology and Measurement in Exercise Performance," *Journal of Applied Sport Science Research* 1 (1987): 1–10.

43. W. J. Kraemer, "Involvement of Eccentric Muscle Action May Optimize Adaptations to Resistance Training," *Sports Science Exchange* (November 1992).

44. W. J. Kraemer and N. A. Ratamess, "Fundamentals of Resistance Training: Progression and Exercise Prescription." *Medicine and Science in Sports and Exercise* 36.4 (2004): 674–688.

45. Ibid.

46. American Academy of Orthopedic Surgeons, *Athletic Training and Sports Medicine,* 2nd ed. (Park Ridge, IL: AAOS, 1991).

47. S. J. Hartley-O'Brien, "Six Mobilization Exercises for Active Range of Hip Motion," *Research Quarterly for Exercise and Sport* 51 (1980): 625–635.

48. D. G. Behm and A Kibele. "Effects of Differing Intensities of Static Stretching on Jump Performance," *European Journal of Applied Physiology* 101.5 (2007): 587–594.

49. D. M. Brody, "Running Injuries: Prevention and Management," *Clinical Symposia* 39 (1987).

50. J. C. Erie, "Eye Injuries: Prevention, Evaluation, and Treatment," *Physician and Sportsmedicine* (November 1991): 108–122.

51. R. C. Wasserman and R. V. Buccini, "Helmet Protection from Head Injuries among Recreational Bicyclists," *American Journal of Sports Medicine* 18 (1990): 96–97.

52. J. Andrish and J. A. Work, "How I Manage Shin Splints," *Physician and Sportsmedicine* (December 1990): 113–114.

53. Brody, "Running Injuries."

54. American Academy of Orthopedic Surgeons, *Athletic Training and Sports Medicine.*

55. B. Q. Hafen and K. J. Karren, *Prehospital Emergency Care and Crisis Intervention,* 4th ed. (Englewood Cliffs, NJ: Prentice-Hall, 1992).

56. J. S. Thornton, "Hypothermia Shouldn't Freeze Out Cold-Weather Athletes," *Physician and Sportsmedicine* (January 1990): 109–113.

57. J. C. Spence, R. C. Plotnikoff, L. S. Rovniak, K. A. Martin Glinis, W. Rodgers, and S. A. Lear. "Perceived Neighbourhood Correlates of Walking among Participants Visiting the 'Canada on the Move' Website," *Canadian Journal of Public Health* 97 (Suppl. 1, 2006) S39–S44.

CHAPTER 5

1. Health and Welfare Canada, "Food Guide Facts: Background for Educators and Communicators" (Ottawa: Minister of Supply and Services, Cat. No. H39-253/101-1992E, 1992).

2. Health Canada: Food and Nutrition, "Canada's Food Guides from 1942 to 1992." Retrieved on May 25, 2006 from www.hc-sc.gc.ca/fn-an/food-guide-aliment/hist/fg_history-histoire_ga_e.html#process.

3. Health Canada: Food and Nutrition, "Revision of Canada's Food Guide to Healthy Eating." Retrieved on May 25, 2006 from www.hc-sc.gc.ca/fn-an/food-guide-aliment/revision/revision_fg-examen_ga_e.html.

4. Ibid.

5. Health Canada, "Eating Well with Canada's Food Guide" (Ottawa: Minister of Supply and Services, HC Pub: 4651; Cat. H164-38/1-2007E; ISBN: 0-662-44467-1). Available online at www.healthcanada.gc.ca/foodguide.

6. S. Laidlaw. "Growing Interest in Sports Nutrition Could Fuel New Market for Milk," *Milk Producer* (October 2007): 25–30.

7. J. Thompson, M. Manore, and J. Sheeska, *Nutrition: A Functional Approach,* Cdn. ed. (Toronto: Pearson Benjamin Cummings, 2007).

8. Ibid.

9. Laidlaw, "Growing Interest in Sports Nutrition."

10. Thompson, Manore, and Sheeska, *Nutrition.*

11. Ibid.

12. Ibid.

13. World Health Organization, "Population Nutrient Intake Goals for Preventing Diet-Related Chronic Disease." Retrieved on April 7, 2009 from www.who.int/nutrition/topics/5_population_nutrient/en/print.html.

14. Janet Christian and Janet Gregor, *Nutrition for Living,* 4th ed. (Benjamin Cummings, 1994), 129.

15. Ibid.

16. D. A. Sedlock, "The Latest on Carbohydrate Loading: A Practical Approach," *Current Sports Medicine Reports* 7.4 (2008): 209–213.

17. M. A. Tarnopolsky, S. A. Atkinson, S. M. Phillips, and J. D. MacDougall, "Carbohydrate Loading and Metabolism in Exercise in Men and Women," *Journal of Applied Physiology* 78 (1995): 1360–1368.

18. Ibid.

19. Thompson, Manore, and Sheeska, *Nutrition.*

20. Ibid.

21. Ibid.

22. University of California at Berkeley Wellness Letter (April 1992): 4–6.

23. Thompson, Manore, and Sheeska, *Nutrition.*

24. S. Conrad, "Current Perspectives on Understanding Fat," Fact Sheet for Canadian Council of Food and Nutrition. Retrieved on September 11, 2008 from www.cfcn.ca/in_action/fact_sheets.asp.

25. Health Canada, "Eating Well with Canada's Food Guide."

26. Conrad, "Current Perspectives."

27. S. Mah, "Current Perspectives on Trans Fat," Fact Sheet for Canadian Council of Food and Nutrition. Retrieved on September 11, 2008 from www.cfcn.ca/in_action/fact_sheets.asp.

28. Ibid.

29. Thompson, Manore, and Sheeska, *Nutrition.*

30. Ibid.

31. Mah, "Current Perspectives."

32. Thompson, Manore, and Sheeska, *Nutrition.*

33. Ibid.

34. A. Tremblay and J-P. Chaput, "About Unsuspected Potential Determinants of Obesity," *Applied Physiology, Nutrition, and Metabolism* 33.4 (2008): 791–796.

35. Christian and Gregor, *Nutrition for Living.*

36. Thompson, Manore, and Sheeska, *Nutrition.*

37. Ibid.

38. Ibid.

39. Ibid.

40. Centers for Disease Control and Prevention, "Food Borne Illnesses," 2002, www.cdc.gov; American Medical Association, "Diagnosis and Management of Foodborne Illness: A Primer for Physicians and Other Health Care Professionals," 2004, www.ama-assn.org/ama/org.

41. Ibid.

42. Ibid.

43. P. Morris, Y. Motarjemi, and F. Kaferstein, "Emerging Food-Borne Diseases," *World Health* 50 (1997): 16–22; Centers for Disease Control and Prevention "Food Borne Illnesses."

44. L. Katzenstein, "Food Irradiation: The Story Behind the Scare," *American Health* (December 1992): 60–80.

45. A. Hechtt, "Preventing Food-Borne Illnesses," *FDA Consumer Magazine.*

CHAPTER 6

1. M. Tjepkema, "Measured Obesity: Adult Obesity in Canada: Measured Height and Weight," *Nutrition: Findings from the Canadian Community Health Survey 1,* 2005 (Statistics Canada no. 82-620-MWE2005001).

2. Ibid.

3. A. M. Thompson, A. D. G. Baxter-Jones, R. L. Mirwald, and D. A. Bailey, "Secular Trends in the Development of Fatness during Childhood and Adolescence." *American Journal of Human Biology* 14.5 (2002): 669–679.

4. P. T. Katzmarzyk, "The Canadian Obesity Epidemic, 1985–1998." *Canadian Medical Association Journal* 166.8 (2002): 1039–1040.

5. Ibid.

6. Health Canada, "Canadian Guidelines for Body Weight Classifications in Adults," 2003. Retrieved July 21, 2004 from www.hc-sc.gc.ca/hpfb-dgpsa/onpp-bppn/weight_book_tc_e.html.

7. R. M. Malina, C. Bouchard, and O. Bar-Or. *Growth, Maturation, and Physical Activity* (Champaign, IL: Human Kinetics, 2004).

8. Ibid.

9. Ibid.

10. A. S. Jackson and M. L. Pollock. "Generalized Equations for Predicting Body Density of Men," *British Journal of Nutrition* 40 (1978): 497–504; A. S. Jackson and M. L. Pollock, "Generalized Equations for Predicting Body Density of Women," *Medicine and Science in Sports and Exercise* 12 (1980): 175–192; A. Sloan and J. Weir, "Nomogram for Prediction of Body Density and Total Fat from Skinfold Measurements," *Journal of Applied Physiology* 28 (1970): 221–222; J. V. G. A. Durnin and J. Womersley, "Body Fat Assessed from Total Body Density and Its Estimation from Skinfold Thickness: Measurements on 481 Men and Women Aged from 16 to 72 Years," *British Journal of Nutrition* 320 (1974): 77–97.

11. R. Ross, T. Berentzen, A. J. Bradshaw, I. Janssen, H. S. Kahn, P. T. Katzmarzyk, J. L. Kuk, J. C. Seidell, M. B. Snijder, T. I. Sorensen, and J. P. Depres, "Does the Relationship between Waist Circumference, Morbidity and Mortality Depend on Measurement Protocol for Waist Circumference?" *Obesity Review* 9.4 (2008): 312–325.

12. C. J. Crespo and E. Smit. "Prevalence of Overweight and Obesity in the United States," in *Obesity: Etiology, Assessment, Treatment and Prevention,* ed. R. E. Andersen (Champaign, IL: Human Kinetics, 2003); B. A. Reeder, A. Senthilselvan, J-P. Després, A. Angel, L. Liu, H. Wang, and S. W. Rabkin, "The Association of Cardiovascular Disease Risk Factors with Abdominal Obesity in Canada," *Canadian Medical Association Journal* 157 (Suppl. 1,1997): S39–S45; CSEP Communique, "Knowledge Translation: Advances in Exercise Physiology Research: The Revision of the Measurement of Waist Circumference in the CPAFLA," November 2008. Retrieved on November 3, 2008 from www.csep.ca.

13. Malina et al., *Growth, Maturation, and Physical Activity.*

14. M. Boyle and G. Zyla, *Personal Nutrition* (St. Paul, MN: West Publishing, 1991) 21.

15. G. Wilson, "Relation of Dieting and Voluntary Weight Loss to Psychological Functioning and Binge Eating," *Annals of Internal Medicine* 119 (1993): 727–730.

16. J. Robison et al., "Obesity, Weight Loss, and Health," *Journal of the American Dietetic Association* 93 (1993): 448.

17. Ibid.

18. Simone French and R. Jeffery, "Consequences of Dieting to Lose Weight: Effects on Physical and Mental Health," *Health Psychology* 13.3 (1994): 195–212.

19. Wilson, "Relation of Dieting and Voluntary Weight Loss."

20. L. Lissner et al., "Variabilities in Body Weight and Health Outcomes in the Framingham Study," *New England Journal of Medicine* 324 (1991): 1839–1844.

21. J. Horm and K. Anderson, "Who in America Is Trying to Lose Weight?" *Annals of Internal Medicine* 119 (1993): 672–676.

22. K. D. Raine, "Determinants of Healthy Eating in Canada: An Overview and Synthesis," *Canadian Journal of Public Health* 96.3 (July/August 2005): S8–S14.

23. T. Rankinen et al., "The Human Obesity Gene Map: 2005 Update," *Obesity* 14 (2006): 529–644.

24. W. Sheldon, S. Stevens, and W. Tucker, *The Varieties of Human Physique* (New York: Harper and Row, 1940) 104.

25. Malina, et al. *Growth, Maturation, and Physical Activity.*

26. A. Stunkard, *Psychiatric Update: American Psychiatric Association* (New York: Harper and Row, 1985) 87.

27. Claude Bouchard et al., "The Response to Long-Term Overfeeding in Identical Twins," *New England Journal of Medicine* 322 (1990): 1477–1488.

28. Ibid.

29. Rankinen et al., "The Human Obesity Gene Map."

30. Ibid.

31. J. Loos and C. Bouchard, "Obesity—Is It a Genetic Disorder?" *Journal of Internal Medicine* 254 (2003): 401–425.

32. Mayo Clinic, "Special Report: Weight Control," 2005, www.mayoclinic.com.

33. A. Tremblay and J-P. Chaput, "About Unsuspected Potential Determinants of Obesity," *Applied Physiology, Nutrition, and Metabolism* 33.4 (2008): 791–796.

34. D. Williams, D. Baskin, and M. Schwartz, "Leptin Regulation of Anorexic Responses to Glucagon-like Peptide-1 Receptor Stimulation," *Diabetes* 55.12 (2006): 3387–3393.

35. Malina, et al., *Growth, Maturation, and Physical Activity.*

36. Ibid.

37. Kelly Brownell, "Comments on the Latest Study on Yo-Yo Diets by Steven N. Blair of the Institute for Aerobics Research in Dallas." Paper presented at the annual research meeting of the American Heart Association, Monterey, CA, January 1993.

38. L. A. Wadsworth, and A. MacQuarrie, "Nutrition Messages on Saturday Morning Children's Television: 1989–1998," *Canadian Journal of Dietetic Practice and Research* 63 (Suppl. 2002): 105; L. A. Wadsworth, and S. Berenbaum, "Textual Analyses of Nutrition Messages on Prime Time Television," *Canadian Home Economics Journal* 51 (2001): 13–18.

39. Philip Elmer-Dewitt, "Fat Times," *Time,* January 16, (1995): 60.

40. S. Lichman et al., "Discrepancy between Self-Reported and Actual Caloric Intake and Exercise in Obese Subjects," *New England Journal of Medicine* 327 (1992): 1894–1897.

41. Statistics Canada, "Health Indicators" (Catalogue no. 82-221-X9), May 2002.

42. North American Association for the Study of Obesity (NAASO), The Obesity Society, "Obesity, Bias, and Stigmatization," 2007, www.naaso.org/information/weight_bias.asp.

43. N. Amy et al., "Barriers to Routing Gynecological Cancer Screening for White and African-American Obese Women." *Journal of Obesity Research* 30 (2006): 147–155.

44. C. J. Cavanaugh and R. Lemberg, "What We Know about Eating Disorders: Facts and Statistics," in *Eating Disorders: A Reference Sourcebook,* ed. Raymond Lemberg and Leigh Cohn (Phoenix, AZ: Oryx Press, 1999).

45. J. M. Jones, S. Bennett, M. P. Olmsted, M. L. Lawson, and G. Rodin. "Disordered Eating Attitudes and Behaviours in Teenaged Girls: A School-Based Study," *Canadian Medical Association Journal* 165.5 (2001): 547–552.

46. National Eating Disorder Information Centre, "Help for Family and Friends." Retrieved on November 4, 2008 from www.nedic.ca/giveandgethelp/helpforfriendsfamily.shtml.

47. Bulimia Anorexia Nervosa Association (Canada), www.bana.ca.

48. National Eating Disorder Information Centre, "Help for Family and Friends."

49. Ibid.

50. Ibid.

51. Jones et al., "Disordered Eating Attitudes."

52. National Eating Disorder Information Centre, "Help for Family and Friends."

53. "Treating Eating Disorders," *Harvard Women's Health Watch* (May 1996): 4–5.

CHAPTER 7

1. MayoClinic.com, "Nurture Relationships: A Healthy Habit for Healthy Aging," 2003, Mayo Foundation for Medical Education and Research (MFMER), www.mayohealth.org; K. Uberg et al., "Supportive Relationships as a Moderator of the Effects of Peer Drinking on Adolescents," *Journal of Research on Adolescents* 15.1 (2005): 1–20.

2. C. Snapp and M. Leary, "Hurt Feelings among New Acquaintances: Moderating Effects of Interpersonal Familiarity," *Journal of Social and Personal Relationships* 18.3 (June 2001): 1344–1350.

3. V. Manusov and J. Harvey, eds., *Attribution, Communication Behavior and Close Relationships* (New York: Cambridge University Press, 2001).

4. J. Caputo, H. C. Hazel, and C. McMahon, *Interpersonal Communication* (Boston: Allyn & Bacon, 1994) 224.

5. Janet D. Woititz, *Struggle for Intimacy* (Pompano Beach, FL: Health Communications, 1985).

6. Sharon S. Brehm, *Intimate Relationships* (New York: McGraw-Hill, 1992) 4–5.

7. "Vanier Institute on the Family Mission Statement," *Canadian Social Trends* (Summer 1993), Statistics Canada (Cat. No. 11-008E), Ottawa: Ministry of Supply and Services.

8. J. Dunn, "Siblings and Development," *Current Directions in Psychological Science* 1 (1992): 6–11.

9. J. Turner and L. Rubinson, *Contemporary Human Sexuality* (Englewood Cliffs, NJ: Prentice Hall, 1993) 457.

10. Ibid.

11. E. Hatfield, "Passionate and Companionate Love," in *The Psychology of Love,* eds. R. J. Sternberg and M. Barnes (New Haven: Yale University Press, 1988) 191–217.

12. R. A. Baron and D. Byrne, *Social Psychology* (Boston: Allyn & Bacon, 1994), 318.

13. E. Hatfield and G. W. Walster, *A New Look at Love* (Reading, MA: Addison-Wesley, 1981).

14. Helen Fisher, *Anatomy of Love: The Natural History of Monogamy, Adultery, and Divorce* (New York: Norton, 1993).

15. A. Toufexis and P. Gray, "What Is Love? The Right Chemistry," *Time* (1993): 47–52.

16. Ibid.

17. Fisher, *Anatomy of Love.*

18. C. McLoughlin, "Science of Love—Cupid's Chemistry," *The Naked Scientists Online,* 2003, www.thenakedscientist.com/HTML/Columnists/clairemcloughlincolumn1.htm.

19. "I Get a Kick Out of You," *The Economist* 370 (8367): 73–75.

20. Deborah Tannen, *You Just Don't Understand: Women and Men in Conversation* (New York: Ballantine, 1990).

21. M. McGill, *The McGill Report on Male Intimacy* (New York: Holt, Rinehart & Winston, 1985) 87–88.

22. Lillian Rubin, *Intimate Strangers* (New York: Harper and Row, 1983).

23. S. Hendricks and C. Hendricks, *Liking, Loving, and Relating,* 2nd ed. (Pacific Grove, CA: Brooks/Cole, 1992).

24. R. Landerman, M. Swartz, and L. George, "The Long-Term Effects of Childhood Exposure to Parental Drinking." Paper presented at the annual meeting of the American Public Health Association, Mental Health session, Washington, DC, 1992; A. Diaz, F. Yancovitz, N. Showers, and I. Epstein, "Predictors and Psychological Consequences of Disclosure of Incest by Female Adolescents." Paper presented at the annual meeting of the American Public Health Association, Mental Health session, Washington, DC, 1992.

25. M. Klausner and B. Hasselbring, *Aching for Love: The Sexual Drama of the Adult Child* (New York: Harper and Row, 1990).

26. Statistics Canada, "Population by Marital Status and Sex." Retrieved on February 23, 2009 from www.40.statcan.gc.ca/cbin/fl/cstprintflag.cgi.

27. Statistics Canada, "Marriages by Province and Territory." Retrieved on February 23, 2009 from www.40.statcan.gc.ca/ cbin/fl/cstprintflag.cgi.

28. Statistics Canada, "Divorces by Province and Territory." Retrieved on February 23, 2009 from www.40.statcan.gc.ca/ cbin/fl/cstprintflag.cgi.

29. Statistics Canada, "Legal Marital Status (6), Common-law Status (3), Age Groups (17) and Sex (3) for the Population 15 Years and Over of Canada, Provinces, Territories, Census Metropolitan Areas and Census Agglomerations, 2001 and 2006 Censuses—100% Data." Retrieved on February 23, 2009 from www12.statcan.gc.ca/english/census06/data/topics/RetrieveProductTable.cfm?ALEVEL=3&APATH=3&CATNO=97-552-XCB2006007&DETAIL=0&DIM=&DS=99&FL=0&FREE=0&GAL=&GC=99&GK=NA&GRP=0&IPS=97-552-XCB2006007&METH=0&ORDER=&PID=88997&PTYPE=88971&RL=0&S=1&ShowAll=&StartRow=&SUB=&Temporal=2006&Theme=67&VID=&VNAMEE=&VNAMEF=.

30. W. Clark and S. Crompton, "Till Death Do Us Part? The Risk of First and Second Marriage Dissolution." Retrieved on February 23, 2009 from www.statcan.gc.ca/pub/11-008x/2006001/9198-eng.htm/.

31. Ibid.

32. Statistics Canada, "Changing Conjugal Life in Canada," *The Daily,* July 11, 2002.

33. R. Friedman and J. Downey, "Homosexuality," *New England Journal of Medicine* 33 (1994): 923–928.

34. Clark and Crompton, "Till Death Do Us Part?"

35. Statistics Canada, "Population by Marital Status and Sex."

36. J. Hirdes and P. Forbes, "Factors Associated with the Maintenance of Good Self-Rated Health," *Journal of Aging and Health* 5.1 (1993): 101–122.

37. Statistics Canada, "Divorces by Province and Territory."

38. Writing Group for the Women's Health Initiative Investigators, "Risk and Benefits of Estrogen Plus Progestin in Healthy Postmenopausal Women: Principal Results from the Women's Health Initiative Randomized Controlled Trial," *Journal of the American Medical Association* 288.3 (2002): 321–333.

39. Friedman and Downey, "Homosexuality."

40. Dorothy Tennov, *Love and Limerence* (Chelsea, MI: Scarborough House, 1989) 45–50.

41. Alex Comfort, *The Joy of Sex* (New York: Simon and Schuster, 1972) 14.

42. R. O'Carroll, "Sexual Desire Disorders: A Review of Controlled Treatment Studies," *The Journal of Sex Research* 28.19: 607–624.

43. National Kidney and Urological Diseases Information Clearinghouse, "Erectile Dysfunction," 2004, http://kidney.niddk.nih.gov/kudiseases/pubs/impotence/index.htm.

44. B. Handy, "The Potency Pill," *Time,* May 4, 1998: 50–57.

45. Arnot Ogden Medical Center, "Frequently Asked Questions," 1998, www.aomc.org/HOD2/general/ViagraFAQ.html.

46. C. Darling and J. Davidson, "Enhancing Relationships: Understanding the Feminine Mystique of Pretending Orgasm," *Journal of Sex and Marital Therapy* 12.19 (1986): 182–196.

CHAPTER 8

1. Centers for Disease Control, *Contraceptive Options: Increasing Your Awareness* (Washington, DC: NAACOG, 1990).

2. University of Southern California School of Medicine, "Noncontraceptive Health Benefits," *Dialogues in Contraception* 3 (1990): 2.

3. D. E. Greydanus and R. B. Shearin, *Adolescent Sexuality and Gynecology* (Philadelphia: Lea & Febiger, 1990) 107.

4. Planned Parenthood, "Chronology of Court Cases: Dr. Morgentaler and Others."

5. Ibid.

6. Childbirth by Choice Trust, *Abortion in Canada Today: The Situation Province by Province* (1995).

7. Planned Parenthood, *Therapeutic Abortions* (1994).

8. Statistics Canada, "Induced Abortions by Province and Territory of Report (Hospitals and Clinics)." Retrieved on February 24, 2009 from www40.statcan.gc.ca/cbin/fl/cstprintflag.cgi; Statistics Canada, "Induced Abortions by Age Group." Retrieved on February 24, 2009 from www40.statcan.gc.ca/cbin/fl/cstprintflag.cgi/.

9. Statistics Canada, "Induced Abortions Statistics." Retrieved on February 24, 2009 from www40.statcan.gc.ca/pub/82-223-x/2008000/5202129-eng.htm.

10. Statistics Canada, "Induced Abortions per 100 Live Births (Hospitals and Clinics)." Retrieved on February 24, 2009 from www40.statcan.gc.ca/cbin/fl/cstprintflag.cgi.

11. Statistics Canada, "Induced Abortions by Age Group."

12. K. Schmidt, "The Dark Legacy of Fatherhood," *U.S. News and World Report* (December 14, 1992): 94–95.

13. U.S. Department of Health and Human Services, *The Health Benefits of Smoking Cessation: A Report of the Surgeon General,* United States Public Health Service, Office on Smoking and Health, Washington, DC: 1990.

14. American College of Obstetricians and Gynecologists, "Nutrition during Pregnancy," Patient Education Pamphlet (AP001), April 1992.

15. D. Hall and D. Kaufmann, "Effects of Aerobic and Strength Conditioning on Pregnancy Outcomes," *American Journal of Obstetrics and Gynecology* 157 (1987): 1199–1203.

16. J. D. Forrest, "Contraceptive Needs through Stages of Women's Reproductive Lives," *Contemporary OB/GYN* (Special Issue on Fertility) (1988): 12–22.

17. W. J. Millar, C. Nair, and S. Wadhera, "Declining Cesarean Section Rates: A Continuing Trend?" *Health Reports* 8.1 (1996): 17–24.

18. Statistics Canada, "Pregnancy Outcome by Age Group (Fetal Loss)." Retrieved on February 25, 2009 from www40.statcan.gc.ca/cbin/fl/cstprintflag.cgi.

19. Public Health Agency of Canada, "Sudden Infant Death Syndrome (SIDS)." Retrieved on February 25, 2009 from file://C:\~1\amthomps\LOCALS~1\Temp\L3PZN9BR.htm.

20. Ibid.

21. Ibid.

22. Ibid.

23. Public Health Agency of Canada, "Canadian Perinatal Surveillance System: Infant Mortality." Retrieved on May 16, 2006 from www.phac.aspc.gc.ca/rhs-ssg/factshts/mort_e.html.

24. University of Southern California of Medicine, *Dialogues in Contraception* 3 (1991): 2.

25. Wikipedia, "Polycystic Ovary Syndrome." Retrieved on February 26, 2009 from en.wikipedia.org/wiki/Polycystic_ovary_syndrome.

26. B. Bruner, K. Chad, and D. Chizen, "Effects of Exercise and Nutritional Counseling in Women with Polycystic Ovary Syndrome," *Applied Journal of Physiology, Nutrition, and Metabolism* 31.4 (2006): 384–391.

CHAPTER 9

1. The FreeDictionary by Farlax. Retrieved on August 27, 2009 from http://medical-dictionary.thefreedictionary.com/addiction.

2. H. F. Doweiko, *Concepts of Chemical Dependency* (Pacific Grove, CA: Brooks/Cole, 1993) 9.

3. C. Nakken, *The Addictive Personality* (Center City, MN: Hazelden, 1988) 23.

4. V. Johnson, *Intervention: Helping Someone Who Doesn't Want Help* (Minneapolis, MN: Johnson Institute, 1986) 16–35.

5. C. M. Beaudoin and B. J. Cox "Characteristics of Problem Gambling in a Canadian Context: A Preliminary Study Using a DSM-IV-Based Questionnaire," *Canadian Journal of Psychiatry* 44.5 (1999): 483–487.

6. Ibid.

7. "Gambling as Addiction," *Science* 307.5708 (2005): 349, www.sciencemag.org/cgi/content/summary.

8. J. W. Welte et al., "Gambling Participation and Pathology in the United States," *Addictive Behaviors* 29.5 (2004): 983–989.

9. N. E. Turner, J. MacDonald, and M. Somerset. "Life Skills, Mathematical Reasoning and Critical Thinking: A Curriculum for the Prevention of Problem Gambling," *Journal of Gambling Studies* 24.3 (2007): 367–380.

10. The Annenburg Public Policy Center, "Card Playing Trend in Young People Continues," press release, September 25, 2005, www.annenbergpublicpolicycenter.org.

11. Canadian Institute for Health Information, *Drug Expenditure in Canada, 1985 to 2007,* CIHI: Ottawa, 2008.

12. Ibid.

13. Ibid.

14. T. Kerr, W. Small, D. Moore, and E. Wood. "A Micro-environmental Intervention to Reduce the Harms Associated with Drug-Related Overdose: Evidence from the Evaluation of Vancouver's Safer Injection Facility," *International Journal of Drug Policy* 18.1 (2007): 37–45.

15. Turner et al., "Life Skills."

16. Annenburg Public Policy Center, "Card Playing Trend."

17. E. Single et al. "The Relative Risks and Etiologic Fractions of Different Causes of Death and Disease Attributable to Alcohol, Tobacco, and Illicit Drug Use in Canada," *Canadian Medical Association Journal* 162.12 (2000): 1669–1675.

18. Canadian Foundation for Drug Policy, *Canada Drug Legislation Update* (Ottawa: 1997).

19. Health Canada, *Canadian Addiction Survey, a National Survey of Canadians' Use of Alcohol and Other Drugs: Focus on Gender,* Health Canada, Ottawa: 2008.

20. Ibid.

21. Canadian Centre on Substance Abuse and the Centre for Addiction and Mental Health, *Canadian Profile 1999,* CCSA and CAMH, Ottawa and Toronto: 1999, 139.

22. World Health Organization, "Other Psychoactive Substances." Retrieved on March 3, 2006 from www.who.int/substances_abuse/ facts/psychoactives/en/print.html.

23. Ibid.

24. Ibid.

25. Canadian Centre on Substance Abuse, "Substance Abuse Policy in Canada," presentation to the House Standing Committee on Health (October 8, 1996).

26. Centre for Addiction and Mental Health (CAMH), "Do You Know . . . Cocaine, 2006." Retrieved on March 2, 2006 from www.camh.net/About_Addiction_Mental_Health/Drug_and_ Addiction_Information/cocaine_dyk.html.

27. Ibid.

28. Health Canada, "Canadian Addiction Survey."

29. Addiction Research Foundation, "Drug Abuse Update: Drugs and Driving" (Spring 1991); Centre for Addiction and Mental Health, "Do You Know . . . Amphetamines, 2004." Retrieved on March 2, 2006 from www.camh.net/About_Addiction_Mental_Health/ Drug_and_Addiction_Information/amphetamines_dyk.html.

30. CAMH, "Do You Know . . . Cocaine."

31. Ibid.

32. Centre for Addiction and Mental Health (CAMH), "Do You Know . . . Amphetamines, 2004." Retrieved on March 2, 2006 from www.camh.net/About_Addiction_Mental_Health/Drug_and_ Addiction_Information/amphetamines_dyk.html.

33. Centre for Addiction and Mental Health (CAMH), "Do You Know . . . Methamphetamines, 2005." Retrieved on March 2, 2006 from www.camh.net/About_Addiction_Mental_Health/ Drug_and_ Addiction_Information/methamphetamine_dyk.html.

34. Centre for Addiction and Mental Health (CAMH), "Do You Know . . . Cannabis, 2005." Retrieved on March 2, 2006 from www.camh.net/About_Addiction_Mental_Health/Drug_and_ Addiction_Information/cannabis_dyk.html.

35. Health Canada, *A National Survey of Canadians' Use of Alcohol and Other Drugs: Prevalence of Use and Related Harms,* Canadian Centre on Substance Abuse: 2004.

36. CAMH, "Do You Know . . . Cannabis."

37. R. Mathias, "Marijuana Impairs Driving-Related Skill and Workplace Performance," *NIDA Notes* 11.1 (January–February 1996): 6.

38. S. MacDonald, R. Mann, M. Chipman, B. Pakula, P. Erickson, A. Hathaway, and P, MacIntyre. "Driving under the Influence of Cannabis or Cocaine," *Traffic Injury Prevention* 9.3 (2008): 190–194.

39. National Institute on Drug Abuse, "NIDA Capsules: Designer Drugs" (August 1989): 17–21.

40. Centre for Addiction and Mental Health, "Do You Know . . . Ecstasy, 2005." Retrieved on March 2, 2006 from www.camh.net/About_ Addiction_Mental_Health/Drug_and_Addiction_Information/ ecstasy_dyk.html.

41. Centre for Addiction and Mental Health, "Do You Know . . . Anabolic Steroids, 2003." Retrieved on March 2, 2006 from www.camh.net/About_Addiction_Mental_Health/Drug_and_ Addiction_Information/anabolic_steroids_dyk.html.

42. Health Canada, "Canada's Drug Strategy" (Cat. No. H390440/ 1998E), 25.

43. Statistics Canada, *The Daily,* Thursday, July 19, 2001.

CHAPTER 10

1. Statistics Canada, "Control and Sale of Alcoholic Beverages," *The Daily,* June 9, 2008. Retrieved on March 20, 2009 from www.statcan. gc.ca/daily-quotidien/080609/dq080609b-eng.htm.

2. Ibid.

3. Health Canada, *Canadian Addiction Survey, a National Survey of Canadians' Use of Alcohol and Other Drugs: Focus on Gender,* Health Canada, Ottawa: 2008.

4. Health Canada, *A National Survey of Canadians' Use of Alcohol and Other Drugs: Prevalence of Use and Related Harms,* Canadian Centre on Substance Abuse: 2004.

5. Ibid.

6. Ibid.

7. Health Canada, *Canadian Addiction Survey.*

8. Statistics Canada, "Control and Sale of Alcoholic Beverages."

9. Ibid.

10. Ibid.

11. Ibid.

12. Ibid.

13. Health Canada, *Canadian Addiction Survey.*

14. Ibid.

15. Health Canada, *A National Survey of Canadians' Use of Alcohol and Other Drugs.*

16. Ibid.

17. World Health Organization, "Trends in Substance Use and Associated Health Problems," WHO Fact Sheet N127, August 1996. Retrieved from www.who.int/inf-fs/en/fact127.html.

18. E. Single et al., "The Relative Risks and Etiologic Fractions of Different Causes of Death and Disease Attributable to Alcohol, Tobacco, and Illicit Drug Use in Canada," *Canadian Medical Association Journal* 162.12 (2000): 1669–1675.

19. J. Rehm, D. Ballunas, S. Brochu, B. Fischer, W. Gnam, J. Patra, S. Popova, A. Sarnochinska-Hurt, and B. Taylor, *The Costs of Substance Abuse in Canada 2002,* Canadian Centre on Substance Abuse, Ottawa: 2006.

20. Addiction Research Foundation, Statistical Information Service.

21. Centre for Addiction and Mental Health, "Do You Know . . . Alcohol, 2003." Retrieved on March 2, 2006 from www.camh.net/ About_Addiction_Mental_Health/Drug_and_Addiction_ Information/alcohol _dyk.html.

22. Addiction Research Foundation, Statistical Information Service.

23. J. Thompson, M. Manore, and J. Sheeska, *Nutrition: A Functional Approach,* Cdn. ed. (Toronto: Pearson Benjamin Cummings, 2007).

24. R. D. Moore and T. A. Pearsons, "Moderate Alcohol Consumption and Coronary Heart Disease: A Review," *Medicine* 65 (1986): 242–267; Y. Okamota et al., "Role of Liver in Alcohol-Induced Alteration of High Density Lipoprotein Metabolism," *Journal of Laboratory Clinical Medicine* 111 (1988): 484–485.

25. W. C. Willett et al., "Moderate Alcohol Consumption and the Risk of Breast Cancer," *New England Journal of Medicine* 316 (1987): 1174–1180.

26. B. Stade, W. J. Ungar, B. Stevens, J. Beyene, and G. Koren, "The Burden of Prenatal Exposure to Alcohol: Measurement and Cost," *JFAS International* 4 (2006): 1–14.

27. Ibid.

28. Ibid.

29. Statistics Canada, "Mortality: Summary List of Causes" (Cat. No. 84-209, 1995), 14–15.

30. Centre for Addiction and Mental Health, "Do You Know . . . Alcohol, Other Drugs and Driving, 2003." Retrieved on March 2, 2006 from www.camh.net/About_Addiction_Mental_Health/ Drug_and_Addiction_Information/alchohol_drugs_driving_dyk. html.

31. Addiction Research Foundation, Statistical Information Service.

32. F. K. Goodwin and E. M. Gause, "Alcohol, Drug Abuse, and Mental Health Administration," *Prevention Pipeline* 3 (1990): 19.

33. Kenneth Blum et al., "Allelic Association of Human Dopamine D2 Receptor Gene in Alcoholism," *AMA* 262 (1990): 2055–2059.

34. Ray and Ksir, *Drugs, Society, and Human Behavior* (St. Louis: Times Mirror/Mosby, 1990).

35. Statistics Canada, "Control and Sale of Alcoholic Beverages."

36. Eric Single, Lynda Robson, Xiaodi Xie, and Jürgen Rehm, *The Costs of Substance Abuse in Canada,* Canadian Centre on Substance Abuse, Ottawa: 1996.

37. J. Kinney and G. Leaton, *Loosening the Grip: A Handbook of Alcohol Information,* 4th ed. (St. Louis: Times Mirror/Mosby, 1991).

38. World Health Organization, Fact Sheet N154, "Tobacco Epidemic: Health Dimensions," revised May 1998.

39. Health Canada, "Canadian Tobacco Use Monitoring Survey (CTUMS)." Retrieved on March 22, 2009 from www.hc-sc.gc.ca/ hl-vs/tobac-tabac/research-recherche/stat/_ctums-esutc_2008/ wave-phase-1_summary-sommaire-eng.php.

40. Ibid.

41. Rehm et al., *The Costs of Substance Abuse in Canada 2002.*

42. U.S. DHHS/Office on Smoking and Health, "Psychological Risk Factors for Initiating Tobacco Use," in *Preventing Tobacco Use among Young People. A Report of the Surgeon General* (Atlanta: 1994).

43. P. Hilts, "Wide Peril Is Seen in Passive Smoking," *New York Times,* May 9, 1990: A25.

44. Ibid.

45. M. Dewey, *Smoke in the Workplace* (Toronto: N.C. Press, 1986) 14.

46. R. M. van Dam, "Coffee Consumption and Risk of Type 2 Diabetes, Cardiovascular Disease, and Cancer," *Applied Physiology, Nutrition, and Metabolism* 33.6 (2008): 1269–1283.

47. J. M. Tunnicliffe and J. Shearer, "Coffee, Glucose Homeostasis, and Insulin Resistance: Physiological Mechanisms and Mediators," *Applied Physiology, Nutrition, and Metabolism* 33.6 (2008): 1290–1300.

48. T. E. Graham, D. S. Battram, F. Deta. A. El-Sohemy, and F. S. L. Thong, "Does Caffeine Alter Muscle Carbohydrate and Fat Metabolism During Exercise?" *Applied Physiology, Nutrition, and Metabolism* 33.6 (2008): 1311–1318; M. A. Tarnopolsky, "Effect of Caffeine on the Neuromuscular System—Potential as an Ergogenic Aid," *Applied Physiology, Nutrition, and Metabolism* 33.6 (2008): 1284–1289; J. M. Tunnicliffe, K. A. Erdman, R. A. Reimer, V. Lun, and J. Shearer, "Consumption of Dietary Caffeine and Coffee in Physically Active Populations: Physiological Interactions," *Applied Physiology, Nutrition, and Metabolism* 33.6 (2008): 1301–1310.

CHAPTER 11

1. World Health Organization (WHO) "10 Facts on the Global Burden of Disease," 2008. Retrieved on November 27, 2008 from www.who. Int/features/factfiles/global_burden/en/index.html.

2. Statistics Canada. "Mortality, Summary List of Causes," 2007. Retrieved on November 28, 2008 from www.statcan.gc.ca/daily-quotidien/o7o427/dq070427b-eng.htm.

3. World Health Organization (WHO) "10 Facts on the Global Burden of Disease."

4. American Heart Association, *Heart and Stroke Facts 1995,* American Heart Association, Dallas, TX: 1995, 1.

5. Ibid.

6. Ibid.

7. Heart and Stroke Foundation of Canada, "Risk Factors: Coronary Heart Disease Risk Factor." Retrieved on June 2, 2004 from http:// ww1.heartandstroke.ca/Page.asp?PageID=110&ArticleID= 589&Src=heart.

8. Heart and Stroke Foundation of Canada and ACTI_MENU, *Do You Have a Healthy Heart?* (Canada: ACTI-MENU, 1999).

9. Ibid.

10. Ibid.

11. Ibid.

12. Canadian Institute for Health Information, *Health Care in Canada 2003,* Canadian Institute for Health Information, Ottawa: 2003.

13. Heart and Stroke Foundation of Canada and ACTI_MENU, *Do You Have a Healthy Heart?*; Heart and Stroke Foundation, "Heart and Stroke Foundation Report Reveals Canadians Don't Get the 9-1-1 on Stroke," press release, June 12, 2008. Retrieved on November 27, 2008 from www.heartandstroke.com/site/apps/nlnet/content2. aspx?c=ikIQLcMWJtE&b=3485819&ct=5466327.

14. Heart and Stroke Foundation, "Heart and Stroke Foundation Report Reveals Canadians Don't Get the 9-1-1 on Stroke."

15. M. Barrow, *Heart Talk: Understanding Cardiovascular Diseases* (Gainsville, FL: Cor-Ed Publishing, 1992).

16. Ibid.

17. A. V. Chobanian, G. L. Bakris, H. R. Black, W. C. Cushman, L. A. Green, J. L. Izzo Jr, D. W. Jones, B. J. Materson, S. Oparil, and E. J. Roccella, "The Seventh Report of the Joint National Committee on Prevention, Detection, Evaluation, and Treatment of High Blood Pressure: The JNC-7 Report," *Journal of the American Medical Association* 289.19: 2560–2572. Erratum 2003: 290.2: 197.

18. S. Scott. "Essential Hypertension: Treatment without Medications (Part 2 of 2)," *ACSM's Health & Fitness Journal* 11.8 (2007): 37–39.

19. Heart and Stroke Foundation, "Has Election Fever Put You under Pressure? World Heart Day Is Sunday, September 28," press release, 2008. Retrieved on November 27, 2008 from www.heartandstroke. com/site/apps/nlnet/content2.aspx?c=ikIQLcMWJtE&b= 3485819&ct=5992163.

20. Statistics Canada, "CANSIM – Results Table 105-0410: High Blood Pressure, by Age Group and Sex, Household Population Aged 12 and Over, Canada, Provinces, Territories, Health Regions (June 2005 Boundaries) and Peer Groups, Every 2 Years." Retrieved on December 1, 2008 from cansim2.statcan.gc.ca/cgi-win/ cnsmcgi.pgm.

21. Heart and Stroke Foundation, "Pressure Rising: High Blood Pressure Rates Still Very High, Particularly for Some Ethnic Groups, Warns Heart and Stroke Foundation," press release, 2008. Retrieved on November 27, 2008 from www.heartandstroke.com/site/apps/nlnet/content2.aspx?c=ikIQLcMWJtE&b=3485819&ct=5365075.

22. Heart and Stroke Foundation, "High-Normal Blood Pressure Puts Canadians in New Cardiac Danger Zone," press release, January 18, 2007. Retrieved on November 27, 2008 from www.heartandstroke.com/site/apps/nlnet/content2.aspx?c=ikIQLcMWJtE&b=3485819&ct=4512791.

23. Ibid.

24. S. Scott. "Essential Hypertension: Treatment without Medications."

25. Heart and Stroke Foundation, "Dietary Sodium Contributes to 17,000 Cases a Year of Stroke and Heart Disease in Canada Study Says," press release, June 11, 2008. Retrieved on November 27, 2008 from www.heartandstroke.com/site/apps/nlnet/content2.aspx?c=ikIQLcMWJtE&b=3485819&ct=5479299; Heart and Stroke Foundation, "Reductions Needed in Sodium Added to Foods: Lowering Dietary Salt Intakes Would Save Lives, Reduce Medical Costs, Health Groups Says," 2007. Retrieved on November 27, 2008 from www.heartandstroke.com/site/apps/nlnet/content2.ikIQLcMWJtE&b=3485819&ct . . .

26. Ibid.

27. M. Barrow, *Heart Talk: Understanding Cardiovascular Diseases.*

28. Heart and Stroke Foundation of Canada and ACTI_MENU, *Do You Have a Healthy Heart?*

29. Canadian Institute for Health Information, *Health Care in Canada 2003.*

30. B. A. Reeder, A. Senthilselvan, J-P. Després, A. Angel, L. Liu, H. Wang, and S. W. Rabkin, "The Association of Cardiovascular Disease Risk Factors with Abdominal Obesity in Canada," *Canadian Medical Association Journal* 157 (Suppl. 1, 1997): S39–S45.

31. Health Canada, *Heart Disease and Stroke in Canada, 1997, a report prepared in collaboration with Health Canada, the Laboratory Centre for Disease Control, Statistics Canada, and the University of Saskatchewan.* Heart and Stroke Foundation of Canada, Ottawa: June 1997, 42.

32. R. Eliot, "Changing Behavior: A New Comprehensive and Quantitative Approach," keynote address at the annual meeting of the American College of Cardiology on "Stress and the Heart," Jackson Hole, WY, July 3, 1987.

33. Statistics Canada, "Mortality, Summary List of Causes, 1995" (Cat. no. 84-209-XPB), Minister of Industry, Ottawa: 1997, 84–209.

34. Heart and Stroke Foundation of Canada, "Risk Factors: Coronary Heart Disease Risk Factor."

35. Ibid.

36. Heart and Stroke Foundation of Canada, "Women and Heart Health," March 1999, www.hc-sc.gc.ca/hl-vs/alt_formats/hpb-dgps/pdf/facts_heart.pdf.

37. H. Gilmour. "Depression and Risk of Heart Disease," Statistics Canada (Catalogue 82-003-XPE), *Health Reports* 19.3 (September 2008).

38. Heart and Stroke Foundation of Canada and ACTI_MENU, *Do You Have a Healthy Heart?*

39. Ibid.

40. National Heart, Lung, and Blood Institute, *Heart Memo: The Cardiovascular Health of Women* (Bethesda, MD: NHLBI, 1995) 5.

41. Statistics Canada, "CANSIM – Results Table 105-0411: Diabetes, by Age Group and Sex, Household Population Aged 12 and Over, Canada, Provinces, Territories, Health Regions (June 2005 Boundaries) and Peer Groups, Every 2 Years." Retrieved on December 1, 2008 from cansim2.statcan.gc.ca/cgi-win/cnsmcgi.pgm.

42. Centers for Disease Control and Prevention, *National Diabetes Fact Sheet: General Information and National Estimates on Diabetes in the United States, 2005* (Atlanta: U.S. Department of Health and Human Services, Centers for Disease Control and Prevention, 2005).

43. H. Brekke et al., "Long Term Effects of Lifestyle Intervention in Type 2 Diabetes Relatives," *Diabetes Research and Clinical Practice* 70 (2005): 225–234.

44. A. M. Kriska, M. Hawkins, and C. R. Richardson, "Physical Activity and the Prevention of Type II Diabetes" *Current Sports Medicine Reports* 7.4 (2008): 182–184.

45. S. T. Johnson, N. G. Boulé, G. J. Bell, and R. C. Bell, "Walking: A Matter of Quantity and Quality Physical Activity for Type 2 Diabetes Management," *Applied Journal Physiology, Nutrition, and Metabolism* 33 (2008): 797–801.

46. Ibid.

47. Canadian Cancer Society, Statistics Canada, Provincial/Territorial Cancer Registries, Public Health Agency of Canada "Canadian Cancer Statistics 2009." Retrieved on Sept 1, 2009 from www.cancer.ca/Canada-wide/About%20cancer/Cancer%20statistics/~/media/CCS/Canada%20wide/Files%20List/English%20files%20heading/pdf%20not%20in%20publications%20section/Stats%202009E%20Cdn%20Cancer.ashx.

48. Ibid.

49. Ibid.

50. Ibid.

51. J. Peto, "Cancer Epidemiology in the Last Century and Next Decade," *Nature* 411 (2001): 390–395.

52. World Cancer Research Fund/American Institute for Cancer Research, *Policy and Action for Cancer Prevention. Food, Nutrition, and Physical Activity: A Global Perspective.* AICR, Washington DC: 2009.

53. Canadian Cancer Society, Statistics Canada, Provincial/Territorial Cancer Registries, Public Health Agency of Canada "Canadian Cancer Statistics 2009."

54. American Cancer Society, *Cancer Facts and Figures 2005,* American Cancer Society, Atlanta: 2005.

55. World Health Organization (WHO) "10 Facts on the Global Burden of Disease."

56. E. Calle et al., "Overweight, Obesity and Mortality from Cancer in a Prospectively Studied Cohort of U.S. Adults," *New England Journal of Medicine* 348.77: 1625–1638; L. Cooney and C. Gufer, "Hyperglycemia, Obesity, and Cancer Risk on the Horizon," *Journal of the American Medical Association* 293: 235–236.

57. T. G. Krontirus, "The Emerging Genetics of Human Cancer," *New England Journal of Medicine* 309 (1983): 404; A. G. Knudson, "Genetics of Human Cancer," *Annual Review of Genetics* 20 (1986): 23.

58. Canadian Cancer Society, Statistics Canada, Provincial/Territorial Cancer Registries, Public Health Agency of Canada "Canadian Cancer Statistics 2009."

59. American Cancer Society, *Cancer Facts and Figures 1994,* American Cancer Society, Atlanta: 1995, 1

60. P. Pisani, *Estimates of Number of Cancer Cases throughout the World Attributable to Infectious Diseases,* International Agency for Research on Cancer, Lyon, France: 2004.

61. Canadian Cancer Society "Human Pappilomavirus (HPV)." Retrieved on December 2, 2008 from www.cancer.ca/Canada-wide/Prevention/Other%20risk%20factors/Human%20papillomavirus%20HPV.aspx?sc_lang=en.

62. Canadian Cancer Society "HPV Vaccines." Retrieved on December 2, 2008 from www.cancer.ca/canada-wide/prevention/other%20risk%20factors/human%20papillomavirus%20hpv/hpv%20vaccines.aspx?sc_lang=en.

63. Ibid.

64. Canadian Cancer Society, Statistics Canada, Provincial/Territorial Cancer Registries, Public Health Agency of Canada "Canadian Cancer Statistics 2009."

65. M. Camus, J. Siemiatycki, and B. Meek "Nonoccupational Exposure to Chrysotile Asbestos and the Risk of Lung Cancer," *New England Journal of Medicine* 338.22 (1998): 1565–1571.

66. National Cancer Institute of Canada "Breast Cancer." Retrieved on November 27, 2008 from www.ncic.cancer.ca/About%20us20and%20news/Cancer%20 statistics/Breast%20cancer . . .

67. National Cancer Institute Statistics, "Breast Cancer Risk," *Health* (May/June 1994): 14.

68. National Cancer Institute of Canada, "Canadian Cancer Statistics 1999."

69. National Cancer Institute of Canada, "Breast Cancer."

70. L.A. Brinton, D.A. Richesson, G. L. Gierach, J. V. Lacey Jr, Y. Park, R. R. Hollenbeck, and A. Schatzkin, "Prospective Evaluation of Risk Factors for Male Breast Cancer," *Journal of the National Cancer Institute* 100.20 (2003): 1477–1481.

71. American Cancer Society, Cancer Facts and Figures 1994.

72. L. A. Brinton et al. "Prospective evaluation of risk factors for male breast cancer."

73. Leslie Bernstein, Brian E. Henderson, Rosemarie Hanisch, Jane Sullivan-Halley, and Ronald K. Ross, "Physical Exercise and Reduced Risk of Breast Cancer in Young Women," *Journal of the National Cancer Institute* 86.18 (September 21, 1994): 1403–1408

74. Canadian Cancer Society/National Cancer Institute of Canada, *Canadian Cancer Statistics 2006,* CCS/NCIC. Toronto.

75. Canadian Cancer Society "Four new genes for colorectal cancer identified," (2008). Retrieved on November27, 2008 from www.cancer.ca/Canada-wide/About%20us/Media%20centre/CW-Media%20releases/CW . . .

76. American Cancer Society, *Cancer Facts and Figures 1994.*

77. Ibid.

78. Canadian Cancer Society, Statistics Canada, Provincial/Territorial Cancer Registries, Public Health Agency of Canada, "Canadian Cancer Statistics 2009."

79. Ibid.

80. Ibid.

81. American Cancer Society, *Cancer Facts and Figures 1994.*

82. Canadian Cancer Society, Statistics Canada, Provincial/Territorial Cancer Registries, Public Health Agency of Canada, "Canadian Cancer Statistics 2009."

83. American Cancer Society, *Cancer Facts and Figures 1994.*

84. Canadian Cancer Society, Statistics Canada, Provincial/Territorial Cancer Registries, Public Health Agency of Canada, "Canadian Cancer Statistics 2009."

85. Ibid.

86. American Cancer Society, *Cancer Facts and Figures 1994.*

87. Ibid.

88. Harvey A. Risch, Meera Jain, Loraine D. Marrett, and Geoffrey R. Howe, "Dietary Fat Intake and Risk of Epithelial Ovarian Cancer," *Journal of the National Cancer Institute* 86.18 (September 1994): 1409–1415.

89. Canadian Cancer Society, Statistics Canada, Provincial/Territorial Cancer Registries, Public Health Agency of Canada, "Canadian Cancer Statistics 2009."

90. American Cancer Society, *Cancer Facts and Figures 1994.*

91. Ibid., 1.

92. Ibid.

93. Ibid.

94. Ibid.

95. Canadian Cancer Society, Statistics Canada, Provincial/Territorial Cancer Registries, Public Health Agency of Canada, "Canadian Cancer Statistics 2009."

96. Ibid.

97. Alberta Cancer Foundation, "The Tomorrow Project within Canada: Canadian Partnership for Tomorrow Project Launch," *Tomorrow's News* 8.2 (2008): 1–4. See also www.thetomorrowproject.org.

98. J. L. Bender, J. Hohenadel, J. Wong, J. Katz, L. E. Ferris, C. Shobbrook, D. Warr, A. R. Jadad, "What Patients with Cancer Want to Know about Pain: A Qualitative Study," *Journal of Pain Symptom Management* 35.2 (2008): 177–187.

99. Ibid.

CHAPTER 12

1. World Health Organization, *Report on Infectious Disease: Removing Obstacles to Health Development,* World Health Organization, 1999.

2. Health Canada, *Prevention and Management of Infectious Diseases* (July 1995).

3. T. Shulman, J. Phair, and H. Sommers, *The Biological and Clinical Basis of Infectious Disease* (Philadelphia: W. B. Saunders, 1992); A. Benenson, *Control of Communicable Diseases in Man* (Washington, DC: American Public Health Association, 1990).

4. K. Nelson, C. Williams, and N. Graham, *Infectious Disease Epidemiology: Theory and Practice* (Gaithersburg, MD: Aspen, 2001) 17–39.

5. Health Canada, "Tuberculosis." Retrieved on March 28, 2009, from www.hc-sc.gc.ca/hl-vs/iyh-vsv/diseases-maladies/tubercu-eng.php.

6. Public Health Agency of Canada,*Canada Communicable Disease Report* 22.18 (September 15, 1996).

7. Health Canada, "Tuberculosis."

8. Health Canada, "Vaccine-Preventable Diseases: Mumps." Retrieved on April 21, 2006 from www.hc-sc.gc.ca/im/vpd-mev/mumps_e.html.

9. Ibid.

10. World Health Organization, "Global Measles Deaths Drop by 74%." Retrieved on December 5, 2008 from www.who.int/mediacentre/news/releases/2008/pr47/en/print.html.

11. World Health Organization, *Report on Infectious Disease.*

12. World Health Organization, "Global Measles Deaths Drop by 74%."

13. Health Canada, "Sexual and Reproductive Health Day." Retrieved on March 29, 2009 from www. hc-sclgclca/ahc-asc/minist/messages/2008_02_12-eng.php.

14. T. Wong and D. Sutherland, "Canadian STI National Goals and Phase Specific Strategies," *Sexually Transmitted Infections* 78 (Suppl. I, 2002): i189–i190.

15. Public Health Agency of Canada, "Reported Cases and Rates of Genital Chlamydia by Age Group and Sex, 1991 to 2007." Retrieved on March 29, 2009 from www.phac-aspc.gc.ca/std-mts/sti-its_tab/chlamydia1991-07-eng.php.

16. Public Health Agency of Canada, "Reported Cases and Rates of Genital Gonorrhea by Age Group and Sex, 1980 to 2007." Retrieved on March 29, 2009 from www.phac-aspc.gc.ca/std-mts/sti-its_tab/gonorrhea1980-07-eng.php.

17. Noni E. MacDonald and Robert Brunham, "The Effects of Undetected and Untreated Sexually Transmitted Diseases: Pelvic Inflammatory Disease and Ectopic Pregnancy in Canada," *Canadian Journal of Human Sexuality* 6.2 (1997); SIECCAN: The Sex Information & Education Council of Canada.

18. "PID: Guidelines for Prevention, Detection, and Management," *Clinical Courier* 10 (1992): 1–5.

19. P. Marchbanks, N. Lee, and H. Peterson, "Cigarette Smoking as a Risk Factor for PID," *American Journal of Obstetrics and Gynecology* 162 (1990): 639–644; J. Kahn, C. Walker, and A. Washington, "Diagnosing Pelvic Inflammatory Disease," *Journal of the American Medical Association* 226 (1991): 2594–2604.

20. Health Canada, "Sexual and Reproductive Health Day."

21. Public Health Agency of Canada, "Reported Cases and Rates of Gonorrhea by Province/Territory and Sex, 1980 to 2006." Retrieved on March 29, 2009 from www.phac-aspc.gc.ca/std-mts/sti-its_tab/gonorrhea_pts1980-06-eng.php.

22. Health Canada, "Reported Cases and Rates of Notifiable STI from January 1 to June 30, 2005 and January 1 to June 30, 2004." Retrieved on April 21, 2006 from www.hc-sc.gc.ca/pphb-dgspsp/std-mts/stdcases-casmts/index/html.

23. Health Canada, *Canada Communicable Diseases Report* 23.12 (June 15, 1997).

24. Health Canada, Bureau of HIV/AIDS and STD and TB Update Series, "Syphilis in Canada," May 1999.

25. Health Canada, *Canada Communicable Diseases Report* 23.12.

26. S. Kroon, "Limiting the Continued Spread of Genital Herpes: Recommendations from the International Herpes Management Forum Management Strategies Workshop," PPS Europe (1994).

27. Marc Steben and Stephen L. Sack, "Genital Herpes: The Epidemiology and Control of a Common Sexually Transmitted Disease," *Canadian Journal of Human Sexuality* 6 (1997).

28. Society of Obstetricians and Gynecologists of Canada (SOGC), "Guidelines for the Management of Herpes Simplex Virus in Pregnancy," SOGC Clinical Practice Guideline, No. 208, June 2008. Retrieved Sept. 1, 2009 from http://www.sogc.org/guidelines/documents/gui208CPG0806.pdf.

29. B. Strong, C. DeVault, B. Sayad, and W. Yarber, *Human Sexuality* (St. Louis: McGraw-Hill, 2005).

30. Health Canada, "HIV/AIDS." Retrieved on August 18, 2004 from www.hc-sc.gc.ca/datapcb/iad/ih_hivadis-e.htm.

31. World Health Organization, "MDG 6 Combat HIV/AIDS, Malaria, and Other Related Diseases." Retrieved on March 30, 2009 from www.who.int/topics/millennium_development_goals/diseases/en/.

32. World Health Organization, "AIDS Epidemic Update" (December 1999): 4.

33. Public Health Agency of Canada, Centre for Infectious Disease Prevention and Control, Surveillance and Risk Assessment Division, *HIV and AIDS in Canada: Surveillance Report to December 31, 2004,* Public Health Agency of Canada, Ottawa: April 2005.

34. Health Canada, "Estimates of the Number of People Living with HIV in Canada, 2005." Retrieved on March 30, 2009 from www.hc-sc.gc.ca/ahc-asc/intactiv/conf/info07-eng.php.

35. Public Health Agency of Canada, Centre for Infectious Disease Prevention and Control, Surveillance and Risk Assessment Division, *HIV and AIDS in Canada: Surveillance Report to December 31, 2004.*

36. Health Canada, "Estimates of the Number of People Living with HIV in Canada, 2005."

37. Public Health Agency of Canada, Centre for Infectious Disease Prevention and Control, Surveillance and Risk Assessment Division, *HIV and AIDS in Canada: Surveillance Report to December 31, 2004.*

38. National Institute of Allergy and Infectious Diseases, "HIV Infection and AIDS: An Overview," 2005. Retrieved from www.niaid.nih.gov/factsheets/hivinf.htm.

39. Health Canada, "Estimates of the Number of People Living with HIV in Canada, 2005."

40. Public Health Agency of Canada, "HIV/AIDS Epi Update: May 2004: HIV/AIDS among Injecting Drug Users in Canada." Retrieved on April 24, 2006 from www.phac-aspc.gc.ca/publicat/epiu-aepi/epi_unpdate_may_04/11_e.html.

41. J. Allen, "Oh, My Aching Head," *Life* (1994): 66–76.

42. National Headache Foundation (NFH), "NFH Headache Fact Sheet," 2004, www.headaches.org.

43. Canadian Diabetes Association, "The Prevalence and Costs of Diabetes." Retrieved on March 30, 2009 from www.diabetes.ca/about-diabetes/what/prevalence.

44. Ibid.

45. Ibid.

46. Health Canada, "Canadian Diabetes Strategy." Retrieved on November 13, 2002 from www.hc-sc.gc.ca/english/media/releases/1999/99135ebk3.htm; currently available online at: www.phac-aspc.gc.ca/ccdpc-cpcmc/diabetes-diabete/english/strategy/index.html.

47. The Arthritis Society, "Defining the Arthritis Crisis: Canadian Arthritis Bill of Rights" (2001).

48. Health Canada National Advisory Council on Aging, "How Many People Have Arthritis?" (1997).

CHAPTER 13

1. World Health Organization, "Public Health and the Environment: Health through a Better Environment." Retrieved on December 8, 2008 from www.who.int/phe/en/.

2. World Health Organization, "10 Facts on Preventing Disease through Healthy Environments." Retrieved on December 8, 2008 from www.who.int/features/factfiles/environmental_health/en/index.html.

3. Ibid.

4. Ibid.

5. Health Canada, "Health and Environment Handbook for Health Professionals" (Cat. No. H46-2/98-211-2E, 1998), v.

6. Ibid.

7. R. Caplan, *Our Earth, Ourselves* (New York: Bantam, 1990) 247.

8. World Health Organization, "World Population Prospects: The 2006 Revision," Population Database. Retrieved on December 8, 2008 from esa.un.org/unpp.

9. Ibid.

10. Ibid.

11. Ibid.

12. World Health Organization, "Air Quality and Health," fact sheet 313, (2008). Retrieved on December 5, 2008 from www.who.int/mediacentre/factsheets/fs313/en/print.html.

13. Environment Canada, "Canadian Environmental Protection Act, 1999 (CEPA, 1999)." Retrieved on May 19, 2006 from www.ec.gc.ca/CEPARegistry/the_act/.

14. Canadian Environmental Assessment Agency, "Introduction and Features: Canadian Environmental Assessment Act." Retrieved on May 19, 2006 from www.ceaa-acee.gc.ca/013/intro_e.htm.

15. Environment Canada, "Agreements." Retrieved on May 19, 2006 from www.ec.gc.ca/cleanair-airpur/Agreements-WS475C5F00-1_En.htm.

16. Environment Canada, "Canadian 1996 NOx/VOC Science Assessment, Executive Summary," www.ec.gc.ca/air/acid-rain_e.html.

17. Canadian Lung Association "Smog Smart Strategies: How to Protect Your Breathing on Smog Days." Retrieved on September 4, 2009 from www.lung.ca/protect-protegez/pollution-pollution/outdoor-exterior/smogsmart-futesmog_e.php.

18. Canadian Lung Association, "Why Care about the Air You Breathe?" (1991).

19. Lester Brown, "A New Era Unfolds," in *State of the World,* 1993, ed. Lester Brown (New York: Norton, 1993).

20. Canadian Lung Association, "Why Care about the Air?"

21. H. F. French, "Clearing the Air," in *State of the World, 1990*, ed. L. R. Brown, A. B. Durning, H. F. French, C. Flavin, J. L. Jacobson, M. D. Lowe, S. Postel, M. Renner, L. Starke and J. E. Young (Washington, DC: Worldwatch Institute, 1990) 109.

22. U.S. Environmental Protection Agency, "Effects of Acid Rain," 2005, www.epa.gov/acidrain.

23. U.S. Environmental Protection Agency, "The Inside Story: A Guide to Indoor Air Quality" (EPA Document # 402-K-93-007), January 2002, http://epa.gov/iaq/pubs/insdet.html.

24. Ibid.

25. Ibid.

26. Health Canada, "Radon Information Sheet" (Minister of Supply and Services, 1989).

27. Environment Canada, "Five-Year Progress Report: Canada-Wide Standards for Particulate Matter and Ozone," Government of Canada,(2006), 1–94.

28. Canadian Lung Association, "Why Care about the Air?"

29. French, "Clearing the Air."

30. L. Thompson, S. El-Solh, and O. McGuire, "Benzene in Canadian Gasoline: Report on the Effect of the Benzene in Gasoline Regulations 2006." Retrieved on September 14, 2009 from www.ec.gc.ca/cleanair-airpur/caol/OGEB/bnz06_eng.html.

31. World Health Organization, "10 Facts about Water Scarcity." Retrieved on December 5, 2008 from www.who.int/features/factfiles/water/en/index.html.

32. Environment Canada, *Water Policy in Canada—Canada's Water* (March 1997).

33. A. Nadakavukaren, *Man and Environment: A Health Perspective* (Prospect Heights, IL: Waveland, 1990), 412–414.

34. R. Griffin Jr, "Introducing NPS Water Pollution," *EPA Journal* 17 (1991): 6–9.

35. J. Naar, *Design for a Livable Planet* (New York: Harper and Row, 1990), 68.

36. A. Nadakavukaren, *Man and Environment: A Health Perspective.*

37. Ibid.

38. World Health Organization, "Q&As: Environmental Health." Retrieved on December 5, 2008 from www.who.int/topics/environmental_health/qa/en/index.html.

39. Ibid.

40. Environment Canada, Toxic Substances Management Policy, Government of Canada, Ottawa: June 1995.

41. D. W. Moeller, *Environmental Health* (Cambridge, MA: Harvard University Press, 1992) 31.

42. C. Flavin, "Slowing Global Warming," in *State of the World, 1990.*

43. Health Canada, "Health and Environment Handbook," 125–126.

CHAPTER 14

1. World Health Organization: "Injuries and Violence Prevention," 1. Retrieved on April 25, 2006 from www.who.int/violence_injury_prevention/violence/en/.

2. Jan J. M. van Dijk, Pat Mayhew, and Martin Killias, *Experiencing Crime across the World* (Deventer, the Netherlands: Kluwer Law and Taxation Publishers, 1990) 38.

3. Ibid.

4. J. Frank, "Violent Youth Crime," *Canadian Social Trends* (Autumn 1992): 3.

5. Ibid.

6. W. Gleberzon, "Ethnicity and Violence: Racial Conflict in Vancouver" (unpublished, undated, on file at the Human Rights Library, Fauteux Hall, University of Ottawa) 7–8.

7. K. Adachi, *The Enemy That Never Was: A History of the Japanese Canadians* (Toronto: McClelland and Stewart, 1991).

8. M. Suderman and P. Jaffe, *Preventing Violence: School and Community-Based Strategies,* Health Canada, 1996.

9. Statistics Canada, "Homicide Offences, Number and Rate, by Province and Territory." Retrieved on February 11, 2009 from www40.statcan.gc.ca/cbin/fl/cstprintflag.cgi.

10. Statistics Canada, "Homicides by Method." Retrieved on February 11, 2009 from www40.statcan.gc.ca/cbin/fl/cstprintflag.cgi.

11. Statistics Canada, "Victims and Persons Accused of Homicide, by Age and Sex." Retrieved on February 11, 2009 from www40.statcan.gc.ca/cbin/fl/cstprintflag.cgi.

12. Ibid.

13. Canadian Firearms Program, "Firearms Licensing." Retrieved on February 11, 2009 from www.cfc-cafc.gc.ca/perform_info/oct-dec-08_e.asp.

14. M. Asberg et al., "Psychology of Suicidal Behaviour," *Annals of the New York Academy of Sciences* 487 (1986).

15. B. L. Tanney, "Mental Disorders, Psychiatric Patients and Suicide," in *Assessment and Prediction of Suicide,* eds. R. Maris et al. (New York: Guilford Press, 1992).

16. I. Sakinofsky, "The Ecology of Suicide in the Provinces of Canada, 1967–71 to 1979–81," in *The Epidemiology of Psychiatric Disorders,* ed. B. C. Cooper (Baltimore: Johns Hopkins, 1987).

17. World Health Organization, "Suicide Prevention (SUPRE)." Retrieved on February 11, 2009 from www.who.int/mental_health/prevention/suicide/suicideprevent/en/print.htm.

18. Statistics Canada, "Suicides and Suicide Rate, by Sex and by Age Group." Retrieved on February 2, 2009 from www40.statcan.ca/cbin/fl/cstprintflag.cgi.

19. Ibid.

20. Health Canada, *Toward a Healthy Future: Second Report on the Health of Canadians,* a public policy report developed by the Federal, Provincial and Territorial Advisory Committee on Population Health (ACPH) in collaboration with Health Canada, Statistics Canada, the Canadian Institute for Health Information and a project team from the Centre for Health Promotion, University of Toronto. Health Canada, Ottawa: 1999, 23.

21. Ibid.

22. Ibid.

23. Child & Family Canada, Fact Sheet on Suicide.

24. World Health Organization, "Self-Directed Violence."

25. Statistics Canada, "Victims and Persons Accused of Homicide, by Age and Sex."

26. Ibid.

27. Dianne Hendrick, "Youth Court Statistics," *Juristat* 19.2, Statistics Canada (Cat. No. 85-002-XPE), 1.

28. K. Stevenson et al., "Youth and Crime," *Canadian Social Trends* (Summer 1999), Statistics Canada (Cat. No. 11-008), 19.

29. Ibid.

30. D. Patel, *Dealing with Interracial Conflict:Policy Alternatives* (Montreal: Institute for Research on Public Policy, 1980).

31. Linda McLeod, *Wife Battering in Canada: The Vicious Circle* (Ottawa: Canadian Advisory Council on the Status of Women, 1980).

32. K. Rodgers, "Wife Assault in Canada," *Canadian Social Trends* (Autumn 1994): 3.

33. Ibid.

34. "Wife Abuse Information," The National Clearinghouse on Family Violence, September 1995.

35. Solicitor General, "Family Violence: Not a Private Problem," RCMP Policy, Public Education Doc. 1966.

36. A. Joerger et al., "Why Men Batter: Why Women Stay," *Community Safety Quarterly* 5 (1992): 22–23.

37. N. West, "Crimes against Women," *Community Safety Survey* 5 (1992): 1.

38. Statistics Canada, *Canadian Crime Statistics, 1995*, 60.

39. Statistics Canada, "Family Violence in Canada: A Statistical Profile 2008" (Cat. No. 85-224).

40. Ibid.

41. Ibid.

42. H. Pan et al., "Physical Aggression in Early Marriage: Pre-relationship and Relationship Effects," *Journal of Consulting Psychology.*

43. G. Wilson et al., *Abnormal Psychology* (Boston, MA: Allyn & Bacon, 1996).

44. Ibid.

45. Ibid.

46. N. Trocomé, B. Fallon, B. MacLaurin, J. Daciuk, C. Felstiner, T. Black, L. Tonmyr, C. Blackstock, K. Barter, D. Turcotte, and R. Cloutier. Canadian *Incidence Study of Reported Child Abuse and Neglect—2003: Major Findings*, Minister of Public Works and Government Services Canada, 2005.

47. World Health Organization: Communications and Public Relations, WHO Fact Sheet N150, March 1997.

48. Statistics Canada, "Family Violence in Canada: A Statistical Profile 2008."

49. World Health Organization, WHO Fact Sheet N150.

50. A. Miller, "Newly Recognized Shattering Effects of Child Abuse," *Empathic Parenting* 1 & 2 (1992).

51. R. M. Malina C. Bouchard, O. Bar-Or. *Growth, Maturation and Physical Activity*, 2nd ed. (Champaign, IL: Human Kinetics, 2004).

52. Statistics Canada, "Selected Violations against the Person, by Gender of Victim and Accused, 1995," *Canadian Crime Statistics* (1995).

53. Health Canada, "Abuse and Neglect of Older Adults" (Cat. No. H72-22/6-1998E).

54. Statistics Canada, "Family Violence in Canada: A Statistical Profile 2008."

55. Ibid.

56. "Sex Offenders," *Juristat* 19.3, Statistics Canada (Cat. No. 85-002-XPE 19), 3.

57. Statistics Canada, "Family Violence in Canada: A Statistical Profile 2008."

58. S. Brennan and A. Taylor-Butts, Canadian Centre for Justice Statistics, Statistics Canada, "Sexual Assault in Canada." Retrieved on February 13, 2009 from www.statcan.gc.ca/pub/85f0033m/85f0033m2008019-eng.htm.

59. Statistics Canada. "Findings." Retrieved on February 13, 2009 from www.statcan.gc.ca/pub/85f0033m/2008019/findings-results-eng.htm.

60. Statistics Canada. "Sexual Assault in Canada." Retrieved on February 13, 2009 from www.statcan.gc.ca/bsolc/olc-cel/olc-cel?lang=eng&catno=85f0033M2008019.

61. Health Canada, "Dating and Violence: Fact Sheet," February 1993.

62. A. Berkowitz, "College Men as Perpetrators of Acquaintance Rape and Sexual Assault: A Review of the Literature," *Journal of American College Health* 40 (1992): 177.

63. Ibid.

64. K.A. Morrison, "Differentiating between Physically Violent and Non-violent Stalkers: An Examination of Canadian Cases," *Journal of Forensics Science* 53.3 (2008): 742–751.

65. P. Gagné and L. Desparois, "Male Erotomania: A Type of Dangerous Sexual Harassment," *Canadian Journal of Psychiatry* 40.3 (1995): 136–141.

66. D. Benson et al., "Acquaintance Rape on Campus: A Literature Review," *Journal of American College Health* 40 (1992): 158.

67. M. Whittaker, "The Continuum of Violence against Women: Psychological and Physical Consequences," *Journal of American College Health* 40 (1992): 151.

68. A. Mathews, "Campus Crime 101," *Eugene Register Guard,* March 1993: 2B.

69. T. Schneider, "Rape Prevention," *Community Safety Quarterly* (1992): 8–13.

70. Ibid.

71. Ibid.

72. Ibid.

73. Health Canada, "Health Aspects of Violence against Women," *Women's Health Forum,* Ottawa, 1996.

CHAPTER 15

1. Canadian Institute for Health Information, *Canada's Health System* (1996).

2. Commission on the Future of Health Care in Canada, press release, "Romanow Report Proposes Sweeping Changes to Medicare," November 28, 2002, available online at: www.hc-sc.gc.ca/english/care/romanow/hcc0403.html.

3. Health Canada, *Toward a Healthy Future: Second Report on the Health of Canadians, a public policy report developed by the Federal, Provincial and Territorial Advisory Committee on Population Health (ACPH) in collaboration with Health Canada, Statistics Canada, the Canadian Institute for Health Information and a project team from the Centre for Health Promotion, University of Toronto.* Health Canada, Ottawa: 1999, 136.

4. Canadian Institute for Health Information, *Health Care in Canada 2005*. Retrieved on May 19, 2006 from www.cihi.ca.

5. Canadian Institute for Health Information, *Health Care in Canada 2007*. Retrieved on April 5, 2009 from http://secure.cihi.ca/cihiweb/dispPage.jsp?cw_page=AR_43_.

6. Ibid.

7. Canadian Institute for Health Information, *Health Care in Canada 2005*.

8. Ibid.

9. Canadian Institute for Health Information, *Health Care in Canada 2007*.

10. Canadian Institute for Health Information, *Health Care in Canada 2007*; Health Canada, "Canada's Health Care System" (Cat. No. H39-502/1999), 7.

11. Public Health Agency of Canada, "Canadian Health Network: Health System." Retrieved on May 23, 2006 from www.canadian-health-network.ca/servlet/ContentServer?cid=1047418085892&pagename=CHN-RCS%2FPage%2FGTPageTemplate&c=Page&lang=En.

12. Canadian Institute for Health Information, *Health Care in Canada 2007*.

13. National Center for Complementary and Alternative Medicine, "Get the Facts: 10 Things to Know about Evaluating Medical Resources on the Web." Retrieved on May 23, 2006 from www.nccam.nih.gov.

14. Health Canada, *Toward a Healthy Future: Second Report on the Health of Canadians.*

15. Ibid.

16. Munroe Anne Johnston, *Gender and Self-Care in Undergraduate Students: A Qualitative Study* (Waterloo, ON: Wilfrid Laurier University, 1993) 12.

17. Health Canada, *Health Human Resources in Community-Based Health Care: A Review of the Literature, a report prepared for the Federal/Provincial/Territorial Conference of Deputy Ministers of*

Health through the Advisory Committee on Health Human Resources (ACHHR). Health Promotion and Programs Branch, Health Canada, Ottawa: 1995, 51.

18. Canadian Institute for Health Information, *Health Care in Canada 2007.*

19. G. Annas, *The Rights of Patients: The Basic ACLU Guide to Patient Rights,* 2nd ed. (Chicago: Southern Illinois University Press, 1989) 105; J. A. Robertson, *The Rights of the Critically Ill* (New York: Bantam, 1983) 32–77.

20. Health Canada, *Health Human Resources in Community-Based Health Care: A Review of the Literature.*

21. Health Canada, *Toward a Healthy Future: Second Report on the Health of Canadians.*

22. Ibid.

23. P. Starr, *The Social Transformation of American Medicine* (New York: Basic Books, 1982) 127, 229.

24. Newfoundland and Labrador Massage Therapy Association, "Frequently Asked Questions about Massage Therapy." Retrieved on May 24, 2006 from www.nlmta.ca/res/index.html.

25. A. Toufexis, "Dr. Jacob's Alternative Mission: A New NIH Office Will Put Unconventional Medicine to the Test," *Time,* March 1, 1993: 43–44, 64–66.

26. Health Canada, "Health Care System." Retrieved on May 24, 2006 from www.hc-sc.gc.ca/hcs-sss/index_e.html.

CHAPTER 16

1. B. Hayslip and P. Panek, *Adult Development and Aging* (New York: Harper and Row, 1992) 21.

2. Statistics Canada, "2006 Census: Portrait of the Canadian Population in 2006, by Age and Sex: Highlights." Retrieved on March 30, 2009 from www12.statcan.ca/census-recensement/2006/as-sa/97-551/p1-eng.cfm.

3. National Advisory Council on Aging, "1999 and Beyond— Challenges of an Aging Canadian Society," 1999-19. Retrieved on September 28, 1998 from http://ncoa.org/.

4. R. M. Malina, C. Bouchard, O. Bar-Or, *Growth, Maturation and Physical Activity,* 2nd ed. (Champaign, IL: Human Kinetics, 2004).

5. National Osteoporosis Foundation, *Physicians' Resource Manual on Osteoporosis: A Decision-Making Guide,* 2nd ed. (National Osteoporosis Foundation, 1991); National Dairy Council, "Calcium and Osteoporosis: New Insights," *Dairy Council Digest* 63 (1992): 1–6.

6. National Advisory Council on Aging. Retrieved on September 28, 1998 from http://ncoa.org/.

7. U.S. Department of Health and Human Services, Public Health Service, National Institutes of Health, Osteoporosis Research, Education, and Health Promotion (NIH Publication No. 91-3216, September 1991) 2.

8. National Research Council, Food and Nutrition Board, *Recommended Dietary Allowances,10th ed.,* a report of the subcommittee on the 10th edition of the FDA's dietary allowances (Washington, DC: National Academy Press, 1989).

9. Ibid.

10. U.S. Department of Health and Human Services, (NIH Publication No. 91-3216, September 1991).

11. Ibid.

12. J. Thompson, M. Manore, J. Sheeska, *Nutrition: A Functional Approach,* Cdn. ed. (Toronto: Pearson, 2007).

13. Health Canada, "Canada's Physical Activity Guide for Older Adults" (Cat. H39-611/2002-1E), 2002.

14. National Kidney and Urologic Diseases Information Clearinghouse, "Kidney and Urologic Diseases Statistics for the United States" (NIH Publication No. 04-3895). Retrieved in February 2004 from www.kidney.niddk.nih.gov/kudiseases/pubs/kustats/index.htm.

15. A. Ferrini and R. Ferrini, *Health in the Later Years* (Madison, WI: Brown and Benchmark, 1993) 281.

16. National Institute of Nutrition, *Food and Nutrition Opportunities in the Seniors' Market: A Situation Analysis – Executive Summary,* March 1996.

17. Philadelphia Corporation for Aging, "Older Adults and Sexuality," *Health Matters* 14.14 (August 2004), www.pcaphl.org/healthmatters/agingsexuality.pdf.

18. National Council on Aging, "Half of Older Americans Report They Are Sexually Active, 4 in 10 Want More Sex, Says New Survey." Retrieved on September 28, 1998 from http://ncoa.org/mews/archives.sexsurvey.htm.

19. National Institute of Nutrition, *Food and Nutrition Opportunities.*

20. Health Canada, Depression Aging Vignettes #78, Division of Seniors and Aging, 1998, www.hc-sc.gc.ca/seniors-aines/seniors/pubs/vigdepre.htm#Dep 2.

21. National Advisory Council on Aging, "1999 and Beyond— Challenges of an Aging Canadian Society," 1999-19. Retrieved on September 28, 1998 from http://ncoa.org/.

22. Health Canada, "Canada's Physical Activity Guide for Older Adults."

23. Thompson, Manore, and Sheeska, *Nutrition.*

24. Statistics Canada, "2006 Census: Portrait of the Canadian Population in 2006, by Age and Sex: Highlights."

25. Health Canada Division of Aging and Seniors, Statistical Snapshot #5, "More Women Than Men," September 1999.

26. Health Canada, *Toward a Healthy Future: Second Report on the Health of Canadians, a public policy report developed by the Federal, Provincial and Territorial Advisory Committee on Population Health (ACPH) in collaboration with Health Canada, Statistics Canada, the Canadian Institute for Health Information and a project team from the Centre for Health Promotion, University of Toronto.* Health Canada, Ottawa: 1999, 166.

27. *Oxford English Dictionary* (Oxford: Oxford University Press, 1969) 72, 334, 735.

28. Canadian Medical Association, "Guidelines for the Diagnosis of Brain Death," *Canadian Medical Association Journal* 136 (1987): 200A.

29. Ibid.

30. Lewis R. Aiken, *Dying, Death, and Bereavement,* 3rd ed. (Boston: Allyn & Bacon, 1994) 4.

31. Elisabeth Kübler-Ross, *On Death and Dying* (New York: Macmillan, 1969) 113.

32. Ibid.

33. Ibid.

34. Ibid.

35. Robert J. Kastenbaum, *Death, Society, and Human Experience,* 5th ed. (Boston: Allyn & Bacon, 1995) 95.

36. K. J. Doka, ed., *Disenfranchised Grief: Recognizing Hidden Sorrow* (Lexington, MA: Lexington Books, 1989).

37. Kastenbaum, *Death, Society, and Human Experience.*

38. J. W. Worden, *Grief Counseling and Grief Therapy: A Handbook for the Mental Health Practitioner,* 3rd ed. (New York: Springer, 2001).

39. The term "quasi-death experience" was coined by J. B. Kamerman; see J. B. Kamerman, *Death in the Midst of Life* (Englewood Cliffs, NJ: Prentice Hall, 1988) 71.

INDEX

esophagus, 107
essential amino acids, 112, 113
essential hypertension, 285
estrogen
in contraceptives, 195, 197–199
menopause and, 122
ovarian cancer and, 306
puberty and, 176, 179–180
replacement therapy for CVD, 287
ethanol, 257
ethyl alcohol, 257
eustress, 56, 57
euthanasia, 431
exercise
see also physical activity
defined, 78, 79
pregnancy guidelines for, 214–215
exercise equipment, 94–95
exercise metabolic rate (EMR), 140–141
exhaustion phase of GAS, 59–60
exhibitionism, 188
exogenous depression, 44, 45
external female genitals, 177–178
external influences, 36
external male genitals, 180–181
eyesight and aging, 418

F
faith, 33
fallopian tubes, 178–179
family
alcoholism and, 269, 270
defined, 162–163
psychosocial health and, 36
smoking and, 274
violence. See domestic violence
family factors
for alcoholism, 266–267
for behaviour, 20
developmental influences of, 36, 102
fast foods, 124–126
fats (lipids)
see also lipoproteins
defined, 115
reducing, 112, 116–117
Federal Standing Committee on Health and Welfare, 207
fellatio, 186–187
female condoms, 200, 201
female hormones, 179–180
female reproductive anatomy and physiology
aging and, 418–419
menopause, 180, 181, 291–292
overview, 177–179
puberty and menstruation, 179–180
female sterilization, 205
fermentation, 258, 259
fertility
see also contraception
cycle, 204

decrease in, 211
defined, 195
overpopulation and, 355
responsibility for, 194
fertility awareness methods (FAM), 203–204
fertility drugs, 223–224
fertilization, 217
fetal alcohol effects (FAE), 264, 265
fetal alcohol spectrum disorder (FASD), 212, 213, 264, 265
fetal alcohol syndrome (FAS), 264, 265
fetishism, 188
fetus, 217
fever, 323
fibre, 113, 114–115
fibrillation, 286, 287
fibrocystic breast condition, 344, 345
fibromyalgia, 348, 349
financial evaluation, 210
firearms, 374
Firearms Act, 374
First Nations
see also Aboriginal Canadians
Canada's health care system and, 406
cardiovascular disease among, 282, 291
ceremonial use of peyote, 247
Oka land dispute, 373
first trimester of pregnancy, 216–217
fitness injuries
causes of, 94
common overuse injuries, 95–97
prevention, 94–95
fixed resistance, 89
flesh-eating strep, 316
flexibility, 81, 91, 94
fluoxetine, 49
follicle-stimulating hormone (FSH), 179
food allergies, 130
food intolerance, 130
food safety
see also healthy eating
chemicals and additives in, 129–130, 298, 300, 369
fat content, 116–117
food-borne illness, 128–129
organically grown, 130
footwear, 94
for-profit (proprietary) hospitals, 406, 407
foreskin, 182, 183
formaldehyde, 360, 361
Forsyth, Heather, 250
Framingham Study, 57
fraud and abuse in health care, 407
freebase cocaine, 242, 243
Freud, Sigmund, 240
Friedman, Meyer, 64
friendships, 163, 164
functional death, 424
fungus, 332
furnaces, 359

infectious diseases
see also bacteria; sexually transmitted infections
body's defences, 321–323
cancer and, 300
emerging, 316
risks factors, 314–315
viruses, 318–321
infectious mononucleosis, 319–320
infertility
definition and causes of, 223
surrogate motherhood, 224
treatment for, 223–224
influenza, 319, 325
inhalants, 248–249
inhalation of drugs, 233
inhibited sexual desire (ISD), 188, 189
inhibition interaction of drugs, 235
injection of drugs, 233
injuries
all-terrain vehicles and, 390
prevention of, 389
unintentional, 389
Inland Waters Directorate, 363
insomnia, 41
insulin, 346, 347
Integrated Pan-Canadian Living Strategy 2005, 10
intelligence and aging, 419
interconnectedness, 33
intercourse, 187
interferon, 318, 319
internal female genitals, 177–178
internal influences, 36–38
internal male genitals, 180–181
International Day for Evaluation of Abdominal Obesity
(IDEA), 290
International Panel on Climate Change, 367
internet
online dating, 186
online medical resources, 394–395
intervention, 269
intimate relationships
see also committed relationships
barriers to, 167–168
characteristics of, 160–162
families, 162–163
friendships, 163, 164
gender issues, 165–167
love, 164–165, 166
partners and couples, 163–164
intolerance interaction of drugs, 235
intramuscular injection, 233
intrauterine device (IUD), 202, 203
intravenous injection, 233
Inuit
cardiovascular disease and, 291
type 2 diabetes and, 295
inunction of drugs, 233
ionizing radiation, 368–369

iron, 122
irritable bowel syndrome (IBS), 346–347
ischemia, 284, 285
isometric muscle contractions, 88
iyengar yoga, 92

J

Japanese Canadians, internment and riots against,
373, 375
jealousy, 168, 169
Johnson, Ben, 249
joints and aging, 416
Journal of the American Medical Association, 424
The Joy of Sex (Comfort), 187

K

ketosis, 144, 145
Kevorkian, Dr. Jack, 431
kissing, 186
Kübler-Ross, Elisabeth, 425–426
Kyoto Protocol, 367

L

labia majora, 177–178
labia minora, 177–178
labour and delivery, 219
land pollution, 366
landfills, 364
late syphilis, 331
latent syphilis, 330–331
laughter and psychosocial health, 42–43
Laval University, 290
laxatives, 238, 239
leaching of metals, 359
lead, 357, 365–366
learned behavioural tolerance, 260, 261
learned helplessness, 37
learned optimism, 37
Legionnaire's disease, 317
legislation
illicit drugs and, 238–239, 244, 250
same-sex marriage, 170
tobacco sales/smoking policies, 274
Lenton, Rhonda, 186
lesbian partnerships, 170
leukemia, 307
leukoplakia, 273
life-and-death decisions, 430–431
life expectancy
average Canadian, 2–3
improved health and, 82
overpopulation and, 355
life span, 38, 82
lifestyle
cancer and, 297
infectious diseases and, 314
obesity and, 148–149
limerence, 184, 185

psychosocial health (*continued*)
    emotional health and, 31–32
    enhancing, 38–43
    factors influencing, 35–38
    managing, 53
    mental health and, 30–31
    mental illness and. *See* mental illnesses
    obesity and, 148
    professional help and, 50–53
    sex issues in, 47–48
    social health and, 32
    spiritual health and, 32–34
    suicide and, 48–50
psychosocial sources of stress, 60–61
psychosocial theories on aging, 416
psychotherapy, 45, 47
puberty, 176, 177, 179–180
pubic lice, 331

Q

quality assurance with health care, 407
quasi-death experiences, 430, 431
Quebec Court of Appeal, 207
Queen's University, 215

R

racial discrimination
    see also prejudice
    anti-Chinese and Japanese riots, 373, 375
    prevention of, 376
radiation
    ionizing, 368–369
    nonionizing, 369
    nuclear power plants, 369
radionuclide imaging, 293
radiotherapy, 308, 309
Radner, Gilda, 310
radon, 360, 361
Rahe, R., 60
rational-emotive therapy, 22
realistic expectations, 39
rebound effects, 236, 237
receptor sites, 231–232
Recommended Nutrient Intake (RNI), 107, 110
recovery principle, 88
recreational drugs, 232, 233
Red Cross, 311
reinforcement, 22
reinforcing factors, 15, 17
relapse
    addiction and, 230, 231
    alcohol and, 270–271
relationships
    see also committed relationships; intimate
        relationships
    building better, 189
    building healthy, 174
    characteristics of good, 171–172

    children and, 172
    communication and, 159–160
    ending of, 173–175
    singlehood, 172
relaxation, 72
reproductive anatomy and physiology. *See* female
    reproductive anatomy and physiology; male
    reproductive anatomy and physiology
resiliency, 38, 39
resistance phase of GAS, 59
resistance training, 89, 93–94
respiratory disorders
    allergies, 340, 341
    asthma, 341–342
    chronic bronchitis, 342, 343
    deaths from, 11, 12
    emphysema, 342, 343
    hay fever, 341
resting metabolic rate (RMR), 140–141
retarded ejaculation, 190, 191
reticular formation, 245
Reuters Health, 229
reversible contraception, 194–203
Rh factor, 221
rheumatic heart disease, 286, 287
rheumatoid arthritis, 348, 349
RICE (rest, ice, compression and elevation), 96, 97
Rio Convention, 367
Road Safety Monitor, 266
Romalis, Dr. Garson, 208
Romanow, Roy, 393
Rosenman, Ray, 64
routes of administration of drugs, 233–234
rubella (German measles), 321
Rudin, Steve, 421
runner's knee, 96
Ryerson University, 381

S

sadomasochism, 188
safety
    with all-terrain vehicles, 390
    on campus, 386
    in the car, 388
    at home, 387–388
    injury prevention, 389
    self-defence against sexual assault, 384, 385, 387
    on the street, 388
saliva, 107
salt, 119, 121
same-sex couples
    committed relationships, 170
    death of a loved one, 428
    having children, 172
    intolerance towards, 376
    marriage legislation, 170
sarcomas, 301
sarcopenia, 422, 423

satiety, 146, 147

saturated fats, 115

schizophrenia, 46–48

screening

for cancer, 299–300, 309

prenatal testing and, 217–218

for sexually transmitted infections, 328

scrotum, 180–181

seasonal affective disorder (SAD), 45

second trimester of pregnancy, 217

secondary headaches, 344

secondary hypertension, 285

secondary prevention, 11

secondary sex characteristics, 176, 177

secondary syphilis, 330

secondhand smoke, 273

sedatives, 236, 237

seizure disorders, 344

selective serotonin reuptake inhibitors (SSRIs), 49

self-assessment, and behaviour change, 23–24

self-care, 396–400

self-concept, and stress, 63–64

self-defence against sexual assault, 385, 387

self-disclosure, 159–160

self-efficacy

control and, 66

defined, 36

developing and maintaining, 38–39

self-esteem

defined, 36–37

developing and maintaining, 38–39, 40

stress and, 63–64

self-nurturance, 171

self-talk, 22–23

semen, 181–182

seminal vesicles, 181

Senate Committee on Social Affairs, Science and Technology, 47

septic systems, 364

serial monogamy, 169

set, and psychoactive drugs, 227

setpoint theory, 148, 149

setting, and psychoactive drugs, 227

Sex and Love Addicts Anonymous, 246

sex and psychoactive drugs, 190–191

sex differences

aging and, 423

alcohol and, 260, 261, 269

in body fat, 135

cancer and, 12–13

cardiovascular disease and, 291

depression and, 48

health and, 11

in intimate relationships, 165–167

in nutritional needs, 122–123

suicide and, 48

sex insensitivity, 11

sexual arousal disorders, 188–190

sexual assault

prevention, 383–387

theories and social assumptions, 382–383

sexual aversion disorder, 188, 189

sexual bias, in mental health diagnosis, 47–48

sexual desire disorders, 188

sexual dysfunction, 188, 189

sexual expression, 185–187

sexual fantasies, 185

sexual identity, 175–177

sexual intimacy, 165

sexual orientation, 183

sexual pain disorders, 190

sexual relationships, 183–185

see also committed relationships; intimate relationships

sexuality

aging and, 418–419

difficulties hindering functioning, 188–191

human sexual response, 182–183

sexual expression, 185–187

sexual orientation, 183

sexual preferences, 184

sexual relationships, 183–185

variant sexual behaviour, 187–188

sexually transmitted infections (STIs)

attitude and belief scale, 327

causes and transmission of, 326–327

communicating about, 337

overview, 323, 325

screening for, 328

signs and symptoms of, 326

sexually transmitted infection (STI) types

candidiasis, 332, 333

chlamydia, 328, 329

general urinary tract infections (UTIs), 333

gonorrhea, 329–330

herpes, 333–334

HIV/AIDS. See HIV/AIDS

pelvic inflammatory disease (PID), 329

pubic lice, 331

syphilis, 330–331

trichomoniasis, 332, 333

venereal warts, 331–332

shaping, 21

Sheldon, William, 145

shelter movement, 376

shin splints, 95–96

shopping, and borrowing, 230–231

sickle cell anemia, 314, 315, 351

significant others, 163–164

Simon Fraser University, 422

simple carbohydrates, 113

singlehood, 172

sinoatrial node (SA node), 282, 283

situational inducement, 22, 23

skin and aging, 416

skin cancer, 305

tension headaches, 343
tension principle, 87
teratogenic effects of drugs, 212–213
tertiary prevention, 11
testes, 180–181
testicular cancer, 305–306
testosterone, 180–181
tetrahydrocannabinol (THC), 243
thanatology, 425
theory of reasoned action, 19
therapists. *See* mental health professionals
therapy
    for addictions, 246
    for alcoholism, 269–270
    expectations, 52–53
    mental health professionals, 50–52
    for orgasm disorders, 190
    for relationship problems, 174
third trimester of pregnancy, 217
thought stopping, 23
thrifty genes, 146
thrombolysis, 293–294, 295
thrombus, 285
thyroid, and obesity, 146
time, for oneself, 39
time management, 73
tobacco. *See* smoking and tobacco
tolerance, 228, 229
touch, and aging, 418
toxic shock syndrome (TSS), 201, 317
toxins, 316, 317
trace minerals, 119
Traffic Injury Research Foundation
    (TIRF), 266
tranquillizers, 236, 237
trans-fatty acids, 117
transient ischemic attacks, 284, 285
transition, 219
transsexualism, 188
transtheoretical model, 16–17
transvestitism, 188
traumatic injuries, 94
treatment programs for alcoholism, 269–270
trial separations, 173
triangular theory of love, 165
trichomoniasis, 332, 333
triglycerides, 115, 289
trihalomethanes, 365
trimesters, 216–217
trust, 163
tubal ligation, 205
tuberculosis (TB), 316, 317–318
tumour, 296, 297
Twain, Mark, 14
12-step programs, 246
Twiggy, 150
twin studies on obesity, 145–146
type 2 diabetes. *See* diabetes

Type A Behavior and Your Heart (Friedman and
    Rosenman), 64
Type A personality, 64, 66
Type B personality, 64, 66
typical-use rate, 195

U

ulcerative colitis, 346, 347
ulcers, 347
ultrafast computed tomography, 293
United Nations
    on climate change, 367
    on family types, 163
    on overpopulation, 355
    on violence against women, 376
United Nations Convention on the Elimination of All
    Forms of Discrimination Against Women, 376
United Nations Framework Convention on Climate
    Change, 367
University of Western Ontario, 215
unsaturated fats, 115
urethral opening, 177–178
urinary incontinence, 417–418
uterine cancer, 307, 309
uterus (womb), 177–180

V

vaccination, 323, 324–325
vacuum aspiration abortion, 208, 209
vagina, 177–178
vaginal intercourse, 187
vaginismus, 190, 191
vaginitis, 332, 333
Vancouver
    anti-Chinese and Japanese riot (1907)
        in, 375
    seasonal affective disorder in, 45
Vanier Institute of the Family, 163
variable resistance, 89
variant sexual behaviour, 187–188
varicella, 320–321, 324
vas deferens, 181
vasectomy, 205
vasocongestion, 182, 183
vegetarianism, 123–124
veins, 282, 283
venereal warts, 331–332
ventricles, 282, 283
very low-calorie diets (VLCDs), 143–144
Viagra, 188–190
victimization
    consequences of, 385
    self-assessment, 382
    sexual. *See* sexual assault
    unintentional injuries and, 389
violence
    alcohol and, 258, 259
    against children, 378–380

violence (*continued*)
 cycle of violence theory, 377
 defined, 373
 domestic, 377–378
 of hate, 375–376
 health and, 388–389
 homicide, 374, 375
 against men, 381
 against older adults, 381–382
 overview, 373
 prevention of, 387–388
 suicide, 374
 against women, 376–377
 youths and, 374–375
Violence Against Women survey, 377
virulent, 314, 315
viruses
 chicken pox, 320–321
 common cold, 318–319
 hepatitis, 320, 321
 infectious mononucleosis, 319–320
 influenza, 319
 measles, 321
 mumps, 320
visualizing, 21
vitamin D
 aging and, 422–423
 importance of, 110, 122
 sources of, 119
vitamin(s)
 benefits and risks of, 121
 defined, 117
 guide, 118–119
 vitamin D. *See* vitamin D
volatile organic compounds, 357
voluntary hospitals, 406, 407
voyeurism, 188
vulva, 177–178

W

waist circumference, 139
Walcher, Werner, 5
Walker, Lenore, 377
warm-up, 93
water, 110–112
water pollution, 363–366
wear-and-tear theory of aging, 415
Webpersonals, 186
Week without Violence, 378
weight loss, 114
weight management
 see also dieting
 body fat assessment, 137–140

calories and, 140
dieting and, 142, 143–144
eating habits and, 142–143
gaining weight, 145
guidelines, 144, 154
long-term weight loss, 140
nutritional planning and, 143
overweight and obesity, 134–140
 see also obesity
physical activity and, 82, 140–142
right weight determination, 135–137
wellness, 3
 see also health
West Nile virus, 316
Western blot test, 338, 339
Wister, Andrew, 422
withdrawal, 202–203, 228, 229
Wolfe, Larry, 215
women
 see also female reproductive anatomy and physiology;
  sex differences
 alcohol and, 260, 261
 alcoholism and, 266, 269
 cardiovascular disease and, 291–292
 disorders related to, 344–345
 nutrition for, 122
 violence against, 376–377
wood stove smoke, 359
Worden, William, 429
Worden's model of grieving tasks, 427, 429
World Health Organization (WHO)
 child abuse statistics, 379
 health definition, 3
 on illicit drugs, 239
 on sugar intake, 113
 suicide rates, 48
 violence definition, 373
world population, 355–356
World Populations Prospects: The 2006 Revision (United
 Nations), 355

X

x-rays and pregnancy, 213
xanthines, 277

Y

yo-yo diets, 148, 149
yoga, 91–92
young-old category, 414, 415
Yukon River Quest, 5

Z

The Zone, 114

PHOTO CREDITS

p. 1 Getty images; p. 2 Stock Boston/David L. Coleman; p.4 CP/Jon Murray; p. 22 Michael Newman/PhotoEdit; p. 23 © Mika/Corbis; p. 28 © Susan Wides/Veer; p. 30 Getty Images/Per Eriksson; p. 37 Copyright © Mark Richards/PhotoEdit; p. 43 Health Canada and Public Health Agency of Canada. Adapted and Reproduced with the permission of the Minister of Public Works and Government Services Canada, © 2009; p. 44 Lawrence Manning/CORBIS; p. 46 Ottawa Citizen/Wayne Cuddington; p. 55 Spike Mafford/Photodisc; p. 57 Digital Vision/Getty Images; p. 63 CandyBox/Dreamstime.com; p. 73 Jason Homa/Getty Images; p. 76 Paul Viant/Getty Images; p. 78 David Stoecklein/CORBIS; p. 79 MACLEANS PHOTO/Phill Snell; p. 80 (left) Gilles Daigle/PhotoCanada Moncton; p. 80 (right) Gilles Daigle/PhotoCanada Moncton; p. 81 (left) Gilles Daigle/PhotoCanada Moncton; p. 81 (right) Gilles Daigle/PhotoCanada Moncton; p. 84 Gilles Daigle/PhotoCanada Moncton; p. 88 Gilles Daigle/PhotoCanada Moncton; p. 90 Gilles Daigle/PhotoCanada Moncton; p. 91 Novastock/GetStock.com; p. 95 Mike Powell/Getty Images; p. 99 Janet Kimber/The Image Bank/Getty Images; p. 101 Peter Cade/Getty Images; p. 106 Michael Keller/CORBIS; p. 111 A. Neste; p. 114 The Image Works/B. Daemmrich; p. 123 Brian Hagiwara/ Foodpix; p. 124 Reg Charity/CORBIS; p. 129 The Image Works/J. Sohm; p. 133 © Jupiterimages Corporation; p. 138 PhotoEdit/David Young-Wolff; p. 138 Life Measurement, Inc.; p. 139 Gilles Daigle/PhotoCanada Moncton; p. 141 © Gabe Palmer/CORBIS; p. 151 © 2009, NMSB/Custom Medical Stock Photo; p. 158 Health Canada and Public Health Agency of Canada. Adapted and Reproduced with the permission of the Minister of Public Works and Government Services Canada, © 2009; p. 160 Charles Gupton/ CORBIS; p. 162 Jose Luis Pelaez/CORBIS; p. 167 Getty Images/ Edgardo Contreras; p. 173 Bruce Ayres/CORBIS; p. 185 Black Star/Lisa Quinones; p. 187 Sarma Ozols/Getty Images; p. 193 Superstock; p. 194 Charles Thatcher/Stone/Getty Images; p. 198 Reuters NewMedia/ CORBIS; p. 199 Reuters NewMedia/CORBIS; p. 200 Dorling Kindersley; p. 202 Allendale Pharmaceuticals, Inc.; p. 210 Bruce Ayres/Getty Images; p. 214 Photo Library/Maxx Images. Inc.; p. 218 Copyright © Tom McCarthy/PhotoEdit; p. 220 Health Canada and Public Health Agency of Canada. Adapted and Reproduced with the permission of the Minister of Public Works and Government Services Canada, © 2009; p. 226 Health Canada and Public Health Agency of Canada. Adapted and Reproduced with the permission of the Minister of Public Works and Government Services Canada, © 2009; p. 234 Copyright © Bill Aron/PhotoEdit; p. 241 SPL/Photo Researchers; p. 249 © Abhay Martin MD, Dermatlas, www.dermatlas.org; p. 254 Health Canada and Public Health Agency of Canada. Adapted and Reproduced with the permission of the Minister of Public Works and Government Services Canada, © 2009; p. 257 Creasource Ltd.; p. 265 Chuck Savage/CORBIS; p. 273 Oral Health America; p. 280 Ron Levine/Getty Images; p. 284 Tom Stewart/CORBIS; p. 289 Copyright © Dennis MacDonald/PhotoEdit; p. 302 Stock Boston/ Jim Pickerell; p. 305 (a) James Stevenson/SP:/Photo Researchers, (b, c) P. Marazzi/SPL/Photo Researchers; p. 319 Don Klumpp/Firstlight.ca; p. 330 SPL/Photo Researchers; p. 332 P. Marazzi.Science Photo Library/Photo Researchers; p. 334 (a) Steven N. Nussenblatt/Custom Medical Stock Photo, (b) ISM/ Phototake; p. 336 Steve Mercer/Getty Images; p. 338 Health Canada and Public Health Agency of Canada. Adapted and Reproduced with the permission of the Minister of Public Works and Government Services Canada, © 2009; p. 339 CP Photo/Chuck Stoody; p. 342 Paul Windsor/ Taxi/Getty Images; p. 343 Elena Dorfman/Offshoot Inc.; p. 351 PhotoDisc; p. 353 Dick Hemingway; p. 355 Richard L'Anson/Lonely Plant Images; p. 359 Will & Deni McIntyre/Photo Researchers, Inc.; p. 368 Gary Buss/Getty Images; p. 372 Mary-Arthur Johnson/Taxi; p. 375 Copyright © Mark Richards/PhotoEdit; p. 377 Bill Aron/PhotoEdit; p. 379 Woodfin Camp/Jacques; p. 383 Jonathan White/iStockphoto; p. 387 William Thomas Cain/Getty Images; p. 392 Dick Hemingway; p. 397 © Epsin/ Anderson/The Image Works; p. 402 Novastock/The Stock Connection; p. 403 © Willie Hill, Jr./The Image Works; p. 411 © Larry Wells/ Maxximages.com; p. 415 John Henley/CORBIS; p. 420 Joe Munroe/ Photo Researchers, Inc.; p. 423 Dan Bosler/Stone Allstock/Getty Images; p. 425 Arvind Garge/Photo Researchers; p. 430 (top) Freddie Lieberman/ Mass Images Inc.; p. 430 (bottom) Copyright © David Young-Wolff/ PhotoEdit